The Shoulder

Surgical and Nonsurgical Management

The Shoulder

Surgical and Nonsurgical Management

Edited by

MELVIN POST, M.D.

Chairman, Department of Orthopaedic Surgery
Michael Reese Hospital and Medical Center
Chicago, Illinois
Associate Professor, Department of Orthopaedic Surgery
Northwestern University Medical School
Chicago, Illinois

LEA & FEBIGER · 1978 · PHILADELPHIA

Library of Congress Cataloging in Publication Data

Post, Melvin, M.D.
    The shoulder.

    Bibliography.
    Includes index.
        1. Shoulder—Surgery.   2. Shoulder—Diseases.
3. Shoulder—Wounds and injuries.   I. Post, Melvin.
[DNLM: 1. Muscular diseases—Therapy.   2. Bone
diseases—Therapy.   3. Joint Diseases—Therapy.
4. Shoulder.   5. Arm injuries—Therapy.   WE810 S559]
RD557.5.S56   617'.572   78-2738
ISBN 0-8121-0617-2

Published in Great Britain by Henry Kimpton Publishers, London

PRINTED IN THE UNITED STATES OF AMERICA

Print Number   3   2   1

To my parents, friends, and teachers
who pointed the way.
But most of all to my wife

PEARL

who has added immeasurably to my life.

Preface

I HAVE HAD a special interest in conditions of the shoulder girdle for many years. Students and colleagues have stimulated this interest by permitting me to follow their patients clinically and to document clinical material for the past 20 years. Thus, it seemed appropriate to assemble a text with the purpose of reviewing older, but still valid ideas, and to convey to the reader newer concepts of treatment based on solid principles and proven clinical experiences in an important, often neglected anatomic region of the body.

The book stresses the need for a thorough examination of the patient, and whenever possible correlates the anatomy and physiology of the region. Rather complete discussions in anatomy, microbiology, rheumatology, and neurology are presented because effective management of shoulder conditions requires an integrated understanding of these subjects.

Each of the authors has been given leeway in expressing his opinions. It is for this reason that there is some duplication of material, as viewed by different disciplines. In any event, each of the suggested treatments for various disorders has been shown to be reliable when judiciously selected.

No attempt is made to discuss all the theories ever written on every subject. These have been reviewed in excellent papers to which the reader is referred. Likewise, although an extensive search of the literature has been conducted, only salient references have been listed. Many of the key references list numerous other excellent papers.

I am deeply indebted to the staffs of the Michael Reese Medical Center and John Crerar Libraries who culled the many references cited in the text. My sincere thanks go to outstanding teachers such as Doctors Jerome Finder, Leonard Weinstein, the late Irving Wolin, and others who allowed me access to their patients over the years.

Much credit must go to those who made this work possible, including Miss June Pedigo who spent countless hours illustrating the book, Mr. Stan Kaval who reproduced almost all of the photographs, often from poorly taken roentgenograms or color slides, Mr. Edward Wickland and the editorial staff and Mr. Thomas Colaiezzi and the production staff of Lea & Febiger, who gave me their invaluable advice. Finally, I wish to express my gratitude to Mrs. Eleanor Mathews, my faithful secretary, who unhesitatingly retyped each edited chapter until completion.

MELVIN POST

Chicago, Illinois

Contributors

MICHAEL H. ELLMAN, M.D.
  Director, Division of Rheumatology
  Michael Reese Hospital and Medical Center
  Chicago, Illinois

  Assistant Professor of Medicine
  Pritzker School of Medicine
  University of Chicago
  Chicago, Illinois

WILLIAM F. ENNEKING, M.D.
  Professor and Chairman
  Department of Orthopaedics
  University of Florida
  Gainesville, Florida

JEROME G. FINDER, M.D.
  Senior Attending, Department of Orthopaedic
    Surgery
  Michael Reese Hospital and Medical Center
  Chicago, Illinois

MARK HAJOST, C.P.
  Research Prosthetist
  Prosthetic Research Laboratory
  Northwestern University
  Chicago, Illinois

SAUL S. HASKELL, M.D.
  Attending
  Department of Orthopaedic Surgery
  Michael Reese Hospital and Medical Center
  Chicago, Illinois

ROBERT D. KEAGY, M.D., M.S.
  Assistant Professor
  Department of Orthopaedic Surgery
  Northwestern University Medical School
  Chicago, Illinois

  Chairman
  Department of Orthopaedic Surgery
  Strauss Surgical Group Association, S.C.

  Louis A. Weiss Memorial Hospital
  Chicago, Illinois

SHERWIN A. KABINS, M.D.
  Chairman, Division of Infectious Diseases
  Vice-Chairman, Department of Medicine
  Michael Reese Hospital and Medical Center

  Associate Professor of Medicine
  University of Chicago
  Chicago, Illinois

HAROLD L. KLAWANS, M.D.
  Director, Division of Neurology
  Michael Reese Hospital and Medical Center
  Chicago, Illinois

  Professor, Department of Medicine (Neurol-
    ogy)
  Pritzker School of Medicine
  University of Chicago
  Chicago, Illinois

BERTRAM LEVIN, M.D.
  Chairman, Department of Diagnostic Radiol-
    ogy
  Michael Reese Hospital and Medical Center
  Chicago, Illinois

Professor of Radiology
Pritzker School of Medicine
University of Chicago
Chicago, Illinois

MELVIN POST, M.D.
Chairman, Department of Orthopaedic Surgery
Michael Reese Hospital and Medical Center
Chicago, Illinois

Associate Professor, Department of Orthopaedic Surgery
Northwestern University Medical School
Chicago, Illinois

ERIC L. RADIN, M.D.
Associate Professor in Orthopaedic Surgery
Harvard Medical School
Boston, Massachusetts

Lecturer in Mechanical Engineering
Massachusetts Institute of Technology
Boston, Massachusetts

ROBERT ROY, M.D.
Chief Resident
Department of Orthopaedics
University of Florida
Gainesville, Florida

SHAHAN K. SARRAFIAN, M.D., F.A.C.S.
Assistant Professor, Department of Orthopaedic Surgery
Northwestern University Medical School
Chicago, Illinois

ROBERT G. THOMPSON, M.D.
Associate Professor, Department of Orthopaedics
Northwestern University and Medical School
Chicago, Illinois

JORDAN L. TOPEL, M.D.
Assistant Professor of Neurology
Department of Neurological Sciences
Rush Medical College
Chicago, Illinois

Contents

1

Historical Reflections

The incentives to write a new book on problems of the shoulder, a field replete with competent authors and texts, are two-fold. Foremost is the goal of presenting the newest concepts and techniques which are exploring and molding the future approaches to problem solving. No less important is the critical reexamination, in perspective, of those existing methods which apparently have stood the clinical test of time. When reassessing the established, the entrenched concepts, the pitfall of accepting them on faith simply because the written word, copied from author to author, through repetition acquires the patina of indisputable authenticity must be avoided.

The collaborating authors whose chapters follow have demonstrated, in my opinion, their familiarity and expertise in the specific areas of their respective subjects. In workmanlike fashion they have competently presented the new and, when appropriate, evaluated the old in balanced perspective.

However, aside from the precise scientific presentations, the traditionalists in medicine and surgery still enjoy the sentimental academic pleasure of the historical review, the transition from the past to the present and, perhaps prophetically, to the future.

As the historical background of certain concepts are reviewed, it is not unusual to rediscover that the ancients recognized pathology and malfunction in a perceptive manner. Often they developed principles and techniques to combat those defects in

an effective manner; the succeeding ages in many instances merely refined the original treatment. This, then, is the warrant for a backward glance into the early ideas about the shoulder as a nosologic entity.

The shoulder particularly lends itself to legend, mythology, and necromancy. The figurative image of the shoulder has subtly invaded the idioms of our culture so that we make daily reference to the shoulder in our speech and writing without conscious awareness of the deep-rooted etiology. The heart, because of its synonymity with love, St. Valentine and courage, is perhaps the only organ complex which sentimentally outrivals the shoulder in our daily thought communication.

The symbolism of the shoulder pervades our very way of life. We are exhorted to shoulder the burden, the responsibility, even the blame. When extra-determined effort is required we must put our shoulder to the wheel. Unity is expressed by marching shoulder to shoulder. Comfort or solace is offered when one is invited to "rest your weary head upon my shoulder." An act of affection and companionship is demonstrated by placing one's arm around the shoulder of a loved one or friend. On the other hand, the lady may reject a lover's advances by giving him the cold shoulder. Indifference, resignation, or equivocation may be indicated by the nuances of an expressive shrug of the shoulders. Soft shoulders carry a hidden or overt reason for caution. If the soft shoulder is feminine, it could lead to tender entrapment. More practically, highway signs warn one of driving danger due to soft shoulders. And so it goes.

The physical attributes of the shoulder are rooted deep in antiquity. In Greek mythology Atlas, a Titan, strove to defeat in war the gods of Olympus. However, he was vanquished and as punishment he was condemned by Zeus to forever stand at the west end of the earth and bear the skies upon his shoulders. The world famous Farnese statue, which stands in the Naples National Museum, depicts him holding the globe of the heavens upon his shoulders.

From the physical aspect the amazing role of the shoulder is obvious. Consider the stress placed upon the shoulder of the athlete who heaves the 16 pound shot more than 70 feet, the trapeze aerialist, the weight lifter, or the powerful anchorman whose fully extended shoulder holds his partner aloft vertically by a tight handgrip. Legend has it that in the ancient Olympic Games, when individual feats of prowess were permissible, one contestant is said to have held his arms abducted at 90 degrees for three days and three nights. Even though one may wonder at the possibility of self-hypnosis or an induced state of catatonia, the demonstration of such raw sustained power of the shoulder girdle leaves one incredulous.

THE SHOULDER IN ORTHOPAEDICS

As one brings specific pathology of the shoulder into focus, the techniques of treatment from the ancient methods of manipulation to the present technology of total shoulder replacement cover a broad spectrum of imagination, rationalization, experiential conclusions, and deductive indications. It is not within the province of this introductory chapter to deal in-depth with the multifaceted subjects concerning the shoulder. This is more properly the prerogative of the individual contributors who have expertly collated the titled subject matter of this volume. Nevertheless, it is not irrelevant to focus attention on some of the classic entities which have challenged and intrigued the early practitioners of medicine.

Dislocation of the Shoulder

Because of its frequency, dislocation of the shoulder probably has been one of the most familiar entities in medicine. Its diagnosis and treatment have fascinated the physician since earliest times; however, although the condition was universally recognized, it was not always treated effectively. The Hippocratic texts described an apparatus for the reduction of shoulder dislocation; a similar design was employed by Paré, as noted in his *Collected Works*.[29] Bick[6] gives an excellent summary of classic writings on the shoulder from the *Corpus Hippocrates*,[12] Greek texts written by various author-contributors between 300 B.C. and A.D. 100.

From the *Corpus Hippocrates*, we know the ancients recognized that shoulders which dislocated easily or repeatedly had laxity of the supporting structures and thus a poor prognosis against further recurrence. When reduction was difficult or attended subsequently by considerable inflammation, the prognosis was considered better because of tighter structures and formation of scar tissue and adhesions which eliminated joint laxity. The use of cautery, placed at the axilla, burned through loose skin into the fibrous and adipose tissue underlying the joint capsule. Subsequent scarification at the weakest part of the capsule produced protective contracture, diminishing the chance of a recurrent dislocation. Injury to the major nerves and vessels was not recorded, although caution was advised to avoid such injury. Modern principles follow a similar logic not only by reefing the capsule, but by shifting musculotendinous support to prevent redislocation. The ancients likewise stressed the need for aftercare: usually prolonged strapping of the arm to the side of the body and application of hot compresses and hand massage.

Of special interest is a paper by Brockbank and Griffiths which provides excellent reproductions of woodcuts taken from books published in 1544, 1607, 1625, 1678, and 1693;[8] they depict 10 crude but ingenious methods of reducing the shoulder dislocation. In effect, these are variations of two techniques. The first, the "Ambe of Hippocrates," relied on a mechanical device which provided traction-abduction of the arm with strong counterpressure against the lateral rib cage. The second was manipulative, the "heel in the axilla" or Hippocratic method, still in practical use today. However, the favorite method advocated by Hippocrates, which he termed "the very best way of restoring a shoulder," was to rest the axilla on a horizontal crossbeam with the patient standing on his tiptoes. Downward traction was then applied to the arm by the physician. Countertraction was supplied by the weight of the patient's body supplemented by the weight of an assistant who suspended himself by locking his wrists around the patient's neck. These points are nicely illustrated in Brockbank and Griffiths' article.

White described two cases of unreduced shoulder dislocations of 2 and 3 months' duration, respectively, seen in 1748 and 1749.[37] Ordinary methods of reduction had failed, which led him to try a new method. Traction was applied to a rope fastened to the wrist on the involved side. The patient was then lifted completely off his feet by means of an overhead pulley. In the first case, the head was mobilized into the axilla, after which White completed the reduction using the Hippocratic heel in the axilla technique.

In the second case, traction on the wrist, pulling the arm vertically upward, was sufficient to get instant reduction as the patient's feet left the ground. A third case, treated in 1760, was more resistant although the duration of the dislocation was only 2 weeks. The author described the humeral head as being beneath the scapula; apparently he was unaware that he most likely was dealing with a posterior dislocation. Again, the overhead traction served to displace the head into the axilla, after which

White was able to manipulate the head into the socket by the heel in the armpit maneuver.

That "there is nothing new under the sun" is exemplified by the suggestion that the ancient Egyptians were employing the Kocher maneuver to reduce the dislocated shoulder 3000 years before the method acquired its eponym. In 1870 Emil Theodor Kocher, a brilliant and perceptive surgeon, described his technique for reducing dislocations of the shoulder, especially long-standing ones.[21,22] His logical manipulative routine is classic and remains today, as then, an effective technique. Of interest, therefore, is the claim of Hussein that wall paintings from the tomb of Rameses II (1200 B.C.) depict a patient's arm being manipulated in one of the positions of the Kocher maneuver.[18]

Excluding the Hippocratic use of cautery by the ancients, open surgery was not attempted until the close of the nineteenth century, when in 1894 Ricord described his method for surgical repair (capsulorrhaphy).[32] Then followed a plethora of surgical procedures, each purporting to solve the problem of recurrent dislocation of the shoulder. Among the early surgeons were Clairmont and Ehrlich, ligamentous sling beneath the neck of the humerus;[11] Clairmont, suspension of head of humerus by tendon transplant passed through drill holes in the acromion process and greater tuberosity;[10] Bankart, rebuilding support of the glenoid labrium;[2,3] Spitzy, suspension of the head of the humerus by silk threads passed through the acromion process;[33] Henderson, fascial sling, or tenosuspension;[17] Gallie and LeMesurier, free tendon and fascial transplants;[14] Nicola, tenodesis by passing the long head of the biceps tendon through the head of the humerus;[27] Magnuson and Stack, lateral transplantation of the subscapularis insertion to the greater tuberosity;[24] Osmond-Clarke, Putti-Platt double-breasting and shortening of the subscapularis;[28] du Toit and Roux, "Johannesburg" staple capsulorrhaphy;[36] Helfet-Bristow, transplantation of distal coracoid tip to the neck of the scapula.[16] These references present but a small fraction of the many innovative procedures designed by a legion of surgeons. Certainly this reflects some of the perplexities of the problem of the habitually dislocating shoulder and the lack of a Utopian surgical "sure-cure."

Resection of the Humeral Head

The published indications for this operation as recently as 35 years ago were traumatic dislocation of the shoulder not reducible by open surgery, and tuberculosis of the shoulder with mixed infection and suppuration. The resection was especially indicated to prevent extension of the abscess into the pleural cavity. The function after resection was often poor because of severe atrophy of the deltoid after removal of the head.

On the other hand, Morton[25] cites the first recorded excision of the head of the humerus by White[38] (1770), who sawed off the upper humeral head because of necrosis. However, the process continued, and later the major portion of the head exfoliated (apparently of a suppurative disease). The remarkable point made by the author was "the entire motion of the limb was preserved."

The foregoing accounts are, of course, mainly of historical interest, yet they emphasize rather dramatically the tremendous strides made in our own lifetime. The sophisticated use of antibiotics, the improved surgical techniques, and the advent of prosthetic replacement arthroplasties now offer reasonably optimistic salvage and restoration of function for joints formerly doomed to permanent disability.

Disarticulation of the Shoulder

It is not improbable that the first disarticulations may have been inflicted punitively in the pre-Christian era, when a victim condemned to death was drawn and quartered by goading four wild horses, each fastened to a separate limb, to pull against each other at 90-degree vectors.

While no objective scientific reports of these grisly events are available as to limb destruction, it seems logical that the shoulder joint, because of its relatively weaker musculoligamentocapsular connections as compared to those of the hip joint, more likely would have been the first to yield to the overwhelming forces.

An authentic case of traumatic avulsion of the entire upper extremity and shoulder is noted and illustrated in *Anatomy of the Human Body* by W. Cheselden.[9] It describes the case of a miller, Samuel Wood, "who in 1737 survived a traumatic amputation of an arm and shoulder, caused by an entwined rope attached to the cogs of a mill wheel. Only slight shock was said to have followed this amputation by avulsion." Little bleeding occurred probably because of the severe overstretch and rebound contraction of the major vessels. The patient had no severe symptoms and was cured by superficial dressings only.

Grimes and Bell have stated the case for elective disarticulation in a practical comment:[15] "The shoulder girdle amputation, although necessarily an extremely mutilating procedure has in certain instances a legitimate place in surgery. Occasionally it must be accepted as the only adequate method of definitive treatment for those tumors unfortunately located in areas not amenable to curative surgery of any lesser degree. Oftentimes because of the surgeon's justifiable reluctance to suggest a necessary shoulder amputation, patients are subjected to multiple inadequate local excisions of malignant lesions about the shoulder area."

It is indicated also as an emergency lifesaving measure in cases of overwhelming irreversible traumatic damage to the shoulder. Massive infection leading to gangrene or a totally useless extremity by reason of major nerve and vascular destruction likewise may justify the procedure.

An English naval surgeon, Ralph Cuming, is credited with having performed the first elective disarticulation, an interscapulothoracic amputation, in 1808, for a gunshot wound.[19,20] Dixie Crosby, in 1836, was the first American surgeon to perform a successful extirpation of the shoulder girdle for tumor.[13] One year later Musey of Cincinnati performed a scapulectomy following a disarticulation of the humerus for sarcoma; the patient survived for 30 years.

However, it remained for Berger to standardize the operation which still bears his name.[4,5] In 1882, Paul Berger, who was surgeon at the Hospital Tenon and Professor of Surgery at the Faculte de Medicine de Paris, amputated the entire upper limb of a patient with an enchondroma of the humerus. In 1883, he reported the result, and in 1887 published his classic work, which was the first detailed monograph on forequarter amputation; in the historical review Ralph Cuming was named originator of the operation. The monograph has continued to be accepted as detailing basic surgical technique and procedure.

Arthrodesis and Arthroplasty

During the past half century there has been an interesting shift in the indications that govern the choice between arthrodesis and arthroplasty of the shoulder, two procedures whose purposes are diametrically opposite: stability versus mobility, respectively.

In 1925, Steindler stated that the principal indication for shoulder fusion was the flail shoulder due to infantile paralysis.[34] He gave credit to E. Albert for having performed the first arthrodesis in 1881.[1] In a later publication Steindler included as indications "tuberculosis, particularly the dry type; arthritis, infantile paralysis with flail shoulder, or peripheral paralysis of the deltoid muscle."[35]

In discussing arthroplasty of the shoulder Steindler stated: "this operation is also very rarely indicated because of the excellent motion obtainable in ankylosis of the shoulder joint by means of the scapulothoracic muscles, provided that the position between humerus and scapula is favorable."[34] Statistics on arthroplasty of the shoulder were meager. Steindler cited a case by W. L. and C. P. Brown (1914) in which a portion of the long head of the biceps was used for inter-

position. He also noted another case by Grange (1920) in which active abduction of 45 degrees, flexion of 45 degrees, and rotation of 60 degrees were finally obtained.

The interposition method was employed in the earlier operations using pedicled muscle flaps, pig's bladder, and chromicized silver-impregnated fascia. Later, more preferred material was free fascia and fat flaps. However, Steindler dismissed the subject by stating categorically that "the joints on which arthroplasty heretofore has not been practiced with any success are: the shoulder, the wrist, the ankle."[35]

There was no significant change in these concepts until the present era, which has witnessed the rapid proliferation of prosthetic replacement arthroplasties. The shoulder joined this revolutionary trend in 1951 when Boron and Sevin successfully implanted an acrylic prosthesis for the shoulder.[7] In the same year Kreuger performed a Vitallium replica arthroplasty of the shoulder for osteonecrosis of the humeral head.[23] In France, Richard, Judet, and Rene in 1952 also reconstructed the proximal end of the humerus for fracture-luxations using an acrylic prosthesis.[31] However, great credit must be given to Neer, who designed a functional prosthesis and pioneered its acceptance in America.[26]

The Neer prosthesis was designed chiefly to replace humeral heads severely comminuted and destroyed by trauma. Its success depended on an intact rotator cuff with preservation of good function of the short rotator muscles and a healthy glenoid surface. If the shoulder stabilizers are nonfunctional due to atrophy, weakness or scarring, for example, the head of the prosthesis cannot be maintained in a stable position as it glides on the shallow glenoid, making it potentially subject to dislocation.

Subsequently, Neer designed a glenoid facing, which expanded the indications for use of the prosthesis to include other pathologic entities involving both the glenoid articular surface and the humeral head, as for example, the arthritides, comminuted fractures, and osteonecrosis.

Various total shoulder prostheses are now

in development. Their function depends on either a nonconstrained principle or a fixed fulcrum design. The Michael Reese fixed fulcrum total shoulder prosthesis, designed by Post and Haskell, added new dimensions to the range of therapeutic usefulness.[30] Because of the fixed fulcrum, stability is intrinsic to the construction of the prosthesis. Thus it is especially useful in those patients without functioning rotator muscles. A good deltoid will suffice to provide useful active shoulder motion. However, relief of pain is the major goal; the prosthesis may achieve this in cases of severe arthritis, traumatically destroyed joints, degenerated glenohumeral joints with nonfunctioning rotator cuffs, old unreduced dislocations or fracture-dislocations of the humeral head, resectable tumors of the proximal humerus, and osteonecrosis of the proximal humerus.

In this brief historical review no attempt has been made for encyclopedic inclusion of all maladies which may afflict the shoulder. Rather, the goal has been to present selected items that, because of antiquity, controversy, uniqueness, or even medical mystery, have captured the imagination and challenged the ingenuity of the physician and surgeon.

The management of a variety of shoulder conditions including posterior dislocation of the shoulder, degenerative painful lesions of the glenohumeral joint, paralytic conditions of the shoulder girdle, and other disease states has undergone a similar evolution. These conditions are discussed in the appropriate chapters.

An effort has been made to maintain perspective in balance. Credit should be given to physicians of old for their acute and accurate observations. One realizes there is no monopoly of intelligence by latter-day physicians and surgeons. In many instances, modern doctors have made great medical strides only because the tools at hand were more sophisticated extensions of brain and hand than were available to the ancients, whose observations, skills, and practices nevertheless fashioned the trellis upon which climbed the vine of scientific knowledge and achievement.

REFERENCES

1. Albert, E.: Zentralbl. Chir., 48, 1881. In Steindler, A.: Operative Orthopedics. New York, D. Appleton and Company, 1925, p. 268.
2. Bankart, A. S. B.: Recurrent or habitual dislocation of the shoulder joint. Br. Med. J., 2:1132, 1923.
3. Bankart, A. S. B.: The pathology and treatment of recurrent dislocation of the shoulder joint. Br. J. Surg., 26:23, 1938.
4. Berger, P.: L'Amputation du membre supérieur dans la contiguité du tronc. Bull. Mem. Soc. Chir. Paris, 9:656, 1883.
5. Berger, P.: L'Amputation du Membre Supérieur dans la Contiguité du Tronc. Monograph. Paris, G. Masson, 1887.
6. Bick, E. M.: History and Source Book of Orthopaedic Surgery. New York, Hospital for Joint Diseases, 1933.
7. Boron, R., and Sevin, L.: Acrylic prosthesis for the shoulder. Presse Med., 59:1480, 1951.
8. Brockbank, W., and Griffiths, D. Ll.: Orthopaedic surgery in the sixteenth and seventeenth centuries. I. Luxations of the shoulder. J. Bone Joint Surg., 30-B:365, 1948.
9. Cheselden, W.: Anatomy of the Human Body, 7th ed. London, H. Woodfall, 1756, p. 321. In Gillis, L.: Amputations, XX. New York, Grune & Stratton, 1954, p. 412.
10. Clairmont, P.: Über neue Operationsmethoden bei habituellen Schulterluxation. Wien. Klin. Wochenschr., 30:1507, 1917.
11. Clairmont, P., and Ehrlich, H.: Ein neues Operations—verfahren zur Behandlung der habituellen Schulterluxation mittels Muskelplastik. Arch. Klin. Chir., 89:798, 1909.
12. Corpus Hippocrates. In Bick, E. M.: History and Source Book of Orthopaedic Surgery. New York, Hospital for Joint Diseases, 1933, p. 13.
13. Crosby, A. B.: The first operation on record for removal of the entire arm, scapula and three-fourths of the clavicle by Dixie Crosby. Med. Rec., Concord, N.H., 10:753, 1875. In Pack, G. T., McNeer, G., and Coley, B. L.: Interscapulo-thoracic amputation for malignant tumors of the upper extremity. Surg. Gynecol. Obstet., 74:161, 1942.
14. Gallie, W. E., and LeMesurier, A. B.: An operation for the relief of recurring dislocation of the shoulder. Trans. Am. Surg. Assoc., 45:392, 1927.
15. Grimes, O. F., and Bell, H. G.: Shoulder girdle amputation. Surg. Gynecol. Obstet., 91:201, 1950.

16. Helfet, J.: Coracoid transplantation for recurring dislocation of the shoulder. The W. Rowley Bristow Operation. J. Bone Joint Surg., 40-B:198, 1958.

17. Henderson, M. S.: Tenosuspension for habitual dislocation of the shoulder. Surg. Gynecol. Obstet., 43:18, 1926.

18. Hussein, M. K.: Kocher's method is 3000 years old. J. Bone Joint Surg., 50-B:669, 1968.

19. Hutchinson, A. C.: Removal of the arm, scapula and clavicle. (The case of Ralph Cuming.) Lond. Med. Gaz., 5:273, 1829.

20. Keevil, J. J.: Ralph Cuming and the interscapulo-thoracic amputation in 1808. J. Bone Joint Surg., 31-B:589, 1949.

21. Kocher, E. T.: Eine neue Reductionsmethode für Schulterverrenkung. Berl. Klin. Wochenschr., 7:101, 1870.

22. Kocher, E. T.: Über die Behandlung veralteter Luxationen im Schultergelenk. Dtsch. Z. Chir., 30, 1890.

23. Kreuger, F. J.: Vitallium replica arthroplasty of shoulder: Case report of aseptic necrosis of proximal end of humerus. Surgery, 30:1005, 1951.

24. Magnuson, P. B., and Stack, J. K.: Recurrent dislocation of the shoulder. J.A.M.A., 123:889, 1943.

25. Morton, L. T.: A Medical Bibliography (Garrison and Morton), 3rd ed. Philadelphia, J. B. Lippincott Co., 1970, p. 509.

26. Neer, C. S. II: Articular replacement for the humeral head. J. Bone Joint Surg. 37-A:215, 1955.

27. Nicola, T.: Recurrent anterior dislocation of the shoulder. A new operation. J. Bone Joint Surg., 11:128, 1929.

28. Osmond-Clarke, H.: Habitual dislocation of the shoulder. The Putti-Platt operation. J. Bone Joint Surg., 30-B:19, 1948.

29. Paré, A.: Collected Works. Translated by Th. Johnson. London, 1634. In Bick, E. M.: History and Source Book of Orthopaedic Surgery. New York, Hospital for Joint Diseases, 1933.

30. Post, J., Haskell, S. S., and Finder, J. G.: Total Shoulder Replacement. A paper presented before The American Orthopaedic Association, Hot Springs, Va., June 24, 1975.

31. Richard, A., Judet, R., and Rene, L.: Acrylic prosthetic construction of upper end of the humerus for fracture-luxations. J. Chir. (Paris), 68:537, 1952.

32. Ricord: Traitement des luxations récidivantes de l'epaule par la suture de la capsule articulaire ou arthrroraphie. Gaz. des hop: 49, 1894. In Bick, E. M.: History and Source Book of Orthopaedic Surgery. New York, Hospital for Joint Diseases, 1933, p. 179.

33. Spitzy: In Bick, E. M.: History and Source Book of Orthopaedic Surgery. New York, Hospital for Joint Diseases, 1933, p. 180.

34. Steindler, A.: Operative Orthopedics. New York, D. Appleton and Company, 1925, pp. 267 and 312.

35. Steindler, A.: Orthopedic Operations. Springfield, Ill., Charles C Thomas, 1940, pp. 315 and 292.

36. du Toit, G. T., and Roux, D.: Recurrent dislocation of the shoulder. J. Bone Joint Surg., 38-A:1, 1956.

37. White, C.: A new method of reducing shoulders without use of an ambe. Med. Obs. Inqu., 2:373, 1762. In Morton, L. T.: A Medical Bibliography (Garrison and Morton), 3rd ed. Philadelphia, J. B. Lippincott Co., 1970, p. 509.

38. White, C.: Phil. Trans. (1769), 59:39, 1770. In Morton, L. T.: A Medical Bibliography (Garrison and Morton), 3rd ed. Philadelphia, J. B. Lippincott Co., 1970, p. 513.

2

Diagnosis

MELVIN POST

Successful treatment of any condition about the shoulder girdle begins with an accurate history. The patient's chief complaint and other symptoms should be meticulously documented in order of their appearance to develop a chronology of the disease state. If the complaint or complaints are few and localized, in actual practice the history can be abbreviated. For example, a patient with a clear-cut acute history of localized pain in the shoulder pointing to a diagnosis of bursitis does not require a complete history and physical examination. On the other hand, a patient who complains of a recurring diffuse ache about the shoulder does require a more stringent examination. There is less likelihood of missing important details if the physician adheres to a systematic method of taking the history, eliciting facts as they relate to the complaint. The object is to gain experience in recognizing a disturbance in function, whether it be local or the result of a distant abnormality.

Each symptom should be fully explored. For a single symptom of pain, its character, frequency, duration, distribution, quality and intensity, indicating what aggravates or relieves it, should be detailed. Was it caused by trauma and is the pain increased by joint motion or stress? As many pertinent questions are asked as are necessary to clarify the cause of the symptoms.

The orthopaedic history is not the only history that should be obtained. The locomotor system often reflects symptoms that start with an internal disorder. A general medical history may impart worthwhile information with elaboration upon diverse systems such as the neurologic, endocrine, or cardiovascular. In essence, when enough relevant information has been gathered the diagnosis will become apparent. At this point, correct interpretation of laboratory data will aid in confirming what is already suspect.

The age of the patient can be important because certain conditions may be more prevalent or may not occur during certain periods of life. The occupation and specific job requirements should be known, not only because there may be a cause-and-effect relationship but also because they may help in planning future treatment. For example, the middle-age person who must use his extremity to reach overhead may require a total shoulder replacement rather than a shoulder fusion or perhaps no treatment following irreparable damage to the glenohumeral joint.

Childhood and adult illnesses, operations, personal habits, exposure to tobacco and drugs, and even family history may be helpful, particularly when such information may have orthopaedic significance. For the child, a data base should be established for such things as when the child first sat and talked and what illnesses had been contracted in the past, because they may have important implications in developing a musculoskeletal history and prognosis.

EXAMINATION

The surgeon should look, palpate, percuss, and listen when examining the shoulder girdle. Detailed parts of the examination are described in ensuing sections as they relate to specific conditions. The examiner must include the rest of the involved upper extremity, especially the hand, in his examination so that a complete picture may be gained.

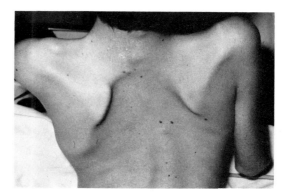

FIG. 2-1. A 13-year-old boy with Duchenne muscular dystrophy. Note the severe atrophy of the back muscles and winging of the scapulae.

Inspection

Examination of the patient starts with inspection of the thorax and shoulder girdle. The general appearance of the skin, general nourishment, posture and attitude of the extremities should be noted. Changes in contour of the shoulder girdle and muscle development or atrophy of the surrounding tissues should receive special attention. The state of the musculature and subcutaneous tissues is influenced by the general nutrition of the patient. Hence, in healthy robust individuals muscle development is generally evident, whereas in undernourished individuals wasting of muscles and subcutaneous tissues may be visible. For example, atrophy of muscles about the shoulders in a boy may suggest a muscle disease, such as muscular dystrophy (Fig. 2-1).

Palpation

Palpation can provide valuable knowledge for the examiner. Skin texture and the extent and condition of any scar about the shoulder should be recorded. A diagnosis of Ehler-Danlos syndrome is suggested by hyperelastic skin. Palpation of subcutaneous tissue, muscle, and the joint capsule in a lean patient may furnish additional clues. A snapping sensation over the long biceps tendon may be detected and suggest subluxation of the tendon from its groove. De-

formities of bone and joints should be described. Tender spots between the acromion and head of the humerus or over the point of the coracoid may be related to a diagnosis of bursitis, whereas tenderness over the intertubercular groove of the humerus may mean that bicipital tendinitis or a rupture of the long head of the biceps is present.

Muscle tenderness can be determined by prudent squeezing, avoiding excessive compression of the structures being tested. Muscle atony secondary to acute denervation recognized by flabbiness and rubbery to woody sensation to palpation suggests muscular dystrophy or polymyositis.

Prolonged immobilization of muscle in a shortened position for weeks or months causes the development of atrophy and contracture of skeletal muscle. The condition may be permanent or reversible and can be determined by careful, passive motion testing of related joints. Contractures are most often found in the adductors and internal rotators of the shoulder. Normally, if the patient is able to place his hands behind his neck with the elbow flat on a table or against a wall, then there is no contracture of the pectoral muscles (Fig. 2-2). Similarly, if the patient can elevate his arm, place his hand behind his head, and touch the opposite side of his neck and can place his hand behind his back, there is full external and internal rotation of the shoulder and no rotator muscle contracture (Figs.

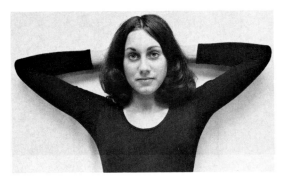

FIG. 2-2. Placing the hands behind the head is a method for demonstrating pectoral muscle contracture. Here, there is no contracture.

2-3 and 2-4). The examination should attempt to differentiate contracture, muscle spasm, and mechanical obstruction, all of which may be present and limit joint motion. Pretreatment differentiation will certainly alter management and help determine what end result can be achieved.

Shoulder joint mobility should include a description of both passive and active ranges of motion. The production of subluxations, pain-producing movements, and grating sensations should be noted. Loose joints associated with relaxed capsules can be easily overlooked. Palpation of peripheral pulses in the upper extremity may give information relating to a diagnosis of thoracic outlet syndrome.

Percussion

Tenderness to percussion can be a source of information in locating points of osseous foci. For example, tenderness can be elicited by gentle tapping over an undisplaced fracture of the clavicle in a child that at first may not be evident on initial roentgenograms.

Auscultation

A stethoscope should be at hand for auscultating masses about the shoulder

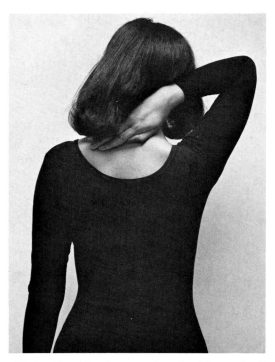

FIG. 2-3. Touching the opposite side of the neck with the hand behind the head indicates full external rotation of shoulder.

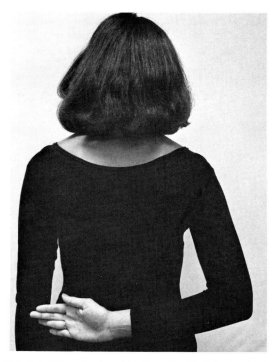

FIG. 2-4. When the hand is placed behind the back at the waist, the degree of internal rotation of the shoulder can be demonstrated. In the picture it is complete.

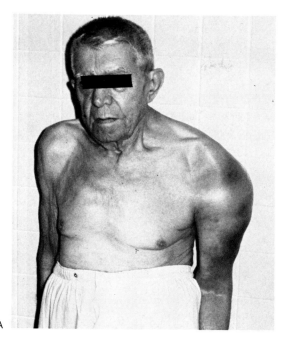
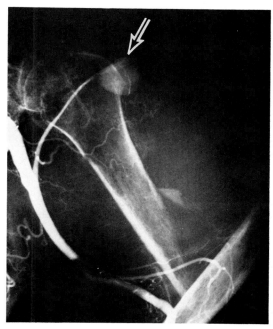

A

B

FIG. 2-5. A, An 82-year-old man fractured the left humeral shaft. The injury was treated with a hanging cast without success. The shoulder continued to swell. A bruit was heard over the shoulder. B, Arteriography was performed several weeks following the injury, and an aneurysm was found (arrow) on the arteriogram. It was subsequently excised and the fracture treated with open reduction.

girdle, particularly when there has been a history of injury. For example, aneurysms may produce an audible bruit which may be confirmed by arteriography (Fig. 2-5).

The examining surgeon should bear in mind that scapulohumeral rhythm is made up of the integrated action of all the joints constituting the shoulder girdle. The sum of the motions of the sternoclavicular, acromioclavicular, and glenohumeral joints and the additional motion of the scapula on the thoracic cage contribute to the synchronous movement of the shoulder girdle. Because a disturbance in normal rhythm can cause a diminution of motion and muscle power during any one phase of movement, it is essential to identify the specific defect. If analysis of the problem causing the shoulder disability is understood, effective treatment is more likely to result.

Muscle Strength

The examiner must learn the method needed to test and grade individual muscle strength. Often, a patient may attribute his inability to elevate the arm to joint stiffness rather than to muscle weakness. When the physician has become skilled in testing muscle strength, minimal disease states that would otherwise have gone undetected will at once become manifest. Improved diagnostic acumen and recording of meaningful observations will permit the easy recognition of psychogenic illness and the progression of a disease state.

From physical examination it must be determined whether or not there is muscle spasm, contracture of muscle groups and pain caused by muscle disease, or nerve involvement before there can be reliable testing of muscle strength; hence, the need for an effective neurologic examination of the abnormal part. The patient should be comfortable and rested and comparison tests of muscles made on the contralateral side. Should differences exist they should be recorded.

Table 2-1 shows the accepted method of grading muscle strengths. A numerical

Table 2-1. *Classification of Muscle Grading*

Grade	Percent	Muscle Strength
0 = Zero	0	No evidence of contractility
1 = Trace	10	Evidence of slight contractility, no joint motion, gravity eliminated
2 = Poor	25	Complete range of motion with gravity eliminated
3 = Fair	50	Complete range of motion against gravity
4 = Good	75	Complete range of motion against gravity with some resistance
5 = Normal	100	Complete range of motion against gravity with full resistance

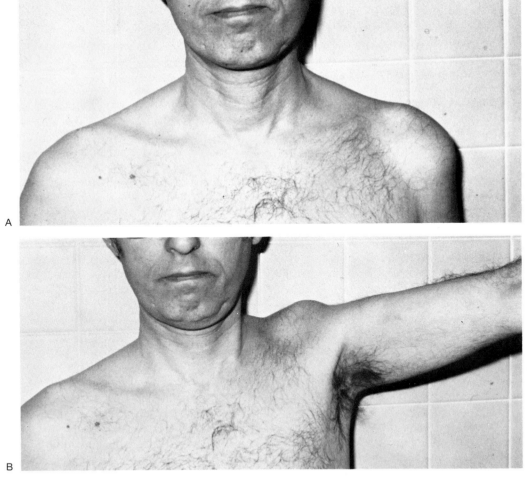

FIG. 2-6. A, This patient had difficulty raising his left upper extremity beyond 45 degrees of abduction. The extremity is shown at rest. B, The patient is holding his arm at 90 degrees of abduction with difficulty. At 45 degrees of abduction the scapula rotated, thereby allowing a greater degree of apparent abduction. Note the severe deltoid atrophy. The cause was not known.

value of 5 represents normal muscle strength, whereas a decreasing value means that strength is accordingly decreased.

If at all possible the same examiner should reexamine the patient each time so as to minimize errors of technique.

Muscles with nearly normal strength can be tested by having the subject attempt to move the part in the direction against applied resistance, or by having the subject hold the part with the muscle contracted while the examiner attempts to move the part against the usual muscle pull.[5] If the muscle is noticeably weak and the patient unable to move the muscle against gravity, it is tested with gravity eliminated. Finally, if it is too weak for movement, contraction can be determined by palpation of the tendon.

Proper positioning and comfort of both the patient and examiner are essential. The actions of multiple muscles may combine to produce the same movement. Therefore, while testing the strength of a muscle it is wise to observe and palpate the muscle and its tendon so as to eliminate the action of neighboring muscles. It is important to observe that the scapula is anchored in position before testing muscle strength about the shoulder girdle. For example, the examiner may mistake weakness of the serratus anterior or trapezius for deltoid weakness. On the other hand, close observation may demonstrate that it is the scapula that is actively rotating, giving the impression that abduction power of the arm is weakened (Fig. 2-6). However, careful testing will permit the examiner to differentiate these fine points. Serratus anterior weakness will permit the shoulder girdle to be passively lifted so that the tip of the acromion is at a level opposite the patient's chin. This condition is occasionally termed "loose shoulder" (Fig. 2-7).

Table 2-2 describes the important muscles about the shoulder girdle, their actions and nerve supply, the effect of paralysis, and the tests used to determine abnormalities.

WINGING OF THE SCAPULA. The combined actions of the trapezius and serratus anterior muscles are necessary to keep the

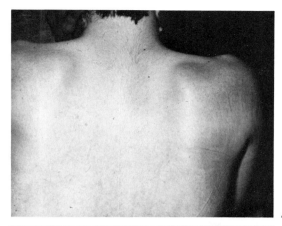

A

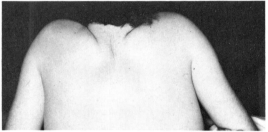

B

FIG. 2-7. A, A 15-year-old boy with Duchenne muscular dystrophy is shown at rest. Even so, note the atrophy of the back muscles and divergence of the scapulae. B, When upward force was placed on the extremities, the shoulder girdle could be displaced so that each acromion lay at the level of the chin. This is termed "loose shoulder" and is caused by serratus anterior weakness.

scapula in a normal position. Paralysis of either muscle leads to winging.

Trapezius paralysis leading to winging of the shoulder blade causes the scapula to be displaced downward and outward (Fig. 2-8C). The upper portion of the scapula is dislocated away from the midline. When winging results from serratus anterior weakness the scapula is displaced inward and upward (Fig. 2-8B). The inferior angle of the scapula in this latter case approaches the spine (Fig. 2-9).

In less pronounced cases of serratus anterior weakness, winging is first manifested when the patient attempts to raise the arm in forward flexion (Fig. 2-10). Scapula winging becomes more conspicuous as the arm is raised against resistance, whereas with complete paralysis of the serratus the scap-

Table 2-2. *Muscles Controlling Shoulder Actions*

Muscle	Nerves	Normal Function(s)	Paralysis	Test(s)
Trapezius	Spinal accessory n. and C3–4	Upper fibers elevate lateral clavicle and scapula; lower fibers brace and press scapula to the thorax	Winging of the scapula; scapula is displaced downward and laterally; superior angle is farther away from vertebral column than inferior angle; scapula bracing, overhead motion, and shoulder elevation are impaired.	Patient shrugs shoulders against resistance; abducts arm against resistance; superior braces shoulder by backward movement and adduction of scapula
Serratus anterior	Long thoracic n. and C5–7	Draws scapula forward keeping it closely applied to the thorax; when shoulder girdle is fixed, muscle acts as an accessory muscle of respiration.	Winging of the scapula, especially the inferior angle, with limited forward movement of the shoulder; elevation of the arm above the head is impaired, and on raising the arm from the side the scapula fails to rotate; scapula is displaced upward and inward.	Patient thrusts outstretched arm against wall or against resistance by examiner; abduction of the arm causes little winging, showing an important difference from effect of trapezius paralysis.
Latissimus dorsi	Thoracodorsal n. and C6–8	Adducts arm by pulling it backward and medially rotates it; upper fibers cause slight bracing and elevation of shoulder whereas lower fibers depress.	No gross changes at rest.	Downward and backward movement against resistance is applied under patient's elbow, resulting in brisk contraction which can be palpated at inferior angle of scapula when patient coughs.
Teres major	Thoracodorsal (lower subscapular) n. and C6–7	Action is same as for latissimus dorsi	Joint capsule cannot be adequately tightened; humeral head fixation inadequate when carrying heavy objects. Adduction can be satisfactorily performed by pectoralis major and latissimus dorsi.	Same as for latissimus dorsi. Muscle is palpable at lower lateral border of scapula.
Rhomboids	Dorsal scapular n. and C4–5	Weak adductors and elevators of shoulder girdle. With serratus anterior and trapezius, rhomboids draw scapula to the thorax and brace scapula.	Impression between vertebral border of scapula and chest wall is deepened, disappearing with raising of the arm.	Patient holds hand on hip, arm back and medial while examiner attempts to force elbow laterally and forward, palpating muscle bellies during test.
Levator scapulae	Dorsal scapular n., C3–5, and direct branches from third and fourth cervical nerves	Elevates shoulder girdle and moves it forward; assists in rotation of the scapula like the rhomboids. When shoulder is lowered, acromioclavicular joint is fixed, it flexes cervical spine laterally.	Isolated paralysis has not been documented.	Same as for rhomboids.
Sternocleidomastoid	Spinal accessory n. and branches from cervical plexus	Tilts head toward shoulder of same side and turns face toward the opposite side; accessory muscle of respiration.	Impairment of rotation of the head; head tilted toward unaffected side and the chin is turned toward the affected side. No important loss of shoulder function.	Turn patient's head to one side and then to other side with resistance over the opposite temporal area.

Muscle	Nerve	Action	Effect of paralysis	Test
Subclavius	Nerve to subclavius and C5–6	Braces sternal end of clavicle against sternum.	Isolated paralysis has not been observed.	None.
Deltoid	Axillary n. and C5–6	Raises arm to horizontal; anterior fibers adduct humerus, acromial fibers abduct and posterior fibers extend arm.	Weakness of abduction but still possible by rotation of the scapula by serratus anterior and trapezius if humeral head is fixed in the glenoid cavity.	With patient's arm abducted to 90°, the examiner resists upward movement.
Subscapularis	Subscapular nerves and C5–7	Medial rotation of humerus; inferior fibers adduct humerus.	Scapula remains in its normal position; isolated paralysis causes little weakness of rotation.	With elbow at side and flexed 90°, the patient resists examiner's attempt to force hand laterally.
Supraspinatus	Suprascapular n. and C4–6	Elevates humerus in anterolateral direction; aids in rotating scapula in sagittal plane; pulls head of humerus upward.	Isolated paralysis causes little change in position of shoulder at rest. Associated with deltoid paralysis, the shoulder joint space will widen.	Abduct arm against resistance (but this is occasionally difficult since trapezius overlies supraspinatus).
Infraspinatus	Suprascapular n. and C4–6	Lateral rotation of humerus and adduction of humerus.	No visible change in position of shoulder; paralysis of both muscles together causes loss of external rotation, whereas paralysis of one muscle makes external rotation difficult.	With elbow at side and flexed to 90°, patient resists examiner's attempt to push hand medially toward abdomen.
Teres minor	Axillary n. and C4–6	Scapula rotates about a vertical axis.		
Pectoralis major	Medial and lateral pectoral nerves and C5–T1	Medial rotation and adduction of humerus; elevates acromial end of clavicle and scapula by contraction of upper fibers; depresses clavicle via lower fibers and depresses head of humerus. Clavicular portion assists in flexion of arm.	Shoulder is elevated and depression of arm weakened; poor adduction; internal rotation of humerus unaffected while subscapularis is intact.	With arm in front of body, patient resists attempt by examiner to force it laterally. Two portions of muscle are visible and palpable.
Pectoralis minor	Medial pectoral n. and C6–8	Draws acromial end of clavicle forward and depresses it; assists serratus anterior in drawing scapula forward.	No important loss of function if paralysis is isolated.	Isolated testing difficult.
Coracobrachialis	Musculocutaneous n. and C5–6	Assists in fixing humeral head in glenoid cavity; rotates scapula slightly and flexes humerus.	Isolated paralysis rare. Subluxation of shoulder will occur if adduction of the abducted arm is attempted against resistance even if long head of triceps is functioning normally.	Isolated testing difficult.
Biceps brachii	Musculocutaneous n.	Most important function is flexion and supination of forearm.	Flexion of forearm is weakened but no significant loss of function in shoulder.	Flexion of supinated forearm against resistance.
Triceps brachii	Radial n. and C6–8	Extends forearm; long head extends the humerus at shoulder joint and in fixing the head of the humerus and is a weak adductor of the humerus.	Loss of extension of the elbow against resistance. Loss of long head, if associated with coracobrachialis paralysis, causes subluxation of the shoulder. Deltoid can extend arm independently.	With forearm in varying positions of flexion, patient resists effort of examiner to flex forearm further.

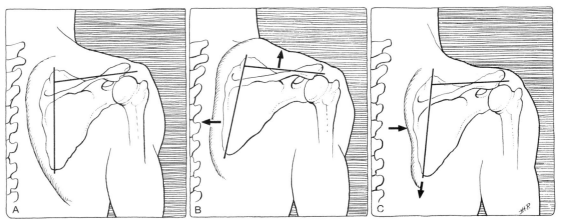

FIG. 2-8. Winging of scapula. A, The normal relationship of the scapula to the spine. B, With serratus anterior weakness the scapula is displaced inward and upward. C, With trapezius weakness the scapula is displaced downward and outward.

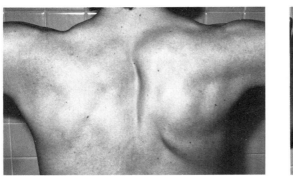

A   B

FIG. 2-9. A, When the extremities were abducted the right scapula was winged, indicating serratus anterior weakness. B, Winging of the right scapula in the same patient is demonstrated as he presses his hands against the wall.

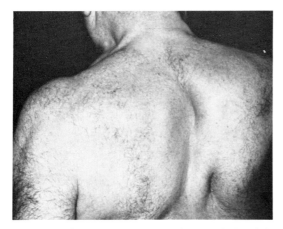

FIG. 2-10. Serratus anterior weakness of the right scapula is shown in a man while he abducts his right arm against resistance. The muscle paralysis started during a viremia.

ula cannot be fixed to the thorax, making it impossible for the patient to raise the arm at all. When there is weakness of both the trapezius and serratus muscles, winging is even more exaggerated than when only one of the muscles is affected. The entire back should be examined because scoliosis may create a false impression of winged scapula.

LATISSIMUS DORSI. When testing the strength of the latissimus dorsi, the cough reflex causes the muscle to contract. In hysterical paralysis, palpation of the muscle may give the impression of weakness or paralysis when the patient is asked to press downward against the examiner's hand, whereas during the act of coughing the muscle is felt to contract quite well.

DELTOID. Movement of the arm to the horizontal and frontal planes is carried out by the deltoid. The second half of movement, from the horizontal plane upward, is carried out mainly by the upper fibers of the trapezius aided by the serratus anterior. The trapezius may compensate to a certain degree for a paralyzed deltoid within the first half of this movement. In deltoid paralysis the second component of overhead motion comes into play from the beginning and confines overhead active movement to 45 degrees (Fig. 2-6).

Joint Motion

The shoulder joint has the most complex motions in the body. The shallow glenoid and the surrounding musculature make possible the observed wide range of motion. For this reason it is necessary to standardize a method of recording motion.[10] The accepted method is based on the principle of the neutral zero, first described by Cave and Roberts.[1] The method for measuring joint motion was approved in 1964 by the Orthopaedic Associations of the English-speaking world. The method is simple, accurate, and reproducible.[3] Most important, it permits comparisons to be made.

With the upper extremity in anatomic position, the starting position is 0 degrees, rather than 180 degrees. In pathologic states the starting point may be other than 0. All motions are recorded with three numbers. Motions that lead away from the body are recorded first on the left side of the starting position, 0 degrees, and motions that lead toward the body are recorded to the right side of the centrally positioned neutral 0-degree starting point.

In all cases of fixed positions, two numbers are recorded, the position in the given plane and the neutral 0-degree starting point. When the value of the fixed joint position is away from the midline, it is recorded to the left of the 0-degree starting point. If the value of the fixed joint position is toward the midline, it is placed on the right of the 0-degree starting point.

Figure 2-11 shows the sagittal (S), frontal

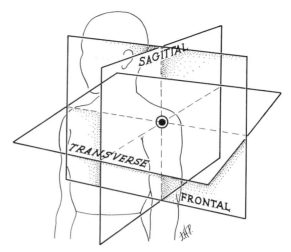

FIG. 2-11. The three planes through the shoulder.

(F), and transverse (T) planes. All rotations are recorded as "R" and not in the planes in which they occur.

Table 2-3 gives the accepted terminology and normal ranges of motions at the shoulder joint. It is important to differentiate glenohumeral from scapulothoracic motion. Whenever possible, motion should be tested with the patient erect, which will allow testing of the greatest possible range of motion.

Figure 2-12 demonstrates the method of measuring motions at the shoulder joint. The sum of the components make up the combined glenohumeral and scapulothoracic motions.

Horizontal flexion is motion of the arm in the horizontal plane anterior to the frontal (coronal) plane across the body, and is measured from 0 to 135 degrees. Horizontal extension is the horizontal motion posterior to the frontal (coronal) plane of the body and measures 0 to 30 degrees (Fig. 2-12A).

Abduction is motion upward and away from the body and measures 0 to 180 degrees, and adduction is the opposite motion of the arm, toward the midline of the body and beyond, and measures 0 to 75 degrees (Fig. 2-12B).

Forward flexion is the forward and upward motion of the arm in the sagittal plane of the body and measures 0 to 180 degrees.

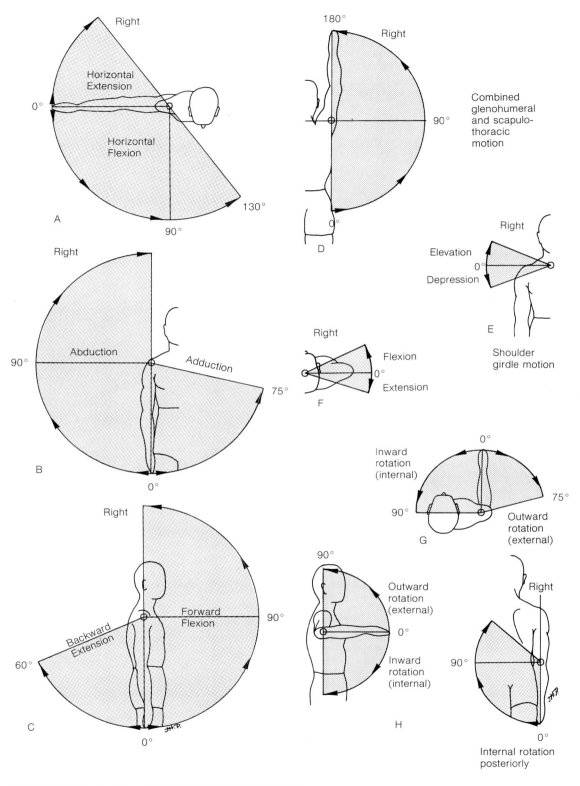

FIG. 2-12. Method of measuring motions at shoulder joint.

Table 2-3. *Shoulder Motions*

Terminology of Motion	Plane of Measurement	Average Range of Motion	Common Name
backward extension	Sagittal	50–0–180	posterior elevation
forward flexion			anterior elevation
abduction	Frontal	180–0–75	lateral elevation-
adduction			medial elevation*
horizontal extension	Transverse	30–0–135	none
horizontal flexion			
with arm at side, external rotation internal rotation		65–0–80	rotation
with arm in 90° abduction (lateral elevation), external rotation-internal rotation		90–0–70	rotation

* In coronal plane neutral to trunk

Backward extension is the upward motion of the arm in the posterior sagittal plane and measures 0 to 50 degrees (Fig. 2-12C).

Combined glenohumeral and scapulothoracic motion entails the rotation of the scapula (Fig. 2-12D).

Shoulder elevation and depression are measured in degrees (Fig. 2-12E).

Forward flexion and backward extension of the shoulder girdle are measured in degrees from a neutral 0-degree starting point. They measure motion of the scapula and the clavicle (Fig. 2-12F).

Inward and outward rotation is recorded with the arm at the side (Fig. 2-12G).

Rotation is measured with the arm abducted 90 degrees (Fig. 2-12H).

Comparison measurements at the shoulder can be more readily made if each examination is recorded by charting motions directly on diagramed sheets of cardboard. This method allows accurate and easy determination of motions at the shoulder.

Deep Tendon Reflexes

Deep reflexes or muscle stretch reflexes are produced by the percussion of the tendons at their insertions. The state of deep reflexes in different disease states can be clinically important. In acute disease of the anterior horn cell, for example, the deep reflexes are lost rapidly, whereas they are more slowly lost with peripheral neuropathic lesions. The following shoulder girdle reflexes are defined as follows:[7,11]

SCAPULOHUMERAL REFLEX. The inferior angle of the scapula is tapped. This normally causes the scapula to move in a medial direction toward the midline along with slight adduction of the arm. Here, the rhomboids are especially active. If the test does not produce results on one side in a very muscular individual, it is not clinically significant.

PECTORAL REFLEX. With the subject's arm semi-abducted, the examiner places his thumb over the pectoralis major tendon near its insertion on the humerus. A sharp blow is struck upward toward the armpit (Fig. 2-13). The contraction of the muscle may be seen and palpated, and causes the arm to internally rotate slightly and adduct.

BICEPS REFLEX. With the subject's arm semiflexed at the elbow and the forearm moderately pronated, the examiner places his thumb over the biceps tendon at the elbow and strikes the tendon. This normally produces a contraction of the muscle and flexion of the forearm.

TRICEPS REFLEX. The patient's elbow is approximately positioned the same as for the biceps reflex test, or it may be held at a right angle. With the subject's arm inter-

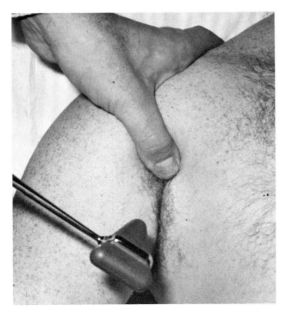

FIG. 2-13. The method for obtaining the pectoral reflex.

nally rotated, the triceps tendon is struck directly just above the olecranon. The triceps muscle contracts and the elbow extends.

CLAVICULAR REFLEX. It is elicited by tapping the lateral portion of the subject's clavicle, resulting in an extensive contraction of various muscles in the upper limb. It may be useful in demonstrating differences in deep reflex irritability between the two upper limbs.

The degree of contraction of the tested muscles may be graded 0, 1, 2, or 3, the higher numbers indicating a greater amount of contraction.

Superficial Reflexes

Superficial reflexes are elicited by stimulating the skin. Muscle responses are produced by way of a reflex arc in which the stimulus is achieved by stroking a sensory zone. Scapular and interscapular reflexes are obtained by scratching the patient's skin over the scapula or interscapular surface, which results in contraction of the scapular muscles.

An important reflex seen in infancy is the Moro reflex (see Fig. 9-10). It is present from birth but usually disappears between 16 and 20 weeks of age. It may not be elicited if the baby has brachial plexus injury, hemiparesis, or fracture of the clavicle. It is elicited in the infant by supporting the infant in the supine position with his neck slightly flexed. The head is dropped briefly, gently, and rapidly through an arc of 30 degrees. A positive response consists of symmetric abduction, extension, and circumduction of the upper extremities, and flexion of the lower extremities.

Clinical Tests for Detection of Neurovascular Compression Syndromes

Rash treatment should not be instituted on the basis of isolated findings. The results of these tests must be correlated with the entire clinical picture before committing the patient to definitive treatment.

ADSON (SCALENE) MANEUVER. With the patient sitting in a relaxed position, hands in lap, the examiner palpates the radial pulse. The patient holds a deep breath, and extends the neck fully, turning the chin to the side being examined. A decrease in or disappearance of the radial pulse is recorded as a positive result of the test. Any part of the test may occlude the subclavian artery.

MODIFIED ADSON TEST. Starting from the same position as that used for the Adson test, the patient's arm is abducted to 90 degrees and externally rotated with the elbow flexed. The subject's head is turned as far as possible to the examined side. The pulse is palpated while the patient holds a deep breath and then coughs. Diminution or disappearance of the pulse represents a positive result of the test.

COSTOCLAVICULAR MANEUVER. The examiner palpates the radial pulse with the patient sitting in a relaxed position. A stethoscope is placed over the midaspect of the clavicle. The patient is asked to extend and depress the shoulders with the examiner exerting pull on the arm in the same direction. Change in the pulse or production of a bruit is recorded.

An alternate method of this maneuver

can be performed if the arm is displaced backward with abduction of the shoulder and flexion of the elbow to 90 degrees. Changes in the pulse or findings of venous obstruction are noted.

HYPERABDUCTION SYNDROME TEST. With the patient sitting in a relaxed position, the examiner palpates the radial pulse and listens for a bruit beneath the clavicle or in the axilla. The patient's arm is then hyperabducted while changes in the pulse are noted. Obstruction in this syndrome is caused by compression of the artery at the level just beneath the insertion of the pectoralis minor tendon. In partial obstruction, a bruit is heard over the subclavian artery. When there is complete obstruction, no bruit is heard.

A modification of this maneuver can be performed with the patient sitting relaxed, arm abducted to 135 degrees and externally rotated, and head turned as far as possible from the examined side. When the patient holds a deep breath, the radial pulse is palpated and changes in the pulse are noted.

USEFUL CLINICAL SIGNS

YERGASON SIGN.[12] The patient's elbow is flexed to 90 degrees with the forearm pronated. While the examiner holds the patient's wrist so as to resist supination, he then directs that active supination be made against resistance. Pain localized to the bicipital groove suggests a disease state of the long head of the biceps as, for example, synovitis of the tendon sheath.

LUDINGTON SIGN.[4] With the patient's fingers interlocked on top of his head and arms abducted, the biceps muscle is actively contracted. Active disease within the bicipital groove may cause pain.

Results of the two aforementioned signs are more likely to be positive in the acute stages of disease. In tendon rupture or advanced degeneration pain may be minimal.

HEUTER'S SIGN.[2] Forearm flexion in pronation is more energetic when the biceps muscle is tense than when the forearm is supinated. In pronation the radius crosses the ulna, so that in flexion the radius is supported and is directed into flexion with only slight exertion. With flexion of the forearm the biceps contracts and its muscle belly swells. Flexion of the forearm in pronation is accomplished primarily by the brachialis muscle, the biceps remaining soft and flabby. However, in forcible movements the biceps also contracts during flexion of the pronated forearm, but forcible forearm flexion in supination causes a striking difference in biceps muscle contraction. Thus, a contraction of the biceps in pronation always causes a movement of supination immediately afterward. With biceps tendon disruptions this sign is absent.

ROENTGEN TECHNIQUE USED IN DIAGNOSIS

The bones and joints comprising the shoulder girdle are among the most difficult in the human body to evaluate by roentgenologic techniques. The numerous curves, recesses, projections, and relationships of the anatomic parts in the shoulder region require exceptional x-ray resolution so that significant normal and abnormal findings are not missed.[6] Not only must the surgeon correctly assess roentgenograms but he must also interpret the findings in relationship to the functional anatomy of the region. X-ray films of normal-appearing structures and the positions employed in obtaining them are demonstrated. It should be remembered that painful injuries may preclude the taking of diagnostic films. The use of special radiologic techniques such as shoulder joint arthrography is discussed in later sections.

Shoulder

ANTEROPOSTERIOR PROJECTIONS. Four different anteroposterior x-ray projections that may be taken are (1) projections of the glenohumeral joint positioning the scapula on a plane parallel with the cassette; (2) an anteroposterior view with the arm externally rotated (Fig. 2-14); (3) an anteroposterior view with the extremity in neutral position; and (4) an anteroposterior view with the extremity in various degrees of internal rotation.

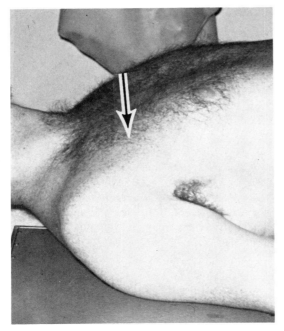

FIG. 2-14. The arm is externally rotated. The arrow indicates the direction of the x-ray beam.

In the first view, the patient is examined when he is in either the erect or supine position. When injury is present, it is less discomforting to take x-ray films of the shoulder in the erect position. The center of the cassette is positioned behind the coracoid. If there is significant curvature of the spine or a true anteroposterior view of the glenoid is desired, the patient is rotated enough to place the scapula parallel with the cassette. The central ray is directed perpendicular to the plane of the film. This view is often needed when taking anteroposterior films of total shoulder replacement.

In the next view, the patient's arm is placed in anatomic position. The arm is slightly abducted and the coronal planes of the humeral epicondyles are placed parallel with the cassette. An x-ray film is made of the glenohumeral joint in this position with the arm in external rotation. The external rotation position permits visualization of the soft-tissue and bone structures of the shoulder in their anatomic positions. It gives a profile of the greater tuberosity, and the site of insertion of the supraspinatus tendon.

Next, the patient rests his hand against his thigh. This rotates the humerus inward so that the epicondyles of the humerus are placed 45 degrees to the cassette. This gives the neutral position. This projection shows the posterior part of the supraspinatus insertion site which can show small calcific deposits.

Finally, the patient flexes the elbow and internally rotates the arm in slight abduction with the back of the hand on the hip. This internal rotation position, in effect, permits a lateral profile of the humerus to be seen. This view demonstrates the region of the subdeltoid bursa and shows a profile of the humerus. It also demonstrates a profile of the subscapularis tendon insertion site.

TRANSTHORACIC VIEW OF THE GLENOHUMERAL JOINT. With the patient erect and the lateral aspect of the shoulder to be examined placed against the cassette, the opposite upper limb is placed above the head with the forearm resting on the vertex of the skull. The central ray is directed perpendicular to the plane of the film just below the level of the coracoid (Fig. 2-15). This projection permits an evaluation of the integrity of the joint, since any break in the normal parabolic curve made up of the humerus and axillary border of the scapula is patho-

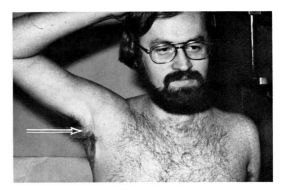

FIG. 2-15. Method for obtaining a lateral transthoracic view of the shoulder. The affected shoulder is placed against the cassette and the unaffected hand is placed upon the head. The arrow indicates the direction of the x-ray beam.

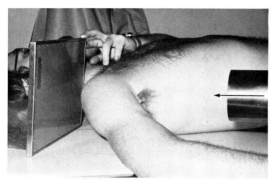

FIG. 2-16. Method for obtaining a true axillary view of the shoulder. The arrow shows the direction of the x-ray beam.

logic, as in shoulder dislocation (see Chapter 20 on shoulder dislocation).

TRUE AXILLARY VIEW (INFEROSUPERIOR AXIAL PROJECTION). The patient's shoulder is elevated 4 inches with the arm abducted, and the cassette is positioned over the top of the shoulder. The central ray is directed through the axilla toward the acromioclavicular joint (Fig. 2-16). When abduction is painful or limited, this view may better be taken with the patient seated. It shows the glenohumeral articulation and coracoid process. The insertion site of the teres minor may also be seen.

MODIFIED AXILLARY VIEWS. A reverse view, the superoinferior projection, may be taken with the patient seated and the arm abducted and resting on a curved cassette. The central ray is directed toward the shoulder at a 5- to 15-degree angle toward the elbow. This view also allows visualization of the glenohumeral articulation.

When the arm cannot be abducted, the patient is placed in a supine position with the cassette behind the shoulder. The central ray is directed at 25 degrees toward the acromioclavicular joint. Although this view demonstrates the glenohumeral articulation it is not a true axillary projection.

An excellent view of the glenohumeral joint can be obtained when the patient's arm is positioned 180 degrees overhead with the back of the shoulder resting on the cassette. The central ray is directed perpendicular to the cassette (Fig. 2-17).

Finally, if only 15 to 20 degrees of arm abduction is possible, the cassette can be placed perpendicularly over the top of the shoulder, and the x-ray beam is directed 25 degrees downward into the open axilla.

SCAPULAR "Y" VIEW.[9] This view is especially useful for determining shoulder dislocations. It avoids additional trauma and pain from positioning. It is easy to reproduce and interpret. Roentgenograms are taken with the patient erect or supine with the injured shoulder in a 60-degree anterior oblique position against the cassette. Arm position may vary without changing the relationship of the humeral head to its glenoid fossa. The central ray passes through the injured shoulder.

The scapula appears as a "Y," with the body forming the vertical limb, and the acromion and coracoid forming the upper limbs. Normally, the humeral head projects directly over the intersection of the three limbs of the "Y." In anterior dislocations the humeral head is seen beneath the coracoid process, whereas in posterior dislocations

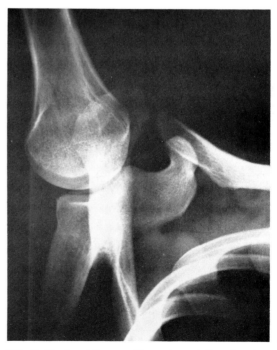

FIG. 2-17. An oblique axillary view of the glenohumeral joint.

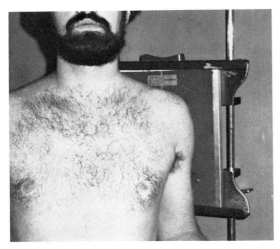

FIG. 2-18. A true anteroposterior view of the glenoid fossa is obtained when the patient is tilted 25 degrees toward the side to be examined, and the x-ray beam is directed perpendicular to the cassette.

the head is under the acromial process (see Fig. 20-33C).

GLENOID FOSSA VIEW. This view can be made with the patient erect or supine. The patient is tilted 25 to 30 degrees toward the side to be examined and the cassette placed centrally behind the shoulder. The central ray is directed perpendicular to the plane of the film. This view demonstrates the gleno-humeral joint space and glenoid fossa (Fig. 2-18). This projection is almost identical with the anteroposterior view with the scapula parallel to the cassette.

BICIPITAL GROOVE VIEW. The patient leans over the table, resting the supinated fore-arms on the table. A cassette is placed on the forearm. After palpating the top of the bicipital groove, the central ray is directed through the groove (Fig. 2-19). This projection gives an axial view of the acromioclavicular joint and the bicipital groove.

ACROMIOCLAVICULAR JOINT. The patient is placed against the cassette in the erect anteroposterior or posteroanterior position. The arms are allowed to hang unsupported or, if possible, equally weighted sandbags are suspended from the wrists. The central ray is directed perpendicular to the midline of the body. By using large film, both joints are projected simultaneously onto one film. This view can demonstrate abnormalities such as separation and dislocation (see section on acromioclavicular sprains).

Similar projections, with the central ray directed upward 15 degrees toward the acromioclavicular joint, will show the relationship of the bones and separate the acromioclavicular joint from the rest of the scapula.

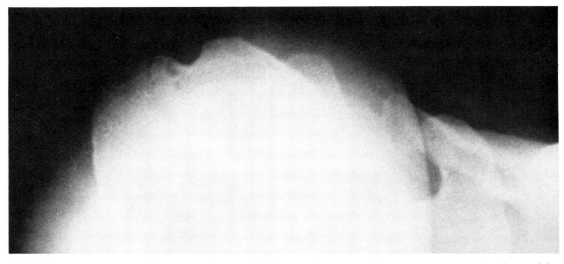

FIG. 2-19. A tangential view of the bicipital groove was obtained while the patient leaned forward and rested the supinated forearms on a table. The cassette was laid on the forearms and the x-ray beam was directed through the palpated bicipital groove.

Clavicle

The anteroposterior view is obtained with the patient in either the prone or the erect position and the central ray directed perpendicular to the plane of the film. This view shows a frontal projection of the clavicle. An axial view of the clavicle can be demonstrated by raising the shoulder on a sandbag, placing the cassette over the superior aspect of the shoulder, and directing the central ray as nearly perpendicular to the plane of the film as possible. Multiple other-angled projections give axial views.

Scapula

The anteroposterior view of the scapula is made with the patient supine or erect. The arm is abducted to draw the scapula outward, the elbow is flexed, and the central ray is directed perpendicular to the middle of the scapula and plane of the film. This

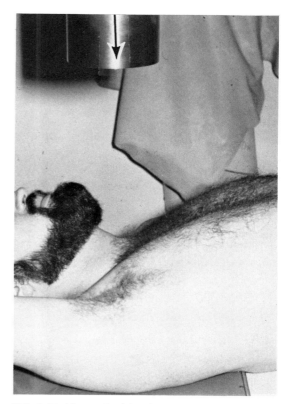

FIG. 2-21. The method for obtaining a tangential view of the scapula. With the arm overhead the body is rotated until the scapula projects free of the rib cage. Arrow indicates the direction of the x-ray beam.

view will show the outer part of the scapula without superimposition of other structures.

The lateral view is made with the patient erect or supine. The patient extends the arm upward, flexes the elbow, and positions the hand beneath the head (Fig. 2-20).

To obtain an oblique lateral (tangential) projection, the patient's arm is placed over the head as described, and his body is rotated until the scapula projects free of the rib cage (Fig. 2-21). The central ray is directed perpendicular to the lateral border of the rib cage at the level of the midscapular region.

Sternum

The sternum, with its underlying soft tissues and bone, makes it difficult to evaluate radiographically.

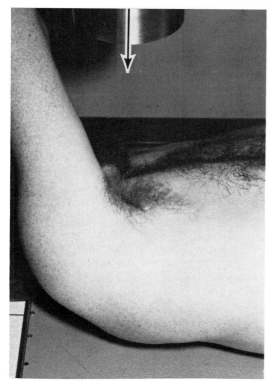

FIG. 2-20. The method for obtaining a lateral view of scapula. The arrow indicates the direction of the x-ray beam.

The left oblique projection is made with the patient prone and the sternum positioned on the center of the table. The left shoulder is elevated just enough to obviate superimposition of the sternum and vertebral column. The patient either holds his breath or stops breathing momentarily during exposure. The central ray is directed perpendicular to the midpoint of the film. This view will show a frontal projection of the sternum.

The lateral view is obtained with the patient standing or in a recumbent position. The shoulders are rotated backward and the hands locked behind the back. The frontal aspect of the sternum should be perpendicular to the plane of the film. The breasts of the female are drawn to the sides. Respiration is momentarily suspended. The central ray is directed horizontal to the midpoint of the film (Fig. 2-22). This projection (anteroposterior view) is obtained when the patient is placed in a prone position with the arms along the sides of the body, palms facing upward and each shoulder is positioned in the same transverse plane. One or both joints may be examined. In the latter case, the head is tilted backward, the chin resting on the table. For unilateral examination, the patient turns his head to the affected side. The central ray is directed perpendicular to the midpoint of the film. This projection demonstrates the sternoclavicular joints and medial ends of the clavicles.

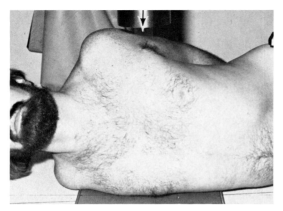

FIG. 2-22. The method for obtaining a lateral view of sternum. Arrow shows the direction of the x-ray beam.

The lateromedial (oblique) projection is made with the patient placed in a position similar to that described previously. The central ray is directed 5 to 15 degrees toward the median sagittal plane, first from one side and then from the other. In this projection the vertebral column is not shown.

Ribs

The initial examination of the ribs following trauma should include anteroposterior and lateral views of the chest cage. This preliminary examination will demonstrate the extent of rib injury and the underlying tissues. When the patient has been stabilized physiologically, additional views that detail the rib cage architecture including its joints can be obtained. Every attempt should be made to position the affected rib(s) parallel with the plane of the film.

The upper anterior ribs are best viewed with the patient erect or recumbent in the posteroanterior position against a large cassette. The central ray is directed perpendicular to the plane of the film. To view the posterior ribs the patient is placed in the anteroposterior position, and the central ray similarly directed.

To view the anterior axillary ribs, the patient is positioned erect or recumbent, back against the cassette and body rotated 45 degrees, the affected side toward the film. The central ray is directed perpendicular to the plane of the film, 4 to 5 inches above the midpoint of the film for the upper ribs and 4 to 5 inches below the midpoint for the lower ribs.

The posterior axillary portion of the ribs are best seen when the patient faces the film (posteroanterior) with the affected side rotated 45 degrees away from the film. The central ray is directed toward the film as in the projection for the axillary portions of the ribs projected free of self-imposition.

XERORADIOGRAPHY

In this electrostatic process,[8] a metal plate coated with pure selenium is electrostatically charged. The plate is exposed by x ray, since radiation decreases the resistance of the charged selenium in proportion to the amount of radiation striking the plate at any given point. Thus, the charge on the surface of the selenium is selectively decreased by a migration of electrons from the metal base through the selenium. At the end of the x-ray exposure a residual electrostatic charge remains on the selenium, the pattern depending on the pattern of radiation that first strikes the plate, and being a function of the various tissue densities.

The residual charge is made visible by exposing the selenium surface to a cloud of powder particles which have been negatively charged. These particles cling to positively charged parts of the plate (see Fig. 20-61C). The powder image then shows the radiodensities of the studied tissue. By changing the charge of the powder particles to positive, image reversal can be achieved.

The advantages of xeroradiography are (1) exceptional resolution, (2) density differences of tissues which can be seen in one image without multiple exposures, and (3) the enhancement of edges of tissues which help delineate overlapping structures such as the sternoclavicular joint region.

ARTERIOGRAPHY

Arteriography is employed for determining vessel abnormalities following trauma and evaluating tumors of bone and soft tissues. Accurate information as to exact site of a lesion and a compromised circulation can be established by this technique (see Fig. 14-15). For example, a swollen part owing to fracture hemorrhage or vascular damage can best be assessed by arteriography (see Fig. 14-17).

The degree of vascularity of a bone tumor can be determined and major feeder vessels identified. This is especially important in tumors at the shoulder. An expert arteriographer can identify abnormal vascular patterns or a lack of any pattern, which can help decide whether a bone tumor is relatively benign or malignant. Thus, the method can be helpful for diagnosis in select cases.

REFERENCES

1. Cave, E. F., and Roberts, S. M.: A method for measuring and recording joint function. J. Bone Joint Surg., 34:455, 1936.
2. Heuter, C.: Zur Diagnose der Verletzungen des M. biceps Brachii. Arch. Klin. Chir., 5:321–323, 1864.
3. Joint Motion, Measuring and Recording. American Academy of Orthopaedic Surgeons, 1965.
4. Ludington, N. A.: Rupture of long head of biceps cubiti muscle. Am. J. Surg., 77:358, 1923.
5. Mayo Clinic and Mayo Foundation: Clinical Examinations in Neurology, 3rd ed. Philadelphia, W. B. Saunders Co., 1971.
6. Merrill, V.: Atlas of Roentgenographic Positions and Standard Radiologic Procedures, Vol. 1. St. Louis, C. V. Mosby Co., 1975.
7. Monrad-Krohn, G. H.: The Clinical Examination of the Nervous System, 8th ed. New York, Paul B. Hoeber, Inc., 1947.
8. Roach, J. F.: Xeroradiography. Radiol. Clin. North Am., 8:271–275, 1970.
9. Rubin, S. A., Gray, R. L., and Green, W. R.: The scapular "Y": A diagnostic aid in shoulder trauma. Radiology, 110:725–726, 1974.
10. Russe, O., Gerhardt, J. J., and King, P. S.: An Atlas of Examination, Standard by Otto Russe. Baltimore, Williams & Wilkins Co., 1972.
11. Steegmann, A. T.: Examination of the Nervous System, 2nd ed. Chicago, Year Book Medical Publishers, Inc., 1962.
12. Yergason, R. M.: Supination sign. J. Bone Joint Surg. 13:160, 1931.

3

Gross Anatomy

SHAHAN K. SARRAFIAN

Topographically the shoulder is divided into three regions:[1] (1) anteriorly, the axillary region; (2) posteriorly, the scapular region; and (3) laterally, the deltoid region.

AXILLARY REGION

The Axillary Space

The axillary space is located between the inner aspect of the glenohumeral joint, proximal humerus, and the thoracic wall. This pyramidal space, located above the armpit, has four walls: anterior, oblique; posterior, oblique; medial, convex; and lateral, narrow. It is supplemented by the base and the summit (Fig. 3-1).

Anterior Wall

The anterior wall is limited above by the clavicle, below by the inferior border of the pectoralis major, laterally by the anterior border of the deltoid, and medially by an imaginary vertical line extending from the middle third of the clavicle to the inferior border of the pectoralis major, passing slightly lateral to the breast.

SKIN. The skin is thin and mobile. The deep layer of the subcutaneous tissue forms a superficial fascia incorporating in its two layers, the inferior fibers of the platysma, a few vessels, and ramifications from the brachial and cervical plexuses.

SUPERFICIAL APONEUROSIS. The superficial aponeurosis originates from the anterior border of the clavicle. This aponeurosis spreads over the anterior surface of the pectoralis major and at the inferior border of the muscle divides into two layers: a superficial layer forming the aponeurosis of the armpit, directed posteriorly towards the inferior border of the latissimus dorsi, and a deep layer covering the posterior surface of the pectoralis major (Fig. 3-2).

SUPERFICIAL MUSCULAR LAYER. The pectoralis major muscle forms the third layer. The lateral border of this muscle delineates, with the anterior border of the deltoid, a deltopectoral space, triangular in contour with the base formed by the clavicle. The cephalic vein and the deltoid branch of the acromiothoracic artery are located in this space (Fig. 3-3).

DEEP MUSCULAR LAYER. Two muscles form the next muscular layer: the pectoralis minor and the subclavius. They are separated by a triangular space, the clavipectoral triangle, with the base directed toward the ribs and the apex toward the coracoid process.

The aponeurosis of the subclavius originates from the anterior border of the clavicle, turns around the muscle, and attaches to the posterior border of the clavicle, forming an osteofibrous gutter. This aponeurosis extends inferiorly and covers the clavipectoral triangle. On the superior border of the pectoralis minor, the clavipec-

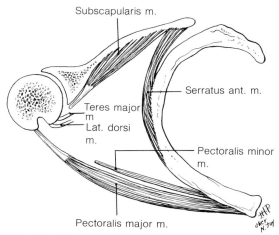

FIG. 3-1. Axillary space.

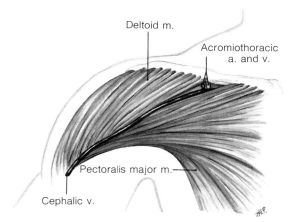

FIG. 3-3. Deltopectoral space.

toral aponeurosis divides into two layers, incorporates the muscle, and continues distally as the axillary suspensory ligament of Gerdy. The distal segment of this aponeurosis is triangular. The base is directed distally and inserts on the axillary fascia, determining the concavity of the axilla. The apex corresponds to the coracoid process. The medial side is formed by the inferior border of the pectoralis minor, and the lateral border is continuous with the coracobrachial fascia (Figs. 3-3 and 3-4).

Posterior Wall

The posterior wall is formed above by the anterior surface of the subscapularis muscle and below by the teres major and latissimus dorsi.

Between the inferior border of the subscapularis and the superior border of the teres major, a triangular space is formed. The base of the triangle corresponds to the neck of the humerus. This triangle is di-

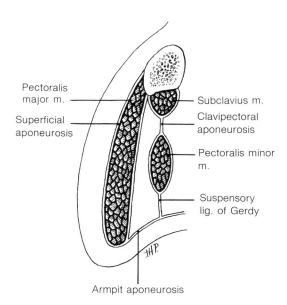

FIG. 3-2. Aponeuroses of the anterior wall of the axilla.

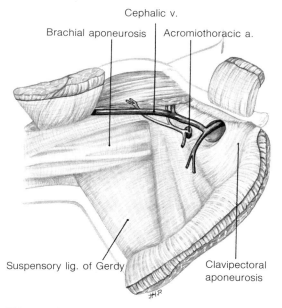

FIG. 3-4. Second layer of the anterior wall is formed by the clavipectoral fascia, the pectoralis minor, and the suspensory ligament of Gerdy.

vided into two subspaces by the long head of the triceps: laterally, the quadrilateral, or humerotricipital, space and, medially, the triangular, or omotricipital, space (Fig. 3-5).

Medial Wall

The medial wall is formed by the thoracic wall reinforced by the superior and middle digitations of the serratus anterior.

The Lateral Wall

The lateral wall is formed below by the coracobrachialis and the two heads of the biceps, and above by the base of the coracoid process and the inner surface of the glenohumeral joint. This wall, located at the convergence of the anterior and posterior walls, is narrow.

The Base

The base is concave transversely and anteroposteriorly. The concavity is determined by the vertical implantation of the suspensory ligament of Gerdy.

The superficial fascia covers the entire

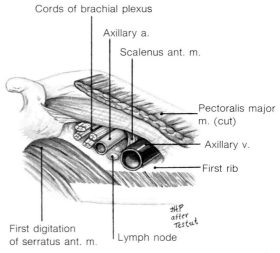

FIG. 3-6. Apex of the axilla. (After Testut and Jacob.[1])

surface and is continuous anteriorly with the fascia of the pectoralis major, posteriorly with the fascia of the teres major and latissimus dorsi. Medially, this fascia fuses with the fascia of the serratus anterior and laterally it blends with the brachial aponeurosis.

The Apex

The apex of the truncated pyramid corresponds to the clavicostal opening. It is limited distally by the first rib and the first digitation of the serratus anterior, proximally by the clavicle and the subclavius muscle, and laterally and posteriorly by the coracoid process and the coracoclavicular ligaments.[1] The apex of the axilla gives passage, from a lateral to medial direction, to the cords of the brachial plexus, the subclavian artery, and the subclavian vein (Fig. 3-6).

Contents of Axillary Region

Neurovascular Bundle

The axillary neurovascular bundle is encased in a tube, the axillary sheath. This sheath derives from the fascia covering the scalene muscles. It is part of the fascia that covers the cervical vertebral column and

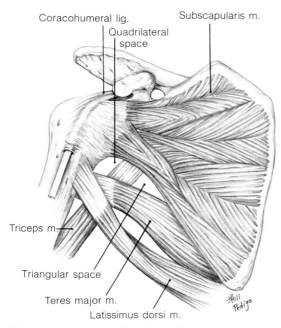

FIG. 3-5. Posterior wall of the axilla.

the pre- and postvertebral muscles of the neck. The axillary sheath is attached to the fascia behind the subclavius.

The neurovascular bundle has an oblique course in the axillary space. It passes from the medial wall to the lateral wall, and at the inferior border of the pectoralis major, the axillary artery becomes the brachial artery (Fig. 3-7).

Regionally, the axillary artery is divided into three portions (Fig. 3-8):

The first portion of the axillary artery is located between the clavicle and the superior border of the pectoralis minor. The axillary vein is medial to the artery. Lateral to the artery are the cords of the brachial plexus. The medial cord crosses the artery from behind. Posteriorly, the artery rests over the costal surface covered by the digitations of the serratus anterior. Anteriorly, the artery is covered by the clavicular head of the pectoralis major and the clavipectoral fascia. The middle of the clavicle corresponds to the origin of the axillary artery.

The superior thoracic artery, inconstant branch, supplies the upper two intercostal spaces. The acromiothoracic artery arises at the superior border of the pectoralis minor,

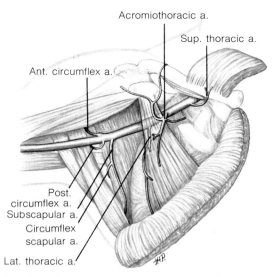

FIG. 3-8. The axillary artery with its 3 portions: first portion is proximal to the pectoralis minor, second portion is behind the pectoralis minor, and third portion is below the pectoralis minor.

pierces the clavipectoral fascia, and divides into four branches: a pectoral branch supplying the pectoral muscles; an acromial branch directed to the upper surface of the acromion, passing under the border of the deltoid; a deltoid branch joining the cephalic vein in the deltopectoral triangle; and a clavicular twig directed to the sternoclavicular joint (Fig. 3-9).

The superior nerve of the pectoralis

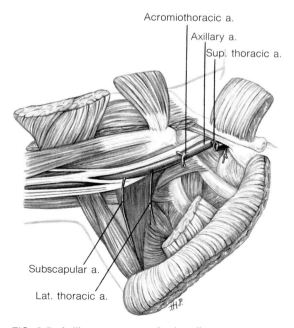

FIG. 3-7. Axillary neurovascular bundle.

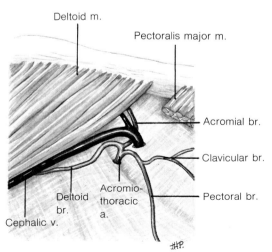

FIG. 3-9. Vessels of the deltopectoral space.

major crosses the axillary artery near its origin and pierces the clavipectoral fascia, innervating the clavicular head of the muscle and the superior portion of the sternal head.

The inferior nerve of the pectoralis major crosses the axillary artery anteriorly, passes under the acromiothoracic artery, and also pierces the clavipectoral fascia to innervate the pectoralis major and pectoralis minor. The nerve of the pectoralis minor crosses the axillary artery posteriorly and appears between the artery and the vein. It innervates the pectoralis minor and gives an anastomotic branch to the inferior nerve of the pectoralis major, forming the ansa of the pectoralis. This nerve loop is located anterior to the axillary artery, under the origin of the acromiothoracic artery. Muscular branches from this loop innervate the pectoralis minor (Fig. 3-10). The inferior nerve to the subscapularis arises from the posterior cord at this level.

The second portion of the axillary artery is located behind the pectoralis minor. The axillary vein and the medial root of the median nerve are on the inner aspect of the artery. Lateral to the artery is the lateral root of the median nerve. Posterior to the artery is the posterior cord. The nerves to the teres major and latissimus dorsi arise at

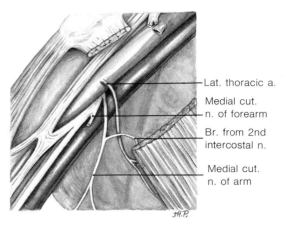

FIG. 3-11. Neurovascular branches correspond to the second portion of the axillary artery.

this level from the posterior surface of the posterior cord. The medial cutaneous nerves of the arm and forearm branch here from the inner aspect of the medial cord.

The lateral thoracic artery, or external mammary artery, arises at the lower border of the pectoralis minor and is directed to the chest wall between the pectoralis major and the serratus anterior (Fig. 3-11).

The third portion of the axillary artery is located below the pectoralis minor. The terminal branches of the brachial plexus surround the artery. The median nerve and the musculocutaneous nerves are anterior to the artery; the ulnar nerve and the medial cutaneous nerves to the arm and forearm

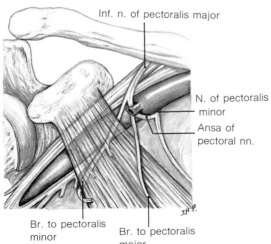

FIG. 3-10. Neurovascular branches correspond to the first portion of the axillary artery.

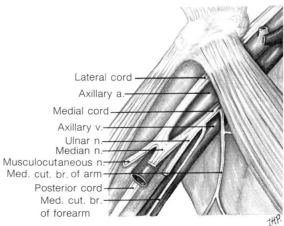

FIG. 3-12. Neurovascular branches correspond to the third portion of the axillary artery.

are medial and posterior in relationship; the radial nerve and axillary nerve are posterior to the artery. The axillary vein is located on the medial and slightly posterior aspect of the artery (Fig. 3-12).

The subscapular artery is the artery of the posterior wall. It follows the inferior border of the subscapularis and sends a large branch, the circumflex scapular artery, through the triangular space. The posterior circumflex artery arises at about the same level, and joined by the axillary nerve, passes posteriorly through the quadrilateral space, encircling the surgical neck of the humerus (Fig. 3-13). During its transverse course, the axillary nerve is situated at about 6 cm. from the origin of the deltoid (see Fig. 3-20). The anterior circumflex ar-

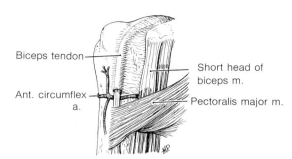

FIG. 3-14. Relationship of the anterior circumflex artery. (After Henry.[3])

Veins

In the axillary region each arterial branch is accompanied by two satellite veins directed toward the axillary vein. This vein is formed by the union of the two humeral veins and the basilic vein. This union occurs near the inferior border of the pectoralis major.

The cephalic vein courses in the deltopectoral triangle and near the clavicle passes under the pectoralis major; it covers the thoracoacromial artery, piercing the clavipectoral fascia to join the axillary vein.

Lymphatics

The axillary lymph nodes are arranged in five groups (Fig. 3-15):

In the *brachial group* (lateral group), the nodes are located along the medial aspect of the axillary vein in its lower segment. They drain the superficial and deep lymphatics of the entire upper extremity. In turn, they drain into the central group, the subclavicular group, and partially into the supraclavicular nodes.

In the *thoracic group* (external mammary group, pectoral group), the nodes are located on the inner wall of the axilla along the lateral thoracic vein (external mammary vein) at the lower border of the pectoralis minor. They drain the breast, the skin of the anterior and lateral aspects of the chest wall, and the supraumbilical portion of the

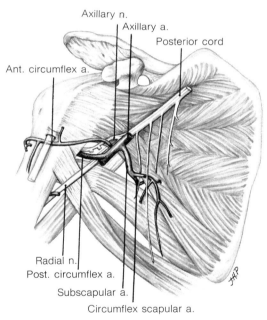

FIG. 3-13. Neurovascular branches of the posterior axillary wall.

tery originates at the level of the inferior border of the subscapularis and reaches the anterior aspect of the surgical neck of the humerus, passing under the conjoint tendon of the coracobrachialis and short head of the biceps (Fig. 3-14).

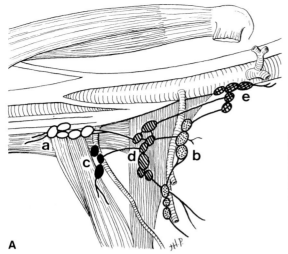

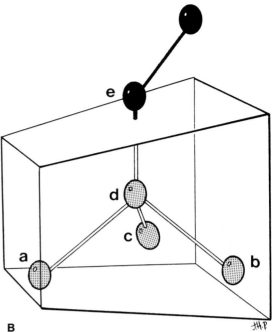

FIG. 3-15. A, Lymphatics of the axillary space. Brachial group (a); thoracic group (b); subscapular group (c); central group (d); subclavicular group (e). B, Diagram of axillary lymph node groups. Brachial group (a); thoracic group (b); subscapular group (c); central group (d); subclavicular group (e).

abdomen. They drain into the central group and a few lymph channels go directly into the subclavicular group.

In the *subscapular group* (posterior group), the nodes are located on the posterior wall of the axilla along the subscapular vessels. They drain the skin and muscles of the superior aspect of the back and posterior aspect of the shoulder. They drain into the central group.

In the *central group,* the nodes are located at the base of the axilla between the chest wall and the arc delineated by the lateral thoracic vein joining the axillary vein. They drain the three preceding axillary lymph node groups. They also drain into the subclavicular group.

In the *subclavicular group* (apical group), the nodes are located along the upper segment of the axillary vein between the pectoralis minor and the clavicle. They drain the central group and also receive lymphatics from the other axillary nodes, the cephalic lymph nodes, and some from the breast directly. They in turn drain into the supraclavicular lymph trunk which ends in the right lymph duct, or the thoracic duct (left side).

SCAPULAR REGION

The scapular region corresponds to the posterior aspect of the scapula. Topographically the region is divided into two regions by the spinous process of the scapula: the supraspinatus fossa and the infraspinatus fossa.

Supraspinatus Fossa

Two muscular layers separated by an aponeurosis are encountered in this fossa.

The first muscular layer is formed by the insertion of the trapezius on the posterior border of the spinous process of the scapula. This flat, relatively thin muscle is covered by a thin aponeurosis.

The supraspinatus aponeurosis covers the entire supraspinatus fossa. It inserts on the posterior border of the spine of the scapula, the superior border of the scapula, and the proximal segment of the medial border of the scapula. This aponeurosis is thick medially and thin laterally. In conjunction with the supraspinatus fossa, it delineates a fibro-osseous space for the muscle.

The second muscular layer is formed by

Trapezial br., post. scapular a.
Suprascapular a.
Suprascapular n.
Posterior
scapular a.

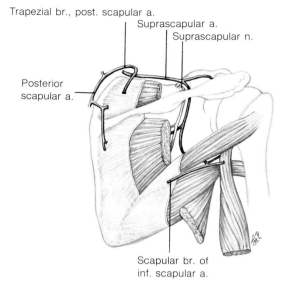

Scapular br. of
inf. scapular a.

FIG. 3-16. Relationship of suprascapular neurovascular bundle in the supraspinatus and infraspinatus fossae.

the supraspinatus muscle arising from the inner two thirds of the fossa and the aponeurosis. Directed transversely, it passes under the acromial process and inserts on the superior surface of the greater tuberosity.

During its transverse course, the supraspinatus muscle passes over the suprascapular nerve and artery (Fig. 3-16). This neurovascular bundle arises from the scapular notch, the nerve passing under the transverse scapular ligament and the artery above it. This neurovascular bundle reaches the infraspinatus fossa by passing through the spinoglenoid notch. During its course, the suprascapular nerve innervates the supraspinatus and infraspinatus muscles from their deep surfaces.

Infraspinatus Fossa

Two muscular layers separated by an aponeurosis are also encountered in this fossa.

The first muscular layer is formed proximally by the posterior segment of the deltoid originating from the posterior border of the spinous process. This muscle covers the superior and lateral aspect of the region and is covered by an aponeurosis. The lower segment of the region is crossed by

the upper fibers of the latissimus dorsi passing over the inferior angle of the scapula. Both muscles forming the first layer are covered by their proper aponeurosis (Fig. 3-17).

The infraspinatus aponeurosis inserts on the medial and lateral borders of the scapula and the posterior border of the scapular spinal process.

At the posterior border of the deltoid, the aponeurosis divides into two layers: a superficial layer, passing on the posterior surface of the deltoid and thus forming the aponeurosis of this muscle, and a deep layer, covering the deep muscles of the fossa up to their humeral insertion. This aponeurosis is thick medially and thin laterally and delineates, with the infraspinatus fossa, a fibro-osseous space for the deep muscles.

The second muscular layer is formed by three muscles: the infraspinatus, the teres minor, and the teres major (Figs. 3-17 and 3-18).

The infraspinatus muscle arises from the inner two thirds of the fossa and the aponeurosis. The muscle is then directed transversely and crosses the suprascapular neurovascular bundle and inserts on the posterior aspect of the greater tuberosity (Fig. 3-16).

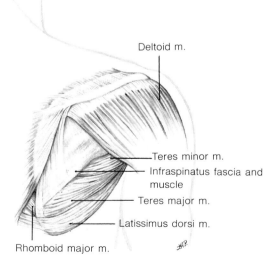

Deltoid m.

Teres minor m.
Infraspinatus fascia and
muscle
Teres major m.

Latissimus dorsi m.

Rhomboid major m.

FIG. 3-17. First muscular layer of the infraspinatus fossa.

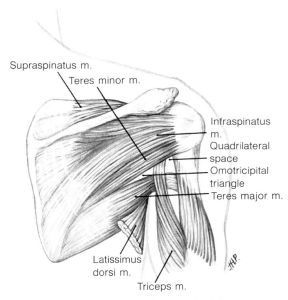

FIG. 3-18. Second muscular layer of the infraspinatus fossa.

The teres minor originates from the axillary border of the scapula, is in close contact with the inferolateral border of the infraspinatus, and quite often fuses with this border of the muscle. It inserts on the inferior surface of the greater tuberosity.

The teres major, located under the teres minor muscle, originates from the inferior angle of the scapula and the lower segment of the longitudinal lateral surface. The tendon of the teres major diverges from the teres minor and is directed laterally and anteriorly, passing in front of the long head of the triceps and inserting into the medial lip of bicipital groove (Fig. 3-18). The omotricipital triangle delineated by the teres minor above, teres major below, and the triceps laterally is penetrated by the circumflex scapular artery.

The teres minor receives its nerve from the posterior division of the axillary nerve passing through the quadrilateral humerotricipital space. The nerve penetrates the muscle from the front. The teres major receives its innervation from the anterior surface, in the axilla.

The scapular arterial blood supply is provided from three sources: the suprascapular artery (superior scapular artery),

the posterior scapular artery branch of the transverse colli artery, and the circumflex scapular artery branch of the subscapular artery (Fig. 3-19).

The suprascapular artery originates from the thyrocervical trunk, crosses the anterior surface of the scalenus anterior, runs a retroclavicular course to the scapular notch, and penetrates the supraspinatus fossa. It then turns through the spinoglenoid notch and, after supplying the infraspinatus muscle, anastomoses with the two other scapular arteries.

The transverse colli artery also arises from the thyrocervical trunk but at a higher level than the suprascapular artery, passes anterior to the scalenus anticus, crosses the floor of the posterior triangle and, on the anterior surface of the levator scapulae, divides into two branches. The superficial branch accompanies the trapezial branch of the accessory nerve, and penetrates the muscle from its anterior surface. The deep arterial branch passes in front of the levator scapulae and turns downward as the posterior scapular artery. This artery is located along the medial border of the scapula in front of the rhomboidei and behind the insertion of the serratus anterior on the

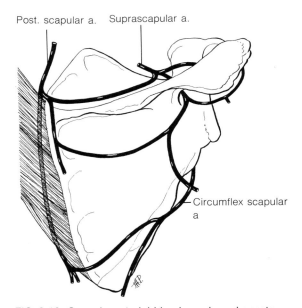

FIG. 3-19. Scapular arterial blood supply and anastomoses.

scapular border. It supplies branches to both the supraspinatus and infraspinatus fossae, and anastomoses with the circumflex scapular artery at the inferior angle of the scapula after turning posteriorly around the inferior border of the rhomboideus major. The nerves to the levator scapulae and rhomboidei accompany the posterior scapular artery.

The circumflex scapular artery penetrates posteriorly through the omotricipital triangle and divides into two branches. One branch penetrates the infraspinatus fossa and anastomoses with the corresponding branches of the suprascapular artery, and another descending branch, directed towards the inferior angle of the scapula, anastomoses with the branches of the posterior scapular artery. These anastomoses establish a collateral circulation between the subclavian artery and the third part of the axillary artery.

DELTOID REGION

The deltoid region is located between the axillary and the scapular regions. It is limited above by the lateral segment of the clavicle and the acromion, below by a horizontal line passing at the inferior border of the pectoralis major, anteriorly by a line running along the anterior border of the deltoid, and posteriorly by a vertical line passing from the posterior corner of the acromial process to the deltoid tuberosity. The posterior deltoid belongs to the scapular region.

Deltoid Muscle

The deltoid muscle is cone shaped, covering the region of the glenohumeral joint. It originates from the lateral third of the clavicle, the lateral border of the acromion, and the posterior border of the spinous process of the scapula. The three portions of the muscle are in continuity and indivisible.

The anterior head arises from the clavicle with direct long longitudinal muscle fibers interspersed among short tendinous fibers.

The posterior head arises from the spinous process of the scapula with a broad tendon and is continued by longitudinal muscle fibers. Both portions insert with corresponding tendons in continuity.

The middle, or acromial, head is multipennate in structure. Four proximal tendinous septa arise from the acromial process, and three distal tendinous septa inserting on the humerus are interposed among the proximal septa. Short muscular fibers arise from the adjacent sides of the proximal septa and insert obliquely into the corresponding surface of the distal septum. The structure resembles that of a feather (see Fig. 4-2).

The three portions of the deltoid insert on the deltoid tuberosity of the humerus in a V-shaped manner. The deltoid V fits into the hollow V of the brachialis muscle.[3]

The superficial deltoid aponeurosis is thin and originates from the spine of the scapula, the acromion, and the clavicle. Posteriorly, it is in continuity with the anterior division of the infraspinatus aponeurosis. Anteriorly, it continues in the deltopectoral triangle and blends with the superficial aponeurosis of the pectoralis major. Distally, it continues with the brachial fascia.

The axillary nerve arises in the axilla and leaves it by passing posteriorly through the quadrilateral humerotricipital space (Fig. 3-20). It runs around the humerus at the level of the surgical neck on the deep surface of the muscle. It divides into two branches. The anterior branch is the longer and runs transversely to supply the anterior and middle deltoid. This branch is located 6 cm. from the lateral border of the acromial process. Ascending and descending nerve branches supply the middle deltoid. Mostly ascending branches innervate the anterior deltoid. The posterior branch is short and runs horizontally to supply the posterior portion with ascending and descending branches. The posterior circumflex artery accompanies the axillary nerve.

The blood supply of the deltoid is essentially from the posterior circumflex artery, which enters the muscle circumferentially and gives off vertical branches. It anasto-

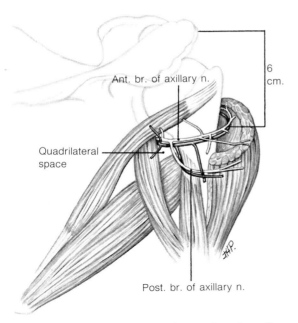

FIG. 3-20. Axillary nerve and posterior circumflex artery.

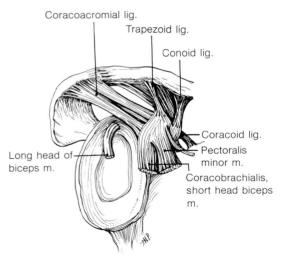

FIG. 3-21. Coracoacromial ligament and coracoclavicular ligaments.

moses with branches from the anterior circumflex artery, the acromial and deltoid branches of the acromiothoracic artery, and the suprascapular artery.

Subdeltoid Space

The reflection of the deltoid brings into view the acromion, the acromioclavicular joint, and the lateral aspect of the clavicle above. Slightly distal and medial to the acromioclavicular joint are the coracoid process with the origin of the short head of the biceps, the coracobrachialis, and the insertion of the pectoralis minor. Obliquely spanning the space between the coracoid and the acromion is the coracoacromial ligament (Fig. 3-21). This ligament is triangular, the base emanating from the posterolateral border of the coracoid process. It runs upward and laterally in an oblique manner and the apex of the triangle inserts on the tip and undersurface of the acromion, anterior to the acromioclavicular joint. A coracoacromial arch is thus formed[2] (Fig. 3-22). This vault acts as a secondary retaining socket for the humeral head. The acromial artery, a branch of the

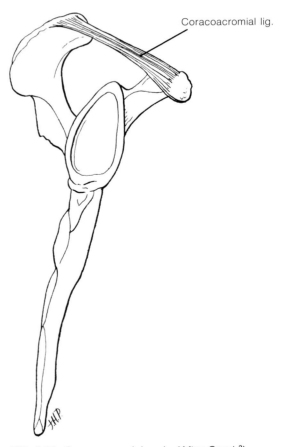

FIG. 3-22. Coracoacromial arch. (After Grant.[2])

acromiothoracic, runs transversely above the coracoacromial ligament and supplies the deltoid. Between the deep surface of the deltoid, the coracoacromial arch, and the underlying rotator cuff lies the subdeltoid, or subacromial, bursa. Normally, this bursa does not communicate with the glenohumeral joint space.

Rotator Cuff (Fig. 3-23)

The reflection of the subdeltoid bursa now reveals the humeral head covered by the rotator cuff. The tendon of the subscapularis is located anteriorly and inserts on the lesser tuberosity of the humerus. This tendon blends with the capsule in the lateral aspect. The inferior border of the subscapularis is identified by the presence of a transverse plexus of vessels. The anterior circumflex artery passes transversely under the short head of the biceps at the lower margin of the subscapularis tendon, under the long head of the biceps, gives off an ascending and a descending branch, and anastomoses with the corresponding branches of the posterior circumflex artery. The ascending branch runs in the bicipital groove and supplies the capsule and humeral head[3] (Fig. 3-14).

The long head of the biceps, located in the bicipital groove, is the guide to the "rotator interval" between the subscapularis and supraspinatus tendon. The insertion of the subscapularis is medial to the long head of the biceps.

The superior aspect of the humeral head is covered by the supraspinatus inserting on the superior facet of the greater tuberosity. This tendon blends with the underlying capsule. The infraspinatus tendon covers the upper posterior aspect of the humeral head and inserts on the middle facet of the greater tuberosity. The teres minor covers the posterior aspect of the humeral head and inserts on the inferior facet of the lesser tuberosity.

The long head of the biceps is located in the bicipital groove, converted into a tunnel proximally by the presence of the transverse humeral ligament. This tendon, originating from the supraglenoid tubercle of the scapula, is intracapsular and extrasynovial. It emerges from the joint into the groove with a tenosynovial sheath.

In the distal segment the bicipital groove gives insertion to the pectoralis major, terminating on the longitudinal crest and forming the outer lip of the groove. The teres major inserts on the inner lip of the groove and the latissimus dorsi, in the groove.

From a topographic point of view, the reflection of the insertion of the pectoralis major reveals the long head of the biceps laterally and the combined short head of the biceps and coracobrachialis muscle. The axillary neurovascular bundle lies under the fascia on the medial aspect of the coracobrachialis and short head of the biceps. The musculocutaneous nerve penetrates the coracobrachialis from its medial aspect, two fingerbreadths below the coracoid process.

Glenohumeral Joint

The proximal part of the humerus is formed by the articular head separated from the greater and lesser tuberosities by the anatomic neck. These tuberosities are separated from each other by the bicipital groove and from the body of the humerus by the surgical neck.

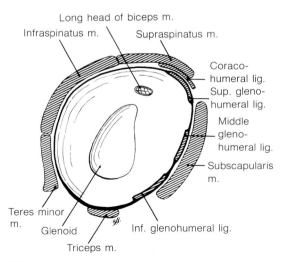

Long head of biceps m.
Infraspinatus m.
Supraspinatus m.
Coraco-humeral lig.
Sup. gleno-humeral lig.
Middle gleno-humeral lig.
Subscapularis m.
Teres minor m.
Glenoid
Inf. glenohumeral lig.
Triceps m.

FIG. 3-23. Rotator cuff.

Articulating Surfaces

The glenohumeral joint is formed by the humeral head and the glenoid surface of the scapula.

HUMERAL HEAD. The humeral head forms one third of a sphere. It is directed medially, upward and posteriorly. It is retroverted in relationship to the transverse axis of the distal humerus. The angle of retroversion averages about 20 degrees (Fig. 3-24).

GLENOID CAVITY. The glenoid fossa is pear-shaped and shallow. The larger segment is inferior to the small segment. A glenoid notch is present on its anterior border in the mid segment.

The surface of the glenoid cavity is directed outward, and anteriorly corresponds to the retroverted position of the humeral head. The glenoid surface represents about a quarter of the humeral surface.

GLENOID LABRUM. The glenoid labrum deepens the glenoid cavity. Triangular in cross section, the labrum attaches by one surface to the periphery of the glenoid. The second surface continues with the surface of the neck of the scapula and gives insertion to the capsule. The third surface is free, articular, and continues with the articular surface.

In the superior segment, the tendon of the long head of the biceps adheres to the labrum or is an integral part of it.

On the anterior aspect, the labrum passes over the glenoid notch and forms an osteofibrous tunnel through which a synovial extension is created that might communicate with the subscapularis bursa.

The inferior segment of the labrum intimately adheres to the tendon of the triceps.

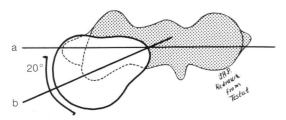

FIG. 3-24. Retroversion of the humeral head. (After Testut and Jacob.[1])

Capsule and Ligaments

CAPSULE. The glenoid attachment of the capsule takes place on the external surface of the labrum and to a lesser degree on the surrounding bone. A larger attachment occurs at the level of the tendon of the biceps which lifts the capsule. The insertion of the latter occurs on the neck of the scapula up to the base of the coracoid process. Anteriorly, at the level of the glenoid notch, the capsular insertion extends over the bone and is continuous with the periosteum. Inferiorly, the capsule blends with the long head of the triceps.

The humeral insertion takes place anteriorly at the lateral border of the anatomic neck. Posteriorly, the insertion is about 1 cm. from the anatomic neck, leaving a bare osseous band which is covered by reflected fibers. Inferiorly, the capsule attaches to the surgical neck and with the synovium forms multiple folds creating an accordion effect.

LIGAMENTS[4] (Figs. 3-23 and 3-25).

Coracohumeral Ligament. This ligament is located on the superior aspect of the glenohumeral joint at the level of the interval formed by the supraspinatus and subscapularis tendons. The ligament originates from the posterolateral border and base of the coracoid, the origin of the coracoacromial ligament, and runs transversely to insert on the greater and lesser tuberosities blending with the adjacent capsule. The anterior border of the ligament is free from the capsule. The posterior border fuses with the capsule.

From the origin of this ligament, some fibers are directed laterally and posteriorly to insert at the superior pole of the glenoid blending with the capsule and the labrum. They form the arciform coracoglenoid ligament.

Glenohumeral Ligaments. These ligaments, reinforcements of the capsule, are not seen from the external surface of the capsule. They come into evidence in anatomic preparations and are best demonstrated when the posterior capsule of the glenohumeral joint and the humeral head

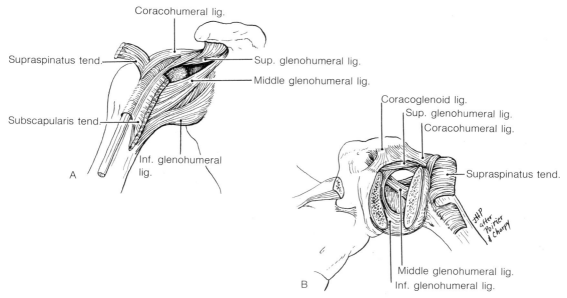

FIG. 3-25. Ligaments of the shoulder joint. A, Anterior view. B, Posterior view. (After Poirier and Charpy.[4])

are removed, bringing into view the deep surface of the capsule and its ligaments.

The *superior glenohumeral ligament,* located under and slightly anterior to the coracohumeral ligament, arises from the superior pole of the glenoid and forms a narrow band inserting in an encroachment of the anatomic neck just above the lesser tuberosity and medial to the bicipital groove. Transverse fibers extend above the groove to the coracohumeral ligament forming the transverse humeral ligament of Gordon-Brodie.

The *middle glenohumeral ligament* arises from the anterosuperior aspect of the glenoid under the origin of the superior glenohumeral ligament. Directed obliquely downward and laterally, it inserts on the lesser tuberosity blending with the subscapularis tendon. Between the superior and middle glenohumeral ligament, a triangular space is formed, covered only by synovium, the foramen ovale of Weitbrecht. This opening is covered by the subscapularis tendon.

The *inferior glenohumeral ligament* arises from the anterior segment of the glenoid

labrum and adjacent bone, from the level of the glenoid notch to the origin of the triceps. The ligament runs quasi-transversely outward and inserts on the inner part of the surgical neck. This is the largest and the strongest of the three ligaments.

The capsuloligamentous complex of the glenohumeral joint is not an effective stabilizer. The posterior capsule is thin and the anterior capsule has a large defect, the foramen of Weitbrecht, with a weak zone between the middle and lower glenohumeral ligaments. The effective static stabilizer is determined by the musculotendinous cuff forming a true cuff posteriorly, superiorly, and anteriorly (Fig. 3-23). The capsular ligament with no tendinous protection such as the inferior glenohumeral ligament becomes strong. The vertical stability of the humeral head, preventing the inferior subluxation, is determined dynamically by the supraspinatus. The subscapularis forms the anterior buttress resisting the protrusion or luxation of the humeral head through the weak zone at the anteroinferior aspect of the capsule. The peri-glenohumeral tendons act as active ligaments.

Acromioclavicular Joint

Articulating Surfaces

The clavicular articulating surface rests on the acromial surface. The joint line is directed anteriorly and medially. The clavicular surface faces downward and laterally, whereas the acromial surface faces upward and medially.

Capsule and Ligaments

The clavicle and acromion are united by a capsule inserting a few millimeters from the articulating surfaces. This loose capsule is reinforced on the superior and inferior aspect by the powerful acromioclavicular ligament which runs transversely over the joint. The posterior fibers are stronger than the anterior fibers. This ligament blends with the insertion of the trapezius and deltoid tendinous fibers. A fibrocartilaginous meniscus is present in the joint (Winslow, 1732). Most frequently, it is a prismatic meniscus descending from the superior aspect into the interior of the joint. Less frequently, it forms a capsular bulge into the interior, or rarely it forms a true meniscus dividing the articular cavity into two chambers.

The lateral stability of the clavicle is mostly determined by the coracoclavicular ligaments: trapezoid and conoid (Fig. 3-21).

Trapezoid Ligament. This quadrilateral ligament is located in a quasisagittal plane. It originates from the posterior segment of the superior surface of the coracoid process and inserts on the inferior surface of the clavicle in its lateral segment along a ridge directed anteriorly and laterally. Of the two surfaces, the superomedial corresponds to the subclavius muscle. The inferolateral surface corresponds below to the supraspinatus muscle. The anterior border is free; the posterior border is in contact with the conoid ligament.

Conoid Ligament. This triangular and curved ligament is located in a frontal plane, posterior to the trapezoid ligament. It originates from the posterior segment of the medial border of the coracoid and inserts on the undersurface of the lateral end of the clavicle at the level of the conoid tubercle and in a semicircular fashion around the tubercle. It forms half of a cone enveloping the trapezoid ligament medially and posteriorly.

Sternoclavicular Joint
(Fig. 3-26, see also Fig. 20-56)

Articulating Surfaces

The medial end of the clavicle is articular only in the inferior half anteriorly. The articulating surface presents a frontal convexity and a slight sagittal concavity. It is saddle-shaped. It articulates with the upper angle of the manubrium and the superior segment of the first costal cartilage.

The sternal articulating surface presents a marked frontal concavity and a slight sagittal convexity.

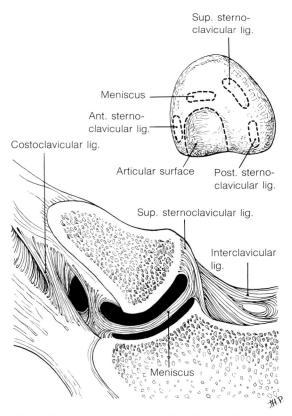

FIG. 3-26. Sternoclavicular joint and ligaments.

Meniscus

A fibrocartilaginous meniscus is present in the joint. It originates firmly from the clavicle above the articulating surface, runs downward and laterally, and inserts at the junction of the first costal cartilage with the manubrium. This disc is attached to the joint capsule and ligament at its periphery and divides the joint space into a meniscoclavicular and meniscosternal compartment.

Ligaments

Anterior Sternoclavicular Ligament. It arises from the clavicular end anterior to the sternal articulating surface, runs over the anterior aspect of the sternoclavicular joint, and inserts on the anterior periphery of the manubrial articulating surface. The superior border of the ligament is nearly horizontal. The inferior border is vertical. The nearly vertical middle fibers are the strongest.

Superior Sternoclavicular Ligament. This ligament originates from the upper segment of the clavicular end and runs transversely to the manubrium. It blends with the interclavicular ligament.

Interclavicular Ligament. It unites the posterosuperior aspects of the clavicular ends passing transversely above the sternal notch. The concave superior border is free. The inferior border attaches to the sternal notch.

Posterior Sternoclavicular Ligament. This ligament extends from the posterior angle of the clavicular end to the manubrium at the periphery of the articular surface. The fibers are short and strong.

Costoclavicular Ligament. This rhomboid ligament originates from the first costal cartilage and the first rib, runs obliquely upward and laterally, and inserts on the inferior surface of the medial end of the clavicle. It has an anterior and a posterior component. A bursa is interposed between these two components. The costoclavicular ligament might be considered the equivalent of the coracoclavicular ligaments.

REFERENCES

1. Testut, L., and Jacob, O.: Traité d'Anatomie Topographique avec Applications Medico-chirurgicales, Vol. 2. Paris, Octave Doin et Fils, 1909.
2. Grant, J. O. B.: A Method of Anatomy: Descriptive and Deductive, 6th ed. Baltimore, The Williams & Wilkins Co., 1958.
3. Henry, A. K.: Extensile Exposure, 2nd ed. Baltimore, The Williams & Wilkins Co., 1957.
4. Poirier, P., and Charpy, A.: Traité d'Anatomie Humaine, Vol. 1. Paris, Masson et Cie, 1899.

4

Biomechanics
and Functional Anatomy

ERIC L. RADIN

In most vertebrates the shoulder represents the most proximal joint of the load-bearing forward extremity. In man the forward extremity has been freed from its weight-bearing function, and has been made into an "upper" extremity which tremendously increases its usefulness as a grasping and carrying organ with great power capable of lifting considerable loads. These functions are further enhanced by the extremely large range of shoulder motion, greatest of any joint in the body. Power, as in throwing or punching, is achieved by rapidly accelerating the upper extremity. Such actions require considerable joint stability. In retrospect, the design specifications of a stable joint with such an extremely large range of motion and with considerable power lead logically to what we find in the human shoulder.

FACTORS INFLUENCING
RANGE OF MOTION

The major constraint to a wide range of motion in diarthrodial vertebral joints is, of course, the bony configuration of the joint and its constraining ligaments. The shoulder is composed of three elements: the clavicle, scapula, and proximal humerus. The glenohumeral (humeroscapular) joint is fashioned with a minimum of bony con-

straint. The glenoid, in most humans, usually approximates 3 cm. in diameter. No other portion of the scapula actually enters into the articulation with the humeral head. The largely spherical humeral head rotates in the shallow, small diameter glenoid deepened by a fibrocartilaginous rim. The attitude of the cup in relation to the centerline of the body may also be elevated and rotated to allow placement of the arm above the head, forward flexed, or abducted. Combined with lateral flexion and extension of the spine, it is quite possible for humans to work with their hands well above or behind their heads.

The ligaments of the glenohumeral joints are so constructed and arranged as to hold the humeral head in a sling fashion. There are no true collateral ligaments in the shoulder to limit motion in the frontal plane.

FACTORS INFLUENCING SHOULDER
POWER

There is considerable functional advantage in having the proximal humerus articulate with a movable bone on the thorax rather than in a socket which would be an intimate part of the rib cage. The first advantage has already been mentioned: the ability to angulate the glenoid socket upward increases the range of glenohumeral motion. A second major advantage has to do with achieving added power in the shoulder. Strength in all diarthrodial joints is achieved by muscle contraction. Power is the relationship of force times the distance per unit of time. Skeletal power, therefore, depends upon the ability of the body to accelerate the upper extremity over a maximal distance at maximum force as quickly as possible. Thus, there is an obvious necessity for a windup when we wish to throw or swing at something with maximum power. We can increase this power by recruiting the spinal and leg muscles, and by moving the mass of our body in the direction we wish our arm to travel.

The problem is that skeletal muscle creates force by contracting, which depends upon a definite strength-length relationship. Physiologists refer to this as the Blix curve (Fig. 4-1). In essence, this means there is a limited range of excursion that muscles can undergo and still remain within their range of maximum power. The relative power of muscle can be further attained by a multipennate rather than a parallel arrangement of the muscle fibers (Fig. 4-2). When the fibers are arranged at an angle there is less overall change in length for a given contraction than occurs with a parallel arrangement of fibers but more force is produced. The powerful deltoid is a fine example of a multipennate muscle. If the deltoid originated directly from the chest

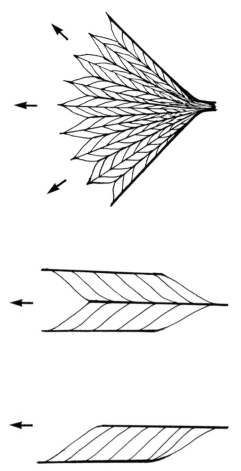

FIG. 4-2. Relative power of muscle can be increased by multipennate arrangement of muscle fibers such as in the deltoid.

wall, it could move the humerus with maximum force but over a relatively small range of motion. Under such an arrangement the deltoid could only be powerful when the humerus was close to the chest, an extreme disadvantage from a functional point of view.

We know that great shoulder strength with the arm above the head is possible. How has this been accomplished? No alteration can be made in the physiologic truism of the length-strength relationship of the muscle. What has been achieved is the mounting of most of the origin of the deltoid on a movable base, the scapula.

The scapula moves in concert with the humerus. Thus, in any attitude of shoulder

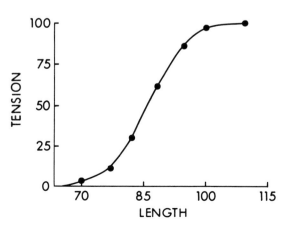

FIG. 4-1. Blix curve.

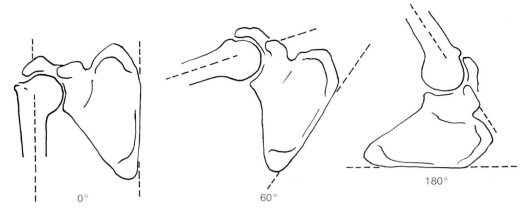

FIG. 4-3. While the arm is overhead the deltoid can act within its resting length.

elevation, the deltoid is for all purposes moved upward so that it may act well within its resting length while the arm remains powerful above the head (Fig. 4-3). This arrangement implies fairly fine control over the scapular movements, and because of the complex curvature of the chest wall, the scapula, in order to follow the humerus upward, must move "up and around." This necessitates a relatively large number of small muscles inserting into the periphery of the scapula, separate and distinct from the control of glenohumeral motion, and also implies that weakness of the scapular muscles will have a weakening effect upon the shoulder.

Not only is muscle strength related to length but muscle strength is also directly related to muscle volume. A large muscle cannot originate from a small tendon on bone, as the stress on the bone would be too great. The humeral "motors" require wide origins, and do originate on the relatively large flat surfaces of the scapula, thus limiting the stress on this bone. Furthermore, the presence of the large spine on the scapula provides several extra surfaces for the origination of muscles. The presence of the acromion also adds to the effectiveness of the deltoid. This "overhang" serves to create additional surface for muscle attachment, as well as to allow the deltoid to act on the humerus at an angle, thereby providing a powerful component of force and abduction which would be absent if the deltoid

originated only from the scapula at a point directly above the humeral head.

STABILITY OF THE SHOULDER DURING POWERFUL CONTRACTION

The stability of the shoulder, particularly during forceful motion, requires dual considerations. First, the bony stability of the glenohumeral joint is lacking. Stability must be maintained by soft-tissue structures. The ligaments of the shoulder are designed to be minimally constrictive, to allow maximum ranges of motion, and to provide only marginal stability, especially anteriorly. The relative clinical frequency of anterior dislocation of the shoulder attests to this fact. It is the rotator cuff that to a great extent provides stability of the humeral head and the glenoid during powerful glenohumeral motion. These muscles contract and maintain the glenohumeral contact. This is especially important because the most powerful of the humeral motors, the deltoid, tends to distract the glenohumeral joint by pulling the humeral head upward and outward from the glenoid (Fig. 4-4). Deprived of its fulcrum, the humerus cannot be forcefully elevated. The rotator cuff, and particularly the supraspinatus, acts to maintain glenohumeral stability during forceful abduction.

Rupture of the rotator cuff limits the ability of the patient to abduct the shoulder against resistance. If the arm is held passively in abduction, the deltoid can effec-

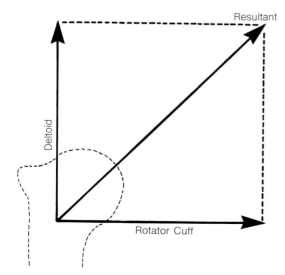

FIG. 4-4. Effective function of the deltoid depends upon the integrity of the rotator cuff.

tively function. Once contracted in abduction, the patient can hold this position even with nonfunctioning cuff muscles.

Not only is stability of the joint important, but its stability in relation to the axial skeleton is also significant. Even with an intact rotator cuff, a powerful deltoid, and powerful scapular motors, an extremely forceful forward acceleration of the humerus is not possible without something to push against. The scapula must be fixed. The scapular muscles have difficulty stabilizing the base of the shoulder, while effecting the necessary motions of the scapula associated with humeral motion. The clavicle acts as a strut between the scapula and the axial skeleton and essentially provides something to push against. The problem is that as the shoulder is abducted the distance between the acromion and the sternoclavicular joint decreases as the scapula moves around the chest wall.

How then can one design a strut that allows for this shortening? The clavicle, constructed of bone, cannot really be made to change length, and the joints at either end of the clavicle cannot be made to sublux, as this would also tend to weaken the strut. This problem has been solved by having the clavicle S-shaped, so that when it is

rotated it is apparently shorter when viewed from an oblique angle. An "S" tends to decrease in overall length. Thus, rotation of the clavicle shortens it. Removal of the clavicle or its instability has some weakening effect upon the shoulder in that scapular fixation is severely compromised.

MECHANICS OF SHOULDER MOTION

As the humerus is elevated there is some gliding and rolling of the large humeral head in the shallow glenoid. With abduction the mechanical center of rotation of the joint moves closer to the anatomic center. As the arm is abducted in internal rotation, it must be placed in external rotation in order for elevation above 135 degrees to occur (Codman's paradox). With the arm in 60 degrees of internal rotation, the greater tuberosity impinges on the anterior and overhanging aspects of the scapula (coracoacromial arch) and blocks abduction beyond 120 degrees. External rotation allows the greater tuberosity to move beneath the arch. Patients with internal rotation contractures of the shoulder will therefore have only limited abduction.

As the arm is elevated the scapula goes through a rather complicated movement, turning counterclockwise as it glides upward on the thoracic cage. With abduction the inferior angle of the scapula swings laterally and forward more than does its medial angle. This rotation of the scapula turns the glenoid cavity upward. In the first 15 to 20 degrees of abduction there is little scapular rotation. The initial movement is primarily glenohumeral. As abduction continues, scapula motion gradually becomes more prominent up to 65 degrees of abduction. According to Saha, the ratio of glenohumeral to scapular motions varies with abduction and is not a constant ratio. This appears to be the case and is in variance with the former concept of a fixed scapular rotation per degree of glenohumeral abduction.

Because of the increasing alignment of the mechanical and anatomic axis of the glenohumeral joint with abduction, the range of excursion of the arm becomes smaller as it is lifted upward. When the arm is close by the side, its range of motion is maximal and decreases progressively as the arm is elevated to full abduction. The arm is able to transcend a rather small radius of circumduction above the head. The flexion-extension range remains considerable in full abduction.

It is difficult to determine the compressive stress across the shoulder joint. Although Saha has made contact studies of the glenohumeral joint surfaces, he was mainly interested in the pattern of contacts. He has not yet published his findings relating to contact area. However, his studies have shown the importance of change in the contact area of the glenohumeral joint and, combined with electromyographic studies of individual muscles, have helped improve our understanding of the functional anatomy of this complex joint. In abduction above shoulder level, the subscapularis acts as an abductor. But above 150 degrees of abduction, this muscle loses its power for further abduction. Since its fibers are no longer aligned with the mechanical axis of the joint, it causes a forward migration of the contact area on the humeral head just at the time most of the articular surface of the humerus is exhausted in the plane of elevation.

Saha has also demonstrated the importance of early migration of the scapula in shoulder flexion as compared to abduction. This scapular migration in flexion, caused by the pectoralis major, subclavius, and serratus anterior, sets the glenoid at an optimal inclination for humeral excursion in the sagittal plane.

Rotation of the clavicle also takes place much earlier in flexion than in abduction. Clavicular rotation occurs during the terminal phase of abduction and is due mainly to subclavius contraction.

MUSCLES INVOLVED IN SCAPULAR MOTION

The fine, coordinated movements of the scapula depend upon coupled individual muscle contraction and release. Scapula elevators are generally considered to be the upper trapezius, levator scapulae, and to some extent the rhomboids. Scapular depression is carried out by the lower trapezius, serratus anterior, and to some extent the latissimus dorsi. Many of these muscles depress the lateral angle of the scapula as well. The combined effect of the upper and lower trapezius is obvious. Downward rotation is controlled by the rhomboid and pectoralis minor muscles while the lower fibers of the pectoralis major and lateral aspect of the latissimus dorsi and levator help. Protraction and lateral and forward movement of the scapula result from contraction of the serratus anterior. Acting together, the pectoralis major and serratus anterior can produce pure protraction without rotation of the scapula. The retraction or adduction of the scapula is caused by the action of the middle and lower trapezius and rhomboids.

MUSCLES INVOLVED IN GLENOHUMERAL MOTION

The main power for abduction of the humerus is, of course, the deltoid. However, it is apparent that deltoid contraction can pull the humeral head upward and outward from the glenoid socket. Acting alone the deltoid cannot effectively abduct the humerus, as it would cause subluxation of the glenohumeral joint (Fig. 4-4). To provide stability, other muscles create a tendinous cap over the top of the shoulder. These muscles are the subscapularis, supraspinatus, infraspinatus, and teres minor. These muscles can also act as rotators of the shoulder but cannot generate the power of larger muscles that originate from the chest wall.

In analyzing the major movers of the arm at the shoulder joint, the elevation of the humerus in a plane parallel with the scapula (abduction) chiefly involves the deltoid and supraspinatus. The long head of the biceps can help if the arm is in supination. The clavicular portion of the pectoralis major and the anterior and posterior deltoid are useful with the arm positioned above the level of the shoulder joint, as are the teres major and minor which neutralize the tendency of the anterior deltoid and upper pectoralis major to flex the arm.

The return of the arm to neutral from the abducted position is principally the work of the latissimus dorsi, teres major, and the sternal portion of the pectoralis major, assisted by the posterior deltoid, coracobrachialis, subscapularis, and the short head of the biceps when the arm is above the shoulder. The long biceps and triceps heads each have relatively powerful, nonrotatory stabilizing components which tend to pull the humerus toward the glenoid. The rhomboids stabilize the scapula, and abdominal muscles and spinal extensors tend to stabilize the trunk during this motion. The spinal muscles also function during full abduction. Man tends to tilt his spine backward as he reaches above the head.

Forward flexion of the humerus (in a plane perpendicular to the scapula) is primarily controlled by the anterior deltoid. The clavicular portion of the pectoralis major is assisted by the coracobrachialis and short head of the biceps, especially when the elbow is extended. The infraspinatus and teres minor act to combat the internal rotation tendencies of the anterior deltoid and pectoralis major. Trapezius and subclavius muscles act to stabilize the scapula. Humeral extension is mainly the work of the latissimus dorsi. The contribution of the sternal portion of the pectoralis major diminishes as the movement progresses. The teres major is assisted by the posterior deltoid, and if the elbow is flexed, it is aided by the long head of the triceps. The posterior deltoid neutralizes the tendency of the pectoralis major and latissimus dorsi to internally rotate the arm. When extension is

forceful, the infraspinatus and teres minor aid in preventing internal rotation. The long head of triceps and coracobrachialis tend to stabilize the shoulder. The rhomboids, the levator scapulae, the abdominal muscles, intercostals, and the sacrospinalis are also involved. The degree to which these muscles are brought into use depends upon the force used in extension.

Backward elevation of the humerus in a plane perpendicular to the scapula (hyperextension) is carried out primarily by the posterior deltoid, latissimus dorsi, and teres major. These muscles acting in concert neutralize any rotatory tendency. The levator scapulae, trapezius, and rhomboids stabilize the scapula while the spinal muscles stabilize the spine. External rotation of the humerus is caused mainly by the contraction of the infraspinatus and teres minor, assisted by the posterior deltoid when the humerus is adducted and extended. The trapezius tends to neutralize the tendency of the rhomboids to elevate the scapula. Internal rotation is principally carried out by the subscapularis and teres major, assisted by the latissimus dorsi, anterior deltoid, and pectoralis major. The coracobrachialis and short head of the biceps also help to reduce the tendency to external rotation. The anterior deltoid, coracobrachialis, and clavicular portion of pectoralis major tend to neutralize extension of the arm by the latissimus dorsi, teres major, and serratus anterior. Forward motion of the humerus in the horizontal plane is a combination of flexion, abduction, and adduction.

It is obvious that recurrent subluxation or dislocation of the glenohumeral joint will destroy the leverage through which the muscles about the joint act, and severely limit both the range of motion and power.

REFERENCES

1. Inman, V. T., Saunders, M., and Abbott, L. C.: Observations on the function of the shoulder joint. J. Bone Joint Surg., 26:1–30, 1944.
2. Jones, L.: The shoulder joint—Observations on the anatomy and physiology, Surg. Gynecol. Obstet., 75:433, 1942.
3. Lucas, D. B.: Biomechanics of the shoulder joint. Arch. Surg., 107:425, 1973.
4. Saha, A. K.: Theory of Shoulder Mechanism. Springfield, Ill., Charles C Thomas, 1961.
5. Saha, A. K.: Mechanics of elevation of the glenohumeral joint. Acta Orthop. Scand., 44:668, 1973.
6. Steindler, A.: Mechanics of Normal and Pathological Locomotion in Man. Springfield, Ill., Charles C Thomas, 1935.

Radiologic Diagnosis

BERTRAM LEVIN

There are numerous variations of the roentgen appearances of normal osseous structures making up the shoulder girdle, many related to secondary ossification centers, some to radiographic projection, others to true variations of normal osseous structures. Only the more common variations, including some that may be mistaken for fractures, will be discussed. For the wide range of normal variations the classic textbook by Köhler and Zimmer is a *must* for anyone who accepts the responsibility of interpreting roentgenograms of bones or joints.[50] More recently, the atlas of the more commonly encountered variations by Keats has proved to be a useful book to be kept at hand while reviewing roentgenograms of any part.[49]

No justice can be done to the broad subjects of bone dysplasias, dysostoses, and dystrophies in this chapter; only a few of the more common are touched upon. These conditions, though varied and numerous in classifications, are rarely encountered. This material is well covered by Wynne-Davies and Fairbank,[102] McKusick,[58] Spranger, Langer, and Wiedmann,[91] and others.

The term "miscellany" is probably more encompassing than is the combination of all other entities that are neatly catalogued and described in other chapters. This chapter deals with that sample of miscellany most often encountered by the orthopaedist and radiologist or, in some instances, presenting unusually interesting radiologic findings, reflecting my biases and experience. Much of the material presented is not "orthopaedic;" that is, there is no need for surgical, manipulative, or fixation treatment. The orthopaedist may, however, come face-to-face or face-to-film with such cases, and familiarity with the clinical and radiologic findings is of importance. Hematologic, endocrinologic, and other systemic diseases may leave their osseous or soft-tissue imprints on shoulder girdle structures. And so may general affections of the skeleton. In addition, there are a number of conditions causing shoulder pain in which the primary pathologic lesion is away from the joint. The roentgen features of some of them merit discussion.

Obviously, space constraints limit the depth of discussion and the number of illustrative radiographs. Fortunately there are reference books of bone radiology of superior quality to which the reader can find in-depth expositions of most bony abnormalities. The books by Murray and Jacobson,[65] by Greenfield,[35] and by Edeiken and Hodes[25] generally suffice as aids in roentgen diagnosis of bone and associated soft-tissue diseases.

NORMAL VARIATIONS

A significant number of normal variations might be mistaken for abnormalities on radiographs of the scapula, clavicle, or upper humerus. Only the more common ones will be illustrated here. The reader is referred to Köhler and Zimmer[50] and to Keats[49] for more detailed discussion.

Scapula

The superior border of the scapula may have an elongated pseudoforamen, its appearance aptly described as clasp-like.[50] This may be mistaken for a fracture (Fig. 5-1).

At the inferior angle of the scapula is a secondary ossification center which usually fuses about age 20 years but may never fuse. This, then, is known as the infrascapular bone (Fig. 5-2).

Vascular grooves and foramina are common and should not be mistaken for fractures or lytic lesions (Figs. 5-3 and 5-4).

Epiphyseal centers and epiphyseal lines may be mistaken for abnormalities unless one is aware of their presence and appearances (Figs. 5-5 to 5-7).

The relatively radiolucent fat stripe of the chest wall may mimic the appearance of a fracture (Fig. 5-8).

When viewed tangentially the free border of the scapula may overlap the body and give an impression of an anteriorly displaced fracture fragment. In this same projection the irregular margins of the body, with varying cortical thicknesses, may create the appearance of an avulsion-type fracture.

Humerus

Depending on the photographic projection, the normal anatomic structure of the head of the humerus may give the impression of abnormality. The porous greater tuberosity and humeral head when projected en face may give the impression of being a lytic or cystic defect.

When seen in internal rotation, the normal proximal humeral epiphyseal line may resemble a fracture of the proximal shaft (see Fig. 18-32).

The crescentic air-density stripe paralleling the articular surface of the humerus is normal. This "vacuum" phenomenon may be seen in any joint of the extremities when

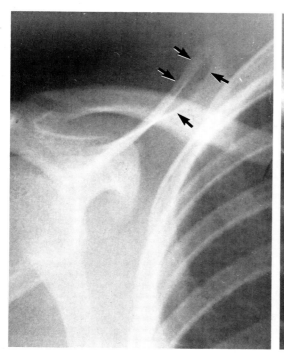 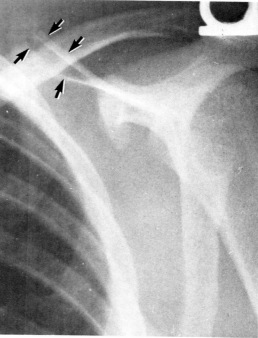

FIG. 5-1. Clasp-like superior margin of scapulae (arrows). Although in this instance the anomaly is bilateral, it is common for it to be unilateral.

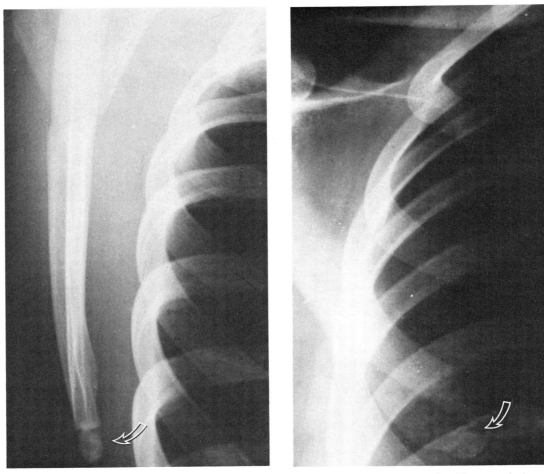

A   B

FIG. 5-2. Infrascapular bone. A, This secondary center of ossification at the inferior angle of the scapula (arrow) may never fuse but persist as a distinct ossicle. B, In the frontal view it is apt to be mistaken for a fracture.

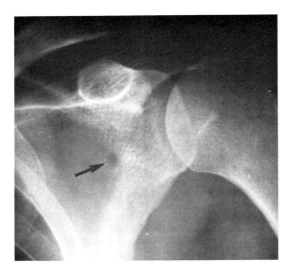

FIG. 5-3. Nutrient foramen (arrow) should not be mistaken for a fracture line. Note also the porosity of the adjacent portion of scapula, a normal appearance.

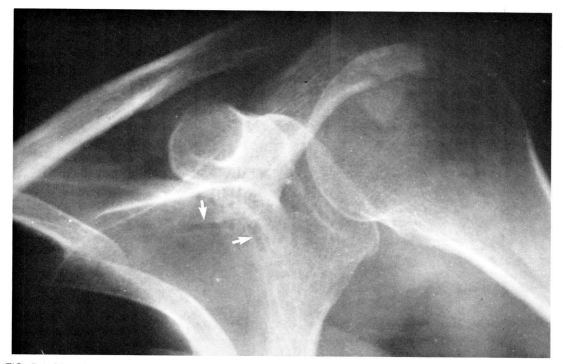

FIG. 5-4. Vascular groove (arrows). This might be mistaken for a fracture line. Note also the porosity of the adjacent portion of scapula, a normal appearance.

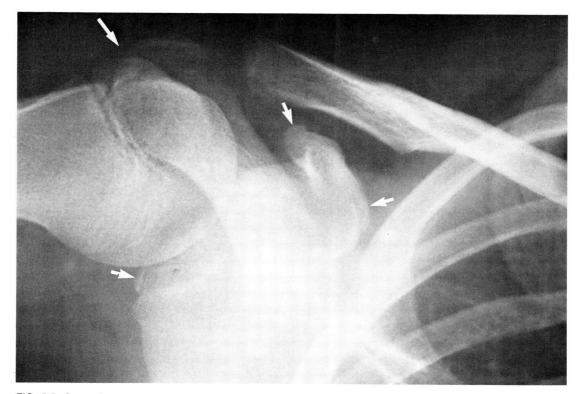

FIG. 5-5. Secondary ossification centers of acromion, coracoid, and glenoid rim of a 13-year-old girl.

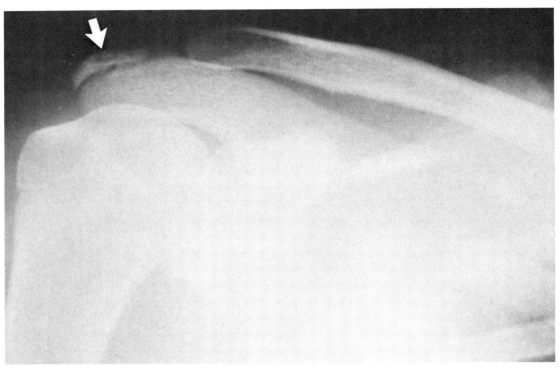

FIG. 5-6. Secondary ossification center of the acromion of a 14-year-old girl.

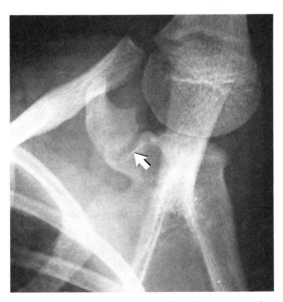

FIG. 5-7. Unfused coracoid ossification center of a 17-year-old girl who had trauma to this shoulder. A fracture was suspected, but the opposite side showed the same finding. This is always seen in adolescence, prior to fusion of the bony parts, on films taken with the arm fully abducted.

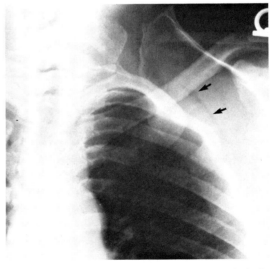

FIG. 5-8. Fat stripe of chest wall. This linear relatively radiolucent shadow may be mistaken for a fracture if one is not aware of its true significance. (This patient has Sprengel's deformity.)

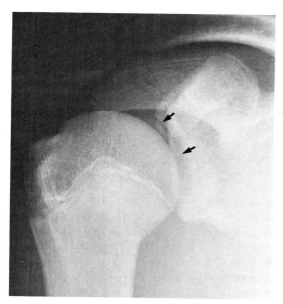

FIG. 5-9. Vacuum phenomenon. The gas stripe marks the joint space. This might be mistaken for a fracture line if one is not aware that this is a normal phenomenon.

the joint is filmed while there is pull on the extremity. Should this project over bone it might be mistaken for a fracture (Fig. 5-9).

Clavicle

NEURAL FORAMEN. In the superior cortex of the middle third of the clavicle there is often a small, round or ovoid radiolucent defect. This is the canal for passage of the middle supraclavicular nerve. Of interest is

the fact that this is infrequently seen bilaterally, even when the contralateral clavicle is seen in multiple projections (Fig. 5-10).

RHOMBOID FOSSA. This is a depression of a few millimeters to over a centimeter in depth, and up to 3 cm. in width on the undersurface of the medial end of the clavicle. It may extend to the medial tip of the bone or be short of it by as much as 2 cm. It represents the site of attachment of the costoclavicular ligament originating on the cartilage of the first rib. The cortex at the depth of the fossa may be sclerotic or may be undiscernible as such; it may be smooth or irregular. Rhomboid fossae are usually bilateral and symmetric but not always so (Fig. 5-11).

IRREGULAR MEDIAL BORDER. Although the medial border of the clavicle is generally smooth and only slightly curved, it may be quite irregular normally. There may be a bayonet, forked, or knobby appearance. These contours are almost always bilaterally symmetric. The adjacent sternal border remains smooth.

EPISTERNAL BONES. Separate ossicles, presumably ununited ossification centers of the manubrium, may be seen above the sternum, just medial to the clavicles (Fig. 5-12).

CORACOCLAVICULAR JOINT. The coracoid tuberosity, a rectangular or truncated triangular projection marking the coracoclavicular ligament attachment, is frequently present. It may be unilateral or bilateral. Its

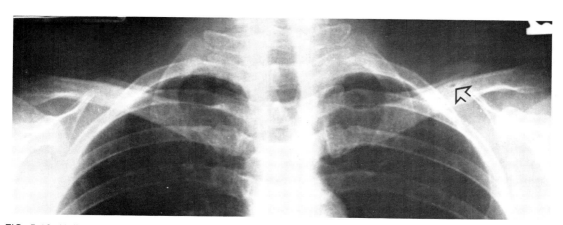

FIG. 5-10. Unilateral left neural foramen (arrow).

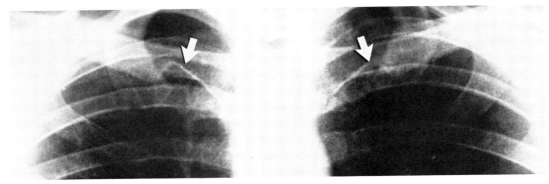

FIG. 5-11. Rhomboid fossae more commonly are sharply grooved but may have a curved border.

surface is usually smooth and flat, unlike that seen in exostosis, though on occasion it may have a pointed configuration. This may exist alone or be associated with an apposing outgrowth from the coracoid process. Bony contact is present only rarely.[99] This may represent a true diarthrosis replacing the normal conoid and trapezoid ligaments.[57,71] The joint may be unilateral or bilateral (Fig. 5-13). It is usually an incidental finding without clinical significance. However, there have been cases reported where pain or limitation of shoulder motion was relieved when the joint was resected.[39,99]

ANOMALIES AND ABNORMALITIES

Sprengel's Deformity

Sprengel's deformity is characterized by congenital elevation of the scapula, usually unilateral (Fig. 5-14). In 10 percent of cases, it is bilateral.[36] This is most often associated with maldevelopment and scoliosis of cervical and upper thoracic vertebrae, sometimes with supernumerary, fused, or absent ribs, and shortened clavicles. The scapula lies cephalad to its normal position, is often widened, and is rotated so as to bring its inferior angle further medial than normal. In about one quarter to one third of the

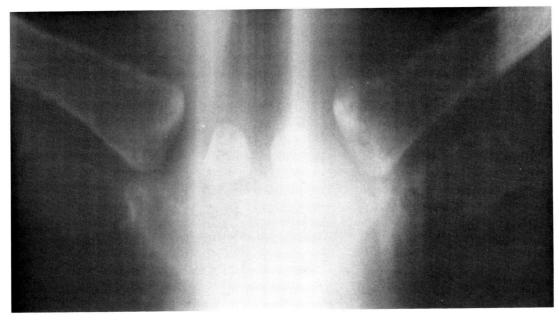

FIG. 5-12. Episternal bones.

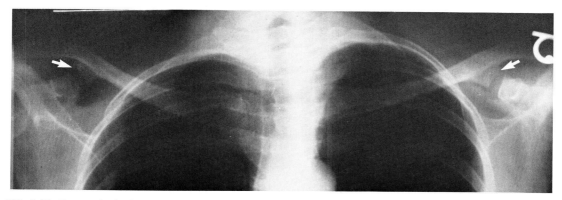

FIG. 5-13. Coracoclavicular joints. These are more often unilateral than bilateral. Note the elongated squared-off outgrowth of the coracoid on the affected sides.

cases, the proximal vertebral border is connected to the cervical spine by a fibrous, cartilaginous, or osseous bridge, the omovertebral body. This may connect with the spinous process, lamina, or transverse process of one or more cervical vertebrae or of the first thoracic vertebra. Of clinical significance is the cosmetic deformity and, of greater importance, the varying degrees of limitation of shoulder abduction. There may also be loss of normal neck rotation, dependent upon the associated cervical spine anomalies and omovertebral bar.

In 1908, Horwitz reported on a careful analysis of 132 cases of Sprengel's deformity.[43] This report is the mother lode which many subsequent investigators have mined because of its comprehensiveness.

Klippel-Feil Syndrome

Klippel-Feil syndrome, clinically manifest by a short neck, consists of a variety of defects involving the bodies, lateral masses, articulations, and posterior elements of the cervical spine (Fig. 5-15). There is generally

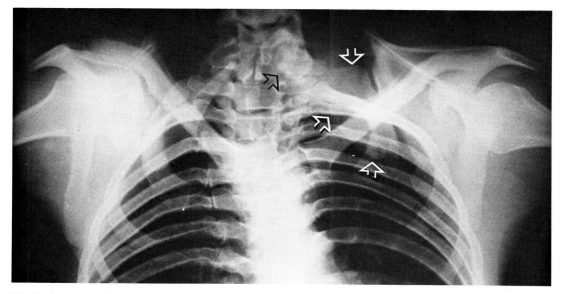

FIG. 5-14. Sprengel's deformity. Both scapulae are elevated. On the left there is a broad omovertebral bone (arrows) extending from the cervical spine to the vertebral border of the scapula. On the right the omovertebral bone is incompletely ossified. Bilateral omovertebral bones are uncommon. The patient has cervical vertebral maldevelopment and thoracic scoliosis, abnormalities commonly found with Sprengel's deformity.

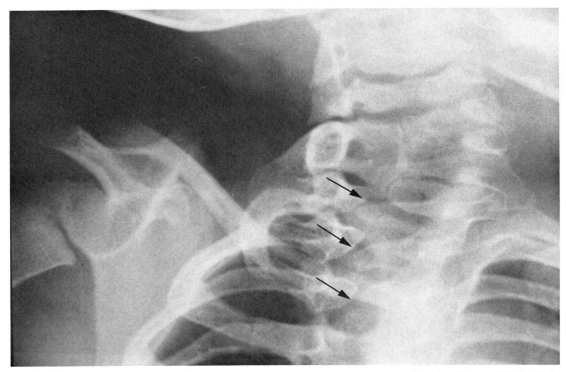

FIG. 5-15. Klippel-Feil syndrome in a 5-year-old girl. Frontal radiograph shows fused vertebrae (C2-3, C5-6), hemivertebrae, neural arch defects (arrows), and elevation of the right scapula (Sprengel's deformity).

restricted motion of the neck. Patients often have other associated anomalies such as thoracic hemivertebrae, fused ribs, or Sprengel's deformity. Feil's original classification is as follows:[38]

Type I: Block fusion of all the cervical and upper thoracic vertebrae;

Type II: Fusion of one or two pairs of cervical vertebrae. This is the most common type. C2-3 (autosomal dominant) is the interspace most often fused; C5-6 fusion (autosomal recessive) is the next most common;

Type III: Combination of Type I or Type II anomalies with either lower thoracic or lumbar intervertebral fusions.

Over 50 percent of persons with Klippel-Feil syndrome have associated genitourinary anomalies including unilateral renal agenesis, malrotation, renal ectopia, renal dysgenesis and renal pelvis, and ureteral duplication.[62,79] Also reported have been a wide variety of associated gastrointestinal,[63] cardiovascular,[63,66] neurologic,[63,66] musculoskeletal,[66,80] and dermatologic[63] abnormalities.

Cleidocranial Dysostosis

Cleidocranial dysostosis appears with a number of clinical and roentgenologic abnormalities. Most common are (1) varying degrees of aplasia of the clavicle, usually bilateral (Fig. 5-16), (2) delayed closures of the fontanelles and suture lines of the skull with occipital wormian bones, and (3) defective ossification of the pubic and ischial bones.[102] In addition, there may be underdevelopment of the facial bones, abnormalities of dentition, unusually long second metacarpals, blunting of the terminal phalanges, coxa vara, and under-modeling of the long bone metaphyses.[7,47] Neural arch defects and cone-shaped thorax are also relatively common associated defects. The

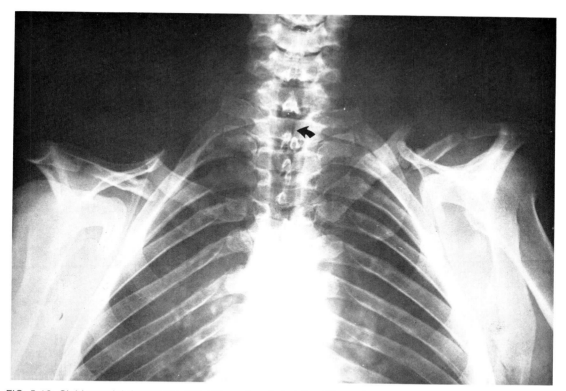

FIG. 5-16. Cleidocranial dysostosis. Tripartite unfused clavicles. The patient has a bell-shaped thorax and spina bifida occulta (arrow).

disease may occur sporadically but there is a high familial incidence.[102]

The clavicular changes consist of defective development. There may be total aplasia (Fig. 5-17), no acromial end or, rarely, no sternal end, or multiple ununited lengths of bone. Both clavicles may present asymmetric maldevelopment. As a result of the clavicular abnormality, the patient has the appearance of drooping shoulders,

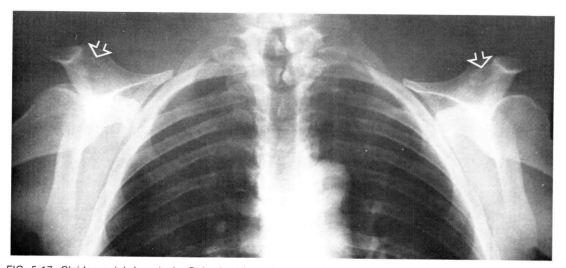

FIG. 5-17. Cleidocranial dysostosis. Only short lateral terminal segments of the clavicles are present.

elongated neck, and a narrow distance between the tips of the shoulders. The patient can approximate his shoulders anteriorly to an unusual degree.

Congenital Pseudarthrosis of the Clavicle

Congenital pseudarthrosis of the clavicle, an entity of obscure pathology, is infrequently encountered. The term implies an antenatal defect which disposes to nonunion of a transverse complete defect in the clavicle, usually in the middle third. Of interest is the "rightsidedness" of the lesion; over 90 percent of the documented cases are of the right clavicle[74] (Fig. 5-18). Bilateralism is unusual[41] (Fig. 5-19). It is clear that the abnormality bears no relationship to congenital pseudarthrosis of the tibia.

The long-held theory that this condition is due to failure of fusion of two ossification centers is not universally accepted.[32,56] There is the possibility that some instances of congenital pseudarthrosis of the clavicle can be transmitted genetically as an autosomal dominant characteristic.[32]

Lloyd-Roberts and associates have proposed and present rather convincing evidence that the effect of exaggerated arterial pulsation on the developing clavicle results in its maldevelopment.[56] Normally, the right subclavian artery lies slightly higher than the left as it passes over the first rib beneath the clavicle. These authors noted a high incidence of cervical ribs or vertically disposed and elevated upper ribs in association with congenital clavicular pseudarthrosis. These would cause the subclavian artery to be brought into closer proximity to the clavicle, and consequently its pulsations could well have a greater mechanical effect on the developing clavicle. In further support of this origin are the cases of left clavicular pseudarthrosis in patients with dextrocardia.[32] Left pseudarthrosis has been reported without dextrocardia, perhaps related to cervical ribs or other cause.

Some patients complain of pain related to activity; most have no pain. Conspicuous swelling caused by angulation of the bony parts is generally the chief complaint. Radiographically, there is complete separation of the two terminal segments of bone at about the middle portion. The medial segment lies above and anterior to the lateral segment. The medial end of the lateral segment almost always is bulbous. The lateral end of the medial segment is usually pointed. Histologically, there is subchondral sclerosis and a well-formed cartilaginous cap over the bone ends at the pseudarthrotic site.[74] Resection of the pseudarthrosis and internal fixation or bone grafting uniformly result in satisfactory union.

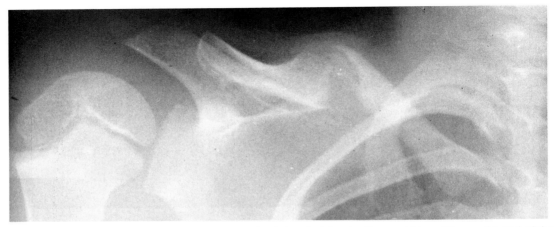

FIG. 5-18. Right unilateral congenital pseudarthrosis of the clavicle of a 5-year-old boy. The medial end of the lateral segment has the typical knobby appearance, whereas the lateral end of the medial segment is pointed. (Courtesy of Dr. Harvey White, Children's Memorial Hospital, Chicago.)

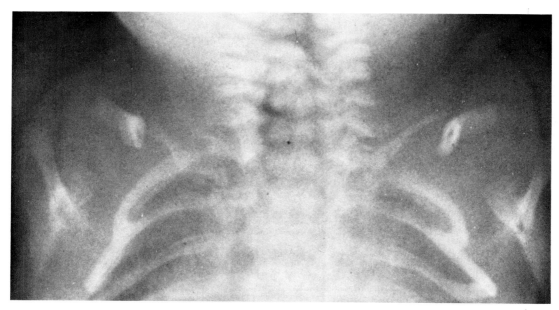

FIG. 5-19. Bilateral congenital pseudarthrosis of the clavicle of a newborn girl. (Courtesy of Dr. Harvey White, Children's Memorial Hospital, Chicago.)

Multiple Cartilaginous Exostoses

Multiple cartilaginous exostoses (diaphyseal aclasis) is an autosomal dominant heritable disorder, its most striking manifestation being numerous cartilage-capped exostoses appearing in different parts of the skeleton.[102] As a result of growth deficiency in the involved bone, there may be a variety of deformities most often discovered in the first decade; males and females are about equally affected. In addition to the cortical exostoses, there are characteristically club-shaped thickenings of the metaphyses. These may project as pedunculated masses varying in size from small to massive and may vary in shape from smooth to cauliflowerlike. The radiographic appearance may suggest that the exostosis is significantly smaller than expected from the clinical appearance. This is easily accounted for; the cartilage cap which may be quite large may not cast a recognizable radiographic shadow.

The tubular bones, iliac crest, and vertebral borders of the scapulae are the most commonly involved sites. In the long bones the more actively growing ends are the most extensively involved. The proximal end of the humerus is involved in about 85 percent of persons with hereditary multiple exostoses.[90] The scapula is less commonly involved.

The most serious complication of the disease is malignant degeneration, variously estimated as occurring in more than 10 percent[54] and as many as 25 percent.[45] Radiologically, the malignant changes may be evident by rapid growth, by spotty densities within the mass, and by poorly defined outlines of the tumor. The scapula is one of the more common sites of malignant transformation.

Osteopoikilosis

Osteopoikilosis is an unusual familial condition characterized by numerous sharply defined circular or ovoid opaque densities in bone, varying in size from 2 to 10 mm.[34] (Fig. 5-20). They appear most abundantly in the epiphyses and adjacent metaphyses, most commonly in long bones and especially tubular bones of the hands and feet. They are usually clustered around the shoulder joint, just as in the pelvic

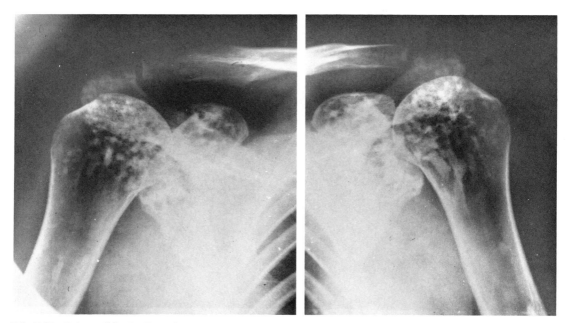

FIG. 5-20. Osteopoikilosis. Round and ovoid dense spots are plentiful closest to the joint. A few have relatively clear centers. Elongated lesions are parallel to the long axis of the bone.

bones they are clustered about the acetabulum, sacroiliac joint, and iliac crest. The lesions are infrequent in the cranium, spine, and ribs. The lesions are medullary and do not distort the cortex or bony configuration.

Microscopically, the lesions consist of thicker than normal trabeculae of varying thickness, regularly arranged. There is no evidence of associated marrow fibrosis.[102]

The abnormality produces no symptoms.

Osteoid Osteoma

Osteoid osteoma represents a benign bone tumor with a nidus of vascularized osteoid tissue and varying amounts of sclerotic surrounding bone (Fig. 5-21). The nidus either may be in the center of the sclerotic bone or may occupy an eccentric position. Angiographic as well as histologic studies have shown the highly vascular nature of the nidus. The patient suffers pain, characteristically at night and of aching nature, increasing with time and almost always relieved by aspirin. The pain may radiate or may be referred to a joint. A small percentage of patients have associated soft-tissue swelling.[27]

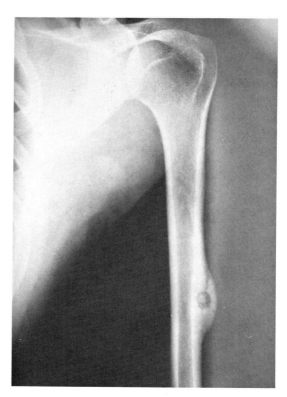

FIG. 5-21. Osteoid osteoma. In the midshaft of the humerus, the lesion exhibits the exuberant cortical new bone formation, the central opacity, and its surrounding zone of radiolucency.

Radiologically, the findings in a long bone are a sclerotic expanded cortex of varying lengths and a central radiolucency varying from 0.5 to 1.5 cm. in diameter. At times the nidus may not be identifiable on plain films and is shown only on tomograms, which at times are invaluable in defining the precise depth of the tumor when surgery is contemplated. Identifying the nidus usually permits differentiating the lesion from chronic osteomyelitis. Angiography is usually not required for the diagnosis but may be of help in demonstrating hypervascularity of the nidus; chronic osteomyelitis, which may resemble osteoid osteoma on plain films, shows no such vascularity. A rare complication of the tumor is overgrowth and/or deformity of the involved bone. Those reported with this complication have had the onset of symptoms before age 5 years.[69]

During operation, it is wise to take films of the surgical specimen to ascertain that the entire tumor, including the nidus, has been removed.

Nonossifying Fibromas

Nonossifying fibromas are asymptomatic benign tumors, usually with incidental radiographic findings, discovered in children or young adults[11,21] (Fig. 5-22). They appear as sharply defined radiolucencies with thin sclerotic margins, located subcortically, most commonly in the diaphyses of the long bones. They are usually solitary but may be multiple. As the child grows older the lesion commonly disappears or it may be carried into the diaphysis as the bone lengthens; it may persist or heal with bone sclerosis. The distal end of the femur is the most common site of the tumor but any long bone may be affected. The radiologic findings are sufficiently distinctive to obviate the need for biopsy.

Solitary Bone Cyst

The solitary bone cyst, a benign neoplasm, has a predilection for the upper end

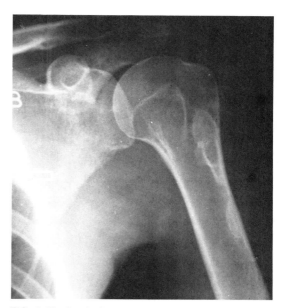

FIG. 5-22. Cortical nonossifying fibromas. These benign cortical defects are of no clinical significance. More commonly they appear singly, but multiple ones are not uncommon.

of the shaft of the humerus where the vast majority of the lesions occur (see Figs. 22-2 to 22-5). The cause is unknown; it occurs more commonly in males and is most often discovered in the first decade of life.[8,30] The solitary cyst is most frequently encountered in the metaphyseal portions of the long bones, often abutting directly against the epiphyseal plate but not crossing it. The lesion varies from 2 to 6 cm. in length when diagnosed, shows destruction of medullary bone, thinning of cortex, often trabeculated lines in the wall of the cyst causing it to appear multicameral, and occasionally some little expansion of the bone. This relatively little expansion is an important feature that distinguishes this lesion from aneurysmal bone cyst. The cortex may narrow to a fine line, accounting for the frequency of fracture of the cyst; it is the pain of fracture that usually calls attention to the otherwise asymptomatic lesion. The cyst migrates into the shaft as the bone grows and usually is replaced by bone as the patient matures.

Infantile Cortical Hyperostosis

The cause of infantile cortical hyperostosis (Caffey's disease) is still obscure; it probably represents a low-grade inflammatory process, though the causative agent remains unknown in spite of extensive studies that have been carried out since it was first described by Caffey and Silverman in 1945.[15] The disease occurs in infants younger than 6 months; it may be present at birth. The triad of manifestations are hyperirritability, swellings of the soft-tissues, and cortical thickening of the underlying bones (Fig. 5-23). Fever is usually present and pseudoparalysis secondary to pain occasionally. The disease is self-limiting, usually lasting but a few weeks, and the cortical hyperostosis, even when marked, generally disappears in a few months. Rarely, deformity of a bone may persist.[12]

Of the flat bones the scapula is one of those most often involved; in the monostotic form the scapula is particularly affected. The mandibles, ribs, parietals, and frontals may also be involved but not the vertebral or tuft bones. The mandible is the most commonly involved bone, in 75 percent of reported cases. Of the tubular bones the clavicles are the most commonly affected. The deformity caused by hyperostosis, particularly of the scapula, may mimic malignant neoplasm, but the clinical appearance, the frequent simultaneous involvement of other bones, and the age of the patient should clearly distinguish infantile cortical hyperostosis from malignancy.

Of interest is the fact that infantile cortical hyperostosis has occurred rarely in the last decade, whereas in the prior 20 years one or two cases were seen monthly in pediatric centers. The cause for this remarka-

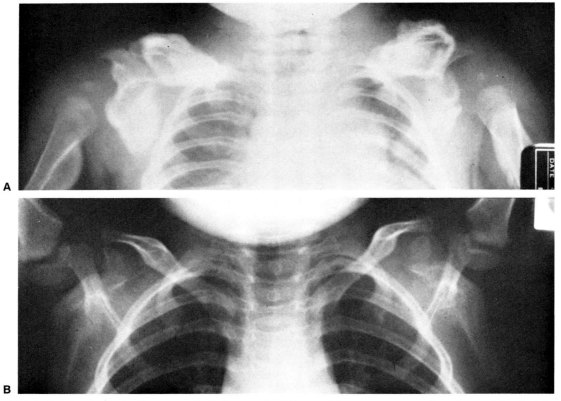

FIG. 5-23. Infantile cortical hyperostosis. A, A 2-month-old infant with exuberant cortical new bone of the clavicles, scapulae, and humeri. B, Twelve months later, no residual deformity is present.

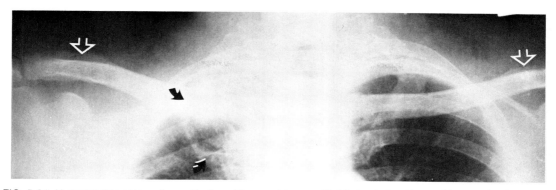

FIG. 5-24. Hypertrophic osteoarthropathy in a 48-year-old man with bilateral shoulder and knee pain. Periosteal new bone is present in the clavicles bilaterally (open arrows). The patient had an abscess in the right upper lung (solid arrows).

ble decrease in incidence of infantile cortical hyperostosis is just as obscure as its cause.

Hypertrophic Osteoarthropathy

Hypertrophic osteoarthropathy is manifested by clubbing of the fingers and periosteal thickening of the diaphyses of long bones, especially of the arms and legs and tubular bones of the hands and feet (Fig. 5-24). The distal ends of the bones are most commonly involved. There is often pain, sometimes referred to adjacent joints, associated painful and tender soft-tissue swelling, and increased warmth of the parts affected. The affection is most often caused by lung cancer, primary or metastatic, or lung abscess. Other intrathoracic diseases, such as benign tumors, mesotheliomas, bronchiectasis, lymphomas, rib tumors, mediastinal tumors, and fungal infections, may also give rise to hypertrophic osteoarthropathy.[40] Less commonly, there are extrathoracic abnormalities, such as ulcerative colitis, amebic and bacillary dysentery, cirrhosis of the liver, Whipple's disease, malignancies of the nasopharynx and of small and large bowel, intestinal tuberculosis, and Hodgkin's disease, leading to the bone changes.[4,37,65]

The cause of the disorder is not known, although most theories relate the changes to increased peripheral blood flow. Following removal of the tumor and effective treatment of the infection, the symptoms commonly disappear and the bones revert to normal.

Radionuclide imaging using ^{99m}Tc-labeled diphosphonate or pyrophosphate will reveal the presence and extent of subperiosteal activity earlier than does radiographic imaging.[23,95] Response to treatment is better determined by the radionuclide imaging than by radiographs.

Superior Sulcus Tumor

Superior sulcus tumor (Pancoast's tumor), arising in the apex of the upper lobe, often invades the brachial plexus and at times the cervical sympathetic chain and may cause destruction of adjacent ribs. Thus, the patient's first complaints may be of shoulder or arm pain, sometimes accompanied by Horner's syndrome.[76] A mass density in the apex of the lung is the earliest radiologic finding; at times it may mimic innocent apical pleural thickening or inflammatory disease of the lung (Fig. 5-25). Rib invasion and destruction may be readily apparent when looked for on plain films; in other instances tomographic studies or nuclear scans are required to yield this information.

Sternocostoclavicular Hyperostosis

In 1975, Köhler and co-workers reported on the findings in three patients, between 32

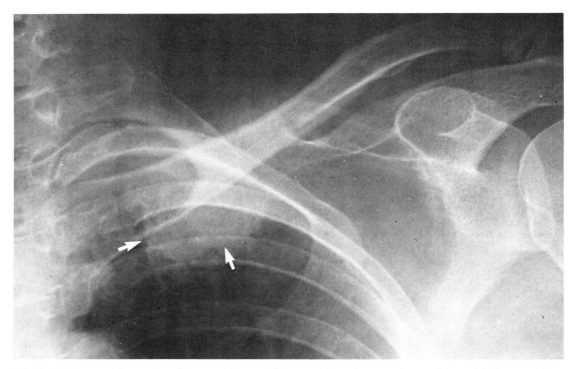

FIG. 5-25. Pancoast tumor in a 57-year-old man with a superior sulcus carcinoma (arrows) but no roentgen evidence of bone invasion. Horner's syndrome, shoulder pain, and symptoms of brachial plexus palsy were present.

and 42 years of age at the onset of symptoms, who complained of persistent pulling pain in the sternum, clavicles, and both first ribs, especially during cold and damp weather[51] (Fig. 5-26). Two had superior vena cava obstruction. Other than high erythrocyte sedimentation rates, no abnormality was confirmed by results of laboratory tests. On physical examination the patients were found to have spindle-shaped swelling of the clavicles. Films showed hyperostosis of the sternal and middle portion of the clavicles, synostosis of the sternoclavicular joints with involvement of the first two ribs bilaterally, and thickening and increase in width of the sternum. The superior vena cava syndrome was caused by subclavian vein obstruction owing to the sternocostoclavicular hyperostosis. Examination of biopsy specimens revealed hyperostotic spongiosclerosis in each case. The pain responded to indomethacin treatment and local x irradiation. The cause for the syndrome is as yet undetermined.

Condensing Osteitis of the Clavicle

Brower and associates gave the name condensing osteitis of the clavicle to an entity with characteristic clinical and roentgenographic appearances[9] (Fig. 5-27). The chief complaint is of pain over the top of the shoulder on abduction. A fusiform swelling over the medial aspect of the ipsilateral clavicle is present. Roentgenograms reveal sclerosis over the medial end of the clavicle and osteophyte formation over the inferior margin of the medial cortex. The histologic findings consist of increased amounts and thickness of cancellous bone and periosteal reaction. The osteophyte reflects periosteal new bone formation. The changes are thought to be the result of increased or altered mechanical stress across the sternoclavicular joint. In the reported cases the symptoms were alleviated by surgical excision of the involved end of the bone.

When first viewing the films one may be

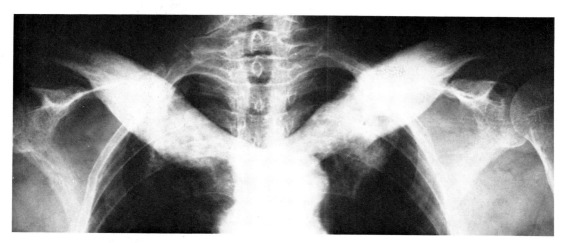

FIG. 5-26. Sternocostoclavicular hyperostosis. There is marked hyperostosis of the sternal and middle parts of the clavicles, synostosis of the sternoclavicular joints, and involvement of the anterior end of the first ribs. Thickening and increase in breadth of the sternum were present as well. (Courtesy of Köhler, H., Uehlinger, E., Kutzner, J., Weihrauch, T. R., Wilbert, L., and Schuster, R.: Sterno-kosto-klavikulare Hyperostose. Dtsch. Med. Wochenschr., 100:1519–1523, 1975. Reproduced with permission of the publisher.)

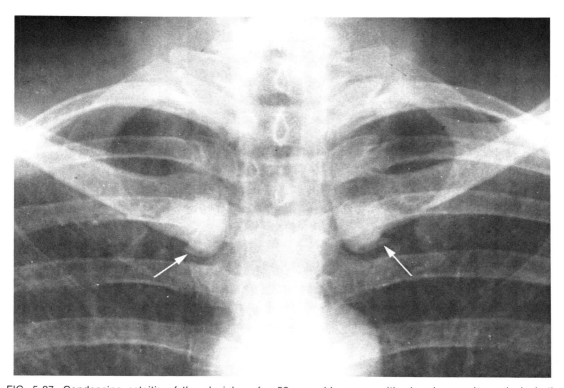

FIG. 5-27. Condensing osteitis of the clavicles of a 53-year-old woman with chronic gnawing pain in both shoulders. There is sclerosis of the medial portion of both clavicles and small exostoses (arrows).

concerned about osteoblastic metastasis, Paget's disease, low-grade osteomyelitis, osteosarcoma, or degenerative arthritis. The roentgen appearance coupled with the clinical findings, however, permits the exclusion of these diseases.

Friedrich's Disease

Friedrich's disease (aseptic necrosis of the clavicle), a rare abnormality, involves only the medial end of the clavicle and usually appears clinically as a painless swelling (Fig. 5-28). Radiographically, there is rarefaction, often with punctate calcification.[28] The adjacent sternum is not involved. In some of the cases reported, trauma to the area calls attention to the preexisting disease; in other instances, earlier trauma may have contributed to the abnormality. Only about a dozen cases have been reported since Friedrich's original description in 1924.

Chondroblastoma

Chondroblastoma has at various times been referred to as Codman's tumor, giant cell tumor variant, enchondromatous giant cell tumor, and epiphyseal chondroblastoma of bone. The tumor, with a predilection for adolescents in the second decade

(nearly 90 percent occur between the ages of 5 and 25 years),[19,44,84] has as one of its major sites of occurrence the head of the humerus. It occurs somewhat more commonly in the lower end of the femur and upper and lower ends of the tibia. It has also been reported as occurring in the acromion, glenoid, and the clavicle, although these are rare sites of involvement.[19] The sex distribution shows a decided predominance of males. Although the lesion sometimes does not cause symptoms there is usually pain with local tenderness and occasionally swelling and limitation of motion of the adjacent joint. Joint effusion may be present, probably related to extension of the tumor through the articular cartilage. The radiographic appearance is that of a round or ovoid area of lucency located eccentrically in the epiphysis, with or without a sclerotic rim (Fig. 5-29). When large enough, the tumor may expand the cortex in more advanced cases, causing periosteal bone production. The lesion may be mottled by calcification or homogeneously radiolucent[59] (Fig. 5-30). Although the tumor generally originates in the epiphyses, it may penetrate into the metaphysis. It may likewise invade the joint. Rarely, the tumor originates in the metaphysis.[3,84]

Curettage with packing of the cavity with bone chips usually is sufficient treatment.

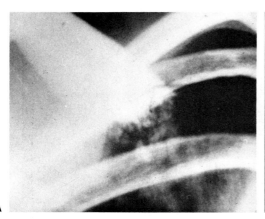

A

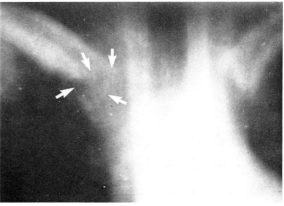

B

FIG. 5-28. Friedrich's disease. A, There is rarefaction of the sternal end of the right clavicle with punctate calcifications. B, A tomogram reveals an osteolytic defect at the sternal end of the right clavicle (arrows). The left clavicle and sternum showed no abnormality. (Courtesy of Fischel, R. E., and Bernstein, D.: Friedrich's disease. Br. J. Radiol., 48:318–319, 1975. Reproduced with permission of the publisher.)

En bloc resection may be required. Amputation may be necessary to treat malignant transformation. Such transformation of the tumor is rare, but has been noted, whether radiation therapy was used[45] or not.[84,89]

Paget's Disease of Bone

No bone of the skeleton is exempt from involvement by Paget's disease (osteitis deformans), and those of the shoulder girdles are not exceptions. The characteristic appearance of coarsened trabeculae, thickened cortex, and expanded bone permits ease of diagnosis in most instances (Figs. 5-31 and 5-32, see also Fig. 19-18). The concurrent appearance of Paget's disease in other bones is of further aid in diagnosis, but of course the disease may be monostotic. The osteolytic form of Paget's disease as seen in osteoporosis circumscripta of the skull has been observed and reported as

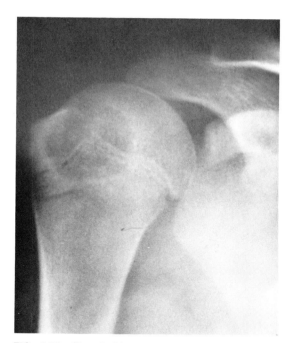

FIG. 5-29. Chondroblastoma. The lesion is sharply defined, entirely lytic, and confined to the epiphysis. That it appears to extend below the epiphyseal plate is related to the projection.

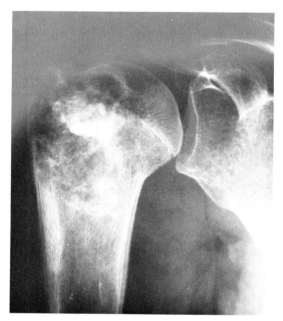

FIG. 5-30. Chondroblastoma. The tumor is mottled by calcification, extends into the metaphysis, and causes expansion of bone. There is a distinct periosteal new bone deposition. (Courtesy of Dr. Alex Norman, Hospital for Joint Diseases and Medical Center, New York.)

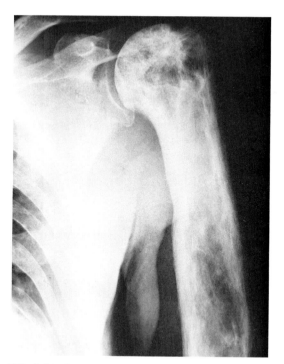

FIG. 5-31. Paget's disease of bone in a 70-year-old man. The left humerus is involved for its entire length. The cortex is thickened, the shaft is expanded, trabeculae are prominent, and areas of osteoporosis are interspersed in the sclerotic bone. The scapula and the clavicle appear normal.

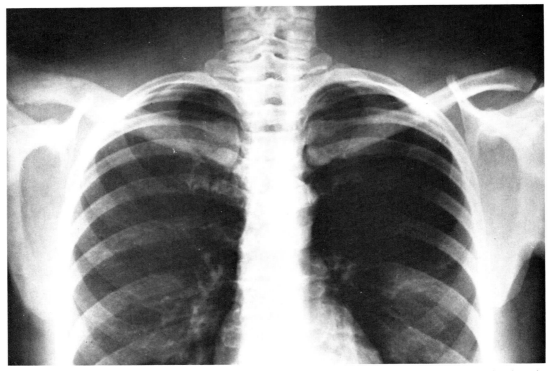

FIG. 5-32. Paget's disease of the clavicle. The right clavicle is widened, the cortex is thickened, and trabeculae are prominent. The patient had similar changes of Paget's disease in the pelvic bones, bilaterally.

occurring in long bones, and might appear in one of the components of the shoulder girdle.[5,101] If there are not the classic findings of Paget's disease in other bones, the lesion may escape correct diagnosis until biopsy. The characteristic findings include (1) abnormally radiolucent bone with obliteration of trabeculae, (2) expansion of the affected bone, (3) a flame- or V-shaped demarcation between affected and normal bone (similar to that seen in fibrous dysplasia), and (4) subarticular extension of the lesion.

Malignant degeneration of Paget's disease into sarcoma is quite rare. When it occurs it is most often in patients with long-standing polyostotic disease but may occur in the monostotic form. Most often only one bone manifests the malignant change, but it is not rare for two or more bones to simultaneously undergo malignant degeneration. Osteogenic sarcoma is the most commonly occurring malignancy, although fibrosarcoma and, even less commonly, chondro-

sarcoma may occur.[101] Sarcomatous change is usually first manifest as a subcortical area of bone destruction; eventually there is destruction of cortex.

When malignant changes appear to be present in pagetoid bone, first consideration should be given to metastasis. Since Paget's disease and cancer most commonly affect the same age group and since there is increased vascularity at the sites of Paget's disease, it is not surprising that metastases may be discovered in pagetoid bone. In fact, metastasis is probably more common than malignant transformation (Fig. 5-33).

Fibrous Dysplasia of Bone

Fibrous dysplasia of bone generally is recognized in the first two decades and may occur in one of three forms:[55] (1) monostotic, the most common, with little associated deformity; (2) polyostotic, in which the distribution of bone lesions may be widespread, often with unilateral predominance

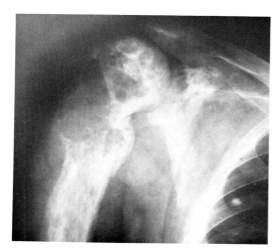

FIG. 5-33. Paget's disease of bone with metastasis. There is thickened cortex, sclerotic bone, and coarsened trabeculae of the humerus and scapula. Examination of biopsy specimens of the lytic and expanded lesion showed metastatic hypernephroma, later demonstrated by pyelograms and confirmed by kidney biopsy.

pearance from that of aneurysmal bone cyst. The latter usually has more cortical than medullary alterations in the early stages, and there is generally a more abrupt junction between the cyst and normal bone than is seen in fibrous dysplasia, in which the dysplastic bone fades gradually into the normal bone.

Although the lesions of fibrous dysplasia usually become static at puberty, they may continue to grow aggressively into the fourth and fifth decades.

Fibrosarcomatous degeneration is a rare complication of fibrous dysplasia.[55] It can be recognized radiographically by enlargement of the local lesion, cortical destruction, and a soft-tissue mass.

(Fig. 5-34); and (3) McCune-Albright's syndrome, a rare entity of polyostotic fibrous dysplasia in females associated with sexual precocity and cutaneous pigmentation (café au lait spots). In either form, pain and deformity may be prominent clinical manifestations; the latter is most commonly seen when the neck of the femur is involved (shepherd's crook deformity). The skull, long bones, flat bones, and vertebrae may be involved.

Radiographically, the lesions appear cystic, often thinning the adjacent cortex and expanding the bone locally. The appearance is often like ground glass. The cystic-appearing lesions may or may not be sharply defined by sclerotic borders. In long bones the lesions are most common in the diaphyses but may appear in or extend into the metaphyses; the epiphyses are not involved, although on occasion there may be early epiphyseal closure owing to extension of the lesion from the metaphysis. In some instances, irregular strands of new bone with flecks of calcification may be interspersed within the "cystic" lesion.[86] When fibrous dysplasia expands bone it may be impossible to differentiate its radiologic ap-

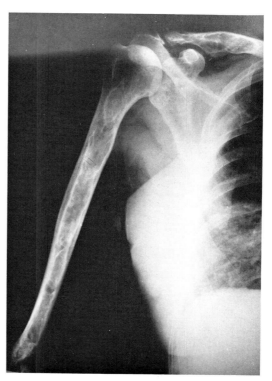

FIG. 5-34. Fibrous dysplasia. The clavicle, fourth rib, and humerus are involved. The right hemipelvis and femur were likewise affected in this 30-year-old woman. The lesions have sclerotic borders and, in the upper humerus, a somewhat ground glass appearance.

Hyperparathyroidism

The osseous changes noted on roentgenograms are the same whether due to primary or secondary hyperparathyroidism (renal osteodystrophy). The earliest roentgenologically recognizable change is the subperiosteal resorption of bone along the radial borders of the middle and distal phalanges of the index fingers which may progress to involve other phalanges as well. To date, this roentgenographic appearance is pathognomonic of hyperparathyroidism. Generalized osteopenia and localized bone abnormalities may also result. The latter include brown tumors, pathologic fractures, and localized resorption of bone. The last-noted condition is often seen about the shoulder girdle.

There are three common sites of local bone resorption in the clavicle.[78] The lateral end frequently exhibits loss of cortical margins and then progressive resorption of bone (Fig. 5-35). The changes appear similar to those that may be seen occasionally in rheumatoid or psoriatic arthritis or following local trauma. Less frequently, the medial end of the clavicle may exhibit bone resorption.[94] The changes at this site in all likelihood occur more commonly than reported, probably because detail in this segment of bone is not well seen on routine radiographs, because it is obscured by mediastinal shadows and the adjacent sternum. Bone resorption likewise commonly occurs at the inferior margin of the clavicle at the junction of the middle and lateral thirds, where the coracoclavicular ligament inserts on the clavicle. Occasionally a normal clavicle may be slightly concave in this location but its cortical margin is intact. Bone resorption leads to loss of cortex, trabecular fuzziness and, in the untreated case, progressive concavity. The predilection for resorption to select this site is probably related to the relatively rich blood supply, coupled with ligamentous forces.

Similar changes occur on the medial bor-

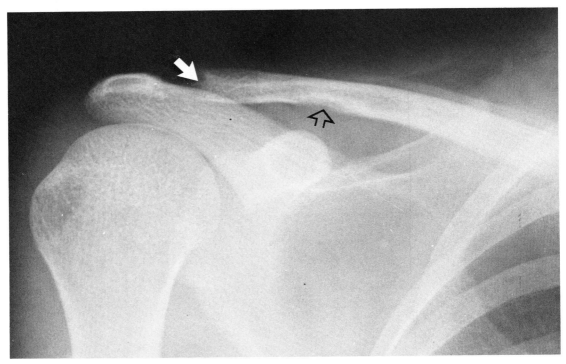

FIG. 5-35. Secondary hyperparathyroidism in a 22-year-old woman with renal osteodystrophy. The right side shows resorption of bone at the distal end of the clavicle (arrow) as well as at the attachment of the coracoclavicular ligament (open arrow). These changes can be present in either primary or secondary hyperparathyroidism.

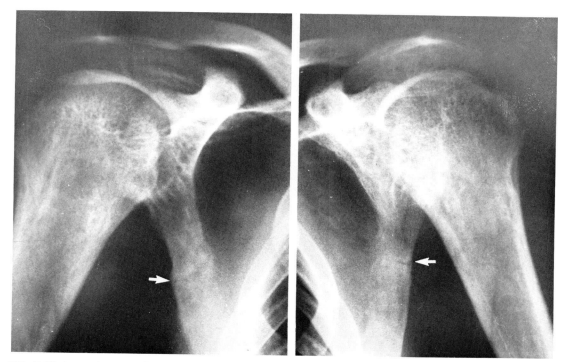

FIG. 5-36. Looser's zones in a 40-year-old woman with chronic renal failure and renal osteodystrophy. The scapulae are common sites of stress fractures (arrows) with inadequate healing response and resultant radiolucent osteoid seams.

der of the neck of the humerus just below the head, forming a notch-like defect. The selectivity of this site is probably related to the abundant local blood supply and the forces exerted by the capsular attachment.

Secondary to the osteopenia, Looser's zones (seams of osteoid with defective demineralization) may appear (Fig. 5-36). In the shoulder girdle they are reported to appear most commonly in the lateral margins of the scapulae and, as elsewhere, are usually symmetric.[98] In my experience the lateral borders are more frequently involved.

Soft-tissue calcification secondary to renal osteodystrophy is probably the most common cause of metastatic calcification. It may occur, but less often, secondary to primary hyperparathyroidism.

Diabetes Mellitus

Diabetic osteoarthropathy has a wide variety of presentations; some are due to neu-

ropathy, some to ischemia, some to infection, and some to a mixture of these causes (Fig. 5-37). The Charcot-type changes occurring in diabetes mellitus are well known and usually are present in the lower extremities. Schwarz and associates have reported purely atrophic resorptive arthropathy in patients with diabetes mellitus and peripheral neuropathy as occurring more commonly in the upper extremities.[86] The roentgen appearance is no different from that in neurotrophic arthropathy of syringomyelia or syphilis (see Chapter 12). Campbell and Feldman have reported that in diabetics marked shoulder osteoarthropathy is characterized by glenohumeral joint space narrowing, humeral head deformity with evidence of bone resorption, varying degrees of subchondral sclerosis, cystic changes, and subluxation.[16] Some bone fragments may be present in the soft tissues, and these may occasionally be resorbed. In less advanced cases, before bone resorption occurs, cystic and sclerotic

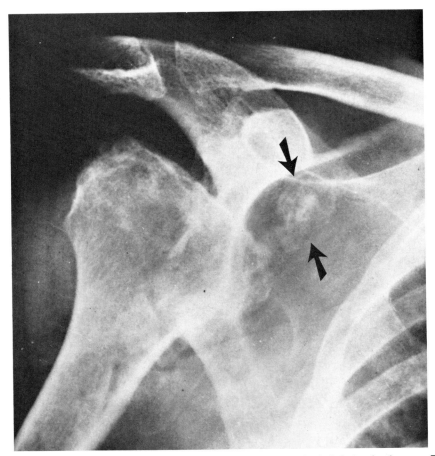

FIG. 5-37. Right shoulder of a 67-year-old man who was known to have had diabetes for 8 years. Bilateral joint space narrowing, productive changes, and marked humeral head deformity are present. The flattened appearance of the right humeral head is a hallmark of the Charcot-type joint. There is relative scarcity of osseous fragments (arrows) caused by resorption. (Courtesy of Campbell, W. L., and Feldman, F.: Bone and soft tissue abnormalities of the upper extremity in diabetes mellitus. Am. J. Roentgen. Rad. Ther. Nucl. Med., 124:7–15, 1975. Reproduced with permission of the publishers.)

changes are present in the humeral head, glenoid, and acromion.

Upper Humeral Notch

Ozonoff and Ziter have claimed that an upper humeral notch may be a relatively common variation of normal.[75] I believe that if it is a variation of normal it must be rare. After careful search of thousands of chest and shoulder films, I have not uncovered a case of a humeral notch unassociated with some generalized abnormality. The defect is a localized notchlike one on the medial aspect of the humerus at the lower margin of the neck, at the capsule insertion (Fig. 5-38). The cortex is irregular in outline, as though undergoing resorption, for a length of 1 to 2.5 cm. The defect is most often seen bilaterally, reflecting its relationship to some generalized disease. Unfortunately, there has been no adequate pathologic study to determine the cause of the notch. It is likely related to stress caused by adductor muscle attachment and to an abundant local blood supply. The humeral notch is most often seen in association with osteopenia secondary to renal osteodystrophy but may be seen in other generalized disorders[77] (Fig. 5-38).

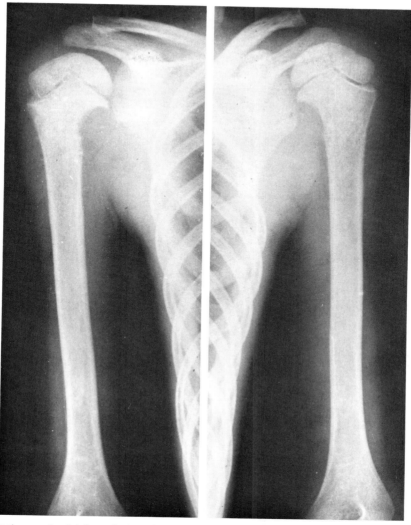

FIG. 5-38. Upper humeral notch in an 8-year-old with widespread metastases from adrenal neuroblastoma. There are bilateral humeral notches. These areas were not examined at autopsy. (Courtesy of Professor A. Schwartz, Hadassah-Hebrew University Medical School, Jerusalem.)

Hematologic Disorders

Hematologic disorders often have widespread soft-tissue, bone, and joint manifestations. In some instances, the abnormalities of soft tissue, for example splenomegaly, or of bone, for example ischemic necrosis, are nonspecific and do not permit differentiation among the blood diseases or from other systemic or local diseases. Usually, however, there are roentgenographic, laboratory, and clinical findings that when taken en toto readily allow specific diagnosis.

Sickle Hemoglobinopathy

Persons with S hemoglobin are often beset with a variety of skeletal changes owing to hyperplasia of the bone marrow erythroblastic elements and to ischemic necrosis from thrombi of sickled cells. Ischemic necrosis commonly involves fingers and toes, especially in children, in whom the roentgen and clinical appearances mimic osteomyelitis (hand-foot syndrome) and the heads of the femora and humeri. In the latter bones, the ischemic necrosis is indistinguishable from that of other causes

(Gaucher's disease, thrombotic thrombocy-topenic purpura, steroid therapy, alcohol-ism, systemic lupus erythematosus, pancre-atitis, trauma, decompression disease, idiopathic). However, in those with S he-moglobinopathy there are generally wide-spread skeletal and soft-tissue changes that permit high-degree accuracy in diagnosis from the roentgen findings alone. These include the almost pathognomonic step de-formity of vertebrae, scattered sclerosis owing to infarction, expansion of the cranial diploe, long bone infarction with marked periosteal reaction, osteomyelitis (Fig. 5-39) (commonly from salmonella infection), and bone expansion with thinned cortices and prominent residual trabeculae due to bone marrow hyperplasia.[64,81] Splenic infarction and renal papillary necrosis are among the more common extraskeletal changes.[81] Ob-viously, the disease can be confirmed by hemoglobin analysis.

Radiologically, the changes in the head of the humerus (or femur) are those of irregu-lar patchy sclerosis, a subchondral crescen-tic fissure representing a fracture through the necrotic subchondral bone and, later, varying degrees of deformity.[61,67,97]

Although the skeletal changes vary in in-cidence among the various S hemoglobi-nopathies, any of the changes can occur in all of them: homozygous (S-S) sickle cell anemia, heterozygous sickle cell trait (S-A), combinations of C hemoglobin and S he-moglobin (S-C disease), sickle cell-thalasse-mia, and sickle cell-hemoglobin D (S-D).

Thalassemia

Changes relating to irregular premature fusion of the proximal humeral epiphysis are relatively common in those suffering from homozygous beta-thalassemia (thalas-semia major, Cooley's anemia), and have a distinctive radiographic appearance re-ported in no other disease. Currarino and Erlandson reported this finding in 23 per-cent of 48 patients over the age of 10 years;[18] none was found in patients below this age. Moseley has reported this finding

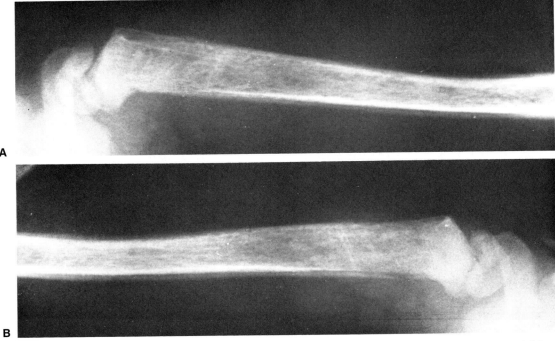

A

B

FIG. 5-39. Sickle cell anemia with osteomyelitis. A, The left arm and, B, the right arm of this young child are involved with destructive and periosteal changes of osteomyelitis.

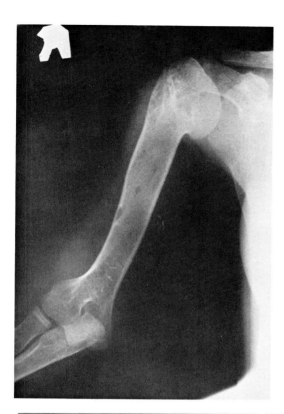

FIG. 5-40. Thalassemia. Varus deformity of the humerus is present and the bone is short. The radiolucent defects probably represent tumorous foci of marrow hyperplasia. (Courtesy of Professor A. Schwartz, Hadassah-Hebrew University Medical School, Jerusalem.)

in patients as young as 8 years.[64] The epiphyseal line fuses prematurely along its medial portion, causing epiphyseal tilt and thus creating a varus deformity which may be quite marked (Fig. 5-40). Because of the growth potential at this epiphyseal line, the premature fusion results in shortening of the humerus by as much as 5 cm. (Fig. 5-41). This finding may be unilateral but is far more commonly bilateral. Although most commonly seen in the proximal end of the humerus, this growth defect may be present at the distal end of the femur and the proximal ends of the tibia and fibula.

It is reasonable to relate these epiphyseal changes to the severe hyperplasia of the bone marrow which accounts for the many other skeletal changes in thalassemia: ex-

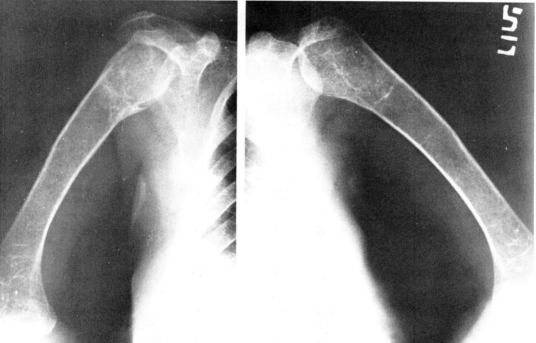

FIG. 5-41. Beta-thalassemia in a 21-year-old man. Humerus varus is severe. On the right, the remnant of the near-vertical epiphyseal plate is barely visible. The humeri are short. A number of growth-arrest lines are evident. (Courtesy of Professor A. Schwartz, Hadassah-Hebrew University Medical School, Jerusalem.)

pansion of the ribs and long bones,[13,14,64,73] sometimes sufficient to cause pathologic fracture,[22] and generalized loss of the secondary trabecular pattern. The peculiar and characteristic changes at the medial portion of the proximal humeral epiphysis probably are the result of marrow hyperplasia with expansion of trabecular bone in the pressure-responsive zone of the metaphysis.[72] In addition to the varus deformity, there may also be a localized area of sclerosis subjacent to the medial portion of the epiphysis. It has been suggested that this represents reparative bone bridging.[72]

Humerus varus may also be caused by trauma (epiphyseal or surgical neck fracture, pathologic fracture as through a cyst of the surgical neck), dysplasia, neuromuscular disorders, osteomyelitis, and metabolic disorders (renal osteodystrophy, hypothyroidism),[72] but in none of these instances is the appearance identical to that of humerus varus of thalassemia.

Acute Leukemia

Bony changes in infants and children with acute leukemia occur with an incidence variously reported as 50 to 90 percent.[6,87,96,100] That the changes are much less frequent in adults with acute leukemia is undoubtedly related to the differences in bone marrow composition and activity. In children the earliest and most common change is a narrow (2- to 6-mm.) band of radiolucency in the metaphysis parallel to and within a few millimeters of the epiphyseal plate[89] (Fig. 5-42). This may appear as early as 1 month after the clinical onset of the disease and is not associated with pain, tenderness, or swelling. In children under 2 years similar changes may rarely be seen in metastatic neuroblastoma and in acute rheumatoid arthritis. Likewise, the radiolucent metaphyseal band may be rarely seen in infants or young children with scurvy and severe debilitating diseases, infectious and otherwise. Over age 2 years, the radiolucent band is almost always secondary to leukemia. It is present in the areas of most rapid growth, especially about

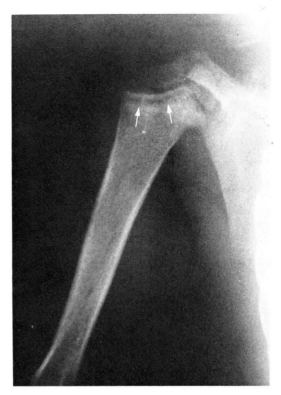

FIG. 5-42. Acute blastic leukemia in a 5-year-old girl. The radiolucent line subjacent to the epiphyseal plate was also present in other long bones.

the knees, proximal femur, and proximal humerus. It is bilateral, symmetric, and most often widespread. (In this regard it should be noted that a similar and at times indistinguishable band may be present about a single joint after immobilization, usually after fracture.) The band is probably not related to local leukemic infiltration; more likely it reflects altered endochondral bone formation. In response to spontaneous, drug-induced, or irradiation-induced remission, these bands will disappear and at times become sclerotic.

The second most common finding is osteolysis which cannot be distinguished from the myriad inflammatory, metabolic, and neoplastic causes of bone lysis. The defects may be focal, multifocal, or diffuse. Since there is often associated bone pain, the defects may be mistaken for osteomyelitis.

Next in order of infrequency is periosteal reaction. This may be single or multilayered and may or may not be in association with lytic lesions. Here, too, there is often associated bone pain and localized tenderness.

The least common bone change noted is osteosclerosis. Only a few such cases in children have been reported.

In adults the bone changes most commonly encountered are osteolytic defects and periosteal elevation with a far lower frequency than in children. In adults the changes are more common in the axial skeleton as opposed to the preponderance of changes in the appendicular skeleton in children, again reflecting differences of bone marrow composition and activity.

Hemophilic Arthropathy

Classic hemophilia due to factor VIII antihemophilic factor deficiency, von Willebrand's disease due to factor VIII globulin deficiency, and Christmas disease due to factor IX plasma thromboplastin deficiency are genetically and hematologically quite different and have some clinical distinctions. However, each can cause arthropathy and what is discussed here can apply to either of the hemophilias.

The most frequent and characteristic clinical feature of hemophilia is bleeding in the joints, usually without a history of trauma. The joints most often affected, in descending order, are the knee, elbow, ankle, hip, and shoulder, although other joints may also be involved. This order probably relates to the vulnerability of joints to trauma, and also to the greater dependency for joint stability on soft-tissue elements than on the bony anatomic configuration.[20] Thus, the joints most commonly involved are hinge joints rather than ball-and-socket joints. Recurring hemorrhages cause significant synovial changes, including vascular proliferation and cell infiltration with raising of the intima and marked villus formation, inflammatory reaction characterized by the presence of granulation tissue in varying stages from capillary neoformation to hypovascular fibrosis, marked siderosis involving the intima and subintima, and dense fibrosis with

synovial hypertrophy.[93] Of greatest importance is the high fibrinolytic activity in walls of the newly formed capillaries and venules of the inflamed synovia. The cathepsin D and lysosome of the injured synovial cells cause collagen destruction and may cause the joint to literally fall apart.[42] This advanced destruction is most common about the knee.

Hemorrhage into the joint may cause widening of the joint space and frank subluxation (see Fig. 20-6). With recurrent hemorrhages and cartilage destruction, the joint space may narrow. The head of the humerus and adjacent glenoid may become quite irregular in outline. Intraosseous cysts may appear (Fig. 5-43, see also Fig. 22-10). These are commonly seen about affected joints and are probably due to subchondral hemorrhage. Radiologically and histologically, they are similar to the subarticular cysts of osteoarthrosis, although they may be more numerous and more variable in size and shape.[42]

Gaucher's Disease

Ischemic necrosis is a relatively common complication of Gaucher's disease. Second only to that in the head of the femur is its occurrence in the head of the humerus.[2,52] Surprisingly, there may be little or no pain associated with the process. The earliest roentgenologic finding is generally subchondral sclerosis of varying degree. This may be followed by a radiolucent crescentic subchondral fissure; on occasion this may precede obvious sclerosis. In the hips this is invariably followed by significant fragmentation of bone with marked irregularity of shape.[24,67] In the head of the humerus, probably because of less stress, the deformity is usually less marked; there is flattening of the normally arcuate humeral head (Fig. 5-44). The cartilage space may or may not be narrowed.

Since the skeletal changes of Gaucher's disease most often are those reflecting proliferation of abnormal cells, the common findings in long bones are those of medullary expansion and cortical thinning. Thus,

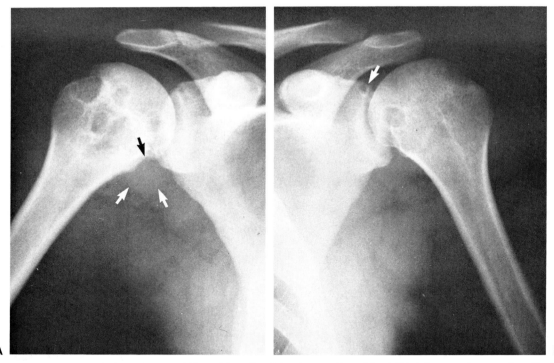

FIG. 5-43. Hemophilia in a 19-year-old boy. There is minimal narrowing of the left joint space. Large subcortical pseudocysts from intraosseous hemorrhage are present bilaterally. A, Intracapsular hemorrhage is evident with erosion of adjacent bone (arrows). B, A single small pseudocyst is present at the cranial margin of the glenoid fossa on the left.

it is not surprising that pathologic fractures may occur[2] (Fig. 5-45). There may also be single, multiple, or myriad patches of osteolysis due to tumoral masses of Gaucher's cells.

Persons with Gaucher's disease may suffer acute episodes resembling those of osteomyelitis.[70] There are localized bone pain and tenderness, often high fever, leukocytosis, and an increased sedimentation rate. Periosteal reaction may accompany or follow the onset of symptoms. The symptoms generally subside spontaneously in 2 to 4 weeks. In some of the reported cases, attempts at examination of biopsy specimens and/or drainage were made without yielding positive findings of osteomyelitis. The temptation to treat suspected osteomyelitis in patients with Gaucher's disease by surgery must be avoided, since such procedures may well lead to chronic osteomyelitis owing to the high susceptibility of Gaucher-involved bone to secondary infec-

tion. The cause of these "bone crises" remains unknown; perhaps it is localized infarction caused by vascular occlusion or vasospasm.[17]

Although the majority of reported cases of Gaucher's disease have been in Jews, there is no exempt ethnic group; the disease may also be seen in blacks, Orientals, and non-Jewish Caucasians.[17,52,64]

Histiocytosis X

Histiocytosis X is the name given by Lichtenstein in 1953 as a general designation to permit an integrated concept of eosinophilic granuloma of bone, Letterer-Siwe disease, and Schüller-Christian disease.[53] Its cause is unknown; Lichtenstein favors infection, conceivably of viral nature.[54] In bone, the expression of this disease is an osteolytic focus which may be solitary or multiple (Fig. 5-46). If the disease is limited to bone, there is none of the constitutional

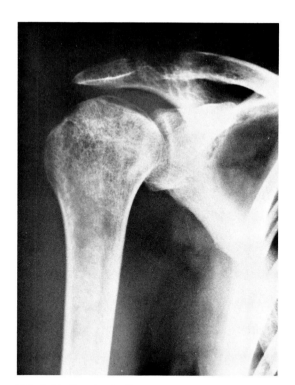

FIG. 5-44. Gaucher's disease in a 35-year-old woman who had shoulder pain. The subchondral crescentic fissure is more prominent than generally seen. Patchy bone sclerosis in the epiphysis, metaphysis, and diaphysis is evident. (Courtesy of Professor A. Schwartz, Hadassah-Hebrew University Medical School, Jerusalem.)

symptoms that accompany the extraskeletal cutaneous, pulmonary, intracranial, and other sites of involvement.

The bone lesion usually has its origin in the diaphyseal medullary cavity, is usually sharply outlined, and radiologically is quite lucent. On occasion, beveling of the edges of lesions creates a "hole within a hole" appearance.[26] The cortex becomes eroded from within, the bone may expand, and there may be periosteal new bone formation even in the absence of fracture. The latter is often laminated and fusiform. Thus, radiologically, the lesion may bear close resemblance to Ewing's sarcoma, osteolytic osteogenic sarcoma, metastatic tumor, and Brodie's abscess, and biopsy is required to confirm the diagnosis.[29,46] The bone defect is often accompanied by pain and, if close enough to the body's surface, by localized

swelling. Although the lesion may be solitary upon discovery, additional lesions may appear later. There is no recurrence, regardless of the form of treatment, whether by curettage, graft, or irradiation.[82]

Multiple Myeloma

The bone changes of multiple myeloma are caused by neoplastic proliferation of plasma cells. The roentgenographic presentation may be that of diffuse osteopenia, of sharply circumscribed (punched-out) lesions, or of areas of poorly circumscribed

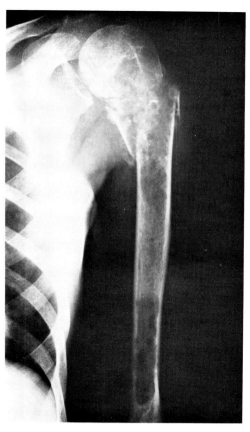

FIG. 5-45. Gaucher's disease in a 50-year-old woman who was first diagnosed as having Gaucher's disease at age 5 years.[24] Tumorous foci of abnormal bone marrow cells created the mottled appearance of the entire length of the humerus. The patient had no discomfort or limitation of motion. At age 50 years, she had suffered a pathologic fracture which healed well. Note the large radiolucent foci in the middle and proximal shaft, reflecting further marrow replacement by Gaucher's cells.

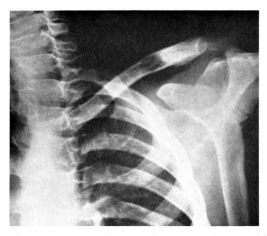

FIG. 5-46. Eosinophilic granuloma in an 18-year-old with pain over the left clavicle. The sharply defined lytic lesion expanded the bone, and there was faint periosteal new bone formation though no fracture. The diagnosis was proved by biopsy examination.

bone destruction of varying size. There is no way of clearly distinguishing these from the lesions of metastatic carcinoma on the basis of radiologic appearances. The facts favoring a diagnosis of multiple myeloma over metastatic cancer are the lack of periosteal new bone and no signs of healing about a pathologic fracture in multiple myeloma, whereas periosteal new bone and signs of healing may be seen more frequently in metastatic carcinoma. About 100 cases of multiple myeloma with sclerotic lesions have been reported.[83] There are three distinct patterns of sclerosis: (1) focal areas of sclerosis similar to those seen in metastatic prostatic cancer; (2) perpendicular spicules of new bone fanning from the bone lesion in much the same fashion as in osteogenic sarcoma; and (3) generalized, fairly uniform sclerosis. Of interest is the fact that approximately 30 percent of patients with sclerotic myelomas have peripheral neuropathic lesions, often severe, but this occurs in only 4 to 10 percent of those with lytic myeloma.[60,83] Periosteal reaction is rare in multiple myeloma. Soft-tissue masses may be identified adjacent to areas of bone destruction; these occur more commonly in myeloma than in metastatic carcinoma but are not a truly distinguishing sign per se.

Moseley has remarked on the frequency of involvement of the outer end of the clavicle and acromion even when the humerus and the remaining portions of the scapula are uninvolved.[64] This has also been my experience. Of course, other portions of the clavicle may be involved, as may be the humerus and ribs.

Soft-tissue Calcification

Soft-tissue calcification may be articular, periarticular, intra-articular, in muscles, subcutaneous tissue, lymph nodes, arteries, or veins.[31,35] Greenfield lists scores of causes of such calcifications;[35] most are uncommon and many others are rare. Certainly the most common cause for soft-tissue calcification about the shoulder is calcific bursitis or peritendinitis.

Circumscribed Myositis Ossificans

Of special concern is the calcification that occurs in circumscribed myositis ossificans, since the radiologic and pathologic appearance may be mistaken for malignancy if one is not aware of the entity and its radiologic presentation (Fig. 5-47). Usually, but not always, there is a clear history of antecedent trauma. Discovery is usually made by roentgen examination because of complaints of a painful tender soft-tissue mass. The roentgenographic appearances have been well described by Norman and Dorfman[68] and by Goldman.[33] A soft-tissue mass is noted most commonly alongside the diaphyseal portion of bone. There is often periosteal reaction of the adjacent bone; this may appear within 2 weeks of trauma and have either a layered or sun-burst appearance. A month or so after trauma (11 days to 6 weeks) flocculent calcification appears within the mass. The calcific densities enlarge and coalesce. By 6 to 8 weeks, calcification takes on a lacy new bone pattern in the periphery of the mass, but the central portion is relatively free of ossification. Often tomographic study is required to delineate this peripheral pattern of opaque density. In addition to this "zonal" pattern,

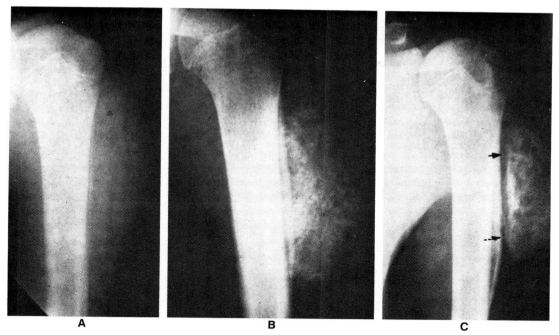

A   **B**   **C**

FIG. 5-47. Circumscribed myositis ossificans in a 13-year-old boy. A, At $3\frac{1}{2}$ weeks after injury there are poorly defined densities in the soft-tissue mass of the deltoid. A periosteal new bone reaction is present along the humerus. B, At $7\frac{1}{2}$ weeks, the mass is heavily ossified and better circumscribed. The periosteal reaction is more apparent. C, At $6\frac{1}{2}$ months, the focus of myositis ossificans is well organized. A peripheral cortex surrounds a relatively less dense center, and a radiolucent cleft (arrows) separates the lesion from the adjacent bone. (Courtesy of Norman, A., and Dorfman, H. D.: Juxtacortical circumscribed myositis ossificans: Evolution and radiographic features. Radiology, 96:301–306, 1970. Reproduced with permission of the publishers.)

within the mass is another important radiographic finding that distinguishes myositis ossificans from malignant tumors arising from bone—a distinct lucent cleft between the lesion and the adjacent bone. Here too, tomography is of importance to ascertain that there is no tumor pedicle between bone and soft-tissue mass. In spite of the periosteal reaction, no cortical disruption occurs in myositis ossificans. Over a period of months the mass shrinks progressively, a further reflection of its benign nature.

If biopsy of the lesion includes only the central relatively radiolucent zone, the histologic appearance may mimic sarcoma because of its cellular fibroelastic tissue and occasional bizarre cell components. Ackerman cautioned that recognition of the zonal pattern of calcification and ossification is of paramount importance in diagnosing this benign reactive process.[1]

Myositis Ossificans Progressiva

The cause of myositis ossificans progressiva, a seriously disabling disease, is unknown. The first manifestations of the disease appear in infancy or early childhood as soft-tissue masses, usually located on the dorsum of the back or neck.[88] These masses may be firm or soft; the overlying skin may ulcerate. After a few days or weeks the masses may regress or become ossified. Characteristically, there is then necrotic reaction with ossification spreading to involve connecting tissue in intermuscular septa, fascial planes, and tendons and resulting in immobility of the upper extremities and trunk. Muscle itself does not ossify.

Associated congenital bone anomalies are almost always present. The great toes are most frequently involved; the most common abnormalities are microdactylia and ankylosis of the interphalangeal joint and the metatarsophalangeal joint with absence of a phalanx.[88] Hypoplasia of metacarpals and phalanges is also a commonly associated defect. Hypoplasia of the middle phalanx of the fifth finger has been reported in a number of cases. Spinal apophyseal joint fusion may occur.[92]

Dermatomyositis

In dermatomyositis, a collagen disorder, females are affected far more often than males. There is generally muscle weakness and pain and sometimes skin changes. Radiologically, there is evidence of tissue calcification of varying degree, probably owing to degeneration of collagen tissue (see Fig. 22-7). The calcification appears in streaky and/or linear form, but there are no radiographic findings that clearly distinguish this from the soft-tissue calcifications of other systemic disorders.

Scleroderma

Scleroderma, another collagen disease, is more generalized than is dermatomyositis. Skin, subcutaneous tissues, bone, the gastrointestinal tract, and lungs are commonly involved. Soft-tissue calcification is common, especially about the joints, but not limited to these areas (Fig. 5-48). The calcification may have a more patchy appearance than that in dermatomyositis but may likewise take on a streaked appearance.

Hyperparathyroidism

Although metastatic soft-tissue calcification may occur in either the primary or secondary (renal osteodystrophy) forms of hyperparathyroidism, it occurs more commonly in the latter.[31] In fact, this is probably the most common cause of metastatic calcification.

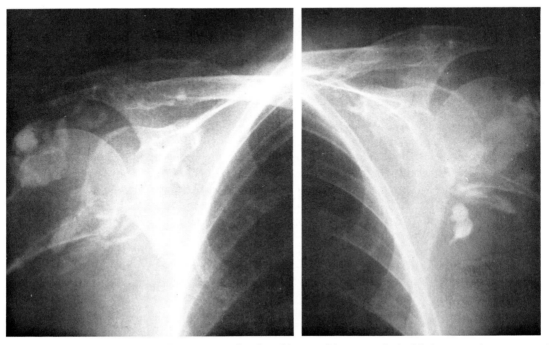

FIG. 5-48. Scleroderma, diagnosed 25 years earlier, in a 60-year-old woman. As in this instance, large areas of periarticular calcinosis may be present in this disease. Calcification about terminal tufts of fingers and adjacent to pressure areas, such as the ischial tuberosity and elbow, is also relatively common.

Calcinosis Interstitialis Universalis

Calcinosis interstitialis universalis is usually recognized in childhood and is of unknown origin. There are extensive calcium deposits both subcutaneously and in deeper connective tissue. The disease is progressive and often leads to death. The deposits are of streaky appearance, arranged longitudinally in the long axes of the extremities. There is no progression to ossification.

Systemic Lupus Erythematosus

In systemic lupus erythematosus not only may there be premature vascular calcification but also calcification in the skin and subcutaneous tissues. The appearance of the calcification, as in other connective tissue disorders, is nonspecific.[48] The calcifications are usually linear or nodular and may be bilateral, unilateral, diffuse, or localized. In some instances, the calcifications may occur in areas involved with skin ulcerations; in most there is no such possible etiologic factor. Some reported cases have had the calcification develop at sites of nonulcerated lupus skin lesions.[10]

Encysted parasites, phleboliths, arterial calcification, tumoral calcinosis, dystrophic calcifications, hypervitaminosis D, sarcoidosis, gout, and paraplegia are among the scores of other causes of soft-tissue calcification.

REFERENCES

1. Ackerman, L. V.: Extraosseous localized nonneoplastic bone and cartilage formation (so-called myositis ossificans). J. Bone Joint Surg., 40-A:279–298, 1958.
2. Amstutz, H. C., and Carey, E. J.: Skeletal manifestations and treatment of Gaucher's disease. J. Bone Joint Surg., 48-A:670–701, 1966.
3. Aronsohn, R. S., Hart, W. R., and Martel, W.: Metaphyseal chondroblastoma of bone. Am. J. Roentgenol. Rad. Ther. Nucl. Med., 127:686–688, 1976.
4. Atkinson, M. K., McElwain, T. J., Peckham, M. J., and Thomas, P. R. M.: Hypertrophic pulmonary osteoarthropathy in Hodgkin's disease. Reversal with chemotherapy. Cancer, 38:1729–1734, 1976.
5. Barry, H. C.: Paget's Disease of Bone. Edinburgh, E. & S. Livingstone Ltd., 1969.
6. Baty, J. M., and Vogt, E.: Bone changes of leukemia in children. Am. J. Roentgenol. Rad. Therapy, 34:310–314, 1935.
7. Bell, J. F., Kuhlmann, R. F., and Molloy, M. K.: Congenital defects of shoulder girdle, sternum, spine and pelvis. Pediatr. Clin. North Am., 14:397–418, 1967.
8. Boseker, E. H., Bickel, W. H., and Dahlin, D. C.: A clinicopathologic study of simple unicameral bone cysts. Surg. Gynecol. Obstet., 127:550–560, 1968.
9. Brower, A. C., Sweet, D. E., and Keats, T. E.: Condensing osteitis of the clavicle: A new entity. Am. J. Roentgenol. Rad. Ther. Nucl. Med., 121:17–21, 1974.
10. Budin, J. A., and Friedman, F.: Soft tissue calcifications in systemic lupus erythematosus. Am. J. Roentgenol. Rad. Ther. Nucl. Med., 124:358–364, 1975.
11. Bullough, P. G., and Walley, J.: Fibrous cortical defect and non-ossifying fibroma. Postgrad. Med. J., 41:672–676, 1965.
12. Caffey, J.: Infantile cortical hyperostosis. J. Pediatr., 29:541–559, 1946.
13. Caffey, J.: Cooley's erythroblastic anemia: Some skeletal findings in adolescents and young adults., Am. J. Roentgenol. Rad. Therapy, 65:547–560, 1951.
14. Caffey, J.: Cooley's anemia: A review of the roentgenographic findings in the skeleton. Am. J. Roentgenol. Rad. Therapy, 78:381–391, 1957.
15. Caffey, J., and Silverman, W. A.: Infantile cortical hyperostosis: Preliminary report on a new syndrome. Am. J. Roentgenol. Rad. Therapy, 54:1–16, 1945.
16. Campbell, W. L., and Feldman, F.: Bone and soft tissue abnormalities of the upper extremity in diabetes mellitus. Am. J. Roentgen. Rad. Ther. Nucl. Med., 124:7–15, 1975.
17. Chang-Lo, M., Yam, L. T., and Rubenstone, A. I.: Gaucher's disease. Review of the literature and report of twelve new cases. Am. J. Med. Sci., 254:303–315, 1967.
18. Currarino, G., and Erlandson, M. E.: Premature fusion of epiphysis in Cooley's anemia. Radiology, 83:656–664, 1964.
19. Dahlin. D. C., and Ivins, J. C.: Benign chondroblastoma. A study of 125 cases. Cancer, 30:401–413, 1972.
20. DePalma, A. F.: Hemophilic arthropathy. Clin. Orthop., 52:145–165, 1967.
21. Devlin, J. A., Bowman, H. E., and Mitchell, C. L.: Non-osteogenic fibroma of bone. A review of the literature with the addition of six cases. J. Bone Joint Surg., 37-A:472–486, 1955.

22. Dines, D. M., Canale, V. C., and Arnold, W. D.: Fractures in thalassemia. J. Bone Joint Surg., 58-A:662–666, 1976.

23. Donnelly, B., and Johnson, P. M.: Detection of hypertrophic pulmonary osteoarthropathy by skeletal imaging with ^{99m}Tc-labeled diphosphonate. Radiology: 114:389–391, 1975.

24. Draznin, S. J., and Singer, K.: Legg-Perthe's disease: A syndrome of many etiologies? With clinical and roentgenographic findings in a case of Gaucher's disease. Am. J. Roentgenol. Rad. Therapy, 60:490–497, 1948.

25. Edeiken, J., and Hodes, P. J.: Roentgen Diagnosis of Diseases of Bone, 2nd ed. Baltimore, Williams & Wilkins Co., 1973.

26. Ennis, J. T., Whitehouse, G., Ross, F. G. M., and Middlemiss, J. H.: The radiology of the bone changes in histiocytosis X. Clin. Radiol., 24:212–220, 1973.

27. Evarts, C. M., and Kendrick, J. I.: Osteoid-osteoma. A critical analysis of tumors. Clin. Orthop., 54:51–59, 1967.

28. Fischel, R. E., and Bernstein, D.: Friedrich's disease. Br. J. Radiol., 48:318–319, 1975.

29. Fowles, J. V., and Bobechko, W. P.: Solitary eosinophilic granuloma in bone. J. Bone Joint Surg., 52-B:238–243, 1970.

30. Garceau, G. J., and Gregory, C. F.: Solitary unicameral bone cyst. J. Bone Joint Surg., 36-A:267–280, 1954.

31. Gayler, B. W., and Brogdon, B. G.: Soft tissue calcifications in the extremities in systemic disease. Am. J. Med. Sci., 249:590–605, 1965.

32. Gibson, D. A., and Carroll, N.: Congenital pseudarthrosis of the clavicle. J. Bone Joint Surg., 52-B:629–643, 1970.

33. Goldman, A. B.: Myositis ossificans circumscripta: A benign lesion with a malignant differential diagnosis. Am. J. Roentgenol. Rad. Ther. Nucl. Med., 126:32–40, 1976.

34. Green, A. E., Jr., Ellswood, W. H., and Collins, J. R.: Melorheostosis and osteopoikilosis: With a review of the literature. Am. J. Roentgenol. Rad. Ther. Nucl. Med., 87:1096–1111, 1962.

35. Greenfield, G. B.: Radiology of Bone Disease, 2nd ed. Philadelphia, J. B. Lippincott Co., 1975.

36. Greville, N. R.: Congenital high scapula (Sprengel's deformity). Mayo Clin. Proc., 31:465–472, 1956.

37. Guenter, C. A., and Hammarsten, J. F.: Hypertrophic osteoarthropathy in cirrhosis of the liver. Am. Rev. Respir. Dis., 101:590–594, 1970.

38. Gunderson, C. H., Greenspan, R. H., Glaser, G. H., and Lubs, H. A.: Klippel-Feil syndrome: Genetic and clinical reevaluation of cervical fusion. Medicine, 46:491–512, 1967.

39. Hall, F. J. S.: Coracoclavicular joint. A rare condition treated successfully by operation. Br. Med. J., 1:766–768, 1950.

40. Hammersten, J. F., and O'Leary, J.: The features and significance of hypertrophic osteoarthropathy. Arch. Intern. Med., 99:431–441, 1957.

41. Herman, S.: Congenital bilateral pseudarthrosis of the clavicles. Clin. Orthop., 91:162–163, 1973.

42. Hilgartner, M. W.: Discussion Paper: Degenerative joint disease. In Recent Advances in Hemophilia. Ann. N.Y. Acad. Sci., 240:340–341, 1975.

43. Horwitz, A. E.: Congenital elevation of the scapula. Sprengel's deformity. Am. J. Orthop. Surg., 6:260–311, 1908.

44. Huvos, A. G., Marcove, R. C., Erlandson, R. A., and Mike, V.: Chondroblastoma of bone. Cancer, 29:760–771, 1972.

45. Jaffe, H. L.: Tumors and Tumorous Conditions of Bones and Joints. London, Henry Kimpton Publishers, 1958.

46. Jaffe, H. L., and Lichtenstein, L.: Eosinophilic granuloma of bone: A condition affecting one, several or many bones, but apparently limited to the skeleton, and representing the mildest clinical expression of the peculiar inflammatory histiocytosis also underlying Letterer-Siwe disease and Schüller-Christian disease. Arch. Pathol., 37:99–118, 1944.

47. Jarvis, J. L., and Keats, T. E.: Cleidocranial dysostosis. A review of 40 new cases. Am. J. Roentgenol. Rad. Ther. Nucl. Med., 121:5–16, 1974.

48. Kabir, D. I., and Malkinson, F. D.: Lupus erythematosus and calcinosis cutis. Arch. Dermatol., 100:17–22, 1969.

49. Keats, T. E.: An Atlas of Normal Roentgen Variants that may Simulate Disease. Chicago, Year Book Medical Publishers, Inc., 1973.

50. Köhler, A., and Zimmer, E. A.: Borderlands of the Normal and Early Pathologic in Skeletal Roentgenology, 3rd Am. ed. New York, Grune & Stratton, Inc., 1968.

51. Köhler, H., Uehlinger, E., Kutzner, J., Weihrauch, T. R., Wilbert, L., and Schuster, R.: Sterno-kosto-klaviculare Hyperostose. Dtsch. Med. Wochenschr., 100:1519–1523, 1975.

52. Levin, B.: Gaucher's disease: Clinical and roentgenological manifestations. Am. J. Roentgenol. Rad. Therapy, 85:685–696, 1961.

53. Lichtenstein, L.: Histiocytosis X. Integration of eosinophilic granuloma of bone, "Letterer-Siwe disease," and "Schüller-Christian disease" as related manifestations of a single nosologic entity. Arch. Pathol., 56:84–102, 1953.

54. Lichtenstein, L.: Diseases of Bones and Joints, 2nd ed. St. Louis, C. V. Mosby Co., 1975.

55. Lichtenstein, L., and Jaffe, H. L.: Fibrous dysplasia of bone. Arch. Pathol., 33:777–816, 1942.

56. Lloyd-Roberts, G. C., Apley, A. G., and Owen, R.: Reflections upon the aetiology of congenital pseudarthrosis of the clavicle. J. Bone Joint Surg., 57-B:24–29, 1975.

57. McClure, J. G., and Raney, R. B.: Anomalies of the scapula. Clin. Orthop., 110:22–31, 1975.

58. McKusick, V. A.: Heritable Disorders of Connective Tissue. St. Louis, C. V. Mosby Co., 1966.

59. McLeod, R. A., and Beabout, J. W.: The roentgenographic features of chondroblastoma. Am.

J. Roentgenol. Rad. Ther. Nucl. Med., 118:464–471, 1973.

60. Mangalik, A., and Veliath, A. J.: Osteosclerotic myeloma and peripheral neuropathy: A case report. Cancer, 28:1040–1045, 1971.

61. Martel, W., and Sitterley, B. H.: Roentgenologic manifestations of osteonecrosis. Am. J. Roentgenol. Rad. Ther. Nucl. Med., 106:509–522, 1969.

62. Moore, W. B., Matthews, T. J., and Rabinowitz, R.: Genitourinary anomalies associated with Klippel-Feil syndrome. J. Bone Joint Surg., 57-A:355–357, 1975.

63. Morrison, S. G., Perry, L. W., and Scott, L. P.: Congenital brevicollis (Klippel-Feil syndrome) and cardiovascular anomalies. Am. J. Dis. Child., 115:614–620, 1963.

64. Moseley, J. E.: Bone Changes in Hematologic Disorders. New York, Grune & Stratton, Inc., 1963.

65. Murray, R. O., and Jacobson, H. G.: The Radiology of Skeletal Disorders: Exercises in Diagnosis. Baltimore, Williams & Wilkins Co., 1972.

66. Nora, J. J., Cohen, M., and Maxwell, G. A.: Klippel-Feil syndrome with congenital heart disease. Am. J. Dis. Child., 102:858–864, 1961.

67. Norman, A., and Bullough, P.: Radiolucent crescent line: Early diagnostic sign of avascular necrosis of femoral head. Bull. Hosp. Joint Dis., 24:99–104, 1963.

68. Norman, A., and Dorfman, H. D.: Juxtacortical circumscribed myositis ossificans: Evolution and radiographic features. Radiology, 96:301–306, 1970.

69. Norman, A., and Dorfman, H. D.: Osteoid-osteoma inducing pronounced overgrowth and deformity of bone. Clin. Orthop., 110:233–238, 1975.

70. Noyes, F. R., and Smith, W. S.: Bone crises and chronic osteomyelitis in Gaucher's disease. Clin. Orthop., 79:132–140, 1971.

71. Nutter, P. D.: Coracoclavicular articulations. J. Bone Joint Surg., 23:177–179, 1971.

72. Ogden, J. A., Weil, U. H., and Hempton, R. F.: Developmental humerus varus. Clin. Orthop., 116:158–166, 1976.

73. O'Hara, A. E.: Roentgenographic osseous manifestations of the anemias and the leukemias. Clin. Orthop., 52:63–82, 1967.

74. Owen, R.: Congenital pseudarthrosis of the clavicle. J. Bone Joint Surg., 52-B:644–652, 1970.

75. Ozonoff, M. B., and Ziter, F. M. H., Jr.: The upper humeral notch: A normal variant in children. Radiology, 113:699–701, 1974.

76. Pancoast, H. K.: Importance of careful roentgenray investigation of apical chest tumors. J.A.M.A., 83:1407–1411, 1924.

77. Preger, L., Sanders, G. W., Gold, R. H., Steinbach, H. L., and Pitman, P.: Roentgenographic skeletal changes in the glycogen storage disease. Am. J. Roentgenol. Rad. Ther. Nucl. Med., 107:840–847, 1969.

78. Pugh, D. G.: Subperiosteal resorption of bone: Roentgenologic manifestation of primary hyperparathyroidism and renal osteodystrophy. Am. J. Roentgenol. Rad. Therapy, 66:577–586, 1951.

79. Ramsey, J., and Bliznak, J.: Klippel-Feil syndrome with renal agenesis and other anomalies. Am. J. Roentgenol. Rad. Ther. Nucl. Med., 113:460–463, 1971.

80. Rechtman, A. M., and Horwitz, M. T.: Congenital synostosis of cervico-thoracic vertebrae (Klippel-Feil Syndrome). Am. J. Roentgenol. Rad. Therapy, 43:66–73, 1940.

81. Reynolds, J.: The Roentgenological Features of Sickle Cell Disease and Related Hemoglobinopathies. Springfield, Ill., Charles C Thomas, 1965.

82. Rodrigues, R. J., and Lewis, H. H.: Eosinophilic granuloma of bone. Review of literature and case presentation. Clin. Orthop., 77:183–192, 1971.

83. Rodriguez, A. R., Lutcher, C. L., and Coleman, F. W.: Osteosclerotic myeloma. J.A.M.A., 236:1872–1874, 1976.

84. Schajowicz, F., and Gallardo, H.: Epiphyseal chondroblastoma of bone. J. Bone Joint Surg., 52-B:205–226, 1970.

85. Schlumberger, H. G.: Fibrous dysplasia of single bones (monostotic fibrous dysplasia). Milit. Surgeon, 99:504–527, 1946.

86. Schwarz, G. S., Berenyi, M. R., and Siegel, M. W.: Atrophic arthropathy and diabetic neuritis. Am. J. Roentgenol. Rad. Ther. Nucl. Med., 106:523–529, 1969.

87. Silverman, F. N.: The skeletal lesions in leukemia. Clinical and roentgenographic observations in 103 infants and children, with a review of the literature. Am. J. Roentgenol. Rad. Therapy, 59:819–844, 1948.

88. Singleton, E. B., and Holt, J. F.: Myositis ossificans progressiva. Radiology, 62:47–54, 1954.

89. Sirsat, M. V., and Doctor, V. M.: Benign chondroblastoma of bone. Report of a case of malignant transformation. J. Bone Joint Surg., 52-B:741–745, 1970.

90. Solomon, L.: Hereditary multiple exostosis. J. Bone Joint Surg., 45-B:292–304, 1963.

91. Spranger, J. W., Langer, L. O., and Wiedemann, H. R.: Bone Dysplasias: An Atlas of Constitutional Disorders of Skeletal Development. Philadelphia, W. B. Saunders Co., 1974.

92. Staple, T. W., Melson, G. L., and Evens, R. G.: Miscellaneous soft tissue lesions of the extremities. Semin. Roentgenol., 8:117–127, 1973.

93. Stoker, D. J., and Murray, R. O.: Skeletal changes in hemophilia and other bleeding disorders. Semin. Roentgenol., 9:185–193, 1974.

94. Teplick, J. G., Eftekhari, F., and Haskin, M. E.: Erosion of the sternal ends of the clavicles. A new sign of primary and secondary hyperparathyroidism. Radiology, 113:323–326, 1974.

95. Terry, D. W., Jr., Isitman, A. T., and Holmes, R. A.: Radionuclide bone images in hypertrophic pulmonary osteoarthropathy. Am. J. Roentgenol. Rad. Ther. Nucl. Med., 124:571–576, 1975.

96. Thomas, L. B., Forkner, C. E., Jr., Frei, E., III,

Besse, B. E., Jr., and Stabenau, J. R.: The skeletal lesions of acute leukemia. Cancer, 14:608–621, 1961.

97. Waldenstrom, H.: First stages of coxa plana. J. Bone Joint Surg., 20:559–566, 1938.

98. Weller, M., Edeiken, J., and Hodes, P. J.: Renal osteodystrophy. Am. J. Roentgenol. Rad. Ther. Nucl. Med., 104:354–363, 1968.

99. Wertheimer, L. G.: Coracoclavicular joint: Surgical treatment of a painful shoulder syndrome caused by an anomalous joint. J. Bone Joint Surg., 30-A:570–578, 1948.

100. Willson, J. K. V.: The bone lesions of childhood leukemia. Radiology, 72:672–681, 1959.

101. Wilner, D., and Sherman, R. S.: Roentgen diagnosis of Paget's disease (osteitis deformans): The usual, the unusual, the complications. Med. Radiogr. Photogr., 42:35–78, 1966.

102. Wynne-Davies, R., and Fairbank, T. J.: Fairbank's Atlas of General Affections of the Skeleton, 2nd ed. Edinburgh, Churchill Livingstone, 1976.

6

Antimicrobial Therapy in Orthopaedic Patients

SHERWIN A. KABINS

This is a selective noncomprehensive review on the use of antimicrobial agents for infections in orthopaedic patients. It represents the approach of one physician interested in infectious diseases. It is meant to provide some principles by which antimicrobials are selected and used to manage common orthopaedic infections. Comprehensive reviews may be found in the literature.[14,19,49,68,97]

ORGANISMS CAUSING INFECTIONS

Table 6-1 provides a partial list of the more common microorganisms causing infections of soft tissue, bone, joint, prosthetic devices, and foreign bodies. The vast majority of infections in most sites are caused by *gram-positive bacterial organisms*. Staphylococcus aureus is the most frequent pathogen.[14,64,90,99] To a lesser extent a variety of streptococci may cause infection.[64,90] S. aureus infections may primarily seed joint or bone by the hematogenous route, particularly in patients with preexistent trauma or deformity such as rheumatoid arthritis. S. aureus may also be directly implanted into tissue by trauma, operations, or procedures such as joint aspirations.[15] Infections of prosthetic devices and foreign bodies are frequently caused by gram-positive organisms other than S. au-

reus.[17,18,101,102] In particular, Staphylococcus epidermidis (S. albus), aerobic and anaerobic diphtheroids, streptococci, and micrococci, all of which are skin organisms, may be implanted at the time of operation.

Gram-negative bacilli are most likely to cause infections in postoperative patients, particularly, those already taking antibiotics or immunosuppressive drugs, or those with an underlying debilitating disease (diabetes mellitus, rheumatoid arthritis, lymphoproliferative disorders, cirrhosis, for example).[32,33,64] These organisms are more difficult to eradicate than gram-positive organisms. They are associated with high frequencies of relapse and tissue destruction. They require the use of one or more antibiotics that have more potential for side effects than the agents used for therapy of gram-positive infections. They may contaminate prosthetic devices and foreign bodies during operative procedures, or later by the hematogenous route from infections arising from intravenous sites, Foley catheters, pneumonia, for example. The more common gram-negative aerobic bacilli encountered in these infections include Escherichia coli, Klebsiella pneumoniae, Proteus, Pseudomonas aeruginosa, and Serratia marcescens.

The drug addict is prone to hematogenous seeding of bone and joint by gram-negative

Table 6-1. *Preferred Antimicrobial Agents for Common Microorganisms**

Organisms	First Choice	Second Choice
BACTERIA		
Gram-positive Cocci and bacilli, excluding *Staphylococcus aureus,*	Penicillin G	Clindamycin‡ or cephalosporins§
resistant to Penicillin G†	Oxacillin, cloxacillin	Clindamycin‡ or cephalosporins§
Enterococci	Ampicillin‖, Amoxicillin	Vancomycin or chloramphenicol
Gram-negative Cocci		
Gonococci and meningococci	Penicillin G	Tetracycline
Gram-negative Bacilli		
Bacteroides		
non-B. fragilis	Penicillin G	Clindamycin or chloramphenicol
B. fragilis	Clindamycin	Chloramphenicol
Brucella	Tetracycline plus streptomycin	Chloramphenicol, trimethoprim with sulfamethoxazole
Enterobacter	Carbenicillin	Gentamicin, kanamycin, or tobramycin
Escherichia coli	Ampicillin	Cephalosporin§, chloramphenicol, gentamicin, kanamycin, or tobramycin
Haemophilus influenzae	Ampicillin or Amoxicillin	Chloramphenicol, tetracycline, trimethoprim with sulfamethoxazole
Klebsiella pneumoniae	Cephalosporin§	Kanamycin, gentamicin, tobramycin
Pasturella multocida	Penicillin G	Tetracycline
Proteus mirabilis	Ampicillin	Cephalosporins§, gentamicin, tobramycin, or kanamycin
Other Proteus	Carbenicillin	Gentamicin, tobramycin, kanamycin
Providencia	Carbenicillin	Gentamicin, tobramycin, kanamycin
Pseudomonas	Carbenicillin‖	Gentamicin, tobramycin
Salmonella	Ampicillin or amoxicillin	Chloramphenicol, trimethoprim with sulfamethoxazole
Serratia	Carbenicillin	Gentamicin, tobramycin, kanamycin
Acid-fast Bacilli		
Mycobacterium tuberculosis	Isoniazid and ethambutol or rifampin#	Streptomycin, cycloserine kanamycin, ethionomide

Table 6-1. *Preferred Antimicrobial Agents for Common Microorganisms* (Continued)

Organisms	First Choice	Second Choice
Atypical mycobacterium	Isoniazid and ethambutol, or rifampin#	Streptomycin, cycloserine, kanamycin, ethionomide
Actinomycetes Actinomycosis	Penicillin G	Clindamycin, tetracycline
Nocardia	Sulfonamide	Trimethoprim with sulfamethoxazole, ampicillin, or erythromycin
FUNGI	Amphotericin B	Flucytosine**

* Because resistance may develop, susceptibility tests should be performed.
† Includes Staphylococcus aureus, non-penicillinase-producing streptococci, pneumococci, clostridium, diphtheroids.
‡ Preferred for penicillin-allergic patients.
§ Includes cephalothin, cefazolin, cephalexin (see footnote † Table 6-6).
‖ Add gentamicin or tobramycin for treatment of bone infections.
Initial therapy, until sensitivity data are available, should be with all three agents.
** For candida or cryptococcus. Also known as 5-Fluorocytosine.

organisms, especially P. aeruginosa, Klebsiella, and Serratia, in addition to becoming infected by S. aureus and Candida.[41,59] Pseudomonas infections of bone commonly follow puncture wounds of the foot. Patients with sickle cell disease or with chronic lymphatic leukemia are prone to infection caused by Salmonella.[20] Salmonella and Arizona bacteria infections of bone or joint frequently appear months after an episode of febrile diarrhea or sepsis. Children under the age of 5 years, and especially between the ages of 6 months and 2 years, are prone to infections of joint or bone by Haemophilus influenzae. Occasionally, H. influenzae may involve the neonate or may hematogenously seed adults who have prior joint disease, such as rheumatoid arthritis.[29,86] Gram-negative bacillary *infections related to animals* include Pasteurella multocida from bites, scratches, or licking of abrasions by cats, dogs, and other domestic animals.[6] Abattoir workers are prone to brucellosis. Salmonella and Arizona bacteria infections can be related to contact with poultry or reptiles.

Gram-negative diplococci, especially Neisseria gonorrhoeae, but on occasion Neisseria meningitidis, usually cause septic arthritis in the otherwise healthy adolescent or young adult.[40]

Anaerobic bacteria, both gram-positive and gram-negative, are more frequently recognized as causes of infection.[34] Wounds are most likely involved, but on occasion joints and bone may be hematogenously seeded from a remote site of infection. Bacteroides fragilis, a gram-negative rod found in feces, has gained special interest because of its resistance to commonly prescribed antibiotics like the penicillins, cephalosporins, and tetracyclines. In orthopaedic patients, B. fragilis infection is most often seen in soft-tissue infections around the groin. Infection of joint and bone is rare except in the feet of diabetics, wherein antibiotic therapy of all types frequently is doomed to failure.

Clues as to the anaerobic etiology of infection include drainage of serosanguineous, bubbly or brownish material, which has either a mousy or putrid odor. Crepitation may be caused by gas-forming anaerobes or facultative anaerobic organisms such as E. coli, K. pneumoniae, enterococci, or a combination of organisms. Progressive synergistic gangrene (frequently due to microaerophilic or anaerobic streptococci and S. aureus) is characterized by a central area of necrosis, surrounded in turn by a bluish-violet area, an erythematous area, and finally an area of induration. Specimens for anaerobic culture should be taken from the advancing red edge of the lesion. Patients usually have low-grade fevers and do not appear toxic. More fulminant anaerobic infections such as myositis and necrotizing fasciitis may cause massive swelling, loss of sensation, jaundice, tachypnea, tachycardia, and toxicity out of proportion to the height of the fever. Immediate examination of gram-stained aspirate of the wound gives vital information as to the bacterial cause or infection. The infections may be due to Clostridium (large gram-positive bacilli) or to a mixture of anaerobic and facultative anaerobic gram-positive or gram-negative bacilli.

Atypical *mycobacterial organisms* or acid-fast bacilli, particularly Mycobacterium fortuitum, Mycobacterium ulcerans, and Mycobacterium marinum, cause superficial infection secondary to trauma. Infections caused by the first two organisms are due to soil contamination, whereas infections caused by the latter relate to abrasions from fish tanks or swimming pools. Atypical mycobacteria like M. kansasii may cause indolent deep destructive infections of bone and joint, and at times tendinitis and bursitis.[80] They produce stiffness and swelling unassociated with warmth and tenderness. Patients with pulmonary tuberculosis may hematogenously seed bone or joints,[9] including the shoulder.[52]

A variety of *Candida species* or, much more rarely, Aspergillus cause opportunistic fungal infections of bone or joints in patients who are debilitated, who have previously received antibiotics or corticosteroids, or have diabetes mellitus.[25,71] These infections frequently occur in patients receiving intravenous therapy (especially parenteral hyperalimentation), in whom the intravenous catheter and fluid serve as a portal and vehicle of entry. The onset of clinical infection may be delayed by weeks or months after the cessation of intravenous therapy. Infection may be manifest only by pain and swelling without evidence of fever or leukocytosis.

Other fungal infections that involve joint or bone in otherwise "normal" persons include coccidioidomycosis,[95] blastomycosis, sporotrichosis[63] and, more rarely, cryptococcosis and histoplasmosis. Coccidioidomycosis deserves some special attention. Joints may be chronically infected and then secondarily involve bone or vice versa.[4] The knee and ends of long bones are most often involved. The onset may be indolent with or without prior or subsequent miliary disease, or the onset may be fulminant as part of a widespread miliary process. In addition, arthralgia and arthritis may be secondary to hypersensitivity reaction early in the course, which is frequently associated with erythema nodosum or erythema multiforme.

Actinomycosis[98] and Nocardia[78] may cause opportunistic or primary infections in joints and bones. Patients may not have obvious underlying diseases and usually appear with chronic problems that often do not suggest infection.

Geographic residence or occupational history may provide helpful clues as to which of these agents is responsible for infection. Residence in the southwestern United States may suggest coccidioidomycosis whereas residence in the Ohio Valley may suggest histoplasmosis. Working with rose bushes or plants may imply sporotrichosis.

EFFICIENT USE OF A MICROBIOLOGY LABORATORY

Isolation of a microorganism and susceptibility tests of the organism to antimicrobial agents augment the chance for successful treatment. Specimens for culture obtained by aspiration or at operation should be sent to the laboratory in both aerobic and anaerobic transport systems. The major limiting factor in isolating anaerobic organisms is the proper use of an anaerobic transport system.[89] The type of specimen submitted may influence the chance of isolation of the offending organism. For certain infections of joints, namely, fungal, tuberculous, or gonococcal, culture of synovial tissue may show positive results more readily than culture of synovial fluid.

Examination of *gram-stained specimens* gives immediate guides to therapy. In addition, a gram-stained specimen showing more than a few organisms without a history of recent antibiotic therapy and in the face of negative results of culture suggests that the laboratory failed to isolate fastidious organisms, rather than to the existence of "sterile" drainage or exudate. By consultation with the microbiologist, better advice can be given in obtaining and processing specimens that may require special nutrients, incubation environment, or rapid processing.

The physician, by providing information as to the nature of the clinical problem, will enhance the chance of isolating organisms that may require special media or incubation conditions. For example, wounds contaminated by soil or aquatic injuries should lead the laboratory workers to a search for atypical mycobacterial organisms which grow at room temperature and not at 37°C, the temperature routinely used for most specimens. In addition, infection secondary to contact with soil or plants may require special cultures and serologic tests for identification of fungi. Wounds, arthritis, or osteomyelitis in an abattoir worker should lead to a search for Brucella by use of special culture media, prolonged incubation of specimens, and serologic tests.

Most laboratories will discard sterile wound or tissue specimens after 48 to 72 hours of incubation and blood cultures after 7 to 14 days of incubation. Prior antibiotic therapy may delay the growth of bacterial organisms. In addition, some organisms such as Brucella or some anaerobic bacteria may take weeks to grow. When pus is obtained from wounds, drainage tracts, or bone of patients who have been taking antibiotics, the laboratory should continue incubation of the specimen for at least 1 week longer than is routine if growth does not occur earlier. At times, the addition of penicillinase (in patients receiving penicillin-type drugs) or use of osmotic-protected media (for cell wall-damaged organisms) may increase the yield of positive results of cultures. The addition of 0.05 percent sodium polyanetholesulfonate to the culture medium may increase the yield (especially from blood), since it is anticomplementary, precipitates immunoglobulins, inactivates leukocytes, and antagonizes the effects of polymyxin and aminoglycoside antibiotics.[5]

Many laboratories will not perform *susceptibility tests* on "normal flora" organisms like S. epidermidis, anaerobic diphtheroids, and the like. Often these organisms are considered as contaminants. Since they may be resistant to first choice antibiotics, the laboratory must be aware that the organisms were isolated from sources that are not likely to be contaminated and may be of clinical importance in order to justify performing susceptibility tests. Therefore, surgical specimens and clean aspirates of tissue, particularly from patients who have prosthetic devices or foreign bodies, should be labeled appropriately to test all isolated organisms for susceptibility to antibiotics.

To ensure that the *specimen* is not contaminated, it should be *obtained,* after a careful surgical preparation and painting of the skin with an antiseptic such as povidone-iodine (Betadine), by aspiration through intact skin or by surgical incision.

Most laboratories discard organisms shortly after isolation and completion of disc sensitivity tests. In treatment of certain infections, particularly of bone, synovial tissue, foreign bodies, and prosthetic devices, it may be necessary to adjust treatment according to quantitative sensitivity studies of the organisms and tests of blood and tissue levels of antibiotics. At this point, it may be impossible to get additional organisms from the patient. Thus, it is advisable to have the laboratory *save organisms isolated from surgical specimens and blood* until it is determined that the patient has responded to therapy.

BLOOD AND OTHER CULTURES. Blood cultures should be obtained for every febrile, infected patient before starting or changing antibiotics. Blood cultures provide valuable information when results of cultures from the site of infection may be negative or the cultures contain a mixture of organisms, some of which may be "skin flora" contaminants. "Skin flora" organisms isolated both from the site of infection and from blood increase the probability of the significance of the organisms as a cause of infection. When wounds contain multiple organisms that would require multiple antibiotics (increasing the likelihood of side effects), a positive result of blood culture allows focusing on the most significant organism(s).

In postoperative febrile patients, specimens for cultures should be obtained from intravenous sites, sputum, urine, and the wound. The antibiotic approach to the treatment of infections involving areas other than bone, joint, or wound will not be reviewed in detail. These infections are frequently caused by gram-negative bacilli. The treatment is based best on results of appropriate culture and susceptibility data. Expectorated sputum is frequently contaminated by mouth flora. At times, transtracheal aspiration is necessary to obtain noncontaminated sputum.[3] Urine should be collected aseptically, either by clean midstream, in and out catheterization, or suprapubic aspiration. In patients with indwelling urinary catheters, urine should be collected by aseptic aspiration from the catheter before it enters the collection bag. Upon aseptic removal of an intravenous catheter, the tip of the catheter may be cut short with sterile scissors and sent for culture. The intravenous sites should be milked to see if pus can be expressed. On occasion, culture of the remaining fluid in the intravenous system will be important. This should be reserved for patients with otherwise unexplained sepsis receiving intravenous fluids which contain additives, for patients from whom the intravenous tubing had not been changed every 24 hours, and for rare cases of unusual gram-negative bacillary bacteremia (i.e., Enterobacter cloacae or Enterobacter agglomerans [Erwinia]), which suggests commercial contamination of the intravenous product.[62]

GUIDES TO ADEQUACY OF ANTIMICROBIAL TREATMENT

To reduce the possibility of recurrence of infection of joint, bone, foreign bodies, and implants, *repeat cultures* of the area of involvement and blood should be performed until results are negative, even in the face of a good clinical response. Antibiotics do not instantly eradicate bacteria. Even with good antibiotic levels, reduction in the number of organisms may not be obvious until 24 to 48 hours, and the infected site may not become sterile until 5 to 7 days after initiation of therapy. In acute joint infections, the synovial fluid white blood cell count should fall significantly by the end of the first week of therapy. If there is persistence of high white blood cell counts, the likelihood of complete recovery of joint function is reduced by as much as two thirds of that achieved in responders.[33] Delayed bacteriologic or clinical resolution of infection may be an indication for alteration of antibiotic therapy and/or surgical intervention.

Repeat blood cultures are especially important for patients who are leukopenic, have a vascular focus of infection, or have an undrained abscess. Such patients may partially improve on antibiotics, but remain bacteremic and require more intense or altered antibiotic therapy and/or surgical intervention.

Blood levels and, if possible, *tissue levels* of antibiotics should be determined if there is persistent clinical infection and/or persistent positive results of cultures. The inhibitory or killing effect of blood or tissue fluid against the affecting organisms provides data as to the adequacy of antibiotic therapy. Data may indicate that an increase in dose of the prescribed antibiotic is necessary. They may indicate that results of tests for synergism between antibiotics to achieve a more optimal bacterial killing should be obtained.

If adequate peak antibiotic levels (equal to or greater than four- to eightfold dilution of blood or tissue fluid inhibits the organism) are achieved, further increased dose of antibiotic or change of antibiotic will probably not help. Instead, surgical intervention is frequently necessary for removal of foreign bodies and/or necrotic tissue. On the other hand, continued or altered antibiotic therapy alone may suffice to eradicate persistent staphylococcal infections. In the face of adequate penicillin therapy, staphylococci may persist (perhaps owing to penicillin's preventing the breakdown of bacterial cell wall structures by inhibition of enzymatic hydrolysis). Bacterial persistence may be due to selection of cell wall-deficient organisms.[56] Frequently, all that is necessary to eradicate these infections is continued treatment, especially if the patient is responding clinically. Alternately, a change to an antistaphylococcal antibiotic that acts at the bacterial ribosome (i.e., clindamycin) may be beneficial. If staphylococcal infection persists for many weeks or recurs, surgical intervention may be necessary.

SELECTION AND DOSAGE OF ANTIMICROBIAL AGENTS

Antibiotic therapy is initiated after cultures of blood and of the site of infection are obtained. The multiple factors that influence the *selection of antimicrobial agents* are:

1. Organism and its susceptibility to the agent.
2. Severity of infection.
3. Convenience and route of administration.
4. Tissue distribution of the agent and the site of infection.
5. Host factors:
   a. Underlying diseases, e.g., sickle cell anemia, and the like
   b. Renal or hepatic failure
6. Side effects of the agent.
7. Whether the agent is bactericidal or bacteriostatic (synergism or antagonism between agents).
8. Interaction of agent with other drugs.

Initial therapy is selected on a clinical basis to cover the most likely causative organisms. Table 6-1 itemizes the antibiotics of choice for treatment of infections caused by specific organisms. Table 6-2 lists the *recommended doses*.

For infections caused by or suspected to be caused by S. aureus, a semisynthetic penicillin such as oxacillin, cloxacillin, or nafcillin is preferred. These agents will also cover most streptococcal infections, except for enterococci and, therefore, can be relied upon as the initial antibiotic in most infections. For penicillin-allergic patients, clindamycin, which is also effective against anaerobic organisms but ineffective against enterococci, is preferred.

Gram-negative bacillary infections are more difficult to treat than gram-positive infections.[32,33,67] Tetracycline, ampicillin, cephalosporins, aminoglycosides (see Table 6-6), trimethoprim with sulfamethoxazole, or chloramphenicol may be given singly or in combinations. For initial therapy before culture and susceptibility data are available, the choice of therapy depends on the index of suspicion and the severity of the process. For example, in sickle cell disease, ampicillin may be initiated to cover Salmonella. In children, especially under the age of 2 years, ampicillin or chloramphenicol may be initiated to cover H. influenzae. Chloramphenicol might be preferred due to the development of ampicillin resistance among strains of H. influenzae (chloramphenicol-resistant strains also occur).

Patients with mild gram-negative infections may be treated with ampicillin or amoxicillin or a cephalosporin until susceptibility data are available. In the more ill patients, a combination of a cephalosporin and aminoglycoside frequently is given until data are available (see Table 6-6). For suspect Pseudomonas infection (i.e., infection in leukopenic or burn patients, in addicts, or in those who had prior cephalosporin therapy), a combination of carbenicillin or ticarcillin and gentamicin or tobramycin may be given. For gentamicin-tobramycin-susceptible P. aeruginosa organisms, tobramycin has a lower minimal inhibitory concentration (MIC) and may be a bit less toxic than gentamicin. Therefore, the therapeutic index (level between MIC

Table 6-2. *Recommended Doses of Preferred Antimicrobial Agents*

Drug	Route	Total Dose/Day*		Dosage Interval† (hr.)
Amikacin	IV or IM	15	mg./kg. (limit 2 gm.)	8
Amphotericin B	IV	0.75	mg./kg. (limit 50 mg.)	24
Ampicillin	IM or IV	200	mg./kg. or 6–12 gm.‡	4–6
Amoxicillin	PO	75	mg./kg. or 4 gm.§ ‖	6
Carbenicillin	IV	500	mg./kg. or 30 gm.‖	4
Cefazolin	IM or IV	50	mg./kg. or 4 gm.	6–8
Cephalothin or Cephaparin	IV	200	mg./kg. or 8–12 gm.	4–6
Cephalexin or cephadrine	PO	50	mg./kg. or 4 gm.	6
Chloramphenicol	IV or PO	50	mg./kg.	6
Clindamycin	IV	20	mg./kg. or 1.8 gm.	8
	PO	10	mg./kg. or 0.9 gm.	8
Cloxacillin	PO	50	mg./kg. or 4 gm.‖	6
	IV	100	mg./kg. or 6–12 gm.	4–6
Ethambutol	PO	15	mg./kg.#	24
5-Fluorocytosine	PO	150	mg./kg.	8
Fusidic acid	PO		3 gm.	8
Gentamicin	IM or IV	4.5–6	mg./kg.**	8
Isoniazid††	PO	5–10	mg./kg. 300–500 mg.	24
Kanamycin	IM	15	mg./kg. (limit 2 gm.)	12
Metronidazole	PO		750–2250 mg.	8
Oxacillin	IV or IM	200	mg./kg. or 6–12 gm.‖	3–4
Penicillin G	IV	100,000	units/kg. or 20–30 million units	4
Penicillin G, buffered	PO	100	mg./kg. or 8–12 gm.‖	6
Penicillin V	PO	50	mg./kg. or 2–4 gm.‖	6
Rifampin	PO	10	mg./kg. or 600 mg.	24
Streptomycin	IM		1–2 gm.	12
Sulfadiazine	PO		6 gm.	4
Tetracycline	PO		2 gm.	6
Ticarcillin	IV	250	mg./kg. or 15 gm.‖	4
Trimethoprim with sulfamethoxazole	PO	640	mg. trimethoprim; 3200 mg. sulfamethoxazole‡‡	6
Vancomycin	IV		2 gm.	6

* For osteomyelitis and foreign bodies. For arthritis and soft tissue, smaller doses ($\frac{1}{2}$ to $\frac{1}{4}$) will suffice after first few days. Doses apply to adults only when expressed in grams. Doses expressed in milligrams/kilograms can be applied to children.

† Total daily dose divided into portions given at the intervals listed. For example, ampicillin 200 mg./kg. total dose, if given at 6-hour intervals, would mean that each dose would be 50 mg./kg.

‡ For Salmonella and some other *Enterobacteriaceae*, 12 to 24 gm./day may be needed.

§ For Salmonella, 100 mg./kg.

‖ At times, 500 mg. of probenecid is also given every 6 hours to double the blood level.

25 mg./kg. for first 2 months.

** Follow blood levels—keep between 4 to 6 mcg./ml.

†† Give pyridoxine, 50 mg. b.i.d.

‡‡ Give same dose for infections of joint. For soft-tissue or urinary tract infections, half the amount should be given, divided into 12-hour dose intervals. Consider concomitant Folinic Acid with prolonged use of higher doses.

and toxicity) of tobramycin for Pseudomonas is greater.

In general, both gentamicin and tobramycin give unpredictable blood levels. Therefore, any patient receiving either of these agents should have periodic peak ($\frac{1}{2}$ hour) and nadir (just before next dose) blood levels determined to ensure achievement of therapeutic and nontoxic levels. Peak blood levels should be between 4 to 8 mcg./ml. Peak and nadir levels should not exceed 10 to 12 mcg./ml. and 2 mcg./ml., respectively. Kanamycin given for nonpseudomonas gram-negative bacillary infections and amikacin produce more predictable blood levels than gentamicin and tobramycin. Nevertheless, a periodic check of peak levels (2 hours after intramuscular dose or $\frac{1}{2}$ hour after intravenous dose) should be made to be sure that the peak level exceeds the MIC of the organism but does not exceed 30 mcg./ml. Nadir levels should not exceed 10 mcg./ml. Total dose should not exceed 500 mg./kg. if possible. Initial aminoglycoside dosage should be based on ideal rather than on actual body weight (especially for obese patients).

For most *anaerobic* gram-positive *infections*, penicillin G is the agent of choice.[34] For anaerobic gram-negative bacillary infections, particularly those due to B. fragilis, clindamycin, chloramphenicol, and possibly even full-dose carbenicillin are useful. Metronidazole (Flagyl), which can only be given orally in the United States, is bactericidal;[72] the aminoglycosides are ineffective against anaerobes. Other bactericidal drugs available against B. fragilis include the aminocyclitol (to be differentiated from aminoglycoside) spectinomycin,[83] and against some strains, carbenicillin or clindamycin. Metronidazole plus clindamycin may provide the best bactericidal therapy for these organisms. Other potential beneficial agents include rifampin, fusidic acid as well as, for some strains, the tetracyclines.[36]

Most organisms have their own intrinsic patterns of sensitivity and resistance to antibiotics. Nevertheless, one cannot rely upon treating an organism based on its taxonomic classification since it may acquire antibiotic resistance. Even organisms like S. aureus may be resistant to the penicillinase-resistant penicillins, i.e., methicillin, oxacillin, cloxacillin, nafcillin, and the cephalosporins. The frequency of resistance to these agents is much higher in S. epidermidis than in other organisms. Therefore, therapy may have to be modified after results of antibiotic susceptibility tests are available.

Once antibiotic *susceptibility data* become available, *therapy should be adjusted on the basis of these data, together with the clinical response of the patient.* Certainly, a change of therapy is indicated for a patient who is not responding to treatment because the organism is resistant to the antibiotics given. A more difficult decision arises when the patient seems to be responding to treatment, but has an organism that appears resistant to the agents being used. Response may be related to surgical drainage, for example, or to normal host factors. For optimal therapy, and to ensure no recurrence, it may be best to change antibiotics, especially for patients with infections of bone or joint. However, before doing so, it should be ascertained that the culture was obtained after careful aseptic preparation of the skin, that more than just an occasional organism was isolated, and that the antibiotic disc susceptibility test is not in error. To ensure that the test is accurate, it may be necessary to have the laboratory repeat the disc test or do a quantitative test of susceptibility by determining the organism's MIC.

PARASURGICAL USE OF ANTIBIOTICS. The goal of parasurgical antibiotic therapy is to achieve blood levels and preferably tissue or hematoma levels higher than the MIC of the infecting organism at the time of procedure. There are few controlled studies showing the efficacy of *prophylactic antibiotics* in orthopaedic surgery.[12,26,65] There are potential dangers in terms of side effects and superinfection. It is impossible and undesirable to cover every potential infecting organism. Since most infections are caused by gram-positive cocci, drugs like oxacillin or cefazolin, in doses of 1 to 2 gm., should be given parenterally 20 to 30 minutes before induction of anesthesia. If an antibiotic is administered after the anesthetic has been started, an anaphylactic reaction may go unrecognized. If it is given more than 12 hours before operation, organisms resistant to the antibiotic can proliferate and invade the hematoma site. In order to prevent side effects and superinfection, it is best to continue antibiotics no longer than 48 to 72 hours after operation. Dose during this period should be 1 gm. every 6 hours. Antibiotic prophylaxis cannot substitute for basic surgical asepsis, appropriate skin preparation with agents like povidone-iodine, and possibly the use of impermeable wound drapes. Some consider that topical antibiotics may be good prophylactic agents and advocate dilute solutions of aminoglycosides.[10] For reasons outlined below, I do not favor the topical use of antibiotics, and medical opinion favors systematic prophylactic therapy.[65] It is important to ensure that good tissue levels are achieved *at all tissue sites*, before organisms are implanted into the wound.

The use of antibiotics before surgery for *established infections* should ensure that the number of organisms is decreased by the time of operation. Therefore, the antibiotic is given for 2 to 3 days prior to surgery. Longer use of antibiotics may be necessary but, if possible, should be avoided to prevent superinfection with resistant organisms. Antibiotics are continued 1 or more weeks after surgery, depending on the nature of the infection and as discussed below.

MYCOBACTERIUM INFECTIONS. Mycobacterium tuberculosis is treated with isoniazid plus ethambutol, usually concomitant with 2 months of streptomycin therapy.[9] Streptomycin can then be discontinued if the organism is susceptible to both isoniazid and ethambutol. Although rifampin has not been approved in the United States for extrapulmonary tuberculosis,[16] it appears to be an effective agent for bone and joint infection, particularly if given with isoniazid for organisms susceptible to both agents. Close observation for hepatotoxicity is necessary. Ethambutol should be given with these two agents, before susceptibility data are available, to ensure that at least two effective drugs are given. Chemotherapy for infections of bone and joint should be continued for at least 24 months. For infections initially treated with isoniazid and rifampin, the last 12 months could be with isoniazid alone. Whenever isoniazid is used in adults, pyridoxine should also be given to lessen the possibilities of side effects.

Atypical mycobacterium infections, particularly M. fortuitum, M. ulcerans, and M. marinum, are difficult to eradicate with antimicrobial therapy and are generally treated surgically. On occasion, M. fortuitum infections may cause an acute cellulitis and require antibiotic therapy. A combination of isoniazid, rifampin, ethambutol, cycloserine, and streptomycin may be necessary. Obviously, such a combination has a substantial risk of side effects and requires careful monitoring. M. kansasii infections should be treated similar to M. tuberculosis infections. Infections limited to tendon and bursa have been eliminated by chemotherapy alone, given for 24 months.[80]

FUNGAL AND ACTINOMYCETES INFECTIONS. Actinomyces is susceptible to high doses of penicillin.[98] Therapy for the first few weeks should be given intravenously in doses of 10 to 12 million units/day and then buffered penicillin G should be given orally in doses of 4 to 6 gm./day. In penicillin-allergic patients, clindamycin or tetracycline may be substituted. Nocardia is susceptible to sulfadiazine or sulfamethoxazole, given in oral doses of 6 gm./day.[78] Peak blood levels (1 to 2 hours after a dose) of 12 to 15 mg./100 ml. should be obtained. Treatment for both of these organisms must be continued for at least 6 months and preferably a year.

Fungal infections frequently require amphotericin B administered intravenously and, at times, intra-articularly and rarely by infusion into bone. A test dose of 1 mg. should be given by slow intravenous infusion over 20 to 30 minutes.[7] In patients who develop hypotension or severe fever or those who are likely to tolerate this reaction poorly, 25 to 50 mg. of hydrocortisone sodium succinate are added to the infusion bottle. For nonacute infection, the dose of amphotericin B can then be slowly increased, by daily 5-mg. increments, to 0.6 mg./kg./day for candidal infection and to 0.75 mg./kg./day for other deep mycotic infections. Infusions should be given slowly over 3 to 6 hours in sufficient 5 percent dextrose and water to provide at least 10 ml. of fluid/mg. of amphotericin B. For acute infections, more rapid daily increments in dose (25 mg./day) should immediately follow the test dose. The maximal daily dose should not exceed 0.75 mg./kg. or 50 mg./day.

Duration of amphotericin B treatment is highly variable depending upon the organism and response, but in most instances should be for at least 2 months, if tolerated. Candidal infections in joints have been cured by as little as 200 mg. given over 2 to 4 weeks (usually with synovectomy).[71] Since joint and bone infections are usually part of a disseminated infection involving other tissue, most physicians like to give a total dose of 1 to 2 gm.[25,71] Some fungal infections, especially coccidioidomycosis, may require 4 to 6 gm. in addition to surgical therapy. Synovectomy is almost invariably necessary,[4] but since dissemination may occur, systemic therapy with at least 2 to 3 gm. of amphotericin B can be justified in noncandidal infections. Even intra-articular therapy may fail unless synovectomy is performed. Nevertheless, cure with local therapy has been reported. For chronic infection of bone, operation plus amphotericin B may fail. For resistant cases, reports of response to amphotericin B supplemented by transfer factor offer some hope.[4]

A water-soluble methyl ester of amphotericin B may provide future advantage.[7] It may prove less toxic and easier to administer than amphotericin B. A relatively new antifungal agent effective against some strains of Candida and cryptococci is 5-Fluorocytosine, or flucytosine.[7] Organisms readily become resistant, particularly if lower than optimal doses are used. Cryptococcal infections may require a combination of flucytosine and amphotericin B. This requires careful monitoring, since side effects may be enhanced. Miconazole is an experimental drug that may be effective for coccidioidomycosis caused by organisms resistant to amphotericin B.

Aspergillus is extremely resistant to therapy. Amphotericin B and flucytosine have individually and in combination frequently been ineffective. A combination of amphotericin B and rifampin holds promise for the therapy of aspergillosis.

DOSAGE INTERVAL OF ANTIMICROBIAL AGENTS

For an antibiotic to be effective, its concentration must be equal to or greater than that of the smallest amount of the agent that will inhibit bacterial growth. Frequently, peak levels several times higher than the MIC must be achieved to eradicate an organism. The inhibitory effect on most organisms will persist if the level is above the MIC for approximately one third of the dosage interval. The interval between doses depends upon the rate of growth of the organism and the half-life of the antibiotic. Rapidly proliferating organisms like staphylococci, streptococci, and gram-negative bacilli require multiple daily doses of drug, in contrast to more slowly proliferating organisms like M. tuberculosis for which once daily or even two to three times weekly therapy may be adequate. The shorter the half-life of the drug, the more frequently must the doses be given. Table 6-2 lists the dosage intervals for the more commonly used antibiotics. I prefer intermittent rather than continuous infusions of intravenous antibiotics, with the possible exception of the aminoglycosides, in severely leukopenic patients (polymorphonuclear leukocyte count less than 500 per mm.[3]).

ROUTES OF ADMINISTRATION OF ANTIMICROBIAL AGENTS

Antimicrobial agents are administered intravenously or intramuscularly, preoperatively, for serious life-threatening infections, and for organisms which have high MICs or are not susceptible to oral agents. Absorption of the drug from the gastrointestinal tract may be delayed or erratic in acutely ill patients. Treatment of P. aeruginosa infections requires parenteral carbenicillin or ticarcillin and/or gentamicin or tobramycin. There are no satisfactory oral preparations that can be substituted for non-urinary tract Pseudomonas infections.

Local instillation of antibiotics is advocated to achieve high levels of antibiotics at the site of infection.[1,44,55,77] This may be essential in rare instances when infection is caused by organisms that are only susceptible to toxic agents which do not adequately get to the site of infection (e.g., amphotericin B or the polymyxins). The argument that routine use of local antibiotics helps when the blood supply is poor is fallacious. Infusion of antibiotic into a wound is unlikely to get to all areas where bacteria are located. Systemic antibiotics will penetrate all viable areas. Areas with a poor blood supply should be debrided and irrigated by nonantibiotic-containing solutions to ensure perfusion of healthy tissue by systemic agents.

Additional problems may preclude the effectiveness of local antibiotics. To ensure that irrigation fluids flow freely, detergents or anticoagulants are often added. Alevaire inhibits penicillin,[70] and heparin interferes with the action of aminoglycosides.[45] In addition, aminoglycosides may be absorbed from the wound and cause deafness, and renal or vestibular damage. Whenever these drugs or the polymyxins are infused into bone or joint, even in dilute solutions, periodic antibiotic blood levels should be determined and results of tests for side effects should be obtained, especially if the same antibiotic is simultaneously given locally and systemically. Many drugs in high concentrations are irritating to tissue; the penicillins, when injected intra-articularly, may cause chronic synovitis. Finally, the irrigation system provides access for bacteria or fungi to cause superinfection, which may be even more difficult to eradicate than the original organism.

Dosage for intra-articular antibiotics should be based on calculations derived from the minimal inhibitory concentration or minimal bactericidal concentration (MBC) of the organism and the estimated volume of joint fluid. Dosage should provide levels in micrograms/milliliters 5 to 20 times the minimal bactericidal concentration of the organisms, and the agent should be given every 12 to 24 hours. Amphotericin B is frequently administered in doses of 5 to 15 mg. daily or 2 to 3 times a week.[71] It is given until the joint fluid is sterile for a week or two. In the rare case in which fungal infection of joint may be due to local invasion (not part of a systemic disease, e.g., candidiasis or sporotrichosis), agents may be given solely by the intra-articular route

to decrease side effects from systemic therapy.[71] Rarely, fungal infections of bone (especially coccidioidomycosis) may require local infusion of 50 mg. of amphotericin B in 500 mg. of sterile water over a 6-hour period on a daily basis.[95] Tests for side effects of amphotericin B should be conducted weekly since systemic absorption may occur.

Various antibiotics have been added to cements, especially methyl methacrylate, for fixation of prosthetic devices.[57] Gram-positive infections induced at the time of operation may be prevented. This therapy is unlikely to prevent infections due to gram-negative bacilli, especially those that may occur secondary to hematogenous spread to the prosthesis, days or weeks after operation. Even delayed gram-positive infections from hematogenous seeding could be expected, since the local antibiotics eventually may become inactive or be metabolized.

TISSUE DISTRIBUTION OF ANTIMICROBIAL AGENTS

EFFECTS OF INFLAMMATION. Antibiotic concentration in tissue is dependent upon vascularity and the "natural barrier" properties of tissue and the "permeability" properties of antibiotics. Inflammation increases permeability, or penetration, of antibiotics to the area of infection. As inflammation subsides, tissue levels of antibiotics fall. This may be critical in acute infections of bone, joint, implants, or foreign bodies. In addition, with increasing duration of therapy, the organisms proliferate less rapidly and are, therefore, less susceptible to antibiotics acting upon the bacterial cell wall (penicillins and cephalosporins). Thus, as improvement occurs, it may be mandatory to continue high dose parenteral therapy for these infections. Prevention of relapse is dependent upon maintaining therapy for weeks to months. In other words, as the patient looks better, feels better, and becomes capable of ambulation, the physician may have to control the temptation to change from parenteral to oral drugs and to reduce the dose of drug.

SITE OF INFECTION. *Soft-tissue or wound* infections are least affected among orthopaedic infections by changes in the state of inflammation. Therefore, almost any antimicrobial agent to which the organism is sensitive will probably be effective. Oral therapy is satisfactory once the patient is stable. Group A Streptococcus pyogenes infections should be treated for at least 10 days. All other soft-tissue infections should be treated for at least 3 days after the disappearance of clinical infection.

Synovial tissue or fluid infections can be treated by multiple antimicrobial agents, as most of them readily penetrate the joint (Table 6-3).[24,42,43,81,85] The ratio between peak serum to joint fluid levels approaches unity for most agents. Major exceptions include the polymyxins (including colistin) and amphotericin B. Antibiotics that penetrate the synovium in adequate amounts, but for which the ratio of peak serum to joint levels is low, include high molecular weight agents like the macrolides (erythromycin) and antibiotics highly bound to protein that are not lipophilic, e.g., cloxacillin.[42] The protein-bound portion of the antibiotic is not bacteriologically active. The antibiotic tissue concentration is often equal to the peak-free (nonprotein-bound) circulating level of drug. In practice, in most instances, there is sufficient antibiotic activity reaching the synovial fluid so that some of the more highly protein-bound semisynthetic penicillins like cloxacillin have been shown to be effective in therapy of staphylococcal septic arthritis.

For most promptly treated acute infections of joints, I prefer parenteral therapy for 3 to 4 weeks, if tolerated. The tendency to con-

Table 6-3. *Antibiotic Levels in Tissues**

Drug	Ratio of Serum to:		
	Joint Fluid	Normal Bone	Infected Bone
Amphotericin B	Borderline		Adequate
Ampicillin	0.75–1		Adequate
Carbenicillin	Good	0.2	Adequate
Cefazolin	0.7–1	0.2–0.3	0.3–1.5
Cephalexin	Good	0.12	Adequate
Cephaloridine	0.5–1	0.2–0.35	
Cephalothin	1	0.25	0.05–0.2
Chloramphenicol	0.5–1		Good
Clindamycin	0.7–0.85	0.4	0.6
Cloxacillin	0.2–0.3		Adequate
Dicloxacillin	Adequate	0.3	0.6
Erythromycin	0.25		
Fusidic Acid	Good	0.5	0.3
Gentamicin	0.4–0.6	0.2–0.5	0.3
Kanamycin	0.5		Adequate
Methicillin	0.7–2	0.25	0.4
Oxacillin	Adequate	0.05–0.2	Adequate
Penicillin G	0.5–1	Poor	Adequate
Penicillin V	2		
Rifampin	Adequate	0.1	0.25
Streptomycin	2		Adequate
Tetracycline	0.5–0.8		Poor†
Vancomycin	0.6–0.8		

* This is a partial list. Ratios are given as ranges reported from different studies. They are ratios of peak levels obtained in blood and tissue. Peak levels in blood and tissue do not occur simultaneously. Levels of antibiotic peak in joint fluid and bone later than in blood. The ratio of peak levels is a better index of tissue penetration than are ratios of levels obtained simultaneously. In those instances in which peak antibiotic levels were not available, qualitative terms—adequate, poor, and good—are used, based on known clinical efficacy studies and on the properties of the antimicrobial agent. Blank spaces indicate lack of sufficient data.
† Accumulates in osteoid instead of infected bone.

tinue with oral therapy for an additional few weeks to several months after initial parenteral therapy has been discontinued is frequently unwarranted. Antibiotic levels decrease as inflammation subsides, although this is less a problem in joints than in bone. There is no good evidence that continued oral therapy (which by comparison to parenteral therapy achieves much lower blood and tissue levels) has anything to offer after completion of a full course of parenteral therapy. When oral drugs are given as the primary mode of therapy, peak blood levels (1 to 2 hours after dose) should exceed the MIC of the organisms by two- to fourfold.

Certain acute joint infections require more or less vigorous chemotherapy.[15] Gonococcal infections may respond to 3 days of intravenous penicillin G in doses of 10 to 12 million units/day, divided into aliquot doses given every 4 hours.[11] I prefer to continue therapy from day 4 to day 14 with oral amoxicillin, prescribing 500 mg. every 6 hours. Lack of prompt response should arouse suspicion of infection caused by a penicillinase-producing strain of gonococcus. Uncomplicated infections due to pneumococci, streptococci (other than enterococcus), and H. influenzae frequently respond to only 2 weeks of parenteral or oral antibiotics. On the other hand, infections caused by Salmonella and Arizona bacteria are extremely difficult to eradicate and may require prolonged therapy.[20] After 3 to 4 weeks of parenteral therapy for these infections, amoxicillin or trimethoprim-sulfamethoxazole can be given orally for 3 to 4 months to a year. For sacroiliac or sacrococcygeal joint infection, antibiotic therapy has been advocated for at least 6 weeks, and possibly for as long as 3 months, especially when infection is caused by S. aureus.[21]

Complete recovery of joint function is highly dependent upon the infecting organism.[33] It approaches 100 percent with gonococci, 88 percent with streptococci and pneumococci, 50 percent with staphylococci, and 33 percent with gram-negative bacilli. Joint infections caused by gram-negative bacilli often respond poorly to therapy or recur.[33]

Results of therapy are worse in joints previously affected by rheumatoid arthritis, sickle cell disease, systemic lupus erythematosus, degenerative joint diseases, Charcot joints, and gout.[33] This is due, in part, to the delayed recognition of infection occurring in the face of disease already capable of causing fever, joint swelling, and pain.[51]

Guides to adequacy of therapy, in addition to clinical response, as indicated previously, are results of repeat synovial fluid culture, white blood cell counts, and measurement of synovial fluid antibiotic concentrations. If the results of culture remain positive and tests show inadequate synovial fluid levels following high dose parenteral therapy, and if there is no suitable alternative antibiotic, intra-articular antibiotic injections or infusions may be justified. Obviously, refractory infections of joints may require surgical intervention. Indeed, early surgical intervention is more effective than intra-articular antibiotic therapy, and should be seriously considered within the first 48 hours to 1 week in poorly responding patients. Nevertheless, some studies indicate that for infections other than those in the hip, patients treated by repeat joint aspiration do as well as, if not better than, those treated initially (early) by open operative procedures.[33] Therefore, open procedures are frequently reserved for patients not responding to repeat aspiration and antibiotics.

Bone infections are more difficult to treat than infections in other tissues since antibiotic levels in bone are usually lower than those obtained in blood (Table 6-3).[27,38,39,43,50,54,73,93,94,100] Generally, more highly vascularized cancellous bone has higher levels than less vascularized cortical bone. Some studies, however, show equivalent levels of antibiotic in these two areas of bone. Antibiotic levels are frequently adequate during the early stage of bone infection.[60] As the infection proceeds, thrombosis of vessels with resultant necrosis of bone ensues, and antibiotic levels in bone fall substantially.

Acute bone infections should be treated initially, if not totally, parenterally. Some would be willing to switch to oral drugs within days after improvement.[35] Even oral therapy with highly protein-bound antibiotics like cloxacillin may frequently be successful, especially if given with probenecid (Benemid), 500 mg. every 6 hours. The use of probenecid raises the blood level of penicillins by a factor of 2. This should be weighed against doubling the dose of the primary drug, since allergic reactions to either drug can occur and pose increased possibility of side effects.

I favor continued parenteral therapy, as long as it can safely be given and tolerated by the patient, to ensure adequate tissue levels. In the therapy of acute staphylococcal osteomyelitis in children, chronic disease occurred in 19 percent of those receiving parenteral antibiotics for 3 weeks or less. Chronic osteomyelitis developed even when oral cloxacillin was administered after parenteral antibiotics were discontinued.[23] In contrast, only 2 percent developed chronic disease among those treated with parenteral antibiotics for longer than 3 weeks. In acute staphylococcal hematogenous osteomyelitis, I prefer to treat from 4 to 6 weeks or until 3 weeks after the patient has become afebrile, whichever is longer. In most instances, there is no need to administer oral agents if the total course of parenteral therapy has been completed. Acute osteomyelitis due to gram-negative bacilli is more difficult to treat.[67] In most instances, the principles of antibiotic therapy are similar to those cited for staphylococcal infections. Parenteral therapy not only may be desirable, but may be the only effective method of antibiotic administration. Surgical intervention is needed more often because of poor response to parenteral drugs. Therapy should be continued for at least 6 weeks, if tolerated.

Oral drugs should be saved primarily for subacute and chronic bone infections caused by organisms with MICs susceptible to antibiotics that can be given by mouth. Most staphylococcal, anaerobic and aerobic streptococcal infections can be effectively treated orally. Peak serum antibiotic levels (1 to 2 hours) should be four to eight times higher than the MIC, or preferably, the MBC of the organisms.

Subacute and chronic infections may not respond as well as acute infections because of reduced access of antibiotics, polymorphonuclear leukocytes and macrophages, and the presence of necrotic debris. Therefore, it is preferable to use bactericidal antibiotics together with debridement for these infections.

Chronic infections of bone and certain acute infections like Salmonella and Arizona bacteria require antibiotics for as long as 4 to 12 months. Therefore, the antibiotics have to be given at least in part by the oral route. Chronic osteomyelitis caused by some gram-negative bacillary organisms (e.g., Pseudomonas) can only be treated by the parenteral route. In such instances, because of patient inconvenience and drug toxicity, therapy is usually discontinued after 6 to 8 weeks. Serial observations over years are necessary to determine the adequacy of antibiotic therapy. Since tissue levels of antibiotics in bone are difficult to obtain, peak blood levels tested against the pathogen(s) are used as guides to the adequacy of the initial therapy, in addition to serial cultures of material draining from bone. The number of organisms should decrease within a week, and the exudate should cease or become sterile within 1 to 2 weeks if therapy is adequate. Persistence of infection in the face of demonstrated adequate antibiotic blood levels should indicate the necessity for surgical intervention.

Infected foreign bodies, necrotic tissue, and abscesses are refractory to treatment in spite of adequate levels of antibiotics at the site of infection. Decreased tissue pH and Po_2 together with a decreased rate of bacterial proliferation interfere with the action of the aminoglycosides. The penicillins and cephalosporins are also less effective against slowly proliferating bacteria. Debridement and drainage are essential, and antibiotics are primarily relied upon to prevent further spread of infection and to eradicate residual organisms after operation.

OSTEOMYELITIS WITH NONUNION FRACTURE

Infection is not often curable during the initial stages of therapy while attempts are being made to achieve bone stabilization.[61,66] Long-term oral antibiotics may suppress infection and thereby help attain or accelerate fracture union. After stabilization is achieved, foreign bodies should be removed and residual infection treated by debridement under parenteral antibiotic coverage. For infections due to organisms not susceptible to oral antibiotics, it may be necessary to leave the infection untreated until stabilization has occurred. At that point, parenteral therapy can be instituted to cover the surgical procedure and the postoperative period. Alternately, since fracture union may not be achieved by these methods, some investigators first remove all necrotic tissue and foreign bodies under parenteral antibiotic coverage with or without suction irrigation, wait for a while, and then attempt to stabilize the bone while continuing antibiotic therapy.[66] To prevent recurrence of infection by whatever method is followed, eventually it is often necessary to give a 4- to 6-week high dose course of parenteral antibiotics (checking serum levels for adequacy of therapy) during and after removal of necrotic tissue and foreign bodies. If necrotic tissue or foreign bodies cannot be removed, there is the possibility of suppressing infections indefinitely by continued use of oral antibiotics.

INFECTION IN AND AROUND PROSTHETIC DEVICES

Infections in prostheses and foreign bodies can seldom be eradicated with antibiotics alone.[17,18,101,102] Occasionally, when infection is caused by a penicillin-sensitive organism like a streptococcus, and is diagnosed within the first 1 to 4 days after operation, a course of 2 to 4 weeks of parenteral or oral therapy may cure the infection.[102] This is true only when there is no evidence of osteomyelitis or accumulation of pus.

Treatment of acute deep wound infections requires adequate drainage in an attempt to avoid persistent colonization of the prosthesis. Frequently, irrigation-suction methods are used for 3 to 4 days to effect drainage. Since these tubes could serve as a source of superinfection, prolonged use should be avoided.

Most often, the infected foreign body serves as a nidus on which bacteria persist in small numbers in crevices too small for white blood cell entry. The persisting organisms remain in a dormant state against which even bactericidal antibiotics are impotent. Therefore, recurrence of infection frequently ensues after cessation of therapy as long as the foreign body is not removed.

The only symptom of chronic infection about a prosthesis may be pain. Fever and systemic symptoms frequently are not present. Culture of material from the area of the prosthetic device obtained by aspiration, if possible, should be sent in an anaerobic transport system to the laboratory with the request that antibiotic susceptibility tests be performed on all isolates.

When it is necessary to leave a prosthesis in an infected bone or a foreign body in place, the best that can be expected from antibiotics is to suppress active infection by indefinite oral therapy. Peak serum levels should be two to four times the MIC of the organism. When replacing an implant in an infected bone, high dose parenteral antibiotic coverage should be given immediately before, during, and for 2 to 3 weeks afterward. At this point, cure may be obtained, and an attempt to stop therapy is warranted. Some believe that oral medication should be continued for an additional 3 to 6 months, or possibly, indefinitely. Recurring infection would require indefinite suppressive antibiotic treatment.

Since prosthetic devices may become infected by the hematogenous route long after operation, some believe that any manipulation (dental, urologic, and the like) in patients with prosthetic devices should be done under antibiotic prophylaxis.[18] A combination of ampicillin, 1 gm. every 6 hours, or procaine penicillin G, one million units every 6 hours, and gentamicin, 1.5 mg./kg. every 8 hours, should be given parenterally just before, during, and for 48 hours after manipulation. In outpatients undergoing minor procedures, this parenteral combination given once an hour prior to the procedure is sufficient.

For treatment of *infections of the lung or urinary tract,* oral or parenteral drugs should be used for at least 10 days, or for 3 to 4 days after the patient has become afebrile, whichever is longer.

HOST FACTORS AFFECTING THERAPY

Certain host factors decrease access or decrease the effectiveness of antimicrobial therapy. In general, bactericidal antibiotics are preferred in the therapy of infection in patients with the following diseases:

Hemoglobinopathy, particularly sickle cell disease, may impair access of antibiotic due to sickling with its consequent interference with perfusion. It may be necessary to give packed red blood cells to raise the hemoglobin to a level of 10 to 11 gm. This will suppress the production of abnormal hemoglobin, which in turn will decrease sickling and increase the access of antibiotics to tissue.

Diabetes mellitus is associated with poor perfusion of tissue and possible altered phagocytosis of organisms. Gangrene and refractory osteomyelitis are well-known problems that often require surgical intervention in diabetics. Intravenous therapy gives more reliable tissue levels than intramuscular or oral therapy in diabetics because of decreased absorption from the latter two sites.

Severe leukopenia (polymorphonuclear leukocytes less than 500/mm.[3]) should be treated with intravenous bactericidal antibiotics and may require leukocyte transfusions.

Antibiotics in Patients with Altered Renal or Liver Function

Table 6-4 lists the antibiotics that are handled primarily by the liver or kidney.

Dosage alteration is necessary in azotemic patients treated by drugs primarily handled by the kidney.[8] This is particularly true when the creatinine clearance is less than 30 ml./min./m[2]. Lesser degrees of abnormal renal function require altered dosage of the aminoglycosides. Details of dosage programs are beyond the scope of this discussion. The single most important principle is to give the usual first dose and follow blood levels to determine maintenance doses. Doxycycline is the only tetracycline that may be safely used in renal failure for the treatment of non-urinary tract infections. Although blood levels do not build up and side effects do not occur, urine levels fall with renal failure.

Table 6-4. *Metabolism and Renal Excretion of Antimicrobial Agents*

Renal Excretion	Hepatic Metabolism
Ampicillin	Amphotericin B
Carbenicillin	Chloramphenicol
Cephalosporins	Chlortetracycline*
Ethambutol	Clindamycin
5-Fluorocytosine	Cloxacillin
Gentamicin	Erythromycin
Kanamycin	Fusidic Acid
Nitrofurantoin	Isoniazid
Penicillin G	Lincomycin
Penicillin V	Methicillin
Polymyxins	Nalidixic acid
Streptomycin	Oxacillin
Sulfonamides	
Tetracyclines†	
Tobramycin	
Trimethoprim-sulfamethoxazole	
Vancomycin	

* Avoid in renal failure because of buildup of toxic metabolites.
† Doxycycline is exception. It can safely be given in renal failure. It is excreted into the gastrointestinal tract.

Advanced liver disease manifested by jaundice, hypoalbuminemia, and prolonged prothrombin time requires dosage alteration of drugs handled primarily by the liver. The normal dose should be given for the first 48 hours; thereafter, maintenance doses of one half to one quarter of the usual dose will suffice.

ANTIBIOTIC SIDE EFFECTS

Table 6-5 lists the more common side effects caused by the frequently employed antimicrobial agents. Any agent is capable of causing fever, or adverse hematologic, renal, or hepatic reactions.[13] A prudent but costly precaution is to check results of blood counts and urinalysis twice weekly and liver function tests once weekly for the first month of treatment. Abnormal urinary sediment should lead to a check of the serum creatinine and electrolytes. The use of aminoglycosides, polymyxins, and amphotericin B requires repeat renal tests for at least 1 week following cessation of treatment.

Allergic side effects can occur with any antibiotic but occur more commonly with the penicillins, cephalosporins, sulfonamides, and streptomycin.[13]

THE PENICILLIN-ALLERGIC PATIENT. Presently, the best means of determining which patients may be allergic to penicillin is by history. Although many patients with a history of penicillin allergy tolerate penicillins without incident, it is wise to avoid penicillins, if at all possible, in patients with any type of "allergy." Anaphylaxis and angioneurotic edema may be immediate life-threatening reactions. Skin tests, resulting in an immediate wheal and flare, using degradation products derived from the specific penicillin prescribed (ampicillin allergy should not be tested for by a penicillin degradation product), can predict persons who will have anaphylactic reactions.[79] Unfortunately, the penicillins have multiple degra-

Table 6-5. *Frequent or Important Side Effects of Antimicrobial Agents**

Drug	Side Effects
Amphotericin B	Azotemia, anemia, hypokalemia, phlebitis, hypotension
Ampicillin	Allergy—rash, interstitial nephritis
Carbenicillin	Allergy, ↓platelet function, hepatotoxicity, ↓K⁺
Cefazolin	Allergy
Cephalexin	Allergy
Cephaloridine	Allergy, renal tubular necrosis
Cephalothin	Allergy
Chloramphenicol	Anemia
Clindamycin	Pseudomembranous and other colitis, rash, allergy, hepatoxicity
Cloxacillin	Allergy
Ethambutol	Optic neuritis, mental confusion, acute gout
5-Fluorocytosine	Hematologic, hepatoxic reactions
Gentamicin	Azotemia, ototoxicity, neuromuscular block
Isoniazid	Hepatotoxicity, SLE-like illness, neuropathy
Kanamycin	Azotemia, ototoxicity, neuromuscular block
Methicillin	Allergy, interstitial nephritis, leukopenia
Metronidazole	Neuropathy, toxic psychosis in alcoholics, especially if receiving disulfiram dark urine, vaginal and urethral irritation, neutropenia
Oxacillin	Allergy, interstitial nephritis, leukopenia
Penicillin	Allergy
Rifampin	Hepatotoxicity, renal reactions, ↓platelets, hemolysis, fever, red urine, or sweat
Streptomycin	Allergy, ototoxicity, neuromuscular block
Sulfadiazine	Allergy, azotemia, rash
Tetracycline	Hepatotoxicity, azotemia, rash, bone lesions, and stain and deformity of teeth in children up to 12 years old and in newborns of mothers who took the drug during the last half of pregnancy.
Tobramycin	Azotemia, ototoxicity, neuromuscular block
Vancomycin	Azotemia, ototoxicity, phlebitis

* All drugs are capable of causing fever, rash, gastrointestinal disorders, and allergic reactions. Each antimicrobial agent has a long list of infrequent or poorly documented side effects which are listed in the package insert that accompanies the antimicrobial agent. Both the physician and the patient should familiarize themselves with the data in the package inserts, especially for infrequently used agents.

dation products that differ from one semi-synthetic penicillin to another. Therefore, it is necessary to use a battery of antigens derived from the specific agent to be used. In clinical practice, this is not feasible, because the antigens are not commercially available. Penicilloyl polylysine is one degradation product of penicillin G that has recently become available commercially.[79] Unfortunately, a negative reaction does not ensure that it is safe to give penicillin G. Some allergists advise that penicilloyl polylysine plus dilute amounts of the prescribed penicillin be used to test the patient. There is disagreement as to whether fresh or older prescribed drugs (more degradation products) should be used for testing. Since kits that provide stable amounts of small doses of antibiotic are not available, the individual physician must make careful dilutions of conventional antibiotics obtained from the pharmacy. Those not familiar with skin testing could get into trouble if dilutions are inaccurate; the tests may give false-positive or false-negative results. Even more important, the highly sensitive patient may have an anaphylactic reaction to minute amounts of penicillin. Intradermal skin tests should only be performed if results of a preceding scratch test are negative.

Thus, it has been my practice to avoid penicillin or any penicillin derivative in any patient with a history suggestive of a past penicillin reaction. When it is absolutely essential to use penicillin, having a qualified allergist test the patient and prescribe a course of action is justified. Some patients with a negative history of penicillin allergy have positive results of skin tests, and it is well known that some patients have anaphylaxis after prior uneventful use of penicillin. Nevertheless, the numbers are small, and the skin tests are sufficiently inaccurate so that routine testing is not justified. It is generally safe to use penicillin without prior skin tests in patients without a history of penicillin allergy. A strong family or personal history of multiple allergies or a personal history of atopy (asthma or eczema) should lead to cautious use of penicillin and prior skin tests. In most instances when there is doubt, it is best to use a non-penicillin drug.

For anaerobic or gram-positive infections, clindamycin is preferred in the penicillin-allergic patient. Erythromycin or tetracycline may be satisfactory for minor soft-tissue infections. For gram-negative infections, an aminoglycoside or chloramphenicol may be used for serious infections, and a tetracycline can be used for minor infections. Trimethoprim-sulfamethoxazole may also be useful for many gram-negative infections.

The cephalosporins have been advocated as safe bactericidal penicillinlike drugs which could be given to patients who are allergic to penicillin. Unfortunately, there is a high incidence of allergic side effects to cephalosporins in patients allergic to penicillin. This is due to the allergic diathesis of the patient, but on occasion is related to cross-allergic reactions between the two agents.[47,82] It has been my practice to avoid the cephalosporins in patients who have a history of anaphylactic or accelerated (urticarial, angioneurotic edema) reaction to penicillin. Those patients having delayed reactions, primarily consisting of a maculopapular rash, which occurred in the distant past, may well tolerate a cephalosporin without problem. The same skin test problems exist for cephalosporins as for penicillin outlined previously.

OTHER ANTIBIOTIC SIDE EFFECTS. *Pseudomembranous colitis*, which may be life-threatening, occurs with variable frequency, from less than 1 to 10 percent of adults receiving clindamycin or lincomycin.[46,96] It occurs less frequently after administration of ampicillin, cephalexin, tetracycline, and chloramphenicol. Its occurrence is unpredictable and sporadic. Its onset frequently occurs during the end of the first week of therapy, or as long as a week after therapy has been discontinued. If diarrhea (five or more liquid stools per day) and/or fever, abdominal pain and distention occur in any patient receiving antibiotics, sigmoidoscopy should be performed for pseudomembranous colitis. If an alternate effective drug can be found, or if sigmoidoscopic examination shows pseudo-membranous changes, the causative antibiotic must be stopped. If diarrhea is mild, there is no evidence of pseudomembranous colitis, and the infection warrants further therapy with the same antibiotic, it may be continued while the patient is kept under scrutiny. Continued diarrhea requires repeat sigmoidoscopic examination at least once a week. Increasing or bloody diarrhea warrants cessation of therapy. Serial abdominal roentgenograms and physical examinations should be done looking for signs of increasing ileus or toxic megacolon. Serial serum albumin should be checked since protein-losing enteropathy may occur. The use of Lomotil and other antidiarrheal agents in therapy of antibiotic-induced diarrhea is controversial. Some believe that these agents enhance the development of pseudomembranous colitis by keeping toxic materials in the bowel, whereas others believe that these agents are beneficial. Cholestyramine, in doses of 4 gm. three times a day, has been advocated for the treatment of established pseudomembranous colitis. Others have advocated corticosteroids particularly, administered by enema for the treatment of colitis. More recent data incriminate a cytotoxin produced by a species of Clostridium as the cause of colitis. Vancomycin, 500 mg. every 6 hours by mouth, seems to offer the best chance of cure.

Patients receiving *aminoglycoside antibiotics* should be monitored for eighth cranial nerve toxicity, especially if azotemic, over the age of 50, or if the drug is continued for more than 10 days. Tests should be done once a week as long as the patient is on therapy and should be repeated one week after therapy has been discontinued. Neuromuscular blockage may occur with the aminoglycosides especially in patients who have myasthenia gravis, parkinsonism, azotemia, or who receive neuromuscular blocking agents during anesthesia or lidocaine administration.

Carbenicillin, a semisynthetic penicillin, is the most effective antipseudomonas antibiotic available (when organisms are susceptible, because acquired resistance has become a problem).[53] In addition to allergic reactions, bleeding diathesis, hypokalemia, and fluid overload may occur owing to the high dose (30 or more gm./day) and blood levels required with this agent. There is approximately 5 mEq. of sodium/gm. of carbenicillin. Hypokalemic metabolic alkalosis occurs in patients who are hyponatremic, because of renal tubular exchange for potassium to preserve hydrogen ions. Carbenicillin may interfere with platelet function especially in patients who have underlying functional abnormalities of platelets (e.g., in azotemia). In addition, carbenicillin may interfere with vitamin K-dependent clotting factors (also true for other antibiotics that eradicate anaerobic gastrointestinal flora). It may rarely cause thrombocytopenia. Obviously, bleeding would be worse in patients receiving prophylactic or therapeutic anticoagulation agents. On occasion, carbenicillin causes marked elevation of liver enzymes which usually return rapidly to normal upon cessation of therapy.

Ticarcillin, a semisynthetic penicillin resembling carbenicillin in spectrum and action, has recently been released for use.[88] It can be used in smaller doses (15 to 20 gm./day) and may therefore have less side effects than carbenicillin. The latter statement remains to be proved.

Semisynthetic penicillins and cephalosporins given in high prolonged doses may be associated with renal side effects. Interstitial nephritis, manifested by abnormal urinary sediment, and azotemia ($\pm$ rash eosinophilia) may occur with any of these agents, but is more frequent with methicillin. Acute tubular necrosis may follow cephalosporin therapy. This is more often related to cephaloridine and much more rarely to cephalothin. Cephaloridine should not be given in doses greater than 4 gm./day in nonazotemic patients and not given at all to azotemic patients. The other cephalosporins appear much safer, but may not be totally free from this potential adverse reaction.

Prolonged high dose penicillin or cephalosporin therapy in azotemic patients may be neurotoxic. These patients may develop seizures, myoclonus, coma, or an altered sensorium. Practically all of the penicillins or cephalosporins may on occasion cause severe leukopenia or hemolytic anemia.

Rifampin, released in the United States for the treatment of pulmonary tuberculosis, is effective for mycobacterium infections, including many atypical organisms involving bone or joint.[16] Hepatotoxicity, with or without fever, is the chief adverse reaction which occurs more frequently in patients receiving concomitant hepatotoxic drugs like isoniazid or halothane anesthesia and/or who have preexisting liver disease.[92] It is unclear whether by obtaining results of serial liver function tests, advanced hepatitis, jaundice, and liver failure would be prevented. If the serum glutamic-oxaloacetic transaminase (SGOT) or serum glutamic-pyruvic transaminase (SGPT) is greater than 200 units, the drugs should be discontinued. Intermittent use of rifampin may be dangerous, owing to antibody formation against the drug. The most common immunologic reactions are fever and flulike symptoms; but thrombocytopenic purpura, hemolytic anemia, and acute renal failure may rarely occur. These reactions are more frequent when adults receive 900 mg. or greater biweekly. Smaller intermittent doses may be safe. Some adult patients receiving daily doses of 600 mg. may develop immunologic reactions if therapy is interrupted. Since rifampin is presently available in the United States only in an oral form, it may have to be stopped at the time of operation. If reinstituted within 48 hours and possibly even within 96 hours, the probability of an immunologic reaction is small. If therapy must be interrupted for a longer interval, serious thought should be given to either discontinuing rifampin, or once reinstituted, carefully following the patient.

Amphotericin B may cause phlebitis, fever, and rigors as well as hypotension because of its myocardial suppressive activity.[7] If these side effects should occur, they can be prevented or ameliorated by corticosteroids given with or before each infusion. Heparin (500 units) added to the infusion may decrease phlebitis. Anemia and azotemia are other well-recognized side effects of amphotericin B. If the creatinine rises above 3.5 mg./100 ml. or if the hematocrit falls below 20, it may be necessary to reduce the dose. Mannitol (25 gm.) given intravenously, simultaneously with amphotericin B, may prevent or ameliorate its renal side effects.[75] Oral sodium bicarbonate has also been advocated to reduce the renal side effects of amphotericin B. Transfusions are rarely necessary.

Superinfection is another side effect of antibiotic therapy. Persistent or recurrent infection requires repeat cultures. The original organisms may have become resistant to the antibiotic, or new organisms may invade tissue. Superinfection is most likely to occur at tissue sites where there is access by organisms from the environment, feces, skin, or the pharynx. Therefore, urinary tract infections, pneumonia, open wounds, or wounds that have a drain or suction device are more prone to superinfection. Sites where easy access to the external milieu is not apparent rarely become superinfected by the hematogenous route, particularly from intravenous infusions. More often, in closed infections, persistence of infection is usually caused by the original organism, which remains sensitive to the original antibiotic and requires surgical intervention. Rarely, persistence of closed infections is due to acquired antibiotic resistance by mutation of the organism.

ANTIBIOTIC ACTIONS AND INTERACTIONS

Bactericidal antibiotics are advocated in the therapy of osteomyelitis and possibly in infections in prosthetic devices and foreign bodies owing to the belief that an agent that kills organisms will be more beneficial in eradicating infection.[14]

The distinction between bactericidal and bacteriostatic antibiotics is to a certain extent arbitrary (Table 6-6). A bactericidal agent is usually defined as one that kills an organism at a concentration close to that which will inhibit it after 18 hours of incubation at 37°C (MBC equal to or only slightly higher than its MIC). By this defini-

Table 6-6. *Bactericidal Versus Bacteriostatic Antibiotics*

Bactericidal Agents	Bacteriostatic Agents
Aminoglycosides*	Amphotericin B
Bacitracin	Chloramphenicol
Cephalosporins†	Clindamycin-lincomycin‡
Isoniazid	Erythromycin
Nalidixic acid	Ethambutol
Penicillins§	5-Fluorocytosine
Polymyxins‖	Sulfonamides
Rifampin	Tetracyclines#
Trimethoprim-sulfamethoxazole	
Vancomycin	

* Aminoglycosides include amikacin, gentamicin, kanamycin, neomycin, streptomycin, tobramycin.
† Cephalosporins include cefazolin, cephradine, cephalexin, cephaloridine, cephalothin, cephapirin.
‡ Clindamycin-lincomycin may have bactericidal action against some organisms.
§ Penicillins include amoxicillin, ampicillin, carbenicillin, cloxacillin, dicloxacillin, flucloxacillin, methicillin, nafcillin, oxacillin, penicillin G, phenethicillin, phenoxymethyl penicillin, ticarcillin.
‖ Polymyxins include colistin, polymyxin B.
Tetracyclines include chlortetracycline, Clomocycline, Demethylchlortetracycline, doxycycline, methacycline, minocycline, oxytetracycline, rolitetracycline, tetracycline.

tion, clindamycin is bactericidal for the streptococci but bacteriostatic for staphylococci. Nevertheless, the ratio between the MBC and MIC for clindamycin against staphylococci is small, as compared to bacteriostatic agents like tetracycline. Bactericidal levels of clindamycin can be achieved against many staphylococci. The rate of killing of organisms is an additional factor that separates the bactericidal efficacy of antimicrobial agents. Clindamycin will kill staphylococci at rates much slower than the penicillins or aminoglycosides. Nevertheless, clindamycin has proved efficacious for the treatment of acute and chronic staphylococcal osteomyelitis.[30,84,99] The penicillins, however, are better bactericidal agents. Other factors such as tissue distribution may equalize the overall effectiveness of clindamycin versus the semisynthetic penicillins. For penicillin G-susceptible organisms, the latter agent is preferred.

Antagonistic or synergistic interactions among antibiotics in most orthopaedic infections are only of theoretical importance. Interactions cannot be accurately predicted.[45] Tests involving the infecting organism with the antibiotics used are necessary to determine if there is an indifferent, additive, synergistic, or antagonistic interaction. Problems of interaction can best be avoided by using single antibiotics. When it is necessary to use multiple agents, of which only one is bactericidal, the possibility of potential antagonistic interaction may be diminished if the bactericidal agent is given 30 to 60 minutes before the bacteriostatic agent. Only a few interactions deserve brief review at this point.

Trimethoprim with sulfamethoxazole (Bactrim, Septra) is approved in the United States for urinary tract infections only, but has proved efficacy in the treatment of salmonellosis and possibly brucellosis.[31] The two bacteriostatic agents cause sequential blockage in the folic acid pathway in bacterial (and some parasitic) cells, the net effect of which is frequently bactericidal. Trimethoprim is a dihydrofolic acid reductase inhibitor, whereas sulfonamides compete with para-aminobenzoic acid. These agents have little or no effect on the folic acid pathway in mammalian cells. Nevertheless, the combination should be avoided in patients who have folate deficiency. Folinic Acid will not interfere with the drug's antimicrobial action.

Enterococcal infections of bone may be refractory to penicillin, since the latter is bacteriostatic against enterococci. Penicillin combined with aminoglycoside may be bactericidal. Similarly, gram-negative bacillary infections of joint or bone may require the combined action of bactericidal agents which act upon the cell wall (penicillin and cephalosporins) and the ribosome (aminoglycosides). Penicillins or cephalosporins alter the cell wall, allowing increased penetration of the aminoglycoside to the cell's interior.[45] This enhances the bactericidal activity, increases the rate of bacterial killing, and possibly delays emergence of resistance. This may be important in eradication of Pseudomonas when carbenicillin or ticarcillin is used with gentamicin or tobramycin, or for more rapid eradication of K. pneumoniae, for which a cephalosporin may be useful when given with gentamicin.

Staphylococcal osteomyelitis is usually treated with a single antibiotic. In attempts to shorten the course of therapy and prevent relapse, investigators have looked at combination antibiotic therapy.[56] Preliminary experimental data indicate that a combination of semisynthetic penicillinase-resistant penicillin, like oxacillin or nafcillin, or a cephalosporin together with an aminoglycoside, like kanamycin or gentamicin, may more rapidly eradicate staphylococcal infections. None of the above antibiotics penetrates into polymorphonuclear leukocytes to kill intracellular bacteria. Rifampin, which is effective against staphylococci, is effective against intracellular organisms. In experimental staphylococcal osteomyelitis of rabbits, rifampin given with a cephalosporin and aminoglycoside kills organisms in bone more rapidly than any individual or two drugs given together.[74] Whether these observations have clinical importance remains to be determined. In addition, indiscriminate use of rifampin may impair its effect against tuberculosis. Whether the benefit from a shorter course of therapy with multiple antibiotics will outweigh the combined antibiotic toxicity remains to be shown. Clindamycin may slow the rate of killing of staphylococci by aminoglycosides or penicillins. This appears to be of minor significance, but the combination should be avoided for proved staphylococcal infections since the risk of side effects in this case outweighs any potential benefit. Clindamycin may also slow the rate of killing by aminoglycosides of gram-negative bacilli with the exception of B. fragilis.

Carbenicillin (or any of the semisynthetic penicillins or cephalosporins) *should not be mixed in the same solution with gentamicin* (or any other aminoglycoside). Such a mixture may lead to a physicochemical interaction which inactivates both agents.[45] Inactivation does not occur under normal circumstances in the body. It will occur when prolonged high tissue levels of both agents develop, such as in the tissue of azotemic patients or in the urine of normal patients.

INTERACTIONS AMONG ANTIBIOTICS AND

OTHER DRUGS. The list of potential drug interactions is growing. Only a few of the interactions that the orthopaedic surgeon may encounter will be covered in this section. Physicochemical incompatibilities of antimicrobial agents are listed in Table 6-7.[45]

Clinical observations suggest that the combination of a cephalosporin and an aminoglycoside may be more nephrotoxic than if the agents are given individually. In contrast, animal studies not only have failed to corroborate this observation but indicate that the cephalosporins may lessen nephrotoxicity, possibly by decreasing renal cortical concentrations of aminoglycosides,[22] or by interfering with the binding of the aminoglycosides to the renal tubular cell membrane. Antibiotic nephrotoxicity and/or ototoxicity may be enhanced by furosemide (Lasix) or ethacrynic acid. Nephrotoxicity is enhanced, especially if there is poor renal perfusion owing to hypotension and/or heart failure.

Coumarin anticoagulation may be altered by antibiotics.[45] Prothrombin times should be closely monitored after the first 4 days of therapy and until 2 weeks after cessation of antibiotic therapy. The peak interaction usually occurs a week after institution and a week after discontinuation of antibiotics. The type of interaction depends upon the

Table 6-7. *Physicochemical Incompatabilities*

Antimicrobial	Incompatible With
Amphotericin B	Normal saline solution
Cephalothin	Lactated Ringer's solution; calcium gluconate; calcium chloride
Chloramphenicol	B complex with vitamin C
Tetracycline	Lactated Ringer's solution; sodium bicarbonate; calcium chloride
Erythromycin	B complex with vitamin C
Methicillin	Normal saline solution or dextrose with pH less than 7
Penicillins	Dextrose or sucrose plus bicarbonate with pH 8 or greater; B complex with vitamin C

antibiotic. Long-acting sulfonamides, chloramphenicol, rifampin,[76] and isoniazid may induce the metabolism of the anticoagulant, causing inadequate levels of the latter during combined therapy. Rebound overcoagulation and hemorrhage may follow cessation of administration of antibiotics. The penicillins, cephalosporins, and aminoglycosides are unlikely to cause this problem. The former agents along with the tetracyclines and clindamycin may interfere with vitamin K-producing anaerobic organisms of the gastrointestinal tract, thereby enhancing the effect of the coumarin anticoagulants. Other drugs that may frequently interact with anticoagulants and antibiotics include phenobarbital, phenytoin (Dilantin), and the oral hypoglycemic agents.

ANTIMICROBIAL AGENTS OF THE FUTURE

NEW AMINOGLYCOSIDES. The new aminoglycosides, including amikacin, Sisomicin, Butirosin, and Netilmicin (SCH 20569), all are effective antipseudomonas drugs.[37,48,58] Some gentamicin-resistant gram-negative bacillary organisms are susceptible to one or another of these agents. Susceptibility tests are required since cross resistance may occur. They must be given parenterally and produce side effects similar to those from other aminoglycosides, although possibly to a lesser degree with some of the newer agents.

Amikacin (recently released for use in patients) should be reserved for infections caused by gram-negative organisms proved or suspected to be resistant to gentamicin or tobramycin.

NEW CEPHALOSPORINS. Cephamandole, Cefuroxime, and Cefatoxin are experimental agents with a wider antibacterial spectrum than the currently available cephalosporins.[28,69,91] This is due, in part, to their effectiveness against some cephalosporinase-producing gram-negative bacilli and/or better penetration through the bacterial cell envelope. Cefuroxime and Cephamandole appear more active than Cefatoxin against Enterobacter and H. influenzae, whereas Cefatoxin appears more active against indole-positive Proteus species and B. fragilis. Being cephalosporins, they are relatively nontoxic and, therefore, have an advantage over the aminoglycosides for the treatment of susceptible Enterobacter, indole-positive Proteus species, B. fragilis, N. gonorrhoeae, and H. influenzae infections.

NEW PENICILLINS. Mecillinam (FL1060) is a novel agent whose mechanisms of action differ from those of the penicillins.[87] It is more effective against gram-negative bacilli, but much less effective against gram-positive organisms. Combined with penicillins or cephalosporins, it may have synergistic effects against Proteus and Klebsiella, respectively, as well as some other gram-negative bacteria.[2]

Although newer and better antibiotics will continue to be developed in the future, present antibiotics used properly can cover most infections. The new antibiotics may decrease toxicity and enhance convenience of therapy, but are unlikely to substantially increase effectiveness. Mainstays of treatment will remain a combination of adequate surgical debridement with appropriate antibiotics given in dosages to achieve adequate levels in blood and tissue for a sufficient length of time.

REFERENCES

1. Anderson, L. D., and Horn, L. G.: Irrigation-suction technic in the treatment of acute hematogenous osteomyelitis, chronic osteomyelitis, and acute and chronic joint infections. South. Med. J., 63:745–754, 1970.
2. Baltimore, R. S., Klein, J. O., Wilcox, C., and Finland, M.: Synergy of methicillin (FL1060) with penicillins and cephalosporins against Proteus and Klebsiella, with observations on combinations with other antibiotics and against other bacterial species. Antimicrob. Agents Chemother., 9:701–705, 1976.
3. Bartlett, J. G., Rosenblatt, J. E., and Feingold, S. M.: Percutaneous transtracheal aspiration in

the diagnosis of anaerobic pulmonary infection. Ann. Intern. Med., 79:535–540, 1973.

4. Bayer, A. S., Yoshikawa, T. T., Galpin, J. E., and Guze, L. E.: Unusual syndromes of coccidioidomycosis: Diagnostic and therapeutic considerations: A report of 10 cases and review of the English literature. Medicine, 55:131–152, 1976.

5. Belding, M. E., and Klebanoff, S. J.: Effect of sodium polyanetholesulfonate on antimicrobial systems in blood. Appl. Microbiol., 24:691–698, 1972.

6. Bell, D. B., Marks, M. I., and Eickhoff, T. C.: *Pasturella multocida* arthritis and osteomyelitis. J.A.M.A., 210:343–345, 1969.

7. Bennett, J. E.: Chemotherapy of systemic mycoses. N. Engl. J. Med., 290:30–32; 320–323, 1974.

8. Bennett, W. M., Singer, I., and Coggins, C. J.: A guide to drug therapy in renal failure. J.A.M.A., 230:1544–1553, 1974.

9. Berney, S., Goldstein, M., and Bishko, F.: Clinical and diagnostic features of tuberculous arthritis. Am. J. Med., 53:36–42, 1972.

10. Bingham, R., Fleenor, W. H., and Church, S.: The local use of antibiotics to prevent wound infection. Clin. Orthop., 99:194–200, 1974.

11. Blankenship, R. M., Holmes, R. K., and Sanford, J. P.: Treatment of disseminated gonococcal infection: A prospective evaluation of short-term antibiotic therapy. N. Engl. J. Med., 290:267–269, 1974.

12. Boyd, R. J., Burke, J. F., and Colton, T.: A double-blind clinical trial of prophylactic antibiotics in hip fractures. J. Bone Joint Surg., 55-A:1251–1258, 1973.

13. Caldwell, J. R., and Cluff, L. E.: Adverse reactions to antimicrobial agents. J.A.M.A., 230:77–80, 1974.

14. Clawson, D. K., and Dunn, A. W.: Management of common bacterial infections of bones and joints. J. Bone Joint Surg., 49-A:164–182, 1967.

15. Cobbs, C. G., and Kaye, D.: Arthritis in infectious diseases. Clin. Orthop., 57:57–67, 1968.

16. Council on Drugs: Evaluation of a new antituberculous agent: Rifampin (Rifadin, Rimactane). J.A.M.A., 220:414, 1972.

17. Coutis, R. D., Schiller, A. L., and Harris, W. H.: Subclinical osteomyelitis of the femoral head. Two cases illustrating a special problem in the use of total hip replacement. Clin. Orthop., 86:68–72, 1972.

18. Cruess, R. L., Bickel, W. S., and vonKessler, L. C.: Infections in total hips secondary to a primary source elsewhere. Clin. Orthop., 106:99–101, 1975.

19. Curtiss, P. H., Jr.: Joint infections: The pathophysiology of joint infections. Clin. Orthop., 96:129–135, 1973.

20. David, J. R., and Black, R. L.: Salmonella arthritis. Medicine, 39:385–403, 1960.

21. Delbarre, F., Rondier, J., Delrieu, F., Evrard, J., Cayla, J., Menkes, C. J., and Amor, B.: Pyogenic infection of the sacro-iliac joint. J. Bone Joint Surg., 57-A:819–825, 1975.

22. Dellinger, P., Murphy, T., Barza, M., Pinn, V., and Weinstein, L.: Effect of cephalothin on renal cortical concentrations of gentamicin in rats. Antimicrob. Agents Chemother., 9:587–588, 1974.

23. Dich, V. Q., Nelson, J. D., and Haltalin, K. C.: Osteomyelitis in infants and children. A review of 163 cases. Am. J. Dis. Child., 129:1273–1278, 1975.

24. Drutz, D. J., Schaffner, W., Hillman, J. W., and Koenig, M. G.: The penetration of penicillin and other antimicrobials into joint fluid. Three case reports with a reappraisal of the literature. J. Bone Joint Surg., 49-A:1415–1421, 1967.

25. Edwards, J. E., Turkel, S. B., Elder, H. A., Rand, R. W., and Guze, L. B.: Hematogenous candida osteomyelitis: Report of three cases and review of the literature. Am. J. Med., 59:89–94, 1975.

26. Ericson, C., Lidgren, L., and Lindberg, L.: Cloxacillin in the prophylaxis of postoperative infections of the hip. J. Bone Joint Surg., 55-A:808–813, 1973.

27. Evaskus, D. S., Laskin, D. M., and Kroeger, A. V.: Penetration of lincomycin, penicillin, and tetracycline in serum and bone. Proc. Soc. Exp. Biol. Med., 130:89–91, 1969.

28. Eykyn, S., Jenkins, C., King, A., and Phillips, I.: Antibacterial activity of Cefuroxamine, a new cephalosporin antibiotic compared with that of cephaloridine, cephalothin and Cephamandole. Antimicrob. Agents Chemother., 9:690–695, 1976.

29. Farrand, R. J., Johnstone, J. M. S., and Maccabe, A. F.: Haemophilus osteomyelitis and arthritis. Br. Med. J., 2:334–336, 1968.

30. Feigin, R. D., Pickering, L. K., Anderson, D., Keeney, R. E., and Shackleford, P. G.: Clindamycin treatment of osteomyelitis and septic arthritis in children. Pediatrics, 55:213–223, 1975.

31. Finland, M., and Kass, E. H.: Trimethoprim-sulfamethoxazole symposium. J. Infect. Dis. (suppl.), 128:S425–S816, 1973.

32. Goldenberg, D. L., and Cohen, A. S.: Acute infectious arthritis. A review of patients with nongonococcal joint infections (with emphasis on therapy and prognosis). Am. J. Med., 60:369–377, 1976.

33. Goldenberg, D. L., Brandt, K. D., Catheart, E. S., and Cohen, A. S.: Acute arthritis caused by gram-negative bacilli: A clinical characterization. Medicine, 53:197–208, 1974.

34. Gorbach, S. L., and Bartlett, J. B.: Anaerobic infections. N. Engl. J. Med., 290:1177–1184; 1237–1245; 1289–1294, 1974.

35. Green, J. H.: Cloxacillin in treatment of acute osteomyelitis. Br. Med. J., 2:414–416, 1967.

36. Hamilton-Miller, J. M. T.: Antimicrobial agents acting against anaerobes. J. Antimicrob. Chemother., 1:273–289, 1975.

37. Heifetz, C. L., Chodubski, J. A., Pearson, I. A., Silverman, C. A., and Fisher, M. W.: Butirosin compared with gentamicin *in vitro* and *in vivo*. Antimicrob. Agents Chemother., 6:124–135, 1974.

38. Herrell, W. E.: Cephalexin in chronic bone infections. Clin. Med., 78:15–16, 1971.

39. Hierholzer, G., Rehn, J., Knothe, H., and Masterson, J.: Antibiotic therapy of chronic post-traumatic osteomyelitis. J. Bone Joint Surg., 56-B:721–729, 1974.

40. Holmes, K. K., Counts, G. W., and Beaty, H. N.: Disseminated gonococcal infection. Ann. Intern. Med., 74:979–993, 1971.

41. Holzman, R. S., and Bishko, F.: Osteomyelitis in heroin addicts. Ann. Intern. Med., 75:693–696, 1971.

42. Howell, A., Sutherland, R., and Rolinson, G. N.: Effect of protein binding on levels of ampicillin and cloxacillin in synovial fluid. Clin. Pharmacol. Ther., 13(5)I:724–732, 1972.

43. Hughes, S. P. F., Dash, C. H., and Field, C. A.: Cephaloridine penetration into bone and synovial capsule of patients undergoing hip joint replacement. J. Antimicrob. Chemother. (suppl.), 1:41–46, 1975.

44. Jones, R. F., Barnett, J. A., and Gregory, C. F.: Regional perfusion with antibiotics for chronic bone infections. Arch. Surg., 106:142–144, 1973.

45. Kabins, S. A.: Interactions among antibiotics and other drugs. J.A.M.A., 219:206–212, 1972.

46. Kabins, S. A., and Spira, T. J.: Outbreak of clindamycin-associated colitis. Ann. Intern. Med., 83:830–831, 1975.

47. Kabins, S. A., Eisenstein, B., and Cohen, S.: Anaphylactoid reaction to an initial dose of sodium cephalothin. J.A.M.A., 193:165–166, 1965.

48. Kabins, S. A., Nathan, C., and Cohen, S.: *In vitro* comparison of Netilmicin, a semisynthetic derivative of Sisomicin and four other aminoglycoside antibiotics. Antimicrob. Agents Chemother., 10:139–145, 1976.

49. Kahn, D. S., and Pritzker, K. P. H.: The pathophysiology of bone infection. Clin. Orthop., 96:12–19, 1973.

50. Kanyuck, D. O., Welles, J. S., Emmerson, J. L., and Anderson, R. C.: The penetration of cephalosporin antibiotics into bone (35414). Proc. Soc. Exp. Biol. Med., 136(3):997–999, 1971.

51. Karten, I.: Septic arthritis complicating rheumatoid arthritis. Ann. Intern. Med., 70:1147–1158, 1969.

52. Kelly, P. J., Coventry, M. B., and Martin, W. J.: Bacterial arthritis of the shoulder. Mayo Clin. Proc., 40:695–699, 1965.

53. Kirby, W. M. M.: Symposium on carbenicillin: A clinical profile. J. Infect. Dis. (suppl.), 122:S1–S116, 1970.

54. Kolczun, M. C., Nelson, C. L., McHenry, M. C., Gavan, T. L., and Pinovich, P.: Antibiotic concentrations in human bone. A preliminary report. J. Bone Joint Surg., 56-A(2):305–310, 1974.

55. Lawyer, R. B., and Eyring, E. J.: Intermittent closed suction-irrigation treatment of osteomyelitis. Clin. Orthop., 88:80–85, 1972.

56. Leading Article: Antibiotics for osteomyelitis. Lancet, 1:153–154, 1975.

57. Levin, P. D.: The effectiveness of various antibiotics in methyl methacrylate. J. Bone Joint Surg., 57-B(2):234–237, 1975.

58. Levison, M. E., and Kaye, D.: *In vitro* comparison of four aminoglycoside antibiotics: Sisomicin, gentamicin, tobramycin and BB-K8. Antimicrob. Agents Chemother., 5:667–669, 1974.

59. Lewis, R., Gorbach, S., and Altner, P.: Spinal pseudomonas chondro-osteomyelitis in heroin users. N. Engl. J. Med., 286:1303, 1972.

60. Lowe, R. W., and Brooks, A. L.: Hematogenous osteomyelitis. South. Med. J., 63:1183–1189, 1970.

61. MacAusland, W. R., Jr.: Treatment of sepsis after intramedullary nailing of fractures of femur. Clin. Orthop., 60:87–94, 1968.

62. Maki, D. G., Rhame, F. S., Mackel, D. C., and Bennett, J. V.: Nationwide epidemic of septicemia caused by contaminated intravenous products: 1. Epidemiologic and clinical features. Am. J. Med., 60:471–485, 1976.

63. Marrocco, G. R., Tihen, W. S., Goodnough, C. P., and Johnson, R. J.: Granulomatous synovitis and osteitis caused by Sporothrix schenckii. Am. J. Clin. Pathol., 64:345–350, 1975.

64. McHenry, M. C., Alfidi, R. J., Wilde, A. H., and Hawk, W. A.: Hematogenous osteomyelitis. A changing disease. Cleve. Clin. Q., 42:125–153, 1975.

65. Medical Letter: Antimicrobial prophylaxis for orthopedic operations. Vol. 17, No. 11, May 23, 1975.

66. Meyer, S., Weiland, A. J., and Willenegger, H.: The treatment of infected non-union of fractures of long bones. J. Bone Joint Surg., 57:836–842, 1975.

67. Meyers, B. R., Berson, B. L., Gilbert, M., and Hirschman, S. Z.: Clinical patterns of osteomyelitis due to gram-negative bacteria. Arch. Intern. Med., 131:228–233, 1973.

68. Miller, J., Brooks, C. E., and Conochie, L. B.: Montreal Symposium. Postgraduate course on "Infection and Orthopedic Surgery" held May, 1972, under auspices of Montreal General Hospital and McGill University.

69. Moellering, R. C., Jr., Dray, M., and Kunz, L. J.: Susceptibility of clinical isolates of bacteria to cefatoxin and cephalothin. Antimicrob. Agents Chemother., 6:320–323, 1974.

70. Moellering, R. C., Jr., Tratt, G., and Weinberg, A. N.: The *in vitro* antibacterial effectiveness of antibiotic-detergent combinations. J. Bone Joint Surg., 53-A:30–36, 1971.

71. Murray, H. W., Fialk, M. A., and Roberts, R. B.: Candida arthritis: A manifestation of disseminated candidiasis. Am. J. Med., 60:587–595, 1976.

72. Nastro, L. J., and Feingold, S. M.: Bactericidal activity of five antimicrobial agents against *Bacteroides fragilis*. J. Infect. Dis., 126:104–107, 1972.

73. Nicholas, P., Meyers, B. R., Levy, R. N., and Hirschman, S. Z.: Concentration of clindamycin in human bone. Antimicrob. Agents Chemother., 8:220–221, 1975.

74. Norden, C. W.: Experimental osteomyelitis. IV. Therapeutic trials with rifampin alone and in

combination with gentamicin, Sisomicin, and cephalothin. J. Infect. Dis., 132:493–499, 1975.

75. Olivero, J. J., Lozano-Mendez, J., and Ghafary, E. M., et al.: Mitigation of amphotericin B nephrotoxicity by mannitol. Br. Med. J., 1:550–551, 1975.

76. O'Reilly, R. A.: Interaction of sodium warfarin and rifampin. Studies in man. Ann. Intern. Med., 81:337–340, 1974.

77. Organ, C. H., Jr.: The utilization of massive doses of antimicrobial agents with isolation perfusion in the treatment of chronic osteomyelitis. Intermediate term results. Clin. Orthop., 76:185–193, 1971.

78. Palmer, D. L., Harvey, R. L., and Whealer, J. K.: Diagnostic and therapeutic considerations in *Nocardia asteroides* infection. Medicine, 53:391–401, 1974.

79. Parker, C. W.: Penicillin allergy. Am. J. Med., 34:747–752, 1963.

80. Parker, M. D., and Irwin, R. S.: *Mycobacterium kansasii* tendinitis and fasciitis. Report of a case treated successfully with drug therapy alone. J. Bone Joint Surg., 57-A:557–559, 1975.

81. Parker, R. H., and Schmid, F. R.: Antibacterial activity of synovial fluid during therapy of septic arthritis. Arthritis Rheum., 14:96–103, 1971.

82. Petersen, B. H., and Graham, J.: Immunologic cross-reactivity of cephalexin and penicillin. J. Lab. Clin. Med., 83:860–870, 1974.

83. Phillips, I., and Warren, C.: Susceptibility of *Bacteroides fragilis* to spectinomycin. J. Antimicrob. Chemother., 1:91–95, 1975.

84. Pontifex, A. H., and McNaught, D. R.: The treatment of chronic osteomyelitis with clindamycin. Can. Med. Assoc. J., 109:105–107, 1973.

85. Rapp, G. F., Griffith, R. S., and Hebble, W. M.: The permeability of traumatically inflamed synovial membrane to commonly used antibiotics. J. Bone Joint Surg., 48-A:1534–1540, 1966.

86. Ravn, H.: Acute hematogenous osteomyelitis due to Type-B *Haemophilus influenzae*. Lancet, 1:517–518, 1966.

87. Reeves, D. S., Wise, R., and Bywater, M. J.: A laboratory evaluation of a novel β-lactam antibiotic Mecillinam. J. Antimicrob. Chemother., 1:337–344, 1975.

88. Rodriguez, V., Inagaki, J., and Bodey, G. P.: Clinical pharmacology of Ticarcillin (α-carboxyl-3-thienylmethyl penicillin, BRL-2228). Antimicrob. Agents Chemother., 4:31–36, 1973.

89. Rosenblatt, J. E., Fallon, A., and Feingold, S. M.: Comparison of methods for isolation of anaerobic bacteruria from clinical specimens. Appl. Microbiol., 25:77–85, 1973.

90. Ruedy, J.: Antibiotic treatment of septic arthritis. Clin. Orthop., 96:150–151, 1973.

91. Russell, A. D.: The antibacterial activity of a new cephalosporin, Cephamandole. J. Antimicrob. Chemother., 1:97–101, 1975.

92. Scheuer, P. J., Summerfield, J. A., Lal, S., and Sherlock, S.: Rifampin hepatitis: A clinical and histologic study. Lancet, 1:421–425, 1974.

93. Schurman, D. J., Johnson, L. B., Jr., Finerman, G., and Amstutz, H. C.: Antibiotic bone penetration. Concentrations of methicillin and clindamycin phosphate in human bone taken during total hip replacement. Clin. Orthop., 111:142–146, 1975.

94. Smilack, J. D., Flittie, W. H., and Williams, T. W., Jr.: Bone concentrations of antimicrobial agents after parenteral administration. Antimicrob. Agents Chemother., 9:169–171, 1976.

95. Stein, S. R., Leukens, C. A., Jr., and Bagg, R. J.: Treatment of coccidioidomycosis infection of bone with local amphotericin B suction-irrigation. Report of a case. Clin. Orthop., 108:161–164, 1975.

96. Tedesco, F. J., Barton, R. W., and Alpers, D. H.: Clindamycin-associated colitis: A prospective study. Ann. Intern. Med., 81:429–433, 1974.

97. Waldvogel, F. A., Medoff, G., and Swartz, M.: Osteomyelitis: A review of clinical features, therapeutic considerations and unusual aspects. N. Engl. J. Med., 282:198–206; 260–266; 316–322, 1970.

98. Weese, W. C., and Smith, I. M.: A study of 57 cases of actinomycosis over a 36-year period: A diagnostic "failure" with good prognosis after treatment. Arch. Intern. Med., 135:1562–1568, 1975.

99. Wharton, M. R., and Beddow, F. H.: Clindamycin for acute osteomyelitis in children. Postgrad. Med. J., 51:166–168, 1975.

100. Wilson, F. C., Worcester, J. N., Coleman, P. D., and Byrd, W. E.: Antibiotic penetration of experimental bone hematomas. J. Bone Joint Surg., 53-A:1622–1628, 1971.

101. Wilson, P. D., Jr., Algietti, P., and Salvati, E. A.: Subacute sepsis of the hip treated by antibiotics and cemented prosthesis. J. Bone Joint Surg., 56-A:879–898, 1974.

102. Wilson, P. D., Jr., Salvati, E. A., Aglietti, P., and Kutner, L. J.: The problem of infection in endoprosthetic surgery of the hip joint. Clin. Orthop., 96:213–221, 1973.

7

Orthopaedic Management of Shoulder Infections

MELVIN POST

Infections of the shoulder must be eradicated quickly so that the normal function of this region can be restored. Different organisms cause varied pathologic conditions, each requiring specific consideration once the germ is identified. This chapter reviews the pathogenesis of infections, and the principles that have been found to be effective in the orthopaedic treatment of shoulder girdle infections. The surgeon should consult the previous chapter on the use of chemotherapeutic agents in order to understand the principles of how chemical agents are selected.

PYOGENIC INFECTION

Nowhere else in the human body is an understanding of the pathogenesis of bone and joint infection more crucial than in the shoulder. At times it is difficult to differentiate in the early stages between long bone and joint infection. Also, it is not enough to presume on statistical grounds that a particular organism is present merely because coagulase-positive Staphylococcus aureus is responsible for bone infections in the child and adult most often, whereas Streptococcus pyogenes causes most acute bone infections in infants (53 percent).[27]

Pathogenesis

Acute Hematogenous Osteomyelitis

Trueta reviewed the literature of the vascular anatomy of long bones, and suggested the fact that the changing vascular pattern of long bones in the first year of life, during childhood, and at puberty is responsible for three types of acute osteomyelitis.[27] He showed, for example, that the epiphyseal plate in the proximal femur acts as a vascular barrier to some vessels traversing the growth plate between the metaphysis and epiphysis between the eighth and eighteenth months. From his definition based upon the vascular anatomy, the infant becomes a child at 1 year of age. The same set of conditions holds true for the humerus.

Trueta also showed that the metaphyseal capillaries next to the growth plate are the final ramifications of the nutrient artery, except for a narrow border at the periphery of the plate.[27] These capillaries form loops and become confluent with a system of large sinusoidal veins. It is here that blood flow slows, creating a medium for pathogenic bacterial growth. Secondarily, spreading infection occludes the smaller arterioles and in time the nutrient artery itself.

Because the metaphyseal sinusoidal veins are effectively blocked by a vicious cycle of infection and increasing edema, the developing transudates reach the thin portion of the metaphysis. After extending up and down the medullary canal, pus creeps beneath the periosteum at the perforated metaphysis and elevates the cambium layer, destroying the vessel connections between this cover and the cortex. Increasing amounts of pus follow this pathway. Eventually, pus may penetrate the periosteum in the untreated case. Within 5 to 7 days in the untreated case, the raised periosteum lays down new bone called the involucrum (Fig. 7-1). At the same time, the loss of the arterial blood supply to the outer cortex and the thrombosis of the nutrient artery which supplies the inner cortex create dead bone, better known as cortical sequestrum (Fig. 7-2). The greater the degree of periosteal

stripping by the infection, the larger will be the sequestrum formation.

Because of the vascular anatomy, the growth plate usually protects both the epiphysis and the joint in the child older than 1 year of age because of the barrier it creates to the vessels that traverse it in the infant younger than 12 months of age. Thus, in the infant the epiphysis and joint are quite susceptible to the damaging effects of infection, whereas in the older child the joint and epiphysis are protected by the vascular barrier of the growth plate. However, toxemia is more dangerous to life in the child than in the infant.

Acute hematogenous osteomyelitis in the adult is uncommon.[16,17] Although it is uncommonly seen in the humerus, an increasing number of cases of hematogenous oste-

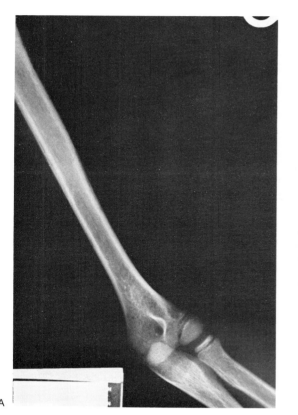
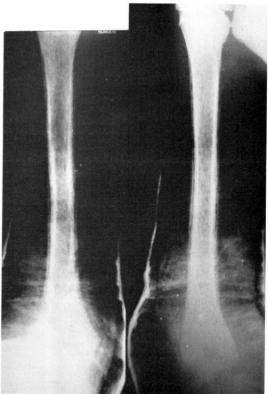

A   B

FIG. 7-1. A, A 9-year-old boy had Staphylococcus aureus infection of the humerus that was untreated for 7 days. Note the circumferential periosteal reaction about the whole humerus. The arm was immobilized in a plaster of Paris cast and intravenous antibiotics started, and the boy was observed. B, Despite this late treatment, note the increasing periosteal reaction formation at 18 days. It took another year for complete resolution of the whole process. Antibiotics were continued for several months.

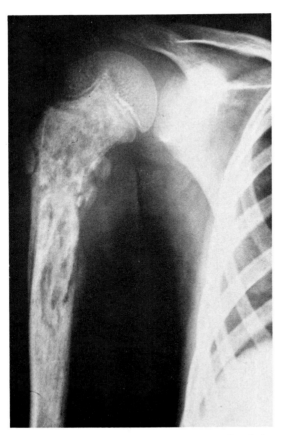

FIG. 7-2. An 11-year-old child developed a Staphylococcus aureus osteomyelitis infection of the humerus. Although correctly diagnosed in the first 24 hours and treated with antibiotics, the disease process progressed. The child was merely observed without surgically draining the shaft. At 6 weeks note the large sequestrum formation which required two late operations and prolonged immobilization of the extremity to stop pus drainage and restore normal function to the extremity.

omyelitis of the humerus, clavicle, and sternoclavicular region are now being seen in heroin addicts. The periosteal cover in the adult is closely adherent to the cortex and less elastic than that in the child or in the infant. Thus, it is unlikely that a large involucrum or sequestrum will form as it does in the infant. Rather, extraperiosteal abscesses and chronic sinuses may result with inadequate treatment.[27] In the adult the whole cortex is usually affected and may lead to chronicity. The sequence of events often leads to septic arthritis.

Curtis and Klein studied the effect of staphylococcal pus and various proteolytic enzymes on the structural integrity of articular cartilage in vitro.[11] They demonstrated that loss of collagen content was necessary for the visible gross destruction of joint cartilage, and that only collagenase causes this situation. Destructive effects of other proteolytic enzymes occur only after thermal denaturation of the cartilage collagen, whereas with physiologic temperatures denaturation of collagen is not seen. Thus, the precise mechanism of cartilage destruction is not yet understood, although it is increasingly likely that lysosomal enzymes may cause the cartilage to break down in septic arthritis. Daniel and associates showed that when septic joints infected with S. aureus are produced in rabbits and the joint is surgically lavaged, there is a delay of collagen loss by temporarily washing out whatever is causing the cartilage destruction.[12]

Diagnosis

Acute Hematogenous Osteomyelitis

Even with the advent of the wide use of antibiotics significant numbers of cases of acute hematogenous osteomyelitis are seen each year. The classic course of the disease is marked by severe pain, muscle splinting of the infected part, high fever, and vomiting. Quite often, a patient will have only mild fever, a history of upper respiratory infection, or trauma.[10] The indiscriminate use of antibiotics may mask symptoms and even hinder the diagnosis. Localized osseous tenderness is an essential feature for establishing an early diagnosis.

As the disease progresses fever tends to rise along with the white blood cell count. Infants seem to be less toxic than the older child. Anemia may appear and increase rapidly, and as toxicity increases electrolyte imbalance supervenes. Thereafter, the osseous lesion may be overlooked as systemic manifestations increase.

Many times, multiple antibiotics are given without knowing the organism, and there is

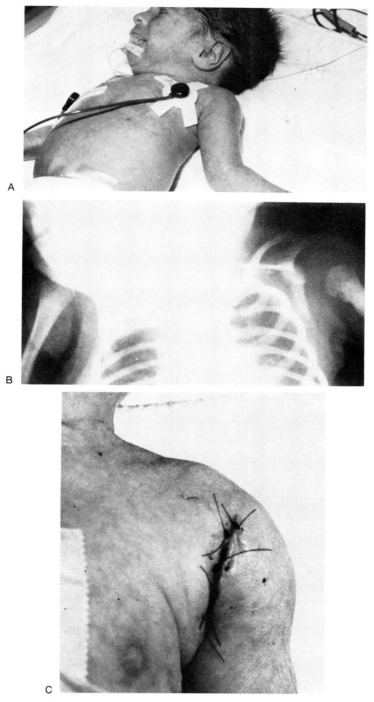

FIG. 7-3. A, A premature girl weighing 1600 gm. developed omphalitis 3 days after birth and 24 hours later a high fever which could not be controlled with intravenous antibiotics. At 6 days, the shoulder swelled dramatically. Pus was obtained from the glenohumeral joint by aspiration. B, Note the subluxation of the infected shoulder joint and the early involvement of the medial humeral metaphysis (S. aureus). It was impossible to state whether the infection started in the joint or the shaft. The joint was drained on the sixth day when the infant became toxic. C, Note the contour of the shoulder 4 days after surgical drainage. The baby became afebrile the next day. Intravenous cephalothin (Keflin) was continued for 3 weeks. Resolution of infection was complete.

some improvement in the systemic status of the patient. Mistakenly, the surgeon may believe he has cured the patient. In these cases, pressure tenderness may persist over the infected area, usually at the metaphysis, even with few visible findings. Thus, the surgeon should persist in searching for the offending organism.

A complete history should be taken. Especially ominous is the development of omphalitis in the first few weeks of life (Fig. 7-3). Acute hematogenous osteomyelitis in infants has a rapid course, and the diagnosis often is discovered too late to prevent irreparable damage to the joint and epiphysis. The diagnosis should not be based on a high fever alone for the temperature may remain in the normal range.[3,4,5] In the older child systemic manifestations are more likely to be present.

The erythrocyte sedimentation rate is consistently elevated and therefore is a more reliable test than is the white blood cell count. Although leukocytosis may at times remain within normal limits, there is usually a left shift of the differential white blood cell count. S. aureus is more likely to be associated with infection in older children in comparison to hemolytic Streptococcus found more often with infections in infants.

Changes on roentgenograms may be observed as early as the end of the fourth day after long bone infection starts in the infant and young child. Certainly, by the fifth to seventh days periosteal reaction is seen in most untreated full-blown cases of acute osteomyelitis.

Septic Arthritis

At times it is difficult to differentiate septic arthritis from acute hematogenous osteomyelitis, especially in the young patient. In septic arthritis the patient may have few symptoms, but most often complains of severe joint pain. The temperature may range from normal to high. The course of the disease in children can be fulminating.

The shoulder joint may swell dramatically in a short period (Fig. 7-3). This finding is related not only to the accumulation of fluid in the joint but to synovial hypertrophy and inflammation. Synovial hypertrophy can be differentiated from joint effusion because hypertrophied synovium erodes adjacent bone even in joint recesses located a distance from the joint.[8] The patient holds the upper extremity in a splinted position with the arm at the side of the body. There appears to be no correlation between the course of the disease and outcome of the infection.

The erythrocyte sedimentation rate usually rises along with the white blood cell count. There is a shift to the left with a predominance of neutrophils. Diagnosis of the offending organism depends upon results of blood cultures and cultures of any aspirated joint fluid. Even in children when the offending organism cannot be discovered, one should look for an occasional gonococcal[15] or brucellar infection.[1] When unusual infections are suspected, special serologic testing may become necessary.[1,21] The range of the white blood cell count varies with the type of infecting organism. For example, in aspirated fluid the cell count of nongonococcal infecting organisms ranged from 11,560 wbc/mm.[3] with 85 percent neutrophils to 104,000 wbc/mm.[3] with 90 percent neutrophils.[3] When fibrin enters the joint fluid the joint exudate may clot, making aspiration difficult or impossible at times.[10]

Roentgenograms show late changes about the joint usually 10 to 14 days after the onset of the infection.[9] Thus, the surgeon should not rely on roentgenograms to establish an early diagnosis. Decalcification of the epiphysis and metaphysis may occur, but only the injured growth plate and epiphyseal cartilage determine the outcome of the infection.[20] It is not unusual to observe shoulder joint subluxation, fragmentation, and periosteal changes including periosteal elevation, especially if there is secondary rupture of a long bone infection into the joint[5,10] (Figs. 7-3 and 7-4).

A significant number of children with septic arthritis may have negative results of cultures, especially if antibiotics have been

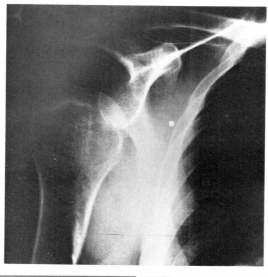

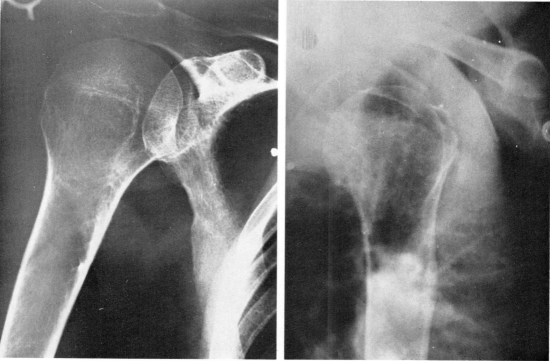

FIG. 7-4. A, A 43-year-old woman developed a septic dislocation of the glenohumeral joint, and high fever. The joint was aspirated and lavaged three times through a large-bore needle. Escherichia coli was obtained and successfully treated with intravenous cephalothin (Keflin). B, Anteroposterior and, C, transthoracic lateral films show the joint 10 days later. At 6 weeks post-treatment, motion was complete.

given previously. These patients are considered to have septic arthritis if joint motion increases pain, the joint is swollen, systemic toxic symptoms are present, fever is present, but no other pathologic processes are present.[23] Moreover, the patient must also have either a positive result of blood culture or two or three conditions including (1) aspirated pus from the joint, (2) a marked increase in the erythrocyte sedimentation rate, or (3) joint changes on roentgenograms.

The differential diagnosis should include diverse conditions such as infantile cortical hyperostosis in the first 3 months of life, and luetic bone infection, especially when it is congenital.

Brodie's Abscess

Brodie's abscess can be recognized as a small, isolated area of destruction of the cancellous bone. It is caused by a chronic attenuated pyogenic infection. Although any organism may cause this lesion Staphylococcus is commonly implicated. It is most often seen in young adult men.

The condition is first noticed when the patient complains of a deep pain in the arm that may be worse at night and might cause the surgeon to suspect osteoid osteoma on clinical grounds. There are no systemic symptoms.

Roentgen examination reveals a central area of bone destruction near the end of the humerus but without periosteal reaction in contrast to Garré's osteomyelitis. In Brodie's abscess a small central radiolucent area may contain a minute central sequestrum surrounded by an area of sclerosis of varying degrees.

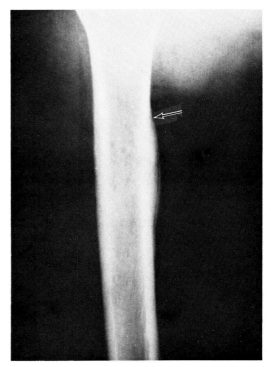

FIG. 7-5. A 19-year-old girl complained of pain in the upper arm for several months but had no other symptoms. There was only slight tenderness over the shaft on deep palpation. A biopsy specimen was obtained at the site beneath the arrow before Garré's nonsuppurative osteomyelitis was differentiated from a bone tumor. At operation, the medullary canal was curetted and specimens for culture and sensitivity studies obtained that later showed S. aureus. The wound was closed tight and antibiotics started. Resolution of the infection was complete.

Garré's Nonsuppurative Osteomyelitis

Garré's osteomyelitis does not suppurate, but is included here in the differential diagnosis because this lesion is characterized by bone production and sclerosis, with interspersed small areas of bone destruction (Fig. 7-5).

The disease is present in youth and in middle age. Temperature may be normal or high. The onset may be insidious, extending over months or even years. Pain with or without swelling may be present.

The most notable roentgen feature is sclerosis of bone (Fig. 7-5). It may even occlude the medullary canal. Interspersed

areas of bone destruction may have a moth-eaten appearance.

Differential diagnosis should include osteogenic and Ewing's sarcoma.

Management

Acute Hematogenous Osteomyelitis

Successful management depends upon early diagnosis and effective treatment. Results of blood culture and antibiotic sensitivities should be obtained in order to establish early bacteriologic diagnosis. Clawson and Dunn have shown that such testing yields a positive result in more than 50 percent of patients.[10] In addition, other sources of possible infection should be sought. As soon as all results of the cultures are obtained, antibiotic treatment should be started. Because the most common organism is S. aureus, antibiotic therapy should be directed toward this germ until the precise organism is known. Large doses of antibiotic by the intravenous route are recommended until symptoms and adverse findings abate, as evidenced by a fall in fever, the erythrocyte sedimentation rate, and the white blood cell count. It is at this point that antibiotics are given by the oral route. For acute joint and long bone infections, I prefer 3 to 4 weeks of intravenous antibiotics in most instances before changing to the oral route from a few weeks to several months, depending on the severity of the infection. If no organism is discovered in the initial cultures and the patient responds satisfactorily, antibiotic treatment is continued.

The infected upper extremity should be immobilized, usually by splinting the arm at the side of the body. This helps to diminish pain and prevent pathologic fracture if the disease process has weakened the bone (Figs. 7-1 and 7-2).

The vast majority of patients do not require surgical treatment if an early diagnosis is established and effective treatment initiated and continued. The primary aim of treatment is to be able to judge when not to open a bone surgically, and yet not defer surgical drainage when it is required. A major goal of treatment is to prevent periosteal stripping. If treatment is delayed for 72 hours, the accumulation of pus increases marrow pressure and causes the periosteal cover to become elevated. In this situation, incision and drainage over the maximum point of tenderness at the metaphysis should be performed early to prevent stripping of the periosteum. The bone should not merely be drilled. A square or core or metaphyseal plug should be removed and the canal curetted. Failure to achieve early drainage leads to progressive involucrum and sequestrum formation (Figs. 7-1 and 7-2). If pus is obtained, specimens for additional cultures and antibiotic sensitivities

are taken. The wound should not be closed tightly. A drain or tube system with continuous irrigation of the infected part should be used to permit residual pus a path of exit.

Chronic Osteomyelitis

When a large amount of sequestrum is present and it appears that it will fail to be absorbed for a long time, sequestrectomy and external immobilization of the weakened humerus should be performed so that the earliest possible return of function may be achieved. If at all possible, sequestrectomy should be deferred until enough new bone involucrum can sustain the length of the shaft without fracture. In this event I use continuous closed-tube drainage with isotonic saline solution. At times more than one such operation may be needed to achieve adequate healing and prevent drainage of pus. The extremity should be immobilized to protect it from fracture. I do not use early skin grafting as advocated by Shannon and associates[25] but wait for subsidence of purulent, draining material and clean granulation tissue before effecting wound closure. I reserve bone grafting procedures for large defects or nonunions when infection has been eradicated. The chief principles in treatment are to rid the bone of infectious material, to preserve the articular cartilage, and to avoid injury to the growth plate.

Pyogenic Arthritis

Most septic joints can be treated with closed methods, but must be opened when more conservative methods fail.[20] The surgeon cannot rely entirely on physical findings in deciding whether or not to surgically drain a joint. For example, the shoulder capsule is more likely to be distended in children than in adults (Fig. 7-3). However, the degree of distension cannot be correlated with which cases should be opened and which merely aspirated one or more times. Compared to other joints such as the hip with little room for distension, the shoulder joint is more elastic and more distensible. In any event, results of appropriate culture and sensitivity studies should be obtained and the shoulder joint aspirated as often as deemed necessary to keep pus from accumulating. I prefer lavage of the joint with physiologic saline solution through a large-bore needle following a surgical preparation of the skin.[12] If there is no response within 48 hours, surgical drainage of the joint is instituted (Fig. 7-3).[3] Other joints such as the hip are not treated in the same manner; arthrotomy is more likely to be performed on these joints. If the shoulder joint is opened, a drain is left in place in order to allow for gravitational drainage. It is removed when no further outflow of pus is present. In an increasing number of cases I have used a continuous closed-tube drainage system with isotonic saline solution as the irrigating fluid. This system has been maintained as long as 3 weeks in a few instances. The tubes are usually removed when results of cultures of the joint effluence become negative. The principle to remember is that pus should not be allowed to accumulate in the shoulder joint, and that it is possible to remove it by needle lavage in a high percentage of cases. However, when this is not possible or an associated osteomyelitis is present that cannot be controlled, opening the joint is preferable to taking chances. Whether one elects to instill antibiotic into the joint at the time depends on individual preference. I rely more on lavage with saline solution and systemic antibiotics.

If the growth plate is injured and shortening of the humerus results, unlike the lower extremity shortening of the arm is compatible with good function.

Brodie's Abscess

Treatment of a Brodie abscess consists of removing a plug or core of bone and curetting the abscess cavity. I have treated these lesions successfully by employing a drain, pack, or Hemovac closed drainage system when pus is found.

Garré's Nonsuppurative Osteomyelitis

More often than not, operation is performed for diagnosis as well as for treatment. In fact, the surgeon may elect to await permanent slide diagnosis before deciding on a course of treatment (Fig. 7-5).

At the time of the initial operation, a plug or core of bone is removed, usually near one end of the lesion in order to obtain some normal bone tissue as well. The medullary cavity is curetted, and culture and sensitivity studies are performed from this tissue. The wound is closed without drains because pus is not ordinarily found in this lesion.

When the diagnosis is made after biopsy, the patient is started on a course of appropriate antibiotic therapy that is continued perhaps for several months, if necessary, until adverse signs and symptoms abate and any abnormal laboratory findings return to normal.

INFECTION IN OPEN FRACTURE OR AFTER OPERATION

Wound sepsis can be avoided in many cases if careful cleansing is practiced. When an open fracture occurs, further contamination of the wound should be prevented. The wound should be covered with a sterile dressing or a sterile compress soaked in aqueous benzalkonium chloride (Zephiran). The surgeon should not be tempted to reduce dirty exposed bone, further introducing filth and organisms into the soft tissues.

The wound must be cleansed in a systematic manner in order to minimize the possibility of infection. The cleansing should be performed in an operating room environment. The wound is sealed with clean sterile dressings and the entire extremity is surgically prepared with pHisoHex. If povidone-iodine (Betadine) is used, it should not be allowed to enter the raw wound. Once the entire extremity and shoulder region are cleaned, a second preparation tray and new sterile gloves are employed. First, the wound is copiously irrigated with sterile saline solution, and the extremity and wound again are surgically cleansed. Finally, the wound and surrounding skin are irrigated with sterile saline solution. If one wishes, the normal skin but not the wound is painted with aqueous Zephiran. Only then is debridement carried out. It must be thorough, even rongeuring dirty surfaces of bone and irrigating the wound repeatedly.

The skin edges should not be closed tightly. In dirty wounds a drain should be used. In some exceptionally contaminated or infected wounds, it is first necessary to eradicate the infection, establishing drainage for the purulent material, immobilizing the extremity, and using correct antibiotic treatment based on results of cultures and antibiotic sensitivity studies if fracture healing is to occur. Eventually, the fracture will heal on the periosteal side opposite the draining bone in many instances.

When internal fixation devices or prostheses are already present in the bone and infection is present, the devices are maintained as long as the infection is contained. Two signs that suggest an infected implant are periosteal formation and progressive bone lysis.[9] Arthrography may demonstrate an infected loosened prosthesis. If an intramedullary rod in the humerus is providing rigid fixation for a fracture, it is not removed as long as it is not causing the persistence of a nonunion. When an implant does predispose to continued infection and tends to become a liability to better shoulder function, it should be removed.

Infection associated with purulent accumulation following operation should be treated vigorously with adequate open drainage and antibiotics. Should a chronic sinus tract develop, it is mandatory to excise the entire tract no matter what its course (Fig. 7-6). A Renografin sinogram will not always show all of the sinuses and closed pockets. At operation, the tracts should be injected with methylene blue to outline as many of the sinuses as possible. The dye will not show all the infected tissues but may provide some idea as to the extent of the sinus tracts. During operation, all sinus tracts, dead bone, and scar tissue should be excised. Most infected wounds can be treated with primary closure and irrigation-suction techniques if the debridement has been adequate. Entry and exit tubes are used with a continuous flow of large amounts of sterile saline solution in the first 24 hours (up to 10 L.). After 24 hours the tubes can become secondarily infected. In this case, I have used a mixture of 0.5 percent acetic acid in sterile saline solution, occasionally adding 20 ml. of Betadine solution/liter of solution in the more superficial wounds. In no event do I employ more than 3 L. of the latter solution in a 24-hour period.

If the effluence remains perfectly clear for 24 to 48 hours, and there is no other systemic evidence of infection, the tubes are removed. Otherwise, the closed irrigation system is maintained for much longer periods or certainly until cultures show no growth. Systemic antibiotics are continued for 3 to 4 weeks, and oral antibiotics for a longer period thereafter, if deemed necessary.

TUBERCULOSIS AND RELATED INFECTIONS

Pathogenesis

Originally, Mycobacterium tuberculosis was the organism associated with tuberculosis in man, while M. bovis and M. avium later became associated with the disease. Later, a number of other pathogenic mycobacteria were found to cause similar disease in various animals. A number of atypical mycobacteria also cause destruction of the joints and the soft tissues about the articulations. However, they do not necessarily produce the classic pathologic lesions described for true tuberculosis.

Hematogenous dissemination of bacilli is the greatest cause of skeletal tuberculosis in the early stages of the infection. In one study in children less than 13 years of age, bone infection occurred with greatest frequency among survivors of miliary tuberculosis.[22] In some cases, the dissemination of infection to the long bones may result from lymphatic spread. Interestingly, lym-

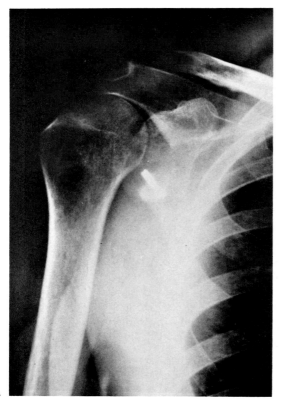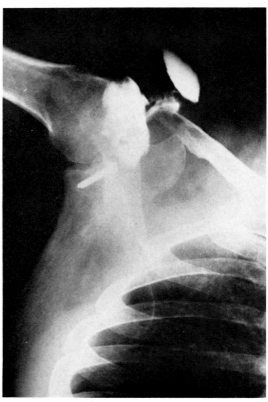

A

B

FIG. 7-6. A, A 31-year-old man developed a sinus tract infection following a Helfet-Bristow repair for recurring shoulder dislocations. Multiple procedures failed to cure the infection. B, A sinogram with the arm in abduction shows the outline of a part of the tract involving the glenohumeral joint. The tract was excised and a synovectomy of the infected lining performed. Although there was no recurrence, severe preoperative stiffness persisted. The infecting organism was identified as S. aureus.

phatics have been observed in all joint tissues except cartilage. It has been noted that trauma may play a significant role in the pathogenesis of bone tuberculosis, since the weight-bearing joints are more often involved than are those of the upper extremity. Smyrnis suggested that severe trauma lowers tissue resistance and facilitates the implantation and growth of tuberculous organisms.[26]

The essential lesion in most cases is a combination of osteomyelitis and arthritis. The joint space is invaded either directly by the hematogenous route or indirectly from lesions in the epiphysis eroding into the joint space. At first a synovitis develops that is followed by the formation of granulation tissue. A synovial effusion forms in which fibrin may precipitate with the formation of "rice" bodies. The pathologic lesions in the soft tissues about bone are the same as those in soft tissues elsewhere.[6,7] The process proceeds from the stages of inflammation to caseation necrosis, then to fibrosis and calcification, and eventually to ulceration with sinus formation after liquefaction occurs in the soft tissues.

Initially, the development of a pannus of granulation tissue causes an erosion and destruction of cartilage, and eventually of the underlying cancellous bone, leading to increasing bone demineralization and increased caseation necrosis (Fig. 7-7). The cartilage is first destroyed peripherally, sparing the joint space for a long time. Proteolytic enzymes are not produced in tuberculous joint infection as they are in pyogenic infections. In any event, paraosseous soft-tissue cold abscesses may result.

In time, the formation of fibrous tissue

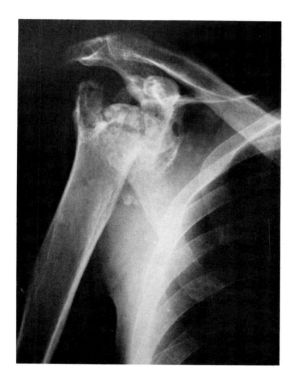

FIG. 7-7. A 44-year-old man was treated for lupus erythematosus with steroids. Shoulder function decreased. Note the collapsed humeral head and destroyed glenoid. At operation, M. tuberculosis caseation was found. The infection was not expected. Necrotic bone fragments were removed and the patient started on chemotherapy. The M. tuberculosis infection was controlled.

causes joint stiffness. Bosworth has suggested that the greatest destruction is caused by abscess formation, pressure effects, and stripping of the blood supply from its osseous structure, resulting in sequestrum in adults and bone dissolution in the younger patient.[6]

Incidence

Although tuberculous infections of the musculoskeletal system are decreasing in the Western World, they still constitute a significant and serious percentage of the infections affecting joints elsewhere. The peak incidence of this infection occurs in older patients.[18] Davidson and Horowitz reported that over a 25-year period in one New York City hospital the bone and joint complication rate was 5 percent in a large

group of children hospitalized with primary pulmonary tuberculosis.[13] Moreover, skeletal tuberculosis eventually developed during follow-up in about 1 percent of children with primary tuberculosis.

Diagnosis

The surgeon must remember to include this disease in the differential diagnosis of shoulder disabilities. Often, there is too much reliance on roentgen examination alone to permit early diagnosis. This is unfortunate, because early in the disease process the articular cartilage and joint space are preserved. Walker showed that of 18 new cases of skeletal tuberculosis seen during 1 year, 9 cases were misdiagnosed, the average delay in diagnosis being 19 months.[28] The time between onset of symptoms until confirmation of the diagnosis ranged from 3 to 48 months in all 18 patients studied.

The symptoms and findings of the tuberculous infection are well known. Night cries, sustained temperature elevation, joint swelling, loss of joint function, and eventually bone destruction, and deformity are salient features of the condition.[7] The surgeon must not await the destructive changes about the shoulder and abscess formation to occur before establishing the diagnosis.

The tuberculin skin test is still valuable in suggesting the diagnosis. A negative result of the skin test does not entirely exclude the diagnosis. In this event, a second strength purified protein derivative test should be performed. A persistently negative result of the skin test is of value in excluding the diagnosis. Culture of the joint fluid or abscess aspirate as well as a routine smear of the material often helps to confirm the diagnosis.

When the tubercle bacillus cannot be found, pyogenic infection, sarcoid, fungi, and even syphilis should be considered in the differential diagnosis.[24]

An abnormal finding on a roentgenogram of the shoulder should lead one to obtain a biopsy specimen of the lesion early if a diagnosis by culture cannot be achieved. Nonspecific roentgen findings of soft-tissue swelling and joint distension of the capsule may be seen. Cartilage destruction later may be manifested by narrowing of the glenohumeral joint space and bone erosion at the articular surface or at the periphery. In addition to bone biopsy, synovial biopsy may be fruitful.

Treatment

In the presence of a positive result of a skin test and a pathology report of granulation tissue compatible with tuberculosis, there is enough evidence to initiate therapy. Appropriate early chemotherapy now controls tuberculosis in most cases. Early joint involvement is best treated by chemotherapy and immobilization. In late stages of the joint disease, synovectomy, debridement, and removal of necrotic bone and pus may be needed to control the disease. If chemotherapy is used and surgical debridement is performed in severe cases, arthrodesis may be avoided. However, surgical fusion may still be necessary.[2] In any event, contemplated surgical treatment should be deferred until the patient has received chemotherapy for 2 to 3 months.

Kelly and co-workers reported 12 cases in which infected soft-tissue lesions resulted from seeding with mycobacteria other than M. tuberculosis.[19] The lesions may be caused by operative incisions, accidental puncture wounds, or injections and lacerations. For their cases, Kelly and associates recommended surgical excision of the diseased tissue. These organisms are not usually susceptible to drug therapy in most of these infections owing to the insensitivity of the organisms to the chemotherapeutic agents. Such infections are not at all rare. When they occur they may be virulent and unresponsive to treatment.

SALMONELLA OSTEOMYELITIS

An increasing number of salmonella osteomyelitis cases have been observed in patients with sickle cell disease in recent years. This apparent rise in the number of cases probably results from patients referred to the tertiary care centers for specialized treatment. Those patients afflicted with hemoglobinopathies and particularly sickle cell disease are most prone to develop this infection because of a number of factors. Most notably, these include thrombosis and bone infarction, the mode of entry of gram-negative organisms via the intestinal tract later spreading through the lymphatics and reticuloendothelial system of the liver, spleen, and bone marrow, and the high concentration of bilirubin or other red blood cell breakdown products within the second portion of the duodenum, which seem to enhance the development of salmonella infection.[14]

Diagnosis

The patient with sickle cell disease and other S hemoglobinopathies often complains of shoulder pain when the humeral head is involved in the disease process. At times salmonella osteomyelitis may develop which has a subacute or an insidious onset.[14] Symptoms include mild fever and bone tenderness at multiple sites that may persist for 1 to 3 weeks before changes of osteomyelitis are observed on roentgenograms. Since the clinical picture of sickle cell crises and the associated symptoms may be confused with the symptoms and signs of salmonella osteomyelitis, the surgeon should rely on results of blood and stool cultures for diagnosis. Most cases show spiking fever, persistent leukocytosis, and extensive roentgen findings, including an abundant involucrum formation and involvement of multiple diaphyseal sites (Fig. 7-8, see also Fig. 5-35).

Occasionally, even when the blood cultures demonstrate no growth, the shoulder joint may swell dramatically and the patient may become toxic (Fig. 7-9).

Treatment

The same principles of treatment hold for salmonella osteomyelitis as for other acute

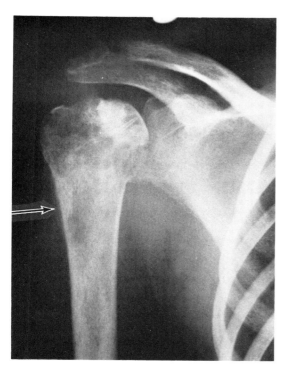

FIG. 7-8. A 24-year-old woman with sickle cell disease. The patient developed a salmonella septic arthritis that was controlled with aspiration and intravenous antibiotics. Nevertheless, 6 months later she developed periosteal reaction changes (arrow) and osteonecrotic areas in the humeral head.

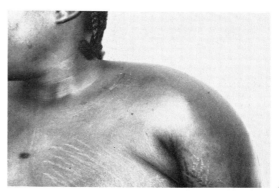

A

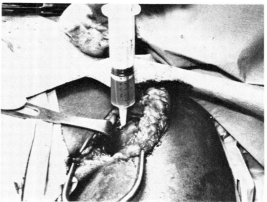

B

FIG. 7-9. A, A 19-year-old girl developed a septic arthritis and was treated with intravenous antibiotics. Her fever rose to 104°F and the shoulder swelled. Cultures showed no growth. B, The glenohumeral joint was incised and drained when the patient failed to respond to closed treatment. At operation, note the pus aspirated from the joint in the syringe. Cultures again showed no growth. Hemovac drainage was instituted with continuous saline irrigation for 10 days. Antibiotic therapy was continued for 4 months. The infection abated and shoulder function was restored.

bone infections. If appropriate antibiotic therapy fails to control the infection, the bone should be decompressed. In bone that shows significant infarction secondary to sickle cell disease, surgical drainage of the bone will fail to preserve the bone. Often, multiple sites of bone are involved so that surgery is fruitless. However, when the shoulder joint itself is involved in the septic process and repeated aspirations fail to control the infection, surgical drainage of the joint is indicated, as it is in any condition of septic arthritis (Fig. 7-9).

REFERENCES

1. Adam, A., MacDonald, A., and MacKenzie, I. G.: Monarticular brucellar arthritis in children. J. Bone Joint Surg., 49-B:652–657, 1967.
2. Allen, A. R., and Stevenson, A. W.: The results of combined drug therapy and early fusion in bone tuberculosis. J. Bone Joint Surg., 39-A:32–42, 1957.
3. Baitch, A.: Recent observations of acute suppurative arthritis. Clin. Orthop. 22:157–165, 1962.
4. Blanche, D. W.: Osteomyelitis in infants, J. Bone Joint Surg., 34-A:71–85, 1952.
5. Borella, L., Goobar, J. E., Summitt, R. L., and Clark, G. M.: Septic arthritis in childhood. J. Pediatr., 62:742–747, 1963.
6. Bosworth, D. M.: Modern concepts of treatment of tuberculosis of bone and joints. Ann. N.Y. Acad. Sci., 106:98–105, 1963.
7. Bosworth, D. M.: Bone and joint tuberculosis in

childhood. Pediatr. Clin. North Am., 1129–1136, November, 1955.

8. Butt, W. P.: The radiology of infection. Clin. Orthop., 96:20–30, 1973.
9. Butt, W. P.: Radiology of the infected joint. Clin. Orthop., 96:136–149, 1973.
10. Clawson, D. K., and Dunn, A. W.: Management of common bacterial infections of bones and joints. J. Bone Joint Surg., 49-A:164–182, 1967.
11. Curtis, P. G., and Klein, L.: Destruction of articular cartilage in septic arthritis. *In vitro* studies. J. Bone Joint Surg., 45-A:797–806, 1963.
12. Daniel, D., Akeson, W., Amiel, D., Ryder, M., and Boyer, J.: Lavage of septic joints in rabbits: Effects of chondrolysis. J. Bone Joint Surg., 58-A:393–395, 1976.
13. Davidson, P. T., and Horowitz, I.: Skeletal tuberculosis. A review with patient presentations and discussion. Am. J. Med., 48:77–84, 1970.
14. Engh, C. A., Hughes, J. L., Abrams, R. C., and Bowerman, J. W.: Osteomyelitis in the patient with sickle-cell disease. J. Bone Joint Surg., 53-A:1–15, 1971.
15. Fink, C. W.: Gonococcal arthritis in children. J.A.M.A., 194:237–238, 1965.
16. Kelly, P. J.: Bacterial arthritis in the adult. Orthop. Clin. North Am., 6:973–981, 1975.
17. Kelly, P. J.: Osteomyelitis in the adult. Orthop. Clin. North Am., 6:983–989, 1975.
18. Kelly, P. J., and Karlson, A. G.: Musculoskeletal tuberculosis. Mayo Clin. Proc., 44:73–80, 1969.
19. Kelly, P. J., Weed, L. A., and Lipscomb, P. R.: Infection of tendon sheaths bursae, joints, and soft

tissues by acid fast bacilli other than tubercle bacilli. J. Bone Joint Surg., 45-A:327–336, 1963.
20. Lloyd-Roberts, G. C.: Suppurative arthritis of infancy. Some observations upon prognosis and management. J. Bone Joint Surg., 42-B:706–720, 1960.
21. Merritt, K., Boyle, W. E., Dye, S. K., and Porter, R. E.: Counter immunoelectrophoresis in the diagnosis of septic arthritis caused by Hemophilus influenzae. Report of two cases. J. Bone Joint Surg., 58-A:414–415, 1976.
22. Milgram, L.: Skeletal tuberculosis in children treated for primary and miliary tuberculosis. Am. Rev. Tuberc., 75:897–911, 1957.
23. Mills, T. J., Owen, R., and Strach, E. H.: Early diagnosis of bone and joint tuberculosis in children. Lancet, 271:57–59, 1956.
24. O'Connor B. T., Steel, W. M., and Sanders, R.: Disseminated bone tuberculosis. J. Bone Joint Surg., 52-A:537–542, 1970.
25. Shannon, J. G., Woolhouse, F. M., and Eisinger, P. J.: The treatment of chronic osteomyelitis by saucerization and immediate skin grafting. Clin. Orthop., 96:98–107, 1973.
26. Smyrnis, P.: Hematogenous infection of closed fracture with Mycobacterium tuberculosis. J. Bone Joint Surg., 39-A:902–904, 1957.
27. Trueta, J.: The three types of acute haematogenous osteomyelitis. A clinical and vascular study. J. Bone Joint Surg., 41-B:671–680, 1959.
28. Walker, C. F.: Failure of early recognition of skeletal tuberculosis. Br. Med. J., 1:682–683, 1968.

8

Neurologic Aspects of the Shoulder

HAROLD L. KLAWANS

JORDAN L. TOPEL

The functionally significant muscles of the shoulder area are innervated primarily from the fourth, fifth, and sixth cervical nerve root segments. Dysfunction in the central nervous system, connections to these nerve roots, the peripheral nerves to the area, or the shoulder muscles themselves may give rise to neurologic symptoms and signs at the shoulder region. The neuromuscular disorders affecting the shoulder girdle can be classified according to the site of neurologic dysfunction:

I. Dysfunction at the Spinal Cord Level
   A. Mass lesions
      1. Spinal cord tumors, including intramedullary, extradural and intradural, extramedullary
      2. Syringomyelia
      3. Epidural abscess
   B. Other infections, including poliomyelitis, tuberculosis, fungi, and syphilis
   C. Motor neuron disease
      1. Werdnig-Hoffmann disease (infantile progressive muscular atrophy)
      2. Kugelberg-Welander disease (a chronic proximal muscular atrophy)
      3. Progressive muscular atrophy
      4. Amyotrophic lateral sclerosis

II. Dysfunction of Nerve Roots
   A. Cervical spondylosis
   B. Cervical disc disease
   C. Tabes dorsalis
   D. Herpes zoster
III. Dysfunction of Peripheral Nerves
   A. Brachial plexus lesions
   B. Brachial plexus neuritis (neuralgic amyotrophy)
   C. Thoracic outlet syndrome
   D. Cervical ribs
   E. Shoulder-hand syndrome
   F. Tumors
   G. Peripheral neuropathies
IV. Dysfunction at the Myoneural Junction
   A. Myasthenia gravis
   B. Eaton-Lambert syndrome (myasthenic syndrome)
V. Neuromuscular Disorders
   A. Dystrophies (inherited myopathies)
      1. Duchenne sex-linked muscular dystrophy
      2. Limb-girdle dystrophy
      3. Facioscapulohumeral dystrophy
      4. Oculopharyngeal muscular dystrophy
      5. Scapuloperoneal atrophy
   B. Inflammatory disorders
      1. Polymyositis
      2. Myositis associated with collagen-vascular disease
      3. Polymyalgia rheumatica

4. Sarcoidosis
C. Other disorders
   1. Carcinomatous neuromyopathy
   2. Thyroid myopathy

The symptoms and signs, arising from the disorders listed, are variable and depend upon the location of the pathologic lesion. For example, a lesion involving the anterior horn cells of the spinal cord (lower motor neuron) will produce atrophy (a decrease in muscle bulk) and fasciculations (fine, rapid, twitching movements appearing with contractions of a bundle or fasciculus of muscle fibers). Involvement of nerve roots or peripheral nerves may give rise to paresthesias (spontaneous tingling, burning, or electric sensations) or dysesthesias (tingling, burning, evoked by stimuli such as rubbing the skin over the affected nerve or nerve root distribution). Pain may be radiating (following a nerve or nerve root distribution) as with cervical disc disease or localized as is often seen with intramedullary spinal cord tumors. Weakness and numbness may also be present, depending on what elements of the nervous system are involved. In addition, specific weakness at the shoulder may be secondary to a tumor in the spinal canal at the fifth cervical level, or the weakness may be a more focal representation of a diffuse process, such as is seen with myasthenia gravis.

This chapter will focus on both the focal and general neurologic processes which can give rise to shoulder girdle dysfunction and pathology, a clear understanding of which will help the physician render better treatment.

DYSFUNCTION AT THE SPINAL CORD LEVEL

Figure 8-1 is a cross section of the spinal cord at the level of the fifth cervical segment. The clinically significant anatomic tracts and divisions are presented in more detail in Table 8-1.

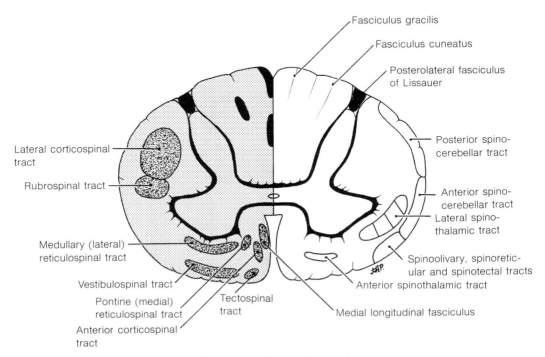

FIG. 8-1. Cross section of the spinal cord at the level of the fifth cervical segment.

Table 8-1. *Clinical Correlation of Significant Spinal Cord Anatomy*

Anatomic Division	Composition	Clinical Features of a Lesion
Anterior horn cells	Cell body of peripheral nerve (lower motor neurons)	Weakness and atrophy of the particular muscles innervated; fasciculations; decreased or no deep tendon reflexes
Corticospinal tract	Continuation of pyramidal tract (upper motor neurons)	Hemiplegia ipsilateral to the lesion; increased deep tendon reflexes; positive Babinski sign
Lateral spinothalamic tract	Relays pain and temperature sensations to thalamus and cerebral hemispheres	Loss of pain and temperature sensations below the level of the lesion, contralateral to the lesion
Decussation of the lateral spinothalamic tract	Relays pain and temperature fibers from the dorsal roots to the lateral spinothalamic tract	Suspended sensory level; loss of pain and temperature sensations bilaterally at the level of the lesion
Posterior columns (tractus gracilis and cuneatus)	Relays position and vibratory sensations to the thalamus	Loss of vibratory and position sensations below the level of the lesion, ipsilateral to the lesion
Intermediolateral cell column	Carries sympathetic nerve fibers (autonomic nervous system)	Ipsilateral Horner's syndrome (ptosis, miosis, enophthalamus, and decreased sweating)

Mass Lesions

Spinal Cord Tumors

Spinal cord tumors may arise from any of the elements comprising the spinal cord or any of its coverings. Spinal cord tumors can be divided into two groups: intramedullary, or within the substance of the spinal cord, and extramedullary, or outside the substance of the spinal cord but still located within the spinal canal. The latter group can be further subdivided into intradural or extradural.

About 10 percent of all spinal cord tumors are thought to be intradural and intramedullary.[24] Ependymomas and astrocytomas account for the majority of these lesions. Although histologically these tumors tend to be relatively benign, their location in the spinal cord often makes definitive surgery impossible and they tend to be locally invasive. The remainder of the intramedullary type are composed of various other tumors, including angiomas and vascular malformations.

Intradural extramedullary tumors account for about 60 percent of all spinal tumors. They are all almost entirely benign. By far, meningiomas and neurofibromas account for the greatest proportion, the latter being slightly more frequent. These tumors usually occur in young or middle-aged adults. Meningiomas are more common in females and are frequently located in the thoracic region. Neurofibromas, like meningiomas, may be found anywhere in the spinal canal, but are more likely located in the lumbar area. They are frequently found in association with von Recklinghausen's neurofibromatosis.

Extradural extramedullary tumors account for approximately 25 percent of all spinal tumors. Metastatic carcinomas, especially from lung and breast, compose the majority of lesions in the group, with other tumors such as lymphomas and chordomas accounting for the rest.

Although the separation of the tumors according to their location is usually helpful to the clinician and surgeon in establishing a diagnosis, the classification does not always hold true. For example, neurofibromas may grow along a nerve root sheath and thus become dumbbell shaped, localizing both intradurally and extradurally (Fig. 8-2). Table 8-2 shows some important differentiating features of intramedullary and extramedullary spinal cord tumors.

SYMPTOMS AND SIGNS. It is important to remember that although spinal cord tumors and spinal cord lesions in general may produce localized pathologic alterations and symptoms in the shoulder girdle area, they almost always will manifest findings of diffuse neurologic involvement of the spinal cord below the level of the tumor.

The symptoms of intramedullary tumors are usually insidious in onset. Pain, although often present, is not radicular in character, but frequently poorly localized. On the other hand, it may be highly localized to the middle of the neck or back at the level of the tumor. Intramedullary tumors arising at the level of the fifth and sixth cervical cord segments may give rise to weakness and atrophy of the deltoid, biceps, and other muscles of the shoulder girdle secondary to involvement of the anterior horn cells (lower motor neurons) at that level. Since spinal cord tumors may extend for several segments, there also may be weakness and atrophy of the muscles of the hand. Fasciculations will eventually appear in the involved muscles. The biceps and brachioradialis reflexes will be diminished or will disappear. Later, involvement of the descending corticospinal tracts will result in spasticity and increased deep tendon reflexes below the level of the lesion. If the tumor does not extend below the level of the sixth cervical segment, the triceps reflex, innervated from the seventh and eighth cervical segments, also will be increased, especially on the side ipsilateral to the decreased biceps reflex. Loss of bladder and bowel functions occurs relatively early with intramedullary tumors.

Sensory symptoms occurring with intramedullary tumors are variable. Tumors situated in the midline produce a dissociated sensory loss. Interruption of the crossing fibers of the lateral spinothalamic tract anterior to the central canal will produce loss of pain and temperature sensation at that level in the upper extremities. Position and vibratory sense will be spared in the upper limbs, whereas all four sensory modalities will be normal in the trunk, lower extremities, and uninvolved dermatomes of the arms. Further encroachment on spinal cord

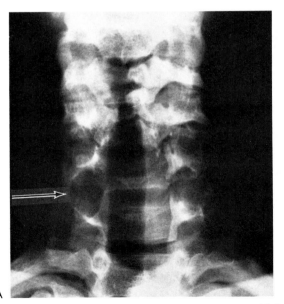
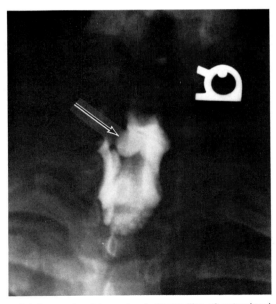

A   B

FIG. 8-2. Two patients with neurofibroma whose chief complaint was shoulder pain. A, X-ray film of extradural tumor eroding pedicle. B, Myelogram of intradural mass.

Table 8-2. *Differentiating Features of Intramedullary and Extramedullary Spinal Cord Tumors*

Features	Intramedullary	Extramedullary
Pain	Often localized to back; may be radiating (especially with hemangiomas)	Radiating (may be localized)
Paresthesias	Infrequent	Common
Sensory loss (pain)	Floating or suspended level (see Table 8-1); sacral sparing until late in the course	No sacral sparing; contralateral loss below level of lesion
Bladder involvement	Early	Relatively late
Abnormalities on plain roentgenograms	Infrequent	Common
Spinal block	Relatively late	Relatively early

structures, however, will produce a more diffuse sensory loss. Involvement of the ascending lateral spinothalamic tracts on one side of the spinal cord will cause loss of pain and temperature sensation below the level of the lesion on the contralateral side of the body. A slowly growing tumor, medially situated, may produce sacral sparing of sensation, because the sacral fibers are the most laterally placed in the lamination of the lateral spinothalamic tract. Eventually, however, even these fibers become involved. As the tumor grows and begins to produce a spinal block, there will be a more complete loss of sensation below the level of the tumor, as well as loss of bladder and bowel functions.

Extramedullary tumors produce significant radicularlike pain secondary to irritation of posterior nerve roots. Pain may radiate from the neck into the shoulder and down the arm into the thumb and index finger, if the fourth, fifth, or sixth cervical segment is involved. It may be exacerbated by coughing or straining. Paresthesias may precede or accompany the pain, usually in the same dermatomal distribution. Shortly after the onset of sensory complaints, weakness, sensory loss, muscle atrophy, and fasciculations will appear in the muscles innervated by the involved nerve roots. Unlike intramedullary lesions, there is no dissociated sensory loss. Deep tendon reflexes may be altered, as they are by intramedullary tumors.

After further compression of the spinal cord by the extramedullary tumor, long tract signs of spasticity and sensory loss will appear below the level of the lesion. Pyramidal tract involvement and spinal block are likely to appear earlier in extramedullary tumors than in intramedullary tumors.

DIAGNOSTIC AIDS. Roentgenograms of the cervical spine are extremely important. Metastatic extramedullary tumors may show vertebral destruction, sclerosis, erosion, or changes in contour of the pedicles (see Fig. 5-25). Neurofibromas classically demonstrate widening of the intervertebral foramina. Meningiomas may show some calcifications. Intramedullary tumors may produce widening of the spinal canal.

Electromyographic nerve conduction studies may help to localize the level of a lesion. They also may help in differentiating a central from a more peripheral lesion, if this is not evident from the clinical examination.

Cerebrospinal fluid (CSF) examination shows an increased level of protein. The protein concentration will be especially high in the presence of a spinal block, up to 1000 mg. percent or even higher (Froin's syndrome). This marked elevation is thought to occur because the protein in the cerebrospinal fluid and that produced by the tumor itself are unable to circulate normally in the subarachnoid space above the level of the lesion. The sugar content of the CSF is normal, a few lymphocytes may be present, and occasionally malignant cells may be seen in the fluid. It should be remembered that lumbar puncture in a patient with a spinal cord tumor is not an innocuous procedure. Exacerbation of symptoms resulting in complete block, quadriplegia, sensory loss, and loss of bladder and bowel functions may necessitate emergency surgical decompression. If a myelogram is to be done, it is often wise to delay CSF examination until that time. Myelography is the definitive investigational procedure for suspected spinal cord tumors, but once again, it should be remembered that these patients may quickly decompensate after the procedure. The risk is lessened if myelography is performed via the lateral cervical approach.

DIFFERENTIAL DIAGNOSIS. Atrophy and weakness causing pain in the shoulder girdle area are nonspecific and may be of peripheral or central (spinal cord) origin. The presence of a dissociated sensory loss or long tract finding places the lesion in continuity to the spinal cord. The differential diagnosis of lower motor neuron findings in the upper extremities coupled with pyramidal tract findings in the lower extremities includes syringomyelia, epidural abscess, amyotrophic lateral sclerosis, transverse myelitis, multiple sclerosis, cervical spondylosis, and subacute combined degeneration. Differentiating factors will be dealt with in later sections.

TREATMENT. Most spinal cord tumors, especially the intradural extramedullary type (meningiomas and neurofibromas), are histologically benign, grow slowly, and produce symptoms by compression and usually not by invasion or destruction. Therefore, complete recovery may follow operation. If the histologic characteristics of the tumor warrant it, radiation therapy may be given after operation.

Syringomyelia

Syringomyelia is a chronic, progressive degenerative process resulting in cavitation and surrounding gliosis of the cervical spinal cord which may extend into the brain stem. Although the cavity (syrinx) may be the only pathologic finding, it is frequently associated with other conditions such as spina bifida, Arnold-Chiari malformation, or von Hippel-Lindau disease. The association of syringomyelia with spinal cord tumors, especially gliomas, hemangiomas, and von Recklinghausen's neurofibromatosis, has been well documented,[38] as has its relationship to trauma.[21]

Syrinxes are most likely to occur in the third or fourth decade, but they can also occur earlier or later in life. Males are affected more often than females.

PATHOLOGY. The most common areas of involvement of a syrinx are the lower medulla and upper cervical cord, and the lower cervical and upper thoracic cord, the latter being more frequent.[7] The spinal cord usually appears swollen and tense over many segments, but in other cases it is atrophic and flattened. There is usually fusiform widening of the cord, and the overlying dura may be thick and fibrotic. The syrinx can be in any area within the spinal cord, but it is most commonly located in the gray substance ventral to the central canal where it may be either symmetric or asymmetric. The cavity contains clear fluid which may be xanthochromic. When it is associated with a tumor, the syrinx tends to be more extensive, may appear to be multiloculated, and the fluid contained in such cavities tends to be more xanthochromic and have a higher concentration of protein.

Microscopically, the cavity walls are lined by glial fibers covered by a thin layer of collagen. Parts of the syrinx may be lined by ependymal cells. Other fiber tracts may be destroyed or displaced.

PATHOGENESIS. Although ischemia, infection, or changes in fluid pressure causing dislocation of ectopic cerebellar tonsils from the foramen magnum (as well as various other mechanisms) have been postulated, the hydrodynamic theory of Gardner is generally accepted as contributing to the origin of congenital syringomyelia.[16] The concept is that the roof of the fourth ventricle fails to perforate during early fetal life, which impairs ventricular drainage. To establish adequate outflow of cerebrospinal fluid from the fourth ventricle, a communication is established between the fourth ventricle and the central canal of the spinal cord. The repeated transmission of the ventricular pressure into the central canal of the spinal cord probably results in the eventual formation of a syrinx.

Acquired syringomyelia may be secondary to softening and resorption within a glioma or from resorption of a hematoma resulting from trauma.

CLINICAL FEATURES. The symptoms and signs produced by a syrinx will obviously depend upon the level of the lesion and the location of the cavity within the spinal cord. Since most congenital syrinxes are situated anterior to the central canal in the cervical region, the clinical presentation for this location will be described.

With destruction of the decussating fibers of the lateral spinothalamic tract, there is loss of pain and temperature sensation in the upper extremities in the dermatomal distribution of the interrupted fibers. As with spinal cord tumors, dissociated sensory loss develops along with a "suspended" or "floating" level of anesthesia, since the ascending lateral spinothalamic tract remains intact until late in the course of the disease. The patient may be totally unaware of the sensory loss and may develop burns, scars, and other evidence of trauma to the anesthetized area. Although the sensory loss is usually bilateral, it may be unilateral.

Pain is often felt centrally in the neck and shoulders. It may, however, be radicular in nature, at times radiating from the shoulder down the arm and into the hand.

When the anterior horn cells are involved in the degenerative process, deep tendon reflexes will be decreased or lost in the upper extremity ipsilateral to the side of the lesion. With bilateral involvement of the anterior horn cells, reflex changes will be symmetric. Involvement of the fifth and sixth cervical segments will cause diminution in the biceps and brachioradialis reflexes, with sparing of the triceps reflex. Seventh and eighth cervical nerve segment involvement will produce diminution in the triceps reflex with sparing of the biceps reflex. Further progression of the cavity will lead to weakness, atrophy, and fasciculations in the muscles supplied from the damaged anterior horn cells. Once again, symmetry and symptoms depend on the location of the syrinx in the spinal cord. Weakness and atrophy usually appear in the intrinsic muscles of the hand, the forearm, and the shoulder girdle muscles.

Further spinal cord involvement leads to spasticity below the level of the lesion secondary to dysfunction of the corticospinal tract. It is an interesting fact that in Barnett's series, stiffness in the legs from spasticity was the most frequent complaint, and not numbness in the hands.[7] Eventually, there will be decreased vibration and position sense below the level of the lesion secondary to posterior column involvement. In lower cervical and upper thoracic lesions, Horner's syndrome (ipsilateral eyelid ptosis, miotic pupil, enophthalmos, and anhidrosis of the face and forehead) may arise secondary to sympathetic dysfunction. Late in the course, bladder and bowel functions become impaired.

Scoliosis is almost always present, usually early in the disease course, owing to damage of the dorsomedial and ventrolateral spinal nuclei.

Almost one quarter of patients with syringomyelia develops neurogenic arthropathies, 80 percent being in the upper extremities.[25] Gross deformities of the shoulder, elbow, or wrist will result (see Figs. 12-7 and 12-8). The occurrence of neurogenic arthropathy in the upper extremities should always raise the possibility of an underlying syringomyelia.

Syringobulbia causes dysfunction of lower cranial nerves resulting in dysarthria, dysphagia, weakness and wasting of the tongue, and a dissociated sensory loss on the face. Involvement is frequently unilateral and asymmetric.

DIAGNOSTIC AIDS. Plain x-ray films will usually show the cervical spine to be normal, but can show a widening of the spinal canal, as is seen with an intramedullary tumor. Plain x-ray films also usually show the skull to be normal, but if associated with other anomalies may show platybasia (flattening of the posterior fossa) or basilar impression (the odontoid process rises above the rim of the foramen magnum).

Cerebrospinal fluid is usually normal, but can have an increase in the protein content. Myelograms may show widening of the spinal cord. On air encephalograms (myelograms) a syrinx can often be differentiated from a solid intramedullary spinal cord neoplasm. If the spinal cord expansion collapses or fluctuates after the placement of air into the subarachnoid space and fourth ventricle, this is indirect evidence that the lesion is a syrinx. If there is an associated Arnold-Chiari malformation, the cerebellar tonsils may be seen descending through the foramen magnum.

DIFFERENTIAL DIAGNOSIS. Differential diagnosis is almost identical to that already given for spinal cord tumors. Intramedullary neoplasms are difficult to differentiate from a syrinx. Growth of a tumor may cause more rapidly progressive symptoms. Bony changes on roentgenograms (erosion or widening of the interpedicular space) are more frequently associated with spinal neoplasms. Collapse of the cavity on air myelograms may suggest a syrinx, but a cavitating tumor may similarly collapse. Surgical exploration often may be necessary in order to establish the diagnosis.

TREATMENT. The treatment of syringomyelia is controversial and not uniformly agreed upon. Each case must be treated individually. Nonsurgical management, decompression laminectomy, and ventriculoatrial shunt have all been advocated.[7]

Epidural Abscess

Epidural abscess is a medical and surgical emergency. The physician must establish a prompt diagnosis and institute therapy as quickly as possible. An abscess may arise by hematogenous spread of bacteria from the tonsils, skin infections, subacute bacterial endocarditis, or even after dental procedures, or it may arise from direct contiguity of lesions near the vertebral column such as furuncles, decu-

biti, or an osteomyelitis. Staphylococcus aureus is the most frequently offending organism.[5] The infection is attended by the signs and symptoms seen with other serious infections, namely, fever, local pain, and elevated white blood cell count and erythrocyte sedimentation rate.

The neurologic symptoms and signs are similar to those of spinal cord tumors, especially those of the extramedullary group, although the progression of the symptoms is often more rapid. There is frequently back pain or spinal ache, followed by radicular pain originating in the neck and radiating into the shoulder and downward into the arm and hand. Weakness, atrophy, and fasciculations of the shoulder girdle muscles and biceps will develop if the nerve roots from the fifth and sixth cervical segments are involved. Paraparesis or quadriparesis and other long tract signs previously discussed will eventually develop and ultimately progress to complete spinal block.

Cerebrospinal fluid examination is an important diagnostic tool, especially valuable in ruling out a concomitant meningitis. However, it must be remembered that lumbar puncture may rapidly decompensate a patient if a complete or near-complete spinal block is present. The spinal fluid pressure is elevated and the protein content is increased. Spinal block is likely if the protein content is high. The sugar content will be normal or low normal unless there is associated meningitis. Early in the course of the illness, there is an increase in the number of polymorphonuclear leukocytes in the spinal fluid, and later in the course there may be an increased number of lymphocytes. Bacteria may be difficult to culture from the cerebrospinal fluid.

If an epidural abscess is strongly suspected, myelography should be performed immediately and spinal fluid can be obtained at that time. High dose intravenous antibiotics, usually a penicillinase-resistant penicillin, should be administered after all appropriate cultures have been obtained. If an extradural mass is found on the myelogram, surgical intervention by evacuation of the abscess is then necessary.

Other Spinal Cord Infections

Various other infectious diseases may give rise to spinal cord pathologic lesions, which result in dysfunction localized to the shoulder girdle region. Tuberculosis, fungi, and syphilis may cause such a picture. Poliomyelitis virus selectively affects the anterior horn cells (lower motor neurons) to produce atrophy, weakness, and fasciculations early in the course of the disease (Fig. 8-3). Long tract findings (upper motor neurons) or sensory findings are usually not seen in poliomyelitis. Postinfectious myelitis, seen following viral illnesses or infectious mononucleosis, is well documented,[13] as is myelitis following vaccination.[39]

Motor Neuron Disease

Motor neuron disease is a group of neurologic disorders in which the primary pathology is in the motor neuron (anterior horn cell), sparing most of the other tracts and neurons in the central nervous system. The separation of these disorders into distinct clinical entities is frequently unclear, but often can be accomplished by taking into account the age at onset, rapidity of progression of the illness, and the degree of central nervous system involvement. What is common to all of the disorders is the result of anterior horn cell loss, i.e., weakness and wasting of muscles, diminution or loss of deep tendon reflexes, and fasciculations. The electromyogram (EMG) characteristically shows denervation, but results of nerve conduction studies are normal.

Werdnig-Hoffmann Disease

Although Werdnig-Hoffmann disease is not a disease process that causes specific localized pathologic changes at the shoulder girdle, it does produce shoulder girdle dysfunction as part of a diffuse, generalized neurologic process. Moreover, it is part of a spectrum of motor neuron diseases affecting the anterior horn cells of the spinal cord which do create specific pathologic lesions at the shoulder area.

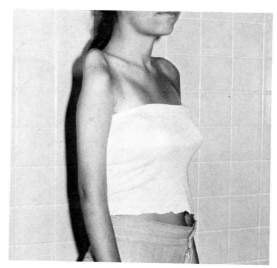

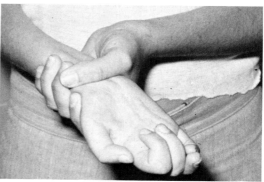

FIG. 8-3. A, Lateral view of shoulder of an 18-year-old girl with poliomyelitis shows severe muscle atrophy of entire upper extremity. B, Palm and back of involved hand.

Werdnig-Hoffmann disease, or infantile progressive muscular atrophy, is a disease of diffuse muscular involvement secondary to the loss of motor neurons in the anterior horn cells of the spinal cord. There is subsequent denervation of the involved muscles and replacement by connective tissue. The peripheral nerves appear atrophic and demyelinated. The progression of the illness is usually rapid, with death occurring by the third or fourth year of life.

Werdnig-Hoffmann disease is an autosomal recessive inherited disease. Two separate groups of Werdnig-Hoffmann patients are now recognized, both with onset early in life, but with different prognoses and progression of symptoms.[32]

Acute Werdnig-Hoffmann disease is manifested soon after birth. Many mothers have noticed decreased fetal movements during their pregnancies as compared with previous pregnancies with normal offspring. All patients have delayed motor milestones by 6 months of age. There are generalized weakness, atrophy, and hypotonia of skeletal muscles and poor head control, along with feeding difficulties. The infant characteristically assumes a "frog" position, lying motionless with abducted hips and flexed knees, expressionless facies, and an open mouth secondary to facial weakness.

Physical examination reveals quadriparesis (floppy baby) with areflexia and a decrease in spontaneous movements. No pyramidal or sensory changes are present. Although no fasciculations are seen in the limbs or trunk, they are often seen in the tongue.

There is a rapid progression of symptoms. Respiratory problems accompanied by bulbar involvement and weakness of the muscles associated with swallowing lead to aspiration pneumonia. Acute Werdnig-Hoffmann disease is almost always fatal by the time the patient is 2 or 3 years of age.

Chronic Werdnig-Hoffmann disease has a later onset in infancy than has acute disease, usually after 1 year of age. In contradistinction to acute Werdnig-Hoffmann disease, there are a slower progression of symptoms and a better prognosis, although ultimately the patients also succumb owing to respiratory and swallowing difficulties. Weakness, although usually generalized, may initially be evident only in the proximal muscles of the lower extremities, and thus may mimic a muscular dystrophy or Kugelberg-Welander disease (see following section). Once again, motor milestones are delayed. Cranial nerve musculature is less affected than limb muscles, although there are weakness of the face and anterior neck muscles, wasting, and fasciculations of the tongue. Deep tendon reflexes are diminished early and eventually lost. Spinal and joint deformities ensue. Survival may continue for several years.

DIAGNOSTIC AIDS. Muscle enzymes, as well as results of cerebrospinal fluid examination, are normal. Electromyograms show neuropathic and not myopathic changes. There is denervation with widespread fibrillation potentials and surviving motor units are increased in amplitude. Nerve conduction velocities are normal.

DIFFERENTIAL DIAGNOSIS. The main problem in Werdnig-Hoffmann disease is to distinguish the disease from one of several muscular dystrophies or congenital myopathies. Electromyographic studies and examination of muscle biopsy specimens may clearly show the disease process to be neuropathic. Chronic Werdnig-Hoffmann disease may mimic Kugelberg-Welander disease, but Kugelberg-Welander disease does not involve the face or the distal parts of the extremities.

Kugelberg-Welander Disease

Kugelberg-Welander disease, or chronic proximal muscular atrophy, is a slowly progressive disease of muscle weakness and wasting. The pathologic condition is similar to that seen in Werdnig-Hoffmann disease, i.e., extensive loss of motor neurons from the anterior horn cells in the spinal cord. Unlike Werdnig-Hoffmann disease, however, it runs a relatively benign course and is more selective in the distribution of the muscular involvement.

The age at onset is anytime in childhood or adolescence. However, it is not uncommon for Kugelberg-Welander disease to have its onset in adult life. Although autosomal dominant inheritance has been documented, it is usually inherited as an autosomal recessive disease.[3] About two thirds of affected patients has a positive family history. Males are affected more frequently than females.

CLINICAL FEATURES. The onset of symptoms and signs is usually between 2 and 20 years of age. There is a slowly progressive and symmetric proximal weakness, usually beginning in the lower extremities and subsequently developing in the shoulder girdle area in later years. Initial symptoms are, therefore, similar to those of a myopathy. The patient first notices difficulty in walking or climbing stairs and a waddling gait may develop. If the onset of the disease is at a young age, there may be some delay in the onset of walking. Subsequently, the patient will have difficulty in raising his arms, and winged scapulae will appear secondary to shoulder girdle muscle weakness. The neck and cranial nerve musculature are almost always spared. Lordotic posture and scoliosis, protuberant abdomen, hyperextended knees, and joint deformities will eventually develop.

Unlike the muscular dystrophies which Kugelberg-Welander disease may closely resemble (especially limb-girdle dystrophy), there are fasciculations in the involved muscles. Fasciculations in the tongue are rare. The deep tendon reflexes at the knees are decreased early, and other reflexes may be eventually diminished or lost. Distal muscles in both upper and lower extremities are rarely affected, in contrast to the distal involvement seen in amyotrophic lateral sclerosis and progressive muscular atrophy. There are no sensory abnormalities.

The course of Kugelberg-Welander disease is usually one of slow, benign progression, although some patients can experience a rapidly deteriorating course of their disease. Normal life span is usually attained. The earlier the age at onset of the symptoms, the worse are the severity and progression of the illness.

DIAGNOSTIC AIDS. Muscle enzymes, particularly creatine phosphokinase, may be minimally elevated.

Electromyograms, as well as muscle biopsy specimens, show neuropathic and not myopathic disease. There are spontaneous fasciculations and evidence of denervation. Results of nerve conduction studies are normal.

DIFFERENTIAL DIAGNOSIS. Kugelberg-Welander disease tends to merge with Werdnig-Hoffmann disease of infants and with amyotrophic lateral sclerosis in adults. Differentiating features are the age at onset, course and progression, and selectivity for proximal muscle involvement. Electromy-

ography and muscle biopsy, along with the clinical finding of fasciculations, will usually enable one to differentiate Kugelberg-Welander disease from the muscular dystrophies. Further differences will be elaborated in subsequent sections dealing with the muscular dystrophies. Thyroid disease must also be ruled out in any patient with proximal muscle weakness, as must polymyositis. These will also be discussed in later sections.

Progressive Muscular Atrophy

Progressive muscular atrophy is another part of the disease spectrum referred to as motor neuron disease (see next section) which is dependent on whether the neuronal involvement is primarily in the lower motor neurons, or in both upper and lower motor neurons. The disease is classified as either progressive muscular atrophy or amyotrophic lateral sclerosis in the adult patient. The pathologic findings in progressive muscular atrophy are exclusively confined to degeneration of the anterior horn cells in the spinal cord. The corticospinal tracts and other ascending, descending, or crossing fibers are spared. There is asymmetric wasting and weakness of muscles, usually beginning in the small muscles of the hand. Later, after the shoulder girdle muscles are affected, there is difficulty in raising the arms or combing the hair. Subsequently, muscles innervated by the lower cranial nerves are involved, followed by muscle dysfunction in the lower extremities. Deep tendon reflexes are diminished. Hyperactive reflexes suggest corticospinal tract involvement and an amyotrophic lateral sclerosis-type picture. There is no spasticity in the "pure" progressive muscular atrophy. Sensory loss is rare. Fasciculations may be present in both upper and lower extremities and in the tongue.

The course of disease in progressive muscular atrophy is one of steady downhill progression leading to respiratory and swallowing difficulties, and ultimately death usually from aspiration pneumonia.

DIAGNOSTIC AIDS. Cerebrospinal fluid and

muscle enzymes are normal. Electromyographic studies show evidence of denervation as in Kugelberg-Welander disease, and findings of denervation are seen in the muscle biopsy specimens. Results of nerve conduction studies are normal.

DIFFERENTIAL DIAGNOSIS. The differentiation of motor neuron disease into progressive muscular atrophy or amyotrophic lateral sclerosis is often difficult and probably unnecessary. Some authors combine the two into one disease entity.[35] Kugelberg-Welander disease usually begins in the lower extremities and does not often involve the distal muscles of a limb.

TREATMENT. Treatment is essentially supportive.

Amyotrophic Lateral Sclerosis

Amyotrophic lateral sclerosis is classified in the disease spectrum of motor neuron diseases, all of which are often considered to be one common disease entity. Amyotrophic lateral sclerosis, in its strict sense, is the most common form of motor neuron disease and shows evidence of both upper motor neuron and lower motor neuron involvement. The pathologic alteration is confined to the motor neurons and their axons in the spinal cord and medulla, and is often greatest in the cervical and lower cranial nerve region. There are neuron loss and gliosis in the anterior horn cell areas of the spinal cord. The pyramidal tracts show demyelination, whereas other tracts show nonspecific changes.

The age at onset is usually in middle life. Males are affected more frequently than females. Most cases are sporadic, with about 10 percent familial and probably of autosomal dominant inheritance.[34] On the island of Guam, amyotrophic lateral sclerosis is associated with a parkinsonism-dementia illness which seems to be an inherited disease, 57 percent of the cases being familial.[26]

CLINICAL FEATURES. Symptoms and signs usually begin in the upper extremities, although they frequently can begin in the lower extremities or in the bulbar musculature. The most common appearance is wasting, weakness, and fasciculations in the muscles of the hands, arms, and shoulders, but usually the signs are more prominent distally in the extremities. Involvement may be either symmetric or asymmetric until it becomes generalized and severe. There may be weakness and wasting and fasciculations of the tongue, along with weakness and wasting of the other bulbar musculature, which produce dysarthria, dysphagia, and facial weakness. Spasticity and stiffness are present in the lower extremities and are frequently associated with severe muscle cramps at night. Deep tendon reflexes are hyperactive and cause clonus, the jaw jerk is increased, and there are bilateral Babinski signs. Results of the sensory examination are normal. Eye muscles are never involved. Bladder and bowel dysfunctions occur late in the disease. There is no intellectual impairment, strictly speaking. The eventual course is of steady, downhill progression over 2 to 3 years. Ultimately, there is inanition with respiratory and swallowing difficulty, leading to aspiration pneumonia and death.

The aforementioned symptoms and signs describe the classic case of amyotrophic lateral sclerosis. There are indeed variations in both the neurologic manifestations and the course of the illness. Spasticity and increased deep tendon reflexes may be the most prominent features of the disease with only minimal wasting and fasciculations. Bulbar musculature dysfunction may be the most prominent sign and suggests myasthenia gravis. Lower motor neuron findings may be the outstanding feature, approaching a picture of progressive muscular atrophy.

DIAGNOSTIC AIDS. Cerebrospinal fluid is usually within normal limits. Serum muscle enzymes, especially creatinine phosphokinase, may be increased, especially during an active phase of the disease.[1] Electromyographic studies show denervation and fasciculations in both the lower extremities and upper extremities. Results of nerve conduction studies are normal until late in the course of the disease. Muscle biopsy specimens similarly show nonspecific evidence of denervation.

DIFFERENTIAL DIAGNOSIS. The presence of upper motor neuron lesions with lower motor lesions necessitates a thorough search for treatable illnesses. The diagnosis of amyotrophic lateral sclerosis is essentially a death sentence. Unfortunately, this search is all too frequently fruitless.

Cervical spondylosis can give lower motor neuron findings in the upper extremities and upper motor neuron findings in the legs. Cervical spine x-ray films and possibly even myelograms may be necessary to rule it out (see later section). Syringomyelia may give similar findings, but almost always produces some type of sensory impairment. Multiple sclerosis usually occurs at an earlier age, and severe motor deficit usually occurs after there are significant eye signs. Heavy metal poisoning, especially lead, can produce a picture like that of amyotrophic lateral sclerosis. If oropharyngeal weakness is prominent, myasthenia gravis may be suggested. Subacute combined degeneration from vitamin B_{12} deficiency can also cause a similar clinical picture.

In general, when full-blown clinical features are present, diagnosis is not difficult.

TREATMENT. No definite therapy is now available and, therefore, treatment is mainly supportive and symptomatic. Guanidine hydrochloride has been shown by some authors to be of some benefit by facilitating the release of acetylcholine at the neuromuscular junction.[28] Its major side effect is that of bone marrow depression.

Other Spinal Cord Problems

Various other conditions produce shoulder girdle dysfunction secondary to pathologic changes in the spinal cord. The most notable of these is trauma. Trauma may cause a transverse myelitis or a syringomyelia-like picture, the latter condition manifesting itself long after the trauma. An associated fractured vertebra or severe cervical osteoarthritis may be related but need not be present. Severe whiplash injury or a severe fall on the head, back, or buttocks is especially prone to produce a traumatic hematomyelia. Symptoms and signs are frequently indistinguishable from those of congenital syringomyelia, although they may have a more rapid onset.

NERVE ROOT DYSFUNCTION

Although many of the extramedullary spinal cord tumors produce symptoms and signs referable to nerve root dysfunction, they have been included in the previous section on spinal cord disease. Cervical spondylosis, on the other hand, is included here, although it, too, can often result in significant spinal cord dysfunction. Most of the initial symptoms of this disorder are related to compression of the nerve roots.

Cervical Spondylosis

Spondylosis describes the degenerative and proliferative changes in the vertebrae that are virtually inevitable in the aging patient as a result of the stresses and strains on the vertebrae over many years. Seventy to 80 percent of people over the age of 50 years shows some degenerative or proliferative changes of cervical osteoarthritis by roentgen examination.[30] It is most pronounced between the fourth and seventh cervical vertebral bodies where the stress from movement is probably the greatest.[27] Since the great majority of the patients remain asymptomatic, the presence of cervical spondylosis on a roentgenogram does not mean that symptoms will appear. It is frequently difficult to distinguish on clinical grounds alone whether a patient's symptoms are related to cervical spondylosis, or whether the changes on roentgenograms are incidental findings.

PATHOLOGY. Cervical spondylosis most likely results from abnormalities that accompany aging. Several aging processes, including a decrease in the water content of the disc, stimulate osteophyte and other fibrous and bony changes. Eventually, these protrude into the spinal canal or adjacent intervertebral foramina. Adhesions around the protrusions and the nerve roots fix the cord and prevent the gliding that normally occurs during cervical movement.[41] The thickened ligamenta flava, bulging anteriorly in cervical extension, causes recurring trauma to the cervical cord by a protruded disc or osteophyte. Thus, trauma and especially sudden hyperextension of the neck will precipitate symptoms in patients with cervical spondylosis.

The development of symptoms attributable to cervical spondylosis relates to the intensity of the process, the size of the spinal canal, and vascular factors. There is a close correlation between severe canal narrowing and signs of myelopathy as well as between severe narrowing of intervertebral foramina and radiculopathy. Compression of the arterial supply by the arthritic changes may produce neurologic dysfunction at a level extending several segments above the level of the cord compression.

CLINICAL FEATURES. The signs of nerve root or spinal cord compression may appear together or separately. The signs and symptoms in the upper extremity vary according to the level of cord compression and spinal nerve roots involved. Impingement upon nerve roots produces localized sensory and motor deficits in a radicular distribution. There will be pain and paresthesias radiating from the neck and shoulder down the arm into the hand, which may be symmetric or asymmetric. As in spinal cord tumors, involvement of the fifth or sixth nerve roots may produce asymmetric weakness, atrophy, and fasciculations in the muscles of the shoulder girdle and upper arm, with biceps and brachioradialis reflexes diminished or abolished but an intact triceps reflex. With spinal cord involvement, the triceps reflex may even be hyperactive. Sensory loss may extend from the shoulder into the arm and downward into the thumb and index finger.

Impingement upon the spinal cord produces pyramidal tract signs in the lower extremities and in the areas in the upper limbs innervated by nerve segments below the level of the lesion. Deep tendon reflexes will be hyperactive in the legs and produce increased tone, clonus, and bilateral Babin-

ski signs. Vibratory and position sense will be diminished below the level of the lesion, the loss being greatest distally in the lower limbs. Because of posterior column involvement, flexion of the neck may produce paresthesias into the arms and down the back (Lhermitte's sign). As the disease progresses and there is further impingement on the spinal cord, there are decreased pinprick and temperature sensation below the level of the lesion, and bladder and bowel dysfunction. Complete spinal block will produce paraplegia or quadriplegia, depending on the location of the lesion, along with sensory loss below the level of the lesion and loss of bladder and bowel function.

DIAGNOSTIC AIDS. Cerebrospinal fluid examination may show a minimally elevated protein content. If a spinal block is present, the protein will be markedly elevated. Glucose and cell count in the fluid are normal.

Roentgenograms of the cervical spine reveal evidence of osteoarthritis with sclerosis and formation of posterior osteophytes and foraminal narrowing. Films of a completely normal cervical spine are strong evidence against the diagnosis of cervical spondylosis.

Electromyographic studies help to localize the level of the lesion. The electromyographic studies may help elucidate whether the atrophy and weakness in the shoulder region are of myopathic or neuropathic origin, if there are no long tract signs.

If the diagnosis is doubtful, myelography should be performed for definitive proof of impingement on nervous structures by the cervical spondylosis.

DIFFERENTIAL DIAGNOSIS. As stated in the previous section, the differential diagnosis of a patient with upper motor neuron findings in the lower extremities and lower motor neuron signs in the upper extremities includes amyotrophic lateral sclerosis, multiple sclerosis, syringomyelia, spinal cord tumors, and subacute combined degeneration.

TREATMENT. Initially, conservative treatment is most often the best choice. Bed rest, heat, analgesics, and intermittent cervical traction and a cervical collar should be tried for 1 to 2 weeks. If conservative treatment fails, surgery should be considered.

Even after operation, marked improvement in spinal cord function is unlikely to occur if the neurologic deficit has been long-standing.[42] The progression of the disease process, however, will usually be stopped. Operation should also be performed in the patients with well-documented progression of spinal cord signs which threaten to produce incapacitation. Foraminal decompression may be necessary to avert complete wasting and weakness of an upper limb.

Cervical Disc Disease

Protruded intervertebral discs produce neurologic dysfunction by impingement upon nerve roots or by spinal cord compression, the former being much more common. The disc lies between two vertebrae and is maintained in its normal position by the anterior and posterior longitudinal ligaments. Since the former is denser and stronger than the posterior ligament, most protrusions occur posteriorly. The posterior ligament itself is stronger in the midline and weaker and more deficient laterally. Protrusions, therefore, are more likely to occur laterally and cause nerve root dysfunction rather than in the midline to produce spinal cord dysfunction.

Disc protrusions most frequently occur in the lumbar region, followed in frequency by the cervical area. They rarely occur in the thoracic region. Most cervical disc protrusions occur at the C6-7 interspace, followed by the C5-6 interspace, and then the C7-T1 interspace.[29] The C6-7 interspace is more prone to damage because of its greater size in comparison to the other cervical interspaces and because its articular facets have assumed an almost vertical position,[4] which permits maximum mobility in the joint space.

Many protruded discs are related to trauma, either from a single or from repeated episodes, with or without predisposing factors. With age, the disc undergoes degenerative changes which may lead to protrusion precipitated by minimal trauma. Skeletal abnormalities, congenital anomalies, and instability of the spine from arthritis, infections, or malignancy also contribute to disc protrusion. Protruded discs are much more common in males and are related to the greater possibility of injury and to the increased stresses and strains in the area.

PATHOLOGY. Protruded discs are composed of dense fibrous tissue. Marked degenerative changes, a decreased water content, and decreased mucopolysaccharide concentration of the disc are seen in some, with some fibrosis at the protruded portion of the disc. Many are also edematous, and long-standing protruded discs may be calcified.

CLINICAL FEATURES. Clinical symptoms and signs, along with their treatment, depend on the relation of the disc to the vertebral column, ligaments, nerve roots, and spinal cord. Bulging discs are an early manifestation of displacement, soon followed by protruded discs (the most common cause of disc disease), and then herniated discs, which occur when there is an actual tear in the annulus fibrosis and posterior longitudinal ligament, allowing escape of part of the nucleus pulposus through the tear.

The onset of symptoms in lateral disc protrusions is frequently observed after a sudden turn of the head and neck. This tends to be followed by severe lateralized neck pain, which persists for a time, and then becomes recurrent. On the other hand, the patient may awaken in the morning with a stiff neck and lateralized neck pain, or the onset of the pain may be vague and difficult to relate to a specific time period or injury. In some patients, the pain is first an aching in the neck, but gradually travels into the shoulder and eventually down the arm, whereas in other patients the pain is immediately radicular in character. Pain is increased by coughing and straining, or caused by motion of the spinal column. There are often periods of relative freedom from pain separating episodes of severe paroxysms of disabling pain.

Paresthesias are frequently present. Pain

or paresthesias in the thumb and index finger indicate compression of the sixth cervical nerve root by the fifth cervical disc. Involvement of the middle finger is indicative of compression of the seventh cervical nerve root by the sixth cervical disc, whereas symptoms in the fourth and fifth fingers suggest compression of the eighth cervical nerve root by the seventh cervical disc.

The head and neck are held in a rigid manner with loss of normal cervical lordosis. The muscles of the neck are in spasm, and motions of the cervical segment of the spinal column are painful and limited. Point tenderness just lateral to the spinous processes at the level of the disc may be present. With impingement on the fifth or sixth cervical root, the biceps and brachioradialis reflexes may be diminished or abolished on that side, whereas the triceps reflex is spared. There may be weakness, atrophy, and fasciculations in the deltoid and other shoulder muscles, and in the biceps and brachialis muscles. Impingement on the seventh cervical root, however, spares the shoulder girdle muscles and biceps but produces weakness and wasting in the triceps and forearm muscles. Sensory changes classically follow the dermatomal distribution for each nerve root.

Midline protruded discs are extremely common and appear as spinal cord compression syndromes. Usually the pain is not radicular but localized to the middle of the neck. Long tract signs and other evidence of spinal cord dysfunction simulating cervical cord tumors, amyotrophic lateral sclerosis, cervical spondylosis, or syringomyelia can eventually develop.

DIAGNOSTIC TESTS.   Roentgenograms of the cervical spine may reveal narrowing of the intervertebral space and straightening of the cervical spine curvature. Calcification in a disc space and narrowing of the intervertebral foramina can also be seen. Roentgenograms of a normal-appearing cervical spine, however, do not rule out the possibility of a protruded disc.

Cerebrospinal fluid may show an elevated protein level. Markedly increased protein content is not consistent with disc disease unless a complete spinal block has occurred.

Myelograms will often demonstrate a protruded disc whether it be lateral or midline.

DIFFERENTIAL DIAGNOSIS.   Clinical examination, neurophysiologic studies, routine cervical roentgenograms, and myelograms may all be needed to distinguish a protruded disc from spinal cord tumor, syringomyelia, cervical spondylosis, amyotrophic lateral sclerosis, multiple sclerosis, and subacute combined degeneration. Differentiating features have been presented in other sections.

TREATMENT.   Protruded cervical discs that are lateral and produce radicular pain respond best to treatment.[23] Initial treatment of lateral protrusions is usually conservative with intermittent cervical traction, bed rest, bed board, heat, and analgesics for 1 to 2 weeks. This is followed by gradual ambulation and substitution of the traction for a cervical collar. If no improvement occurs after an adequate trial of conservative management, operation should be performed. Moreover, if initial neurologic dysfunction is significant, operation should be performed without delay.

Midline disc protrusions respond poorly to conservative treatment. Operation should be performed, especially if symptoms and signs of spinal cord dysfunction are present.

Tabes Dorsalis

Tabes dorsalis is one of the neurologic complications of syphilis. Involvement in the upper extremities in this disorder is rare but at times can result in the development of a Charcot joint. This results from repeated trauma because of the absence of the normal sensory appreciation of pain and position sense, and because of ligamentous laxity. Charcot joints in the upper extremity, even in the presence of positive results of serologic tests, are almost never related to syphilis. On the other hand, they are usually secondary to syringomyelia, and less frequently, to diabetes mellitus (see Fig. 5-45). Therefore, a Charcot shoulder joint should alert one to a search for either of the two diseases mentioned previously, even if definite evidence of active or latent syphilis is present.

Herpes Zoster

Herpes zoster infection is usually a benign illness with affinity for the dorsal root ganglions. It produces a characteristic vesicular skin rash that follows along the nerve root distribution. Although most commonly seen in the thoracic region, it is not uncommonly seen in either the cervical or lumbar areas. It is also common along the ophthalmic division of the trigeminal nerve.

Severe pain is almost always present, and often precedes the skin eruption. Stinging, burning, or crushing sensations may also be present. Sensory loss is variable, in that it may follow the dermatomal distribution or may be patchy and involve other dermatomal areas.

Frequent motor paralysis occurs after the skin eruption. This is more commonly seen in male patients and can occur from days to months after the rash. The deltoid is the most frequently involved muscle in the upper extremity.[40] Serratus anterior paralysis has been observed in this disease. Incomplete recovery of function is usually the outcome.

Cerebrospinal fluid examination may show an increased number of lymphocytes and an elevated protein content but a normal glucose content. Isolation of the virus from the cerebrospinal fluid is extremely difficult, but it has been isolated from trigeminal nerve ganglions.[8] No specific treatment is yet available. Supportive treatment in the form of external support for a severely paralyzed muscle (serratus anterior) will improve shoulder function in the recovery phase.

DYSFUNCTION OF PERIPHERAL NERVES

Brachial Plexus Lesions

The brachial plexus extends a length of 15 cm. in the adult. The fifth cervical to the first thoracic nerve roots contribute to the formation of the plexus. Contributions from the fourth cervical nerve root or the second thoracic nerve root result in a prefixed or postfixed plexus, respectively. In the supraclavicular fossa, the trunks are in close relation to the subclavian artery, and both are closely adjacent to the cupola pleurae. In the axilla (infraclavicular area), the cords are positioned and named relative to the axillary artery. As a general rule, supraclavicular lesions produce damage in a dermatomal distribution, whereas infraclavicular lesions are nonsegmental and produce a deficit secondary to the specific patterns of the cords that are involved.[36]

Open injuries to the brachial plexus are uncommon. Because of the close approximation of the subclavian arteries and the apex of the lung, they are often lethal. Knives, broken glass, and bullets are the usual causes of open injuries.

Closed injuries to the brachial plexus, on the other hand, are common. The majority of these are traction lesions involving the supraclavicular part of the plexus.[6] Traffic accidents account for a large percentage of these injuries.[36] The mechanism involved is forceful distraction of the head from the shoulder. The distribution of damage to the plexus in traction injuries is determined by the position of the arm relative to the body at the time of impact.[22] An abducted arm produces greater stress on the lower roots, and an adducted arm produces greater stress on the upper roots. Other traction injuries, however, may produce infraclavicular damage.

Other common causes of brachial plexus injuries are those occurring postoperatively, after either general or regional anesthesia. This is most likely related to positioning on the operating table during prolonged thoracic or abdominal surgery. The neurologic deficit is rarely permanent, and recovery usually occurs within several months.

Brachial plexus injuries are not uncommon as a result of birth and delivery problems. Signs are usually evident immediately after birth. Most injuries are of the upper plexus, although the entire plexus may be involved.

CLINICAL FEATURES. The majority of lesions are of the upper trunk (Duchenne-Erb), and involve the fifth and sixth cervical roots. Lesions of the lower trunk (eighth cervical and first thoracic nerves, Dejerine-Klumpke) are rare in the adult and most occur from birth injuries. They appear as mixed median and ulnar nerve palsies. Lesions of the middle trunk by itself are extremely rare.

Lesions of the upper trunk produce adduction and medial rotation of the humerus. There is paralysis of the deltoid and lateral rotators of the humerus and other muscles of the shoulder girdle such as the supra- and infraspinatus and subscapularis, with an inability to abduct the arm. Dysfunction of the biceps results in the inability to flex the elbow or supinate the forearm. The forearm, therefore, is extended and pronated with the palm facing backward and outward, producing the "Porter's-tip" hand (Fig. 8-4). Musculature in the hand remains unaffected.

The biceps and brachioradialis reflexes are markedly diminished or abolished, but the triceps reflex will be spared. Sensory loss is variable, but may involve the thumb and index finger, radial side of the forearm, and the lateral portion of the arm and deltoid region of the shoulder.

A combination of upper and middle trunk lesions produces, in addition to the previously mentioned features, paralysis of the triceps and the extensors of the wrist and fingers. All the deep tendon reflexes in the affected limb will be diminished or abolished.

DIAGNOSTIC AIDS. Cervical spine roentgenograms should be taken and fractures or dislocations searched for. Two to three weeks after the injury, electromyographic and nerve conduction studies should be

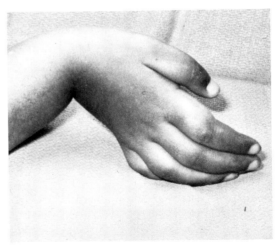

FIG. 8-4. "Porter's tip" hand.

performed, which can be used to determine motor activity and note progression of recovery. Electromyographic study is probably superior to clinical examination to assess recovery.

If no recovery has occurred after 3 months, myelography and histamine response tests and possibly even surgical exploration should be undertaken.[22] Postganglionic lesions, but not preganglionic lesions, alter the wheal and flare response to histamine, since the cell body is not separated from the dendrite reaching the skin. A preganglionic lesion as seen by the histamine response test implies a poor prognostic sign.[10]

PROGNOSIS. The average rate of nerve regeneration is 1 mm./day,[37] and the length of time required for reaching the muscle and connecting with the motor end-plates is a prime factor for recovery. On the average, 20 to 24 months is the maximum period for reinnervation still compatible with useful recovery of the muscle function.[36] After this period, the motor end-plates fibrose and are unable to receive the axons. Thus, the prognosis for the intrinsic muscles of the hand is worse than for proximal muscles of the arm because of their location, tendency to atrophy, and exquisite functional requirement.

A preganglionic lesion, seen when the spinal roots are avulsed from the cord, has a hopeless prognosis for recovery.[22] A postganglionic lesion, on the other hand, always has the possibility for recovery, provided the structural elements persist. Preganglionic lesions can be demonstrated by the presence of denervation in the posterior cervical musculature on electromyograms, a Horner's syndrome, fractured vertebral transverse process, or dislocation of intervertebral joints which facilitates disruption of the plexus from the cord, sympathetic dysfunction as in severe burning pain, and the axon reflex test with histamine.

TREATMENT. Treatment in the first week requires immobilization of the shoulder on an abduction splint or splinting by pinning the shirt sleeve in a position of 60-degrees abduction, forward flexion, and external rotation.[36] Vigorous physiotherapy with range of motion exercises must be given frequently to prevent contractures. Treatment of pain with analgesics may be necessary. Multivitamins and thiamine should supplement an adequate diet. After 4 to 6 weeks, immobilization may be gradually discontinued, and full physiotherapy begun.

Compressive lesions such as those caused by encroachment from a fractured clavicle are indications for surgery. On patients who show progression of the neural deficit or reversal of recovery, neurolysis of scarred nerves should be performed. In addition, patients who show no signs of reinnervation and recovery after 3 months may require explorative operation.

Brachial Plexus Neuritis

Brachial plexus neuritis (*neuralgic amyotrophy*) is a disease of unknown etiology, although trauma, vaccination, infection, and other autoimmune mechanisms have been postulated as precipitating factors.[18] Usually there are no constitutional symptoms. Pain is usually the predominant early symptom. Its onset is sudden, and it is usually localized to the shoulder and lateral aspect of the upper arm. The pain is most often a constant severe ache, but can be burning and stabbing in nature. It is aggravated by movement of the arms at the shoulder, but not by neck movement. Considerable muscle tenderness may also be present.

The pain lasts from a few hours to 2 weeks. As the pain decreases in intensity, muscle weakness and paralysis appear in one or more of the muscles of the shoulder girdle, followed by atrophy of the involved muscles. The serratus anterior, deltoid, and spinales muscles, respectively, are the most frequently affected,[31] although muscles of the arm and forearm may occasionally be involved. Involvement of the other shoulder with pain then by weakness and paralysis may follow, although not usually to the same degree.

Sensory loss is usually minimal. Most often, there is loss of sensation only in the distribution of the circumflex nerve (small strip over the outer side of the upper arm) which may be an important diagnostic clue. It is rare to have a significant sensory loss in the arm, forearm, or hand.

The prognosis for recovery is usually good, and is often rapid. Some cases may not show recovery until months after onset, and may show continued recovery for as long as 2 years after onset of the disease.

There is no specific treatment for neuralgic amyotrophy. Analgesics and physical therapy with full range of movements are often necessary. As with other disease entities, steroids are frequently tried, but their efficacy in this condition has not yet been proved.

Thoracic Outlet Syndrome

See Chapter 14.

Shoulder-Hand Syndrome

See Chapter 14.

Peripheral Nerve Tumors

Tumors of any of the peripheral nerves of the shoulder region will produce symptoms and signs in the respective muscles which they innervate. Neuromas, neurofibromas, ganglioneuromas, and lipomas are some of the more common types of tumor.

Peripheral Neuropathies

Diabetes mellitus is a major cause of peripheral neuropathy. With loss of pain and joint position sense, repeated trauma may produce a Charcot joint, resulting in diabetic pseudotabes (see section on Tabes Dorsalis). Although most commonly seen in the lower extremity, the Charcot joint can occur in the shoulder in diabetes mellitus (see Fig. 5-45). As previously stated, a Charcot joint at the shoulder is usually due to syringomyelia or diabetes mellitus, the former being more common, and almost never is it related to tabes dorsalis.

DISORDERS OF THE MYONEURAL JUNCTION

Myasthenia Gravis

Myasthenia gravis is a disease of defective nerve impulse transmission characterized by excessive fatigability and weakness of muscles. The symptoms and signs are usually worse at the end of the day after muscle activity and less severe during and after rest. Limb-skeletal muscles or muscles innervated by cranial nerves may be affected, the latter being more common.

The origin of myasthenia gravis remains a mystery. It is relatively certain that the problem is at the myoneural junction, that is, where the axonal extensions of the nerve meet the respective muscle fibers that they innervate. Whether the defect is before (neural) or after (myo) the synaptic junction is unresolved at this time. Acetylcholine is liberated from vesicles at the terminal bouton areas of the nerve into the synaptic cleft region, where it is either bound to receptor sites on the postsynaptic membrane or hydrolyzed by cholinesterase. Recordings of microelectrodes in patients with myasthenia gravis reveal miniature end-plate potentials of much less amplitude than normal,[19] presumably related to some problem with acetylcholine.

CLINICAL FEATURES. Myasthenia gravis may begin at any age, but is especially prominent in young adults. Females predominate in the young age groups, but in older ages the frequency of men with the disease approaches that of women.

The onset of symptoms may be sudden or insidious. The initial symptoms most commonly involve the muscles innervated by cranial nerves, especially the extraocular muscles and levator palpebrae, and result in ptosis or diplopia. Involvement of oropharyngeal muscles produces dysarthria, dysphagia, weakness of facial expression, difficulty in chewing, or changes in phonation.

Involvement of the limb muscles is common, especially the proximal muscles in the upper extremities. Difficulty in lifting objects or raising the hands over the head ensues, and eventually there may be difficulty in walking or climbing stairs. When the weakness in the extremities is in the proximal musculature, it is usually symmetric, whereas distal weakness may be more asymmetric. Myasthenia gravis can cause only limb weakness without ocular or bulbar symptoms, but this is indeed uncommon.

The characteristic findings in a patient with myasthenia gravis is that the weakness and fatigue fluctuate from day to day and possibly from hour to hour, and usually improve with rest. Thus, a patient may be able to comb her hair upon awakening in the morning, but will be unable to lift her arms over her head after physical exertion. This should improve with rest.

Deep tendon reflexes are usually normal. Hyperactive reflexes or persistently decreased or abolished deep tendon reflexes suggest other diseases, the latter especially suggesting the myasthenic syndrome (Eaton-Lambert syndrome). Atrophy, usually minimal, may occur, but no fasciculations are seen unless the patient is on anticholinesterase therapy. Results of sensory examination are normal.

Eaton-Lambert Syndrome

The Eaton-Lambert syndrome, or myasthenic syndrome, is also a disease of impaired nervous impulse transmission. Although most patients have an associated malignancy (especially oat cell carcinoma of the lung, but certainly not limited to this particular neoplasm), the Eaton-Lambert syndrome can be present in some patients for many years without any evidence of a concomitant neoplasm. The neurologic defect is similar to that seen in botulism poisoning and is most likely secondary to a decrease in the amount of acetylcholine released by a nervous impulse.[18] In contrast to myasthenia gravis, the vesicles containing the acetylcholine are normal in size but too few in number to be effective in nerve transmission. The pathologic alterations seen in muscle biopsy specimens are relatively nonspecific changes.

CLINICAL FEATURES. The neurologic symptoms may precede the development of the neoplasm by several months, but most often appear after a primary tumor is known to be present. There is progressive weakness, fatigability, and wasting in the proximal muscles of the limbs. Initially, usually the muscles of the pelvic girdle and thigh are involved, and difficulty walking, climbing stairs, or rising from a sitting position result. Eventually, the shoulder girdle and arm muscles are involved, and the patient has difficulty in raising the arms over the head. Ptosis, diplopia, and other involvement of cranial nerve musculature are rare, but may be fleetingly present. The involved muscles tend to produce severe aching.

The weakness may indeed fluctuate, but this is much less pronounced than in myasthenia gravis. A temporary increase in muscle power after brief exercise is frequently noted. One can demonstrate increased hand grip strength during contraction sustained for several seconds. The deep tendon reflexes at the knee are the earliest reflexes to be decreased, but subsequently all reflexes will be diminished or abolished. There are no fasciculations, but atrophy is present in the involved muscles.

The removal of the neoplasm probably has no effect on the myasthenic syndrome.[35] Spontaneous remissions can occur. Death usually results from the neoplasm and not from the neurologic dysfunction, strictly speaking.

NEUROMUSCULAR DISORDERS

The Muscular Dystrophies

The three most commonly seen inherited muscular dystrophies are the Duchenne sex-linked muscular dystrophy, facioscapulohumeral dystrophy, and limb-girdle dystrophy. Other, less frequently seen dystrophies are oculopharyngeal muscular dystrophy and scapuloperoneal atrophy. Some of the differentiating features of the more common dystrophies are presented in Table 8-3.

Duchenne's Sex-linked Muscular Dystrophy

Duchenne's muscular dystrophy is a sex-linked recessive inherited disease manifesting itself in young age groups and usually running a subacute course. Death occurs in adolescence or young adulthood. Unlike many of the other dystrophies, it does involve other systems in the body.

Males are usually affected before the third or fourth year of life but occasionally the onset is later in childhood. Rare cases of Duchenne's dystrophy with Turner's syndrome have been reported.[15] The disease has a high rate of mutation, with as many as 30 percent of cases occurring spontaneously without a family history or detectable carrier.[35] Another one third will not have a family history, but carriers can be found by biochemical or histochemical techniques.

PATHOLOGY. Skeletal muscle biopsy specimens reveal a decrease in the number of muscle fibers, and muscle necrosis and replacement of the diseased muscle by fat and connective tissue. Phagocytosis of degenerating muscle fibers is present, as is evidence of abortive regeneration of muscle fiber.

CLINICAL FEATURES. The weakness usually begins proximally and symmetrically in the pelvic girdle musculature. Initial symptoms are, therefore, difficulty in walking and a tendency to fall. Although the onset of walking is often delayed, in some patients walking may be normal until the third or fourth year of life. There will be difficulty in

Table 8-3. *Differentiating Features of The Common Muscular Dystrophies*

	Duchenne Sex-linked Dystrophy	Limb-girdle Dystrophy	Facioscapulo-humeral Dystrophy
Inheritance	Sex-linked recessive	50% Autosomal recessive	Autosomal dominant
Age at onset	Usually by 4th year	Variable	Late 1st or early 2nd decade
Sex	Male	Equal frequency of males and females	Equal frequency of males and females
Initial distribution	Pelvic girdle	Shoulder or pelvic girdle	Shoulder girdle
Pseudohypertrophy	Common	Rare	Rare
Involvement of face	Usually spared	Rare	Common
Rate of progression	Relatively rapid, except for Becker type	Intermediate	Variable, usually slow or abortive
Contractures and deformities	Common	Occasional	Rare
Serum enzyme elevation	Significantly elevated, especially early in the course; carriers show increased enzymes (especially creatinine phosphokinase)	May be mildly elevated; no increase in carriers	Usually normal

climbing stairs and rising from the floor. Gower's sign will be positive, in that the patient will tend to climb his own legs when asked to rise from the floor. His gait becomes waddling, he tends to stand with his feet wide-based, and his abdomen protrudes.

Subsequently, the proximal muscles of the upper extremity are involved, and the patient experiences difficulty in raising the arms over the head and in lifting objects (Fig. 8-5). Eventually, there are severe wasting and contractures of most skeletal muscles, especially in the lower extremities. Cranial nerve musculature is usually spared except for the lower facial muscles. Swallowing and phonation usually remain unaffected.

Physical examination relatively early in the course of the disease reveals symmetric weakness in the proximal muscles of the lower extremities. Shoulder girdle muscle weakness can usually be demonstrated early in the course of the disease even though the patient may be asymptomatic in regard to the upper extremities. Eventually, distal muscles will become involved. Initially, there is hypertrophy of some muscles, usually the calves, followed by pseudohypertrophy of the muscles when the necrotic muscle fibers are replaced by fat and connective tissue. Lumbar lordosis and scoliosis develop. Deep tendon reflexes are diminished and eventually disappear, except for the preservation of the ankle reflexes until relatively late. Despite severe atrophy, no fasciculations are seen.

Cardiac involvement is frequent, but chronic congestive heart failure is rare. This is secondary to replacement and fibrosis of some of the heart musculature, mainly in

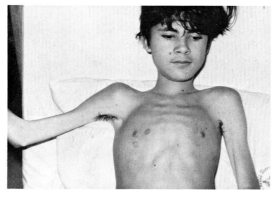

FIG. 8-5. With the arm abducted, note the contractures of the adductors and the pectoral muscles of a 14-year-old boy with Duchenne's muscular dystrophy.

the left ventricle.[33] Abnormalities seen on electrocardiograms include tachycardia and classically tall R waves in the right precordial leads and deep Q waves in the limb leads and left precordial leads.[33] Atrial and ventricular arrhythmias may occur.

Skeletal abnormalities are manifested by decreased skeletal growth, narrowing and rarefaction of the shafts of the long bones, and impaired development of some flat bones.[45] Severe decalcification, scoliosis, and gross distortion of the skeletal system ensue. Minimal trauma produces fractures. These changes are most likely secondary to disuse of the limbs and the absence of normal muscular stress and strain.

COURSE. The Duchenne type of muscular dystrophy follows a continuous, relentless, downhill course. In general, the patients are unable to walk by about 10 years of age, and are limited to a wheelchair existence not long thereafter. Severe contractures, usually beginning in calf muscles and hip flexors and later in muscles of the upper extremities, develop. Immobility and bed rest rapidly accelerate the weakness and the development of contractures. By adolescence or early adult life, death occurs secondary to respiratory difficulties and infections, and rarely from cardiac failure.

DIAGNOSTIC AIDS. Serum muscle enzymes, especially creatinine phosphokinase, are invariably increased, often to exceedingly high levels early in the course. The enzyme levels are highest in infancy and markedly decrease as age increases, paralleling the change in muscle pathology. Seventy to seventy-five percent of adult carriers will show an increased serum creatinine phosphokinase.[43] Serum pyruvate kinase has recently been shown to be helpful in revealing carrier states.[2]

Electromyograms show findings consistent with myopathic disease, i.e., decrease in size and amplitude of motor unit potentials without an increase in spontaneous activity (fasciculations and fibrillations). Muscle biopsy results are as stated above.

VARIANTS. Becker muscular dystrophy (benign sex-linked recessive muscular dystrophy) is a relatively benign sex-linked inherited form of muscular dystrophy.[9] Onset is usually later in childhood than in the Duchenne form of dystrophy and can even have its onset in young adult life. The progression of the illness is much slower and less severe. There are gradual weakness and wasting of the proximal muscles of the lower limbs followed by the same in the upper extremities. Although a normal life span is possible, a wheelchair existence is usually reached in middle adult life. There are no cardiac deformities, contractures, or skeletal abnormalities. Creatinine phosphokinase may be increased but not nearly as high as is that seen in Duchenne's muscular dystrophy.

DIFFERENTIAL DIAGNOSIS. The diagnosis of Duchenne's muscular dystrophy in a patient with a positive family history, high creatinine phosphokinase, and progressive muscular weakness is easy to make. Other cases must be distinguished from other congenital myopathies, thyroid disease, and childhood onset of some form of spinal muscular atrophy. Examination of electromyograms and muscle biopsy specimens, stained by special techniques, can enable the differentiation.

TREATMENT. Treatment at the present time is symptomatic and supportive. Ambulation is important in early stages in light of rapid deterioration once the patient becomes bedridden. Orthopaedic procedures may be necessary to relieve the deformities. Defining carrier states is important for genetic counseling.

Limb-girdle Dystrophy

Limb-girdle dystrophy is another of the muscular dystrophies characterized by weakness either of shoulder girdle muscles or of the pelvic girdle musculature, usually with eventual spread to the other after a variable amount of time. Females are affected as frequently as males. Many cases are sporadic, but about one half of the affected patients shows autosomal recessive inheritance.[35] This group of muscular dystrophy patients is much less well defined than the other groups, and there tends to be overlap into other forms of dystrophies, as well as difficulty in separating this disease from some of the neuropathic disorders.

The age at the time of onset is extremely variable. Symptoms usually begin in the second or third decade, but cases can occur in the fourth decade. Those appearing in the first decade manifest a disease similar to the benign form of sex-linked muscular dystrophy (Becker type).

CLINICAL FEATURES. Initial features depend on whether the shoulder or pelvic girdle musculature is the first area to be involved. Weakness of the muscles of the shoulder girdle produces difficulty in lifting the hands over the head and the development of sloped shoulders. Muscles of the shoulder girdle commonly affected are the rhomboids, trapezius, serratus anterior, and latissimus dorsi.[43] The involvement may subsequently spread to the more distal muscles of the upper extremity. Eventually both the shoulder girdle and pelvic girdle are involved. Lower limb involvement produces dysfunction in the psoas, gluteus maximus, quadriceps, and adductors. Anterior tibial muscles and peroneal muscles may also be affected, but the calf muscles are spared until late. The dysfunction is symmetric and wasting soon becomes evident. There may be mild calf hypertrophy in some cases. The cranial nerve musculature is spared, but the neck muscles are affected at about the same time the disease appears in the shoulder girdle.

The biceps and brachioradialis reflexes, along with the knee reflex, are decreased or abolished, but the ankle jerks are preserved. Wasting will be pronounced, but there are no fasciculations. Muscle contractures and skeletal deformities appear late in the disease as the patient becomes bedridden. Cardiac involvement is rare.

COURSE. The course of the illness is extremely variable, but in general this disorder is more benign than the Duchenne muscular dystrophy. Some families may show the illness restricted to only a small group of muscles in apparent arrest for many years. The severity and rate of progression vary greatly, but usually by the middle of adult life the patient will assume a wheelchair existence. Life span is probably somewhat decreased. Usually the prognosis is better if the shoulder girdle muscles are involved first, because ambulation is allowed for a longer period of time.

DIAGNOSTIC AIDS. Serum muscle enzymes, especially creatinine phosphokinase, may be elevated, but certainly not as high as in Duchenne's muscular dystrophy. Carriers do not have an increase in their serum muscle enzymes.

Changes on electromyograms are consistent with a myopathic process (see previous section). Results of nerve conduction studies are normal. Muscle biopsy specimens reveal nonspecific evidence of myopathy.

DIFFERENTIAL DIAGNOSIS. As stated previously, the group of limb-girdle dystrophies are not as well defined as the other groups of dystrophies, and differentiation from other myopathic and even neuropathic processes may also be difficult. Symptoms of proximal muscle weakness and wasting are also common to many acquired myopathies of some systemic diseases, such as sarcoidosis, thyroid disease, or collagen-vascular disease. Others to be distinguished are the benign sex-linked muscular dystrophy (Becker type), polymyositis, and Kugelberg-Welander disease. Clinical examination, neurophysiologic and biochemical studies, and muscle biopsy specimens specially stained for fiber group types may all be needed to achieve an accurate diagnosis.

TREATMENT. As of yet, no specific therapy is available. Treatment is mainly supportive and to prevent a wheelchair existence, because the muscle contractures and weakness will rapidly progress once the patient is unable to walk.

Facioscapulohumeral Dystrophy

Facioscapulohumeral dystrophy is an autosomal dominant inherited muscular dystrophy that is seen as frequently in males as in females.[42] Some sporadic cases do occur, and rarely there have been cases documented with an autosomal recessive type of inheritance. Onset is at any time from childhood to adult life, but most commonly in the late first or early second decades. Weakness early in infancy is rare. Slow progression of symptoms is usually the rule, and the patients usually live a normal life span.[42]

CLINICAL FEATURES. The onset of facioscapulohumeral dystrophy is similar to that of limb-girdle muscular dystrophy. Weakness begins insidiously in the shoulder girdle, often asymmetrically, and results in difficulty in raising the arms and produces elevation and winging of the scapulae. At times, the biceps and triceps muscles may be weaker and more wasted than the deltoid muscles on the same side of the body. Distal musculature in the upper limbs is usually spared. Unlike limb-girdle muscular dystrophy, however, the shoulder girdle weakness is followed by facial weakness. Thus, there will be lack of facial expression, difficulty in pursing the lips, and trouble with speech. A characteristic pouting expression and transverse smile appear. There will be difficulty in closing the eyes tightly. There is subsequent spread of the weakness to the muscles of the pelvic girdle and lower limbs.

Unlike many of the other dystrophies and neuropathic diseases, the dysfunction in facioscapulohumeral dystrophy is frequently patchy and asymmetric. Another peculiar characteristic is early involvement of anterior tibial muscles which produces footdrop and a flapping gait. Eventually there may be truncal weakness and lumbar lordosis.

There is no involvement of the levator palpebrae, extraocular muscles, pharyngeal muscles, or muscles of mastication. There are no skeletal nor specific cardiac abnormalities, and skeletal deformities and contractures are rare.

COURSE. The course of facioscapulohumeral dystrophy is one of variable severity and rate or progression of disease. Although some patients are severely disabled, in most patients the disease follows an insidious course with prolonged periods of apparent arrest.[42] Most patients survive and are active to a normal age. Variation in the severity of the disease expression from family to family can be seen. In the more rapidly progressive cases, death usually results from respiratory infection.

DIAGNOSTIC AIDS. Serum muscle enzymes are usually normal. Occasionally, creatinine phosphokinase may be slightly elevated. Electromyograms and muscle biopsy specimens reveal nonspecific changes of a myopathic process. Results of nerve conduction studies are normal.

DIFFERENTIAL DIAGNOSIS. Limb-girdle muscular dystrophy is similar to facioscapulohumeral dystrophy at its onset by causing proximal weakness in the upper limbs, but involvement of facial musculature in limb-girdle dystrophy is not common. Elevation of the scapulae on abduction of arms is thought to be characteristic of facioscapulohumeral dystrophy.[43] Furthermore, asymmetry of signs and symptoms and the early involvement of anterior tibial muscles are rare in early limb-girdle dystrophy. Polymyositis, thyroid disease, and the spinal muscular atrophies should also be considered.

TREATMENT. As with the other dystrophies, treatment is symptomatic and supportive. Care is taken to prevent development of contractures and thus to continue the ambulation of the patient.

Oculopharyngeal Muscular Dystrophy

Oculopharyngeal muscular dystrophy is an autosomal dominant inherited degenerative disease which occurs more frequently in people of French-Canadian descent.[11] Onset of the disease is late in life, usually around 40 years of age. Males and females are affected equally in frequency.

Symptoms usually begin with dysphagia followed by bilateral ptosis. Extraocular muscle movements are not affected. Weakness of the shoulder girdle and other proximal muscles of the upper extremities may be significant. There are no sensory abnormalities or upper motor neuron signs. Progression is relatively slow and benign, and the life span is usually not significantly altered.

Electromyographic studies and muscle biopsy specimens are nonspecific for a myopathic disorder. Serum muscle enzymes are normal.

Scapuloperoneal Atrophy

Scapuloperoneal atrophy is a slowly progressive neuromuscular disorder inherited as an autosomal dominant disease.[20] It is rare in frequency compared to other dystrophies and neuropathic processes. There is still some debate whether this is a primary neuropathic or myopathic process, and the syndrome tends to merge with Kugelberg-Welander disease, limb-girdle dystrophy, and Charcot-Marie-Tooth disease (peroneal muscular atrophy).[35]

Onset is usually in late adolescence or early adult life, and progression of symptoms is slow. There are symmetric weakness and wasting of the long extensor muscles of the toes and ankles. Subsequently, weakness begins in the shoulder girdle muscles and produces winged scapulae. The weakness in the legs spreads to involve the more proximal muscles. In several cases, facial weakness, dysphagia, and dysarthria have been present. Deep tendon reflexes are decreased in the arms, whereas knee and ankle reflexes are usually abolished. Results of sensory examination are normal.

Electromyograms reveal myopathic changes, but, in addition, there are spontaneous fibrillation potentials suggesting a neuropathic process. Results of nerve conduction studies are normal. Muscle biopsy specimens show nonspecific changes. The distribution of weakness and atrophy of the face and shoulder muscles are similar to those of facioscapulohumeral dystrophy. The distal weakness and atrophy in the legs resemble Charcot-Marie-Tooth disease. Other features suggest Kugelberg-Welander disease. As yet, too few cases have been studied, and scapuloperoneal atrophy may yet turn out to be a variant of one of the previously named diseases and not a specific disease entity in itself.

Inflammatory Muscle Disorders

Polymyositis

See Chapter 22.

Myosilis Associated with Collagen-vascular Disorders

A variant of polymyositis is the myositis associated with the connective tissue diseases. This includes rheumatoid arthritis, systemic lupus erythematosus, Sjögren's syndrome, scleroderma, and rarely polyarteritis nodosa. Polyarteritis nodosa probably does not produce a true myositis, but more likely microinfarctions in the muscle with secondary inflammation.

The myositis present in the aforementioned disorders is similar to that seen in "pure" polymyositis. There are no antinuclear antibodies, anti-DNA antibodies, and rheumatoid factor in the sera of patients with polymyositis. Sera conversion of patients being followed as true polymyositis to positive antibodies or rheumatoid factors suggests one of the overlap syndromes. Since most patients with active collagen-vascular disease are treated with high dose corticosteroids, the plan of treatment is essentially the same.

Although not a collagen-vascular disease, sarcoidosis is a chronic inflammatory condition which can occasionally produce a myositis.[17] Progressive muscle wasting and weakness resembling polymyositis or an adult muscular dystrophy will be present. Once again, treatment is with corticosteroids.

Polymyalgia Rheumatica

Polymyalgia rheumatica is encountered in patients 55 to 60 years of age and older.[19] Myalgias, arthralgias, and stiffness in the muscles of the shoulder girdle, neck, and back are present. Occasionally, the pelvic girdle and lower limbs are involved. Muscle tenderness is prominent. A significant point of differentiation from other muscular and neurologic disorders is that true weakness is usually not significant. Constitutional symptoms of fever, malaise, and weight loss may be present.

The erythrocyte sedimentation rate is invariably elevated, almost always over 60, and often over 100. Anemia is often present. Results of electromyography, nerve conduction studies, serum muscle enzymes, and muscle biopsy specimens are all normal. Low dose corticosteroid therapy is employed unless there is a concomitant temporal arteritis.

The association of temporal arteritis with polymyalgia rheumatica is well known.[19] Temporal arteritis is a medical emergency, and immediate treatment with corticosteroids is imperative to prevent blindness which results from the arteritis in the ophthalmic artery. Any patient over the age of 50 with multiple aches and pains and new complaints of headache needs an immediate determination of sedimentation rate whether or not the temporal arteries are palpable or thickened. If the sedimentation rate is significantly elevated, temporal artery biopsy and high dose corticosteroid therapy should be implemented immediately.

Carcinomatous Neuromyopathy

As one of the remote effects of carcinoma on the nervous system, a neuromyopathy may develop in patients with cancer without evidence of metastatic involvement of the central nervous system, peripheral nerves, or muscles.[14] In an adult patient with an unexplained, acquired myopathy, an underlying neoplasm must be searched for.

The pathogenesis is unknown, but it is likely that the tumor is producing a neuro-humeral substance that indirectly affects the nerves and muscles. Findings are most commonly seen in males and those with oat cell carcinoma of the lung. The cancer may precede or follow the onset of the myopathy.

There are weakness and wasting of the proximal muscles of the upper extremities and usually of the lower limbs as well. Clinical examination and electromyographic studies do not reveal polymyositis or the myasthenic syndrome (Eaton-Lambert syndrome). Muscle biopsy specimens reveal nonspecific changes. There is no specific treatment for the myopathy.

Thyroid Disease

Thyrotoxic myopathy must always be ruled out in a patient with an unexplained myopathy. In greater than 50 percent of hyperthyroid patients, there is electromyographic and often clinical evidence of a myopathy.[12] The cause is probably secondary to the effects of thyroid hormone.

Symptoms and signs are really no different from those of the other myopathies except that signs of hyperthyroidism may be present. Another point of differentiation is that deep tendon reflexes are normal. Pain is not a prominent feature, though there may be some degree of muscle aching. Weakness and atrophy are prominent in the proximal muscles of both upper and lower limbs, and fasciculations may be present. Respiratory muscles are rarely involved. Muscle biopsy specimens may be normal or show nonspecific evidence of a myopathy.

Treatment is management of the underlying hyperthyroidism. It should be recalled from a previous section that 5 to 10 percent of myasthenia gravis patients develops hyperthyroidism, which could significantly contribute to the muscle weakness.

REFERENCES

1. Achari, A. M., and Andersen, M. S.: Serum creatine phosphokinase in amyotrophic lateral sclerosis: Correlation with sex, duration, and skeletal muscle biopsy. Neurology (Minneap.), 24:834–837, 1974.
2. Alberts, M. C., and Samaha, F. J.: Serum pyruvate kinase in muscle disease and carrier states. Neurology (Minneap.), 24:462–464, 1974.
3. Armstrong, R. M., Fagelson, M. H., and Silberberg, D. H.: Familial spinal muscular atrophy. Arch. Neurol., 14:208–212, 1966.

4. Austin, G.: The diagnosis and treatment of intervertebral disc disease. In The Spinal Cord: Basic Aspects and Surgical Considerations. Edited by G. Austin. Springfield, Ill., Charles C Thomas, 1972.

5. Baker, A. S., Ojemann, R. G., Swartz, M. N., and Richardson, E. P.: Spinal epidural abscess. N. Engl. J. Med., 293:463–468, 1975.

6. Barnes, R.: Traction injuries of the brachial plexus in adults. J. Bone Joint Surg., 31-B:10–16, 1949.

7. Barnett, H. J. M., Foster, J. B., and Hudgson, P.: Syringomyelia. Philadelphia, W. B. Saunders Co., 1973.

8. Bastian, F. O., Rabson, A. S., Yee, C. L., and Tralka, T. S.: Herpes virus hominis: Isolation from human trigeminal ganglion. Science, 178:306–307, 1972.

9. Becker, P. E., and Keiner, F.: Eine neue X-chromosomale Muskeldystrophie. Arch. Psychiatr. Nervenkr., 193:427, 1955.

10. Bonney, G.: Prognosis in traction lesions of the brachial plexus. J. Bone Joint Surg., 41-B:4–41, 1959.

11. Bray, G. M., Kaarsoo, M., and Ross, R. T.: Ocular myopathy with dysphagia. Neurology (Minneap.), 15:678–684, 1965.

12. Buchthal, F.: Electrophysiological abnormalities in metabolic myopathies and neuropathies. Acta Neurol. Scand. (suppl. 43), 46:129, 1970.

13. Cotton, P. B., and Webb-Peploe, M. M.: Acute transverse myelitis as a complication of glandular fever. Br. Med. J. 1:654–655, 1966.

14. Dayan, A. D., Croft, P. B., and Wilkinson, M.: Association of carcinomatous neuromyopathy with different histological types of carcinoma of the lung. Brain, 88:427–434, 1965.

15. Emery, A. E., and Walton, J. N.: The genetics of muscular dystrophy. Prog. Med. Genet., 5:116, 1967.

16. Gardner, W. J.: Hydrodynamic mechanisms of syringomyelia: Its relationship to myelocoele. J. Neurol. Neurosurg. Psychiatry, 28:247–259, 1965.

17. Gardner-Thorpe, C.: Muscle weakness due to sarcoid myopathy. Neurology (Minneap.), 22:917–928, 1972.

18. Gathier, J. C., and Bruyn, G. W.: Neuralgic amyotrophy. In Handbook of Clinical Neurology. Amsterdam, North-Holland Pub. Co., 1970, Vol. 8.

19. Hunder, G. G., Disney, T. F., and Ward, L. E.: Polymyalgia rheumatica. Mayo Clin. Proc., 44:849–879, 1969.

20. Kaeser, H. E.: Scapuloperoneal muscular atrophy. Brain, 88:407–426, 1965.

21. Klawans, H. L.: Delayed traumatic syringomyelia. Dis. Nerv. Syst., 29:525–528, 1968.

22. Leffert, R. D.: Brachial plexus injuries. N. Engl. J. Med., 291:1059–1067, 1974.

23. Love, J. G.: Protruded intervertebral discs. In Clinical Neurology. Edited by A. B. Baker and L. H. Baker. Hagerstown, Md., Harper & Row, 1971, Vol. 3.

24. Merritt, H. L.: A Textbook of Neurology. Philadelphia, Lea & Febiger, 1973.

25. Meyer, G. A., Stern, J., and Pappel, M. W.: Rapid osseous changes in syringomyelia. Radiology, 69:415–418, 1957.

26. Mulder, D. W., and Espinosa, R. E.: Amyotrophic lateral sclerosis: Comparison of the clinical syndrome in Guam and the United States. In Motor Neurone Diseases. Edited by F. H. Norris and L. T. Kurlan. New York, Grune & Stratton, 1969.

27. Muller, N.: Spondylosis of the cervical vertebral column. In Handbook of Clinical Neurology. Edited by P. J. Vinken and G. W. Bruyn. Amsterdam, North-Holland Pub. Co., 1970, Vol. 7.

28. Norris, F. H.: Guanidine in amyotrophic lateral sclerosis. N. Engl. J. Med., 288:690–691, 1973.

29. Odom, G. L., Finney, W., and Woodhall, B.: Cervical disc lesions. J.A.M.A., 166:23–28, 1958.

30. Pallis, C., Jones, A. M., and Spillane, J. D.: Cervical spondylosis: Incidence and implication. Brain, 77:274–289, 1954.

31. Parsonage, M. J., and Turner, J. W. A.: Neuralgic amyotrophy. The shoulder girdle syndrome. Lancet, 1:973–978, 1948.

32. Pearn, J. H., Carter, C. O., and Wilson, J.: The genetic identity of acute infantile spinal muscular atrophy. Brain, 96:463–470, 1973.

33. Perloff, J. K., Roberts, W. C., de Leon, A. C., and O'Doherty, D.: The distinctive electrocardiogram of Duchenne's progressive muscular dystrophy. Am. J. Med., 42:179–188, 1967.

34. Pratt, R. T. C.: Genetics of Neurological Disorders. London, Oxford University Press, 1967.

35. Rowland, L. P., and Layzer, R. B.: Muscular dystrophies, atrophies and related diseases. In Clinical Neurology. Edited by A. B. Baker and L. H. Baker. Hagerstown, Md., Harper & Row, 1971, Vol. 3.

36. Schaafsma, S. J.: Plexus injuries. In Handbook of Clinical Neurology. Edited by P. J. Vinken and G. W. Bruyn. Amsterdam, North-Holland Pub. Co., 1970, Vol. 7.

37. Seddon, K. J.: Nerve lesions complicating certain closed injuries. J.A.M.A., 135.691–694, 1947.

38. Sloof, J. L., Kernohan, J. W., and MacCarthy, C. S.: Primary Intramedullary Tumors of the Spinal Cord and Filum Terminale. Philadelphia, W. B. Saunders Co., 1964.

39. Spillane, J. D., and Wells, C. E. C.: The neurology of jennerian vaccination. Brain, 87:1–44, 1964.

40. Taterka, J. H., and O'Sullivan, M. E.: The motor complications of herpes zoster. J.A.M.A., 122:737–739, 1943.

41. Taylor, A. R.: Mechanism and treatment of spinal cord disorders associated with cervical spondylosis. Lancet, 1:717–720, 1953.

42. Walton, J. N.: Clinical aspects of human muscular dystrophy. In Muscular Dystrophy in Man and Animals. Edited by G. H. Bourne and N. Golarz. Basel, Karger, 1963.

43. Walton, J. N., and Gardner-Medwin, D.: Muscular dystrophy and myotonic disorders. In Disorders of Voluntary Muscles. Edited by J. N. Walton. Edinburgh, Churchill Livingstone, 1974.

44. Walton, J. N., and Warwick, C. K.: Osseous changes in myopathy. Br. J. Radiol., 27:1–15, 1954.

9

Orthopaedic Management of Neuromuscular Disorders

MELVIN POST

In past years it was thought that with the disappearance of poliomyelitis and improved methods of obstetric care the need for stabilizing procedures about the shoulder, such as arthrodesis and muscle-tendon transfers, would be greatly minimized. Especially in the Western World this happy thought was short-lived because of the increase of automobile, industrial, and athletic injuries. There is still a need for the surgeon to assess accurately functional neuromuscular deficits, and to understand what methods are best suited to restore function about the shoulder girdle after an irreparable loss of muscle. The surgeon must decide whether to perform an arthrodesis with its greater chance for success, and its production of strength and power but diminished motion, or a muscle transfer with the possibility of a greater range of shoulder motion. If muscle transfer fails, an arthrodesis can still be performed, at least in cases of deltoid paralysis.

This section reviews the principles, indications, and methods for stabilization and restoration of shoulder function.

EVALUATION OF SHOULDER GIRDLE FUNCTION

Each patient must have a thorough examination including (1) a peripheral nerve evaluation; (2) strength testing of the muscles of the upper extremity and the back as they affect the shoulder girdle; and (3) motion testing of all three joints of the shoulder girdle (glenohumeral, acromioclavicular, and sternoclavicular) and the scapulothoracic articulation, as well as active motion testing of the distal joints. A comparison should be made with the opposite side. It is essential to know if a muscle is partially or completely paralyzed, the time of onset, and to what degree spontaneous recovery is still possible. For example, is loss of abduction merely caused by paralysis of the anterior and middle deltoid or serratus anterior, or a combination of both? Can a precise level of nerve involvement be determined by clinical examination?[54] Is the loss of multiple muscle groups so great that there is no possibility of restoring overhead motion by any muscle transfer? Often, muscle paralysis enhances the possibility of subluxation of the humeral head from the glenoid. Can this be effectively controlled? With increased paralysis of shoulder muscles, there is a greater burden placed upon the scapulothoracic muscles. In this event, the surgeon should recognize how a contemplated substitution of one muscle may affect the integrated action of other muscle groups. Preoperatively, the end result should be predictable to a reasonable degree.

Steindler has shown that the acromioclavicular joint permits (1) backward and forward movement, (2) pendulum motion about the horizontal transverse axis, and (3) gliding movement backward and forward about a vertical axis.[59] He stated that the sternoclavicular joint moves 20 to 25 degrees in a vertical axis, 30 degrees about a horizontal axis, and up to 60 degrees in an up and down sagittal plane. The glenohumeral joint abducts 120 degrees when external rotation of the arm is normal beyond 90 degrees of arm abduction. Full overhead 180 degree motion results when the scapulothoracic articulation rotates 60 degrees. Thus, any defect in the mechanisms responsible for the component motions, whether caused by trauma, contracture, or loss of muscle power, does interfere with normal scapulothoracic rhythm. Contractures must be overcome before muscle transfer is performed in those patients who are not candidates for arthrodesis. A transplanted muscle not only loses significant strength but cannot move a joint that is stiff or whose articular surfaces are severely damaged. Moreover, the muscle must be large and strong enough to accomplish its intended purpose.[48] In effect, the surgeon must formulate a workable plan of treatment in order to achieve the best result.

Deltoid Paralysis

The literature is replete with papers regarding restoration of function of the paralyzed deltoid about the shoulder.[19,25,32] In 1867, Duchenne reasoned from electrophysiologic experiments that the most powerful action of the deltoid was produced by the anterior fibers, with a decreasing ability to elevate the arm to 90 degrees toward the posterior fibers. In 1903, Bunts reported 7 of 19 patients with deltoid paralysis who had spontaneous recovery in abduction, although 4 of these failed to regain deltoid power.[7] In 1910, Lewis reported on his method of restoring abduction power at the shoulder by transferring the trapezius into the glenohumeral capsule, and oversewing the detached origin of the paralyzed deltoid.[32] Using anatomic models, Pollock showed the supplementary muscle actions about the shoulder with deltoid paralysis.[42] Staples and Watkins confirmed Pollock's observation that full active shoulder abduction could be regained in the absence of deltoid power if the other supplementary muscles were functioning.[56] Dehne and Hall agreed with these findings, although they noted a persistently disturbed scapulothoracic rhythm.[11]

In 1927, Mayer described his method of trapezius transfer to restore deltoid function. The trapezius is detached from its bony insertion and lengthened by construction of an artificial tendon made of fascia lata, and the rolled end is sutured to the humerus near the deltoid insertion.[35] Later experience showed that results could be improved by keeping the fascial transplant as a flat sheet, corresponding in shape to the deltoid, rather than as rolled cord[36] (see Fig. 9-3). Mayer showed that sufficient healing occurred between muscle and fascial transplant to justify its use.

In 1955, Bateman modified the trapezius transfer by moving the acromion and part of the scapular spine with its trapezius attachment to the lateral humerus.[3] Saha believed that the leverage was too short by this method and wasted available power.[46] He completely mobilized the upper and middle trapezius from its insertion, gaining 5 cm. of length without traumatizing the neurovascular supply to the muscle. The muscle with the detached distal clavicle, the capsule of the acromioclavicular joint, the acromial process, and the adjoining portion of the posterior border of the spine were rerouted and attached to the humeral shaft as far distally as possible (see Fig. 9-4).

Other methods have been devised to accomplish active abduction at the shoulder. In 1928, Reidel transferred both the origin and insertion of the teres major to the acromion and posterior humeral shaft, respectively, for posterior deltoid paralysis.[44]

In 1932, Ober[40] (see Fig. 9-5), in 1936, Davidson[10] and in 1950, Harmon[22] transferred the heads of the short biceps and the long triceps to the anterior and posterior edges of the acromion to restore deltoid function.

Hildebrandt,[25] in 1906, and Haas,[19] in 1935, transferred the origin of the pectoralis major to restore deltoid power.

For paralysis of the anterior, middle, or posterior parts of the deltoid Harmon transferred the active anterior deltoid posteriorly, for example, for paralysis of the respective portion of the deltoid muscle[21,22] (see Fig. 9-6).

Scapular Instability

Adequate shoulder function cannot be achieved without scapular stability. In 1932, Whitman described his method of repair of serratus anterior paralysis in which the vertebral border of the scapula is attached to the spinous processes of the fourth to seventh thoracic vertebrae by four fascial strips[64] (see Fig. 9-7). In 1937, Dickson fixed the scapula to the paravertebral cervical muscles and to the first thoracic spinous process with a strip of fascia lata.[13] He used the same method to fix the inferior angle of the scapula, using fascial strips to the active pectoralis major and latissimus dorsi to stabilize and yet allow active pull on the hypermobile scapula, which results from the paralyzed serratus anterior and rhomboids. In 1939, Brockway,[5] and in 1932, Lowman[34] used interscapular fascial transplants to provide stability of the affected scapula.

Brunnstrom showed the importance of the muscles that attach to the scapula, and stressed the significance of scapular stability.[6]

Spira reported his method of stabilizing the dropped shoulder resulting from paralysis of the shoulder girdle muscles in which the inferior angle of the scapula is fixed to the sixth rib.[55] Although this fixes the shoulder blade, it eliminates useful accessory movement during humeral elevation.

Serratus Anterior and Associated Muscle Paralyses

Normal upper extremity movement depends to a large extent upon the integrity of the muscles that attach to the scapula. The two most important muscles that control scapular movement and stability are the serratus anterior and trapezius. Others, including the rhomboids and levator scapulae, are also important for normal shoulder blade function. In 1938, Horwitz and Tocantins described the anatomy of the serratus anterior, and showed how the long thoracic nerve was susceptible to damage by its morphologic relationship to surrounding structures, to trauma, and to a variety of noxious agents.[26,27] They stressed the importance of scapular derotation in restoring tonicity of the paralyzed serratus by flexing the elbow, and thereby decreasing the pull of the biceps and coracobrachialis on the glenoid part of the scapula. Wolf used an appliance to control winging after permanent serratus paralysis when operative treatment could not be undertaken.[66] It allowed complete arm freedom, and pressed the winged scapula against the chest cage while preventing scapular rotation. Although the patient should be encouraged to wear external devices such as this even during periods of sleep in the stage of recovery from paralysis, the devices are not well tolerated.

In 1904, Tubby described his method of restoring serratus function by utilizing the sternal portion of the pectoralis major. He freed its humeral attachment, divided the sectioned pectoralis into several fasciculi, and sutured the pectoralis into as broad an expanse of serratus anterior as possible.[63]

For permanent serratus anterior paralysis, Hass, in 1931, described his method of transferring the teres major insertion to the fifth and sixth ribs, after the cut tendon is divided for each of the rib attachments and passed deep to the latissimus.[23]

In 1945, Durman restored serratus anterior function by transfer of the lower third of the pectoralis major insertion to the inferior angle of the scapula using a strip of fascia lata.[15] Chaves,[8] in 1951, and Rapp,[43] in 1954, used the pectoralis minor, extending the cut tendon with a strip of fascia lata and suturing it near the vertebral margin of the scapula (see Fig. 9-8).

In 1951, Herzmark attempted to improve residual rhomboid function by reattaching the rhomboid insertion to the posterior surface of the scapula and overlapping the trapezius.[24]

In 1954, Steindler recommended transferring the levator scapulae to the acromion to substitute for paralysis of the upper trapezius, and transferring the pectoralis major and/or minor to the inferior scapula angle to effect rotational control of the scapula in the anteroposterior axis when necessary.[61]

PHYSIOLOGIC BASIS FOR RESTORATION OF SHOULDER FUNCTION

It remained for Saha, in 1967, to clarify the understanding of appropriate methods of treatment for paralytic conditions about the shoulder. He organized the shoulder muscles into three groups based upon their physiology[46] (Table 9-1).

Prime Movers

Prime movers consist of the deltoid and the clavicular portion of the pectoralis major. They give the most active power in shoulder abduction, and act in three directions. By inserting the greatest distance from the glenohumeral joint, lifting power is enhanced. When they are paralyzed, surrounding muscle substitution is insufficient to restore adequate function. In this instance, muscle transfer is needed to restore active shoulder abduction.

Steering Group

The subscapularis, supraspinatus, and infraspinatus muscles (the short rotators) are the steering group. Their chief action is to stabilize the humeral head in the shallow glenoid and to steer the head by rolling and gliding movements. They also assist in shoulder abduction.

According to Saha, the infraspinatus acts mainly to control posterior gliding of the humeral head in the end stage of overhead elevation, an action similar to that of the subscapularis in the same position.[46] Retroversion of the humeral head is converted into relative anteversion in the overhead position. To prevent anterior subluxation, infraspinatus muscle function is needed. Supraspinatus and subscapularis action is necessary for shoulder abduction, steering the humeral head during abduction in various planes through a 150-degree arc. Extremes of the arc are aided (30 degrees on each side), simultaneously, when the scapula moves anteriorly and posteriorly and rotates vertically. Saha emphasized that control of vertical gliding of the humeral head is accomplished by the muscle fibers acting in the plane of motion, while the anterior and posterior muscle fibers cause the humeral head to glide in the horizontal plane with consecutive stages of shoulder abduction. Although the supraspinatus and subscapularis are essential for elevation, minor vertical gliding during elevation backward by the infraspinatus does not occur. The steering muscles fix the humeral head in the glenoid during each increment of elevation.

Depressor Group

The muscles of the depressor group are made up of the sternal head of the pectoralis major, latissimus dorsi, teres major, and teres minor. The last-named muscle is included here because electromyographic evidence has shown that it participates in this group action.[46] These muscles rotate the humerus during abduction and depress the humeral head, helping to effect the last few degrees of abduction. They also have a minimal steering action on the humeral head. When the power of these muscles is eliminated, the ability to lift heavy objects is correspondingly reduced.

Scapulothoracic rotation and trunk sta-

Table 9-1. *Possible Tendon Transfers to Restore Power at the Glenohumeral Joint*

Muscle Requiring Replacement or Reinforcement	Action	Choice of Muscles for Transfer in Order of Preference
Subscapularis	Posterior glider	1. Upper two digitations of serratus anterior 2. Pectoralis minor 3. Pectoralis major (whole or part). Muscles 1 to 3 act almost in the same direction as that of fibers of subscapularis 4. Levator scapulae 5. Scalenus anterior 6. Scalenus medius 7. Splenius capitis 8. Sternocleidomastoid Muscles 4 to 8 act from above and are second class substitutes
Infraspinatus	Posterior glider (acting from behind)	1. Latissimus dorsi 2. Teres major
Supraspinatus	Superior glider	1. Levator scapulae 2. Sternocleidomastoid 3. Scalenus anterior 4. Scalenus medius 5. Splenius capitis All these muscles act from above and, therefore, are good substitutes
Deltoid and clavicular head of pectoralis major	Prime mover (lifting)	1. Trapezius (as far down as possible on the shaft)

From Saha, A. K.: Surgery of the paralyzed and flail shoulder. Acta Orthop. Scand. (Suppl.), 97:40, 1967.

bility are necessary components in influencing humeral placement. Scapular stability during humeral elevation is also important and is provided by gravity, the lower fibers of the serratus anterior and rhomboids.

The classification of the shoulder muscles into their component functions now allows the surgeon to analyze the patient's problem more clearly, and to institute effective treatment. In paralysis of the prime movers, the importance of the steering group of muscles must be considered when performing tendon transfers to restore shoulder abduction. With paralysis of the steering muscles, transfer of a muscle, such as the trapezius, or of several muscles to a common attachment permits arm lifting only to 90 degrees and results in a loss of synchronous scapulohumeral rhythm.[9] Therefore, the preservation of the steering

muscles is crucial for the functioning of prime movers. When any two of these are paralyzed, tendon transfers should be performed to restore function.

Table 9-1 gives Saha's recommendations for possible tendon transfers to restore power at the glenohumeral joint. Although his work was based on the postpoliomyelitis patient, it can be applied to muscle paralyses resulting from multiple other causes.

The goal of any tendon transfer is to allow the patient to lift a reasonable amount of weight and place the hand in a number of positions needed for daily living. Saha believes that deltoid paralysis is best restored by trapezius transfer (see Fig. 9-4). Subscapularis paralysis may be treated by transfer of the upper two digitations of the serratus (Fig. 9-1). Levator scapulae transfer may be used for paralysis of the supraspinatus (Fig. 9-2), and pectoralis minor trans-

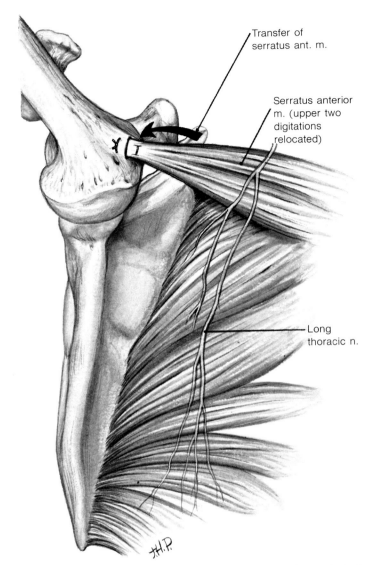

FIG. 9-1. Saha's transfer of upper two digitations of serratus to restore subscapularis function. The superior portion of the vertebral border of the scapula and the levator scapulae insertion are exposed by a saber-cut incision. The trapezius is reflected superiorly and backward. With the superior part of the vertebral border of the scapula pulled backward, the upper two digitations of the serratus anterior are identified and hooked with a vein retractor close to the superior scapular angle between the serratus and subscapularis. The upper digitations are freed from the superior vertebral scapular border to the level of the base of the spine. The cut tendinous portion is folded and held with a heavy suture. With the patient's arm elevated 130 degrees, the end of the cut tendon is rerouted through the axillary floor near its posterior boundary, and injury to the thoracodorsal nerve to the latissimus dorsi and the long thoracic nerve to the serratus anterior is avoided. The neurovascular bundle is retracted superiorly and laterally and the cut tendon pulled anteriorly into the axilla. With blunt dissection posterior to the neurovascular bundle, the lesser tuberosity is exposed. The cut tendon is rerouted to the lesser tuberosity and fixed with heavy sutures as shown. (Modified from Saha, A. K.: Surgery of the paralyzed and flail shoulder. Acta Orthop. Scand. (Suppl.), 97:5–90, 1967.)

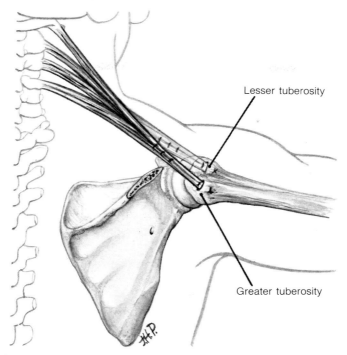

Lesser tuberosity

Greater tuberosity

FIG. 9-2. Saha's transfer of levator scapulae to restore supraspinatus or subscapularis function. With the identical surgical approach described in Figure 9-1 for the transfer of the upper two digitations of the serratus anterior for subscapularis paralysis, the superior and inferior borders of the levator scapulae are identified and the muscle's insertion is freed from the vertebral border of the scapula. The levator muscle belly is exposed to its mid-portion. The end of the cut tendon is folded and sutured. For paralysis of the supraspinatus it is rerouted to the greater tuberosity, and for subscapularis paralysis it is anchored to the lesser tuberosity as required. (Modified from Saha, A. K.: Surgery of the paralyzed and flail shoulder. Acta Orthop. Scand. (Suppl.), 97:5–90, 1967.)

fer can be performed for paralysis of the subscapularis. He employs sternoclei-domastoid transfer for supraspinatus paralysis, and either latissimus dorsi or teres major transfer, or both, for subscapularis paralysis.

PRINCIPLES OF MUSCLE TRANSFER ABOUT THE SHOULDER

The main purpose of muscle transfers about the shoulder is to restore function in paralyzed muscles in order that the upper extremity can work effectively. For example, isolated deltoid paralysis is not an indication for tendon transfer when scapulothoracic rhythm is not greatly disturbed. Transfer operations should be performed only if there is adequate function in the elbow and hand. Obviously, they should not be done if the distal parts are flail.

Certain prerequisites are needed for successful muscle transfer.[48,59] They are as follows: (1) contractures first must be overcome; (2) transferred muscles should have an action similar or related to the muscle they replace; (3) the integrity of the muscle should be protected by avoiding the splitting of a tendon or muscle which lets one half act independently of, or even antagonistically to, the other half; (4) the transferred muscle must be of sufficient size and strength to provide effective work; (5) the transferred muscle should pull in a relatively straight line; (6) tension on the transferred muscle should be enough to avoid any slack when the joint is in the correct position, i.e., it should be snug; (7) the new tendon attachment must be secure, preferably attaching it to bone; (8) passive joint motion should be excellent; and (9) joint surfaces should be congruous and smooth so that work force by the muscle is not expended. Obviously, the integrity of the nerve and blood supply of the transferred muscle must be maintained.

Early Management of Paralyzed Muscles

Rapid recovery of paralyzed muscle is favorable for early return of function. A weakened muscle that stretches has less chance for recovery. Thus, early treatment should consist of (1) immobilization in a functional position, (2) stimulation in an attempt to reduce atrophic changes, and (3) exercises to rebuild viable weakened muscle fibers.[20] These facts are especially important when it is realized that it is possible for atrophic skeletal muscle to regenerate itself through the activation of special, normally dormant cells, called satellite cells.

IMMOBILIZATION. For deltoid paralysis the arm should not be allowed to hang in the acute phase, especially if the shoulder cannot be actively moved. The extremity should be immobilized in a sling or an immobilizer, and the arm should be supported when at rest.

Serratus anterior paralysis requires a brace, such as described by Wolf[66] and Johnson and Kendall,[28] that presses the scapula to the thorax and derotates it downward and inward. Similarly, a brace for trapezius paralysis should give upward support while holding the scapula to the thorax. The actual construction and material selected may have to be modified for each individual patient, as the device is not ordinarily well tolerated. The patient should be encouraged to wear the brace even during rest periods.

STIMULATION. To prevent overstretching during the immobilization phase, and if the patient is cooperative, stimulation by heat, and more efficiently with electric stimulation of the muscle, can be tried in hope of retarding atrophy of denervated muscle.[4] The deltoid best lends itself to this treatment. In the future technical advances may allow the implantation of neuromuscular assistive electronic devices that stimulate paralyzed muscles in select cases and restore function.

EXERCISES. Every paralyzed muscle may contain the ability to regain at least some strength if the injured tissue is nurtured. Exercises may significantly contribute to the nourishment of the tissue. According to Wright, when a muscle is not used its circulation decreases further increasing atrophy.[68]

At least several times each day the patient should attempt to contract the paralyzed muscle voluntarily. For example, for the paralyzed serratus, the shoulder blade is brought forward, perhaps by pushing against a wall. In the beginning the patient may not be able to perform exercises against gravity.

Late Management of Paralyzed Muscles

When the surgeon contemplates an operation to restore function in a paralyzed muscle, he must be certain that the tendon transfer and not spontaneous muscle recovery is the reason for return of function. For example, although return of function in muscles paralyzed from nerve compression may take 3 to 6 months, it may require as long as 15 months in other cases, as observed in one patient with serratus anterior paralysis afflicted with herpes zoster. During this period the patient wore a brace and performed exercises. If recovery is not apparent and the patient complains of pain in the neck and shoulder region, loss of strength, stiffness, restricted motion about the shoulder, or deformity, surgical treatment can be considered.

OPERATIONS TO RESTORE LOST FUNCTION AT THE SHOULDER

A variety of different operations have been used over the years to restore function for paralyzed muscles about the shoulder. The accumulated experience of many authors shows that certain procedures are worthwhile if the criteria already set forth are present. Table 9-2 summarizes the oper-

Table 9-2. *Operations to Improve Function After Paralysis*

Muscle Paralysis	Author and Year	Muscle Transferred or Method of Stabilization
Deltoid	Mayer, 1927, 1939	Trapezius to humerus (Fig. 9-3)
	Ober, 1932	Heads of short biceps and long triceps to acromion (Fig. 9-5)
	Harmon, 1947, 1950	Shift backward or forward of active anterior or posterior deltoid (Fig. 9-6)
	Bateman, 1955	Trapezius to humerus
	Saha,* 1967	Trapezius to humerus (Fig. 9-4)
Deltoid-supraspinatus, associated with rhomboid weakness	Brockway, 1939	Interscapular fascia lata strips
Serratus anterior		*Anchoring Methods*
	Whitman, 1932	Fascia lata strips to spine (Fig. 9-7)
	Dickson, 1937	Fascia lata tubes to inferior border of pectoralis major and latissimus dorsi
	Spira, 1948	Scapular inferior angle fixation to rib
		Muscle Transfers
	Tubby, 1904	Pectoralis major to serratus anterior
	Durman, 1945	Pectoralis major to scapula
	Hass, 1931	Teres major insertion transfer to fifth and sixth ribs
	Chaves-Rapp, 1951, 1954	Pectoralis minor to inferior angle of scapula (Fig. 9-8)
	Herzmark, 1951	Rhomboid advancement
Upper trapezius	Steindler, 1954	Pectoralis major and/or minor to inferior scapula
Trapezius	Dewar-Harris, 1950	Fascia lata sling fixation of scapula and lateral transfer of levator scapulae (Fig. 9-9)
Levator scapulae	Dickson, 1937	Fascia lata tubes anchor scapula to cervical muscles and to spinous process of first thoracic vertebra

* See Table 9-1 for recommendations of Saha.

ations used to improve shoulder function that have been proved effective.

The prerequisites for successful outcome are that (1) shoulder girdle muscles are active and the scapula is stabilized; and (2) the glenohumeral joint must be reduced and have good passive motion.

Deltoid Paralysis

Mayer's Transfer of Trapezius[35,36]

The incision is directed from the base of the spine of the scapula laterally to the outer aspect of the clavicle, overlying the trapezius attachment to the bone. The full-thickness medial skin flap is dissected upward for 7.5 cm. over the surface of the trapezius (Fig. 9-3A).

The insertion of the trapezius is elevated, and then by blunt dissection lifted from its bed until its neurovascular supply is viewed on the deep surface about 7.5 cm. from the acromion (Fig. 9-3B). Posterior dissection is carried out between the trapezius and supraspinatus, and anteriorly between the trapezius and sternocleidomastoid.

A second incision, 5 cm. long, is made externally over the region of the deltoid

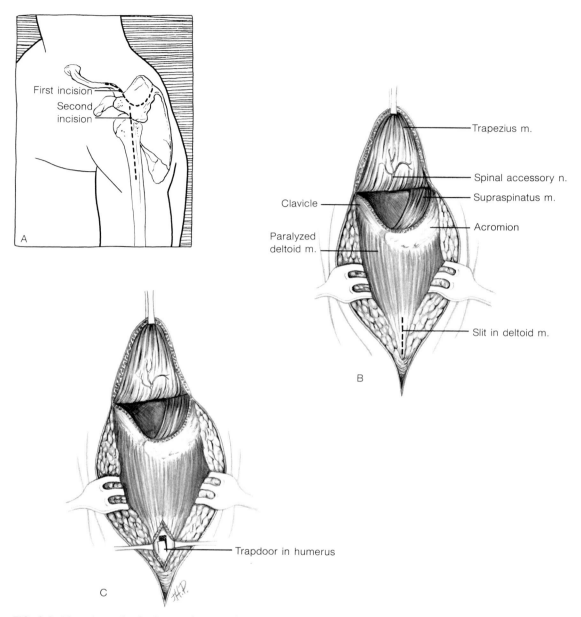

FIG. 9-3. Mayer's method of trapezius transfer to restore deltoid abduction power. (See text for discussion.) (Modified from Mayer, L.: Transplantation of trapezius for paralysis of abductors of arm. J. Bone Joint Surg., 9:412–420, 1927; and Mayer, L.: Operative reconstruction of the paralyzed upper extremity. J. Bone Joint Surg., 21:377–383, 1939.)

muscle insertion. The muscle fibers are slit for a distance of 3.8 cm. and the bone is exposed. A bone flap is elevated from the humerus, measuring 1.5 × 1.0 cm. (Fig. 9-3C).

A fascia lata sheet of adequate length, measuring 10 cm. in width above and tapered to a point below, is taken through a 22.5-cm.-long lateral thigh incision (Fig. 9-3D). The graft must reach from the cut edge of the trapezius to the bone window below. The broad upper end is attached with interrupted sutures as far proximally as possible on the undersurface of the trapezius with the rough surface of the fascia facing the

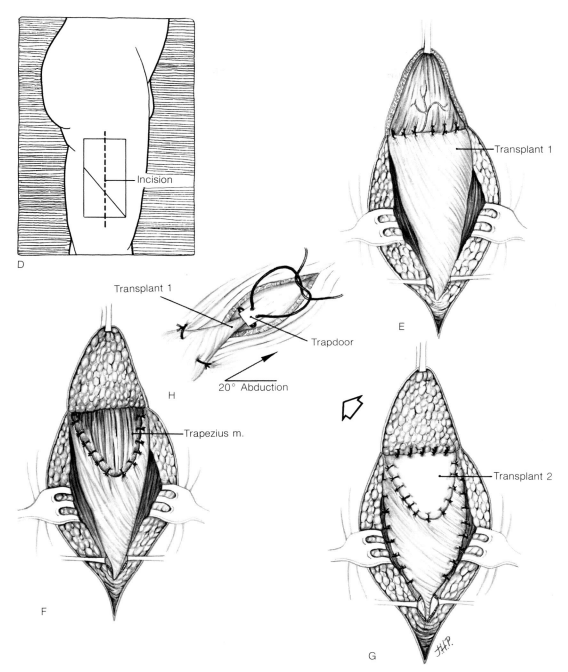

FIG. 9-3. Continued.

muscle. The distal edge of the trapezius is sutured to the fascia (Fig. 9-3E).

A second fascia lata sheet, measuring 7.5 cm. on each side, is fastened over the anterior surface of the trapezius to its cut lateral edge, the rough surface facing downward, and sutured to the first fascial graft, thereby enclosing the trapezius (much like the envelopment of the tensor thigh muscle between two layers of fascia) (Fig. 9-3F). The patient's arm is pulled over the acromion, and the front and back edges of the fascial graft are sutured to the anterior and posterior deltoid borders. With the help of heavy nonabsorbable suture, the lower end of the graft is placed through the bone window and fastened. It should be taut when the arm is held in abduction (Fig. 9-3H).

Whenever fascia lata grafts are used as extensions of a transferred muscle, there is danger that the fascia will eventually stretch and thereby diminish work effort by the transferred muscle.

AFTERCARE. The arm is laterally elevated 45 degrees and flexed 20 degrees and maintained in this position for 4 or 5 weeks in a plaster spica cast. Thereafter, gentle exercises are begun. However, for at least 4 additional months the arm is never permitted to drop to the side of the body so that immobilization must be continued when the extremity is not being exercised.

Bateman's Transfer of Trapezius[3,4]

The prerequisites are the same as those for Mayer's procedure.

The incision is begun over the medial spine of the scapula and continued along the spine to the lateral acromion and anteriorly along the outer third of the clavicle. A 6.3-cm. vertical incision is made over the lateral shoulder extending downward from the curved upper incision. The flaps are dissected to expose the spine of the scapula, the proximal lateral surface of the humerus, and the distal inch of the clavicle. The soft tissues are dissected free from the undersurface of the acromion and the spine of the scapula. An oblique osteotomy of the spine is performed, directed downward and laterally, mobilizing much of the trapezius.

The lateral 1.9 cm. of clavicle, lateral to the coracoclavicular ligament, is excised. The patient's arm is abducted to 90 degrees and a site on the lateral humerus scarified to which will be attached the trapezius. A few screws are used to fix the acromion to the lateral humerus at its new site.

AFTERCARE. A shoulder spica cast is applied for 4 to 6 weeks with the arm in 90 degrees of abduction. Thereafter, the cast is bivalved and cautious active exercises of the arm are started. At 8 weeks postopera-

tively, the cast is replaced within an abduction brace. Active exercises are gradually increased, during which time the arm is slowly allowed to fall to the side of the body.

Saha's Transfer of Trapezius[46]

A saber-shaped incision is started just above the level of the anterior axillary fold and extended slightly below the base of the spine, 2.5 cm. lateral and parallel to the vertebral border of the scapula. The incision is carried over the top of the acromion to the area just medial to the acromioclavicular joint.

The skin flaps are widely dissected to expose the whole origin of the paralyzed deltoid and upper shaft of the humerus. The deltoid origin is freed in its entirety.

An osteotomy of the clavicle is performed just lateral to the coracoclavicular ligament. The scapular notch is palpated, and with a Gigli saw an oblique osteotomy is performed on the base of the scapular spine (Fig. 9-4A). The cut clavicle with its attached trapezius, capsule of the acromioclavicular joint, acromial process, and adjoining part of the posterior border of the spine is elevated and mobilized from its bed. Thus, the upper and middle trapezius is mobilized from its insertion almost its entire length without affecting its neurovascular supply. The parts of bone still attached to the elevated trapezius are made raw. These bones are broken with pliers to facilitate easy placement at the new, raw site on the lateral humeral shaft (Fig. 9-4B). The acromion is fixed with two screws while the muscle is kept in a relaxed position so that the arm may be lowered later without difficulty.

AFTERCARE. Immobilization and exercises are the same as those described for the Bateman method.

Ober's Transfer of Triceps and Biceps to Acromion[10,40]

Ober described his method for complete deltoid paralysis. However, the best end

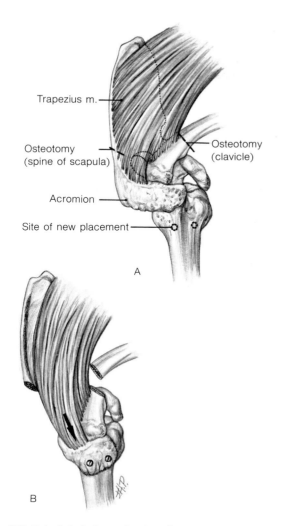

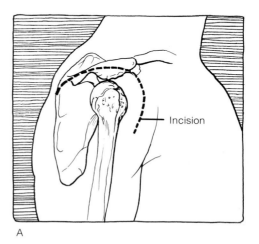

bony part with its short head of the biceps detached. This muscle is carefully freed to its nerve supply to avoid injury to its neurovascular supply.

Next, the long head of the triceps is exposed posteriorly at its origin on the scapula. It is removed along with a piece of bone and freed from the upper fourth of the humerus.

FIG. 9-4. Saha's trapezius transfer to restore deltoid abduction power. The crushed raw acromion is fixed to the lateral humerus. (See text for discussion.) (Modified from Saha, A. K.: Surgery of the paralyzed and flail shoulder. Acta Orthop. Scand. (Suppl.), 97:5–90, 1967.)

result can be expected when there is some residual power in the deltoid, and there is good power in the triceps, biceps, the pectoralis major, and all the scapular muscles.

A saber-shaped incision is made over the shoulder, the anterior limb extending downward over the deltopectoral groove for 7.5 cm. The posterior limb of the incision extends downward 7.5 cm. over the back of the shoulder (Fig. 9-5A).

The coracoid process is exposed and the

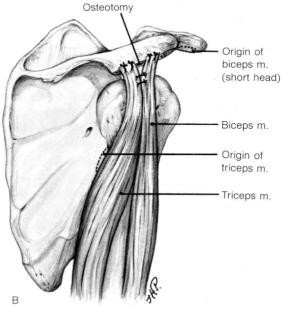

FIG. 9-5. Ober's transfer of short head of the biceps and long head of the triceps to the acromion. (See text for discussion.)

Two cuts are made in the acromion, anteriorly for the biceps tendon, and posteriorly for the triceps tendon. The transferred muscles are passed through separated fibers of the deltoid and emerge near the acromion opposite the denuded areas on the acromion. The patient's arm is abducted and the transferred muscles are anchored with heavy sutures (Fig. 9-5B).

AFTERCARE. Postoperative management is the same as that already described for trapezius transfer.

Harmon's Transfer of Deltoid[21,22]

When the anterior deltoid is paralyzed, as in obstetric palsy, the posterior portion of the deltoid can be transferred anteriorly with good results.

A semicircular incision is made around the shoulder just beneath the edge of the acromion. It extends from the outer third of the clavicle laterally around the acromion to the middle of the spine of the scapula. The flaps are reflected to expose the entire deltoid origin (Fig. 9-6A). The active posterior part of the deltoid is detached from its origin and an osteoperiosteal bone cuff is removed. The upper half of this part of the muscle is freed, care being taken not to injure its nerve and blood supply. The lateral third of the clavicle is made raw, and the functioning posterior muscle flap is transferred anteriorly and anchored against the raw clavicle with stout nonabsorbable sutures (Fig. 9-6B). The sutures are placed through the anterior periosteum.

AFTERCARE. The extremity is placed in a shoulder spica cast with the arm abducted 75 degrees for 3 or 4 weeks. The cast is then bivalved and gentle active exercises are initiated. At the end of 6 weeks the whole cast is removed, and an abduction brace is worn for at least 4 months, during which time active exercises are continued. The arm is brought down slowly to the side.

Serratus Anterior Paralysis

Paralysis of scapular muscles such as the serratus anterior causes disturbed shoulder

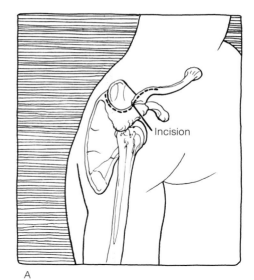

A

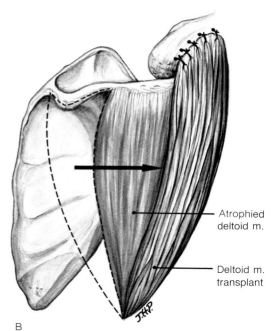

Atrophied deltoid m.

Deltoid m. transplant

B

FIG. 9-6. Harmon's transfer of the posterior deltoid to restore deltoid function. (See text for discussion.) (Modified from Harmon, R. H.: Surgical reconstruction of the paralytic shoulder by multiple muscle transplantations. J. Bone Joint Surg., 32-A:583–595, 1950.)

function.[28] When scapular instability is severe surgical stabilization may be indicated in select cases. Each patient must be evaluated, since there is no large series of cases to confirm the true merit of these operations.

Whitman's Fascial Fixation of Scapula to Thoracic Spine[64]

An incision is extended from the posterior acromial tip medially and downward along the vertebral border of the scapula. The periosteum and attached muscles are elevated to expose the bone of the superior and vertebral borders of the scapula. Four holes are drilled through the scapula at the superior angle, at the junction of the spine and vertebral border in the middle of the vertebral border, and at the inferior angle. Similarly, after subperiosteal stripping, holes are made in the spinous processes of the fourth through the seventh thoracic vertebrae.

Four strips of fascia lata are taken, 20 cm. long and 0.6 cm. wide. Each is passed through its corresponding hole in a spinous process and scapula, and tied and sutured while the scapula is held downward and inward (Fig. 9-7). The periosteum is sutured back in place over the fascial strips.

AFTERCARE. The extremity is held in a shoulder spica cast with the arm abducted 45 degrees. The cast is removed at 4 weeks and gentle exercises are started. Full activity is gradually increased after 8 weeks.

Dickson's Fixation of Scapula to Pectoralis Major and Latissimus Dorsi[13]

Dickson believed that weakness of the muscles attaching to the scapula was associated with the promotion of high thoracic and cervicothoracic curves. He employed methods of scapula fixation to relieve spinal curvature, while improving shoulder function by stabilizing the scapula with tubes of fascia lata grafts in contradistinction to Lowman's method of using flat fascia lata strips.

Primarily, for serratus anterior weakness, a small slot is made in the lower axillary border of the scapula through an incision overlying this region. A fashioned tube of fascia lata, smooth side facing outward, is passed through the hole, sutured, and its distal end split after passing it subcutane-

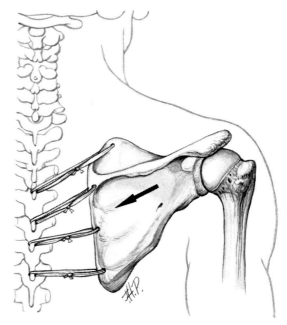

FIG. 9-7. Whitman's method for stabilizing the scapula. (See text for discussion.) (Modified from Whitman, A.: Congenital elevation of the scapula and paralysis of serratus magnus muscle. J.A.M.A., 99:1332–1334, 1932.)

ously, one end to the lower fibers of the pectoralis major and the other end to the anterior border of the latissimus dorsi. The split ends are sutured in place to the respective muscles with the scapula drawn forward, the pectoralis major origin being reached through a small incision made at the lateral thorax. If the fascial grafts are held under tension movement of the scapula toward the vertebral column may cease. In theory, the transmitted tension through the fascial strips to the pectoralis major and latissimus dorsi might create an extra active pull on the scapula.

AFTERCARE. The extremity is held in 45 degrees of abduction in a plaster shoulder spica for 4 weeks. Gentle exercises are started, and after 6 weeks all support is discontinued.

Brockway's Interscapular Fixation[5]

Brockway's operation attempts to improve lifting power of the arm by overcoming the paralyzed deltoid and weak rhomboid muscles. Before operation, adduction contractures should be stretched or released. Performed early, this operation may prevent adduction contractures in patients with poliomyelitis.

Through short incisions the periosteum is stripped over both scapulae along the vertebral borders at the level of the spines. One end of a 1.9-cm. width of fascia lata strip is passed through a hole placed 2.5 cm. lateral to the vertebral border of the scapula just below the spine. The fascia is sutured back on to itself; the other end is passed subcutaneously and fastened to the opposite scapula in the same manner. Sufficient tension should be obtained so that the vertebral borders of the scapulae are almost parallel to each other. Rotations of the scapulae are not hindered.

AFTERCARE. The arm should be immobilized in 40 degrees of abduction for 4 weeks. Thereafter, a brace is used for at least several months with the arm in wide abduction to avoid stretching the graft, and to allow muscle reeducation during exercises. The brace is removed. Abduction power of the shoulder is improved because there is stabilization of the scapulae against which the weakened deltoid can work.

Spira's Fixation of Scapula to Rib Cage[55]

When extensive paralysis of shoulder muscles is present, function of the shoulder girdle is seriously impaired. This operation fixes the scapula, and curtails scapular rotation. It is preferred to fascial grafting when it appears that the weight of the extremity without active muscles will allow continued scapular stability without stretching of the fascial grafts.

The principle is to fasten the inferior angle of the scapula to the sixth rib by (1) biting a section from the lower angle of the scapula and allowing the rib to rest within the recessed portion of the scapula, or (2) creating a hole in the inferior angle, cutting the sixth rib at the posterior axillary

fold, crushing the rib and passing it through the hole.

In one method, Spira removed a 2-cm. portion of bone from the inferior angle of the scapula. The sixth rib is cautiously spread and the rib allowed to rest within the recess of the inferior scapula.

In a second method, the sixth rib is exposed subperiosteally, and an osteotomy performed at the posterior axillary fold. The dorsal part is crushed and the pliable rib then passed through a 2-cm.-diameter hole made in the inferior angle of the scapula. The two ends of the cut rib are sutured together.

AFTERCARE. The extremity is supported in Velpeau position for 5 weeks. Thereafter, gently active motion exercises are started.

Tubby's Transfer of Pectoralis Major to Serratus Anterior[63]

A 7.5- to 10-cm. incision is made in the anterior axilla and the sternal portion of the pectoralis major widely exposed by retracting the dissected flaps. The humeral insertion of the muscle is freed and the muscle itself separated from the surrounding tissues. By dividing the cut end of the pectoralis major into several fascicles, it is possible to suture them into a large width of the serratus anterior corresponding to the five digitations of the serratus when the paralyzed serratus is drawn forward.

AFTERCARE. The extremity is immobilized in Velpeau position for 6 weeks. Active exercises are then started to improve motion and to reeducate the muscles about the shoulder.

Durman's Transfer of Pectoralis Major to Scapula[15]

The patient is placed on the unaffected side and the affected arm draped free. An incision is made from the anterior border of the deltoid, across the inferior edge of the tendon of the pectoralis major, along the anterior axillary fold to the chest wall. The upper medial flap is retracted to allow exposure of one third of the anterior surface of the pectoralis major. The lower third of the muscle is separated from the upper two thirds of the pectoralis major. The lower third is mobilized from the chest wall to the humerus, and its tendon is cut closely from the humerus.

A second 10-cm. longitudinal incision is made over the inferior angle of the scapula with the patient's arm abducted. The posterior periosteum of the inferior angle of the scapula is stripped and a one half inch hole made in the bone.

A fashioned strip of fascia lata, measuring 7.5 by 15 cm., is rolled about the cut tendon portion of the pectoralis major to create several thicknesses of tubing. The free end is passed subcutaneously to the posterior incision over the scapula tip and looped through the hole, pulled taut, and sutured upon itself for a distance of 2.5 cm. During the suturing of the graft the scapula should be held depressed against the chest wall and rotated anteriorly.

AFTERCARE. The arm is immobilized at the side for 3 weeks in Velpeau position. Thereafter, gentle motion exercises are started and gradually increased.

Chaves' and Rapp's Transfer of Pectoralis Minor to Scapula[8,43]

The patient is positioned on the table with the side to be operated upon elevated 30 degrees on a sandbag behind the back. The affected chest wall and the upper extremity are surgically cleansed and draped free. A Mayo stand is placed beside the table to permit the extremity to rest upon it in abduction. A S-shaped incision is started at the middle portion of the clavicle and curved around the coracoid process toward the direction of the anterior axilla (Fig. 9-8A). The pectoralis minor is identified and detached from the coracoid. It is dissected free from the surrounding soft tissues to its mid-belly, care being taken to preserve its nerve supply. Thereafter, the skin incision is continued toward the inferior angle of the scapula, but stopped at the posterior axil-

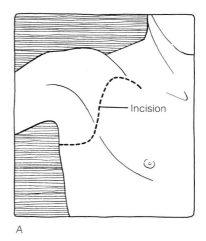

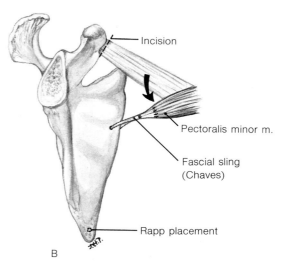

FIG. 9-8. Chaves-Rapp's methods for restoring serratus anterior function. (See text for discussion.) (Modified from Chaves, J. P.: Pectoralis minor transplant for paralysis of the serratus anterior. J. Bone Joint Surg., 33-B:228–230, 1951; and Rapp, I. H.: Serratus anterior paralysis treated by transplantation of the pectoralis minor. J. Bone Joint Surg., 36-A:852–854, 1954.)

lary line. A tunnel is created beneath the pectoralis major, and the pectoralis minor tendon is passed backward.

A strip of fascia lata, measuring 5 by 10 cm., is removed from the thigh and then attached to the pectoralis minor tendon. Chaves placed the fascial sling through a hole made in the middle portion of the vertebral border of the scapula,[8] whereas

Rapp, after the bone is cleared by subperiosteal dissection, placed the fascial strip through a hole made in the inferior angle of the scapula[43] (Fig. 9-8B). In either procedure, the fascial prolongation is reflected upon itself and sutured.

AFTERCARE. The upper extremity is immobilized in Velpeau position for 6 weeks. Thereafter, gentle active exercises are started.

Trapezius Paralysis

Dewar-Harris's Fascial Sling and Levator Scapulae Transfer[12]

Through a L-shaped incision placed over the upper dorsal spine and transversely over the scapula, the insertion of the levator scapulae is transferred laterally (Fig. 9-9). A 5-cm. width of fascia lata is passed through a hole in the scapula near its vertebral border and through foramina created in the spinous processes of the second and third thoracic vertebrae. The levator scapulae is transferred to the lateral scapular spine (Fig. 9-9).

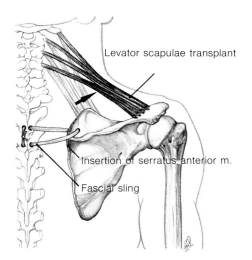

Levator scapulae transplant

Insertion of serratus anterior m.

Fascial sling

FIG. 9-9. Dewar-Harris's method for restoring trapezius function. (See text for discussion.) (Modified from Dewar, F. P., and Harris, R. L.: Restoration of function of the shoulder following paralysis of the trapezius by fascial sling fixation and transplantation of the levator scapulae. Ann. Surg., 132:1111–1115, 1950.)

The anchor created by the fascial graft substitutes for the action of the middle part of the trapezius, and the lateral shift of the levator scapulae serves as the substitute for the superior trapezius.

AFTERCARE. The extremity is held in moderate abduction for 2 months. Thereafter, gentle active motion exercises are started.

Levator Scapulae and Spinal Muscle Weakness[13]

Dickson's Procedure

When there is paralysis of the spinal and scapular levator muscles the shoulder blade may drop, and a high cervicothoracic curve may develop, according to Dickson.[13] At least for the dropped shoulder, his method of stabilizing the shoulder when considered desirable seems worthwhile in select cases.

A 10-cm. longitudinal incision is made over the spine of the scapula also exposing the acromial end. A hole is made in the lateral part of the spine near the acromion. A second incision is placed over the posterior aspect of the cervical spine. A fascia lata tube graft, smooth side facing outward, is looped through the hole in the scapular spine and laced into the cervical muscles at the apex of the curve, elevating the dropped shoulder as much as possible. Each end is sutured in place.

A third incision is made over the spinous process of the first thoracic vertebra, and a hole is made through its base. Another fascial tube graft is looped through a second hole made near the vertebral end of the spine of the scapula, passed subcutaneously to the first thoracic vertebra, and sutured at each end under tension.

AFTERCARE. The extremity is held in a shoulder plaster spica with the arm abducted 45 degrees. At the end of 4 weeks gentle active exercises are begun. At the end of 6 weeks all support is discontinued and active exercises are increased.

PARALYSIS DUE TO BIRTH INJURY

Paralysis of the muscles of the upper extremity result from obstetric trauma to the brachial plexus or to the nerves passing to it. Smellie first described the condition in 1764.[53] Duchenne, in 1872, described it in infants,[14] and Erb, in 1874, reported the condition in adults.[16] Thus, the most common type of birth paralysis became known as Erb-Duchenne palsy. In 1885, Klumpke reported another uncommon type.[29] Three distinct types based on injury to specific nerve components are now recognized: (1) Erb-Duchenne, (2) whole arm, and (3) Klumpke types, each producing classic findings.

Incidence and Etiologic Factors

The sex incidence slightly favors males over females. In a large series of cases, Sever reported that the right side was involved a greater number of times than the left,[49] whereas Wolman's series showed left-sided palsy to be slightly higher than right-sided palsy.[67] In any event, the consensus indicates that more males than females are affected.

Birth injury is now accepted as the causative factor, and occurs in offspring of primigravida more often than in those of multiple pregnancies. Statistics prove that brachial plexus injury occurs most often with vertex presentation in comparison to breech delivery, although the latter occurs twice as often as in the general population. From one report, presumably the use of forceps was a relevant factor. Another striking factor is the unquestionably large size of most babies, averaging 5.2 kg. in Wolman's report.[67]

Adler and Patterson showed that new patients with Erb's palsy had a decreasing incidence of the condition from 1939 to 1962, from 1.56 to 0.38 per thousand live births, owing to the improved recognition of cephalopelvic disproportion and improved obstetric management techniques.[1]

Pathologic Anatomy and Pathogenesis

Upper Arm Palsy (Erb-Duchenne)[14,16]

Taylor,[62] in 1907, and Osterhaus,[41] in 1908, believed that birth injury was due to overstretching of the nerves. In 1916, Sever confirmed these views, from infantile cadaver experiments, by showing that forcible lateral bending and traction of the head and neck to the contralateral side produced injury to the fifth and sixth cervical nerves.[49] He concluded that these nerves were overstretched and torn in varying degrees just above their junction where the suprascapular nerve arises, known as Erb's point. The classic clinical picture depends upon the specific nerves injured and the degree of stretching or tearing.

In Erb-Duchenne palsy, by far the most common type, C5 and C6 nerve roots are injured. The poorest prognosis results when the nerve roots are avulsed from the spinal cord. At first, the entire shoulder girdle may be paralyzed. As recovery ensues, the abductor and external rotator muscles may remain partially or completely paralyzed and allow the arm to lie in an attitude of internal rotation and adduction. Weakness or complete paralysis may persist in the deltoid, the short rotators of the shoulder, the biceps, supinator, and occasionally, the serratus anterior and coracobrachialis. With growth, anterior joint capsule contracture involving the subscapularis, the pectoralis major, and their fascial coverings results. After 5 years of age, in the more severe cases, posterior subluxation of the humeral head may occur from the unopposed pull of the contracted unparalyzed latissimus dorsi, teres major, and subscapularis. Obviously, some muscle fibers in the subscapularis are not paralyzed and cause the shortening, unlike the completely paralyzed muscle which does not contract.

Sever stated that, except for the clavicle, birth fractures at the shoulder region were rare and true Erb's palsy was not associated with proximal humerus trauma.[49] Scaglietti believed that obstetric joint trauma was the most frequently observed lesion leading to epiphyseal separation at the proximal humerus with characteristic clinical and roentgenologic findings.[47] Early roentgenograms show no changes because of the cartilaginous upper end of the humerus. The first positive roentgen signs appear with the formation of periosteal callus secondary to trauma after the first week of life. Toward the third month, when the first ossification center appears in the head of the humerus, a diagnosis of partial or complete epiphyseolysis with or without displacement of the upper end of the humerus can be made. This sequela of obstetric shoulder trauma must be differentiated from pure birth palsy. Wickstrom and associates showed that if the shoulder remains in a position of marked internal rotation, deformity of the glenoid can increase with growth.[65] It does appear that a significant number of these patients may sustain injury to the cartilaginous humeral head and epiphyseal plate in addition to developmental abnormalities. It does not follow that proximal humeral birth trauma is usually associated with nerve injury. Other bone deformities are observed such as the elongation of the coracoid process due to the pull of its attached muscles.

Liebolt and Furey,[33] in 1953, and Babbitt and Cassidy,[2] in 1968, reported anterior infantile dislocation of the shoulder with obstetric trauma to the nerves wherein there was no apparent abnormality at birth. However, between birth and 4 to 6 months dislocation occurred. The dislocation may be related to severe muscle weakness about the shoulder which permits humeral head displacement when the extremity is placed in abduction and external rotation, and may require open reduction. The scapula may appear winged, and if the winging is observed early in infancy shoulder dislocation should be suspected.

Other joint abnormalities may occur, especially in older children. These include elbow joint deformities, elbow contractures, and radial head dislocation.

Whole Arm Palsy
(Erb-Duchenne-Klumpke)

The seventh, eighth, and possibly the first thoracic nerve roots, as well as the fifth and sixth nerve roots, are injured in whole arm palsy, the next most common type. Anisocoria and narrowing of the palpebral fissure are not unusual with this type. These symptoms are related to injury to the eighth cervical or first thoracic nerves which have communicating fibers with the cervical sympathetics. In addition to those developments which may occur with injury to the upper roots, wristdrop and paralysis of the flexors and extensors of the fingers are common, as well as paralysis and atrophy of the intrinsic muscles of the hand. These injuries carry a poor prognosis in view of the fact that while some of the muscles of the upper arm may partly recover, the lower arm muscles almost never recover. Thus, the entire extremity may remain flaccid, the scapula winged, and diaphragmatic paralysis from phrenic nerve injury may occur.

Lower Arm Palsy (Klumpke)[29]

When the seventh and eighth cervical roots are injured, weakness occurs in the muscles of the wrist and finger flexors as well as in the intrinsic hand muscles in lower arm palsy, the least common type. With sensory deficit the prognosis is poor. However, there may be little sensory loss. The terminal part of the Moro reflex may be normal with an inability of the digits to spread, and the thumb and index digits to flex. The grasping reflex is lost.

Diagnosis

When the infant is first observed in the first few days or weeks of life, the affected arm lies limp at the side, extended, internally rotated, with the forearm pronated (Fig. 9-10). The paralysis is usually flaccid. On attempted testing of the Moro reflex there is inability to abduct, elevate, and externally rotate the arm or supinate the

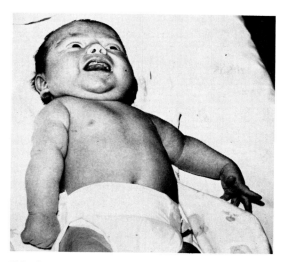

FIG. 9-10. A 4-week-old infant with Erb's palsy is shown during the Moro test. Note the external rotation and abduction of the normal left arm as well as the spreading of the fingers. The affected right arm lies motionless at the side in internal rotation with the forearm in pronation.

forearm. With Erb's type the lower arm is not affected, wrist and finger extension and flexion being unaffected.

At this moment it is crucial to differentiate pseudo-paralysis due to infection or fracture of the clavicle, humerus, or forearm bones, congenital abnormalities such as rare shoulder dislocation, and arthrogryposis. As complete a neurologic examination as possible should be performed at each visit, carefully recording any abnormalities and change in the findings.

Roentgenograms of the cervical spine and pertinent portions of both upper extremities should be taken. If bony trauma is suspected but not seen, repeat examination is indicated within 7 to 10 days following delivery, and the fact that the humeral epiphysis is not ossified at birth kept in mind.

Electromyography has not proved fruitful in infants, except perhaps to document clinical findings and to follow recovery. Of far greater value is a careful, well-documented clinical reexamination by the same person.

On rare occasions myelography in infants may be needed to determine whether root avulsions from the spinal cord have occurred. If there is dye leakage the prognosis is exceptionally poor. In general, this testing is not usually required.

When a definite diagnosis of birth palsy is made, it takes only a few weeks before wasting of the limb muscles and flattening of the shoulder appear. Soon, internal rotation at the shoulder becomes apparent owing to paralysis of the external rotators and unopposed pull of the internal rotator muscles. There may be a rapid onset of contractures about the shoulder. Precise localization of the anatomic lesion may be difficult in the beginning, and necessitate additional periodic examinations.

Early Treatment

In the first 2 years of life treatment should be conservative. The chief goal of treatment should be to prevent muscle and joint contractures, especially internal rotation deformity. Unparalyzed muscles should be positioned so that they cannot become contracted, whereas paralyzed muscles should be placed in a relaxed functional position in order to prevent shoulder joint deformity. This will allow them to regain whatever power is possible. Wickstrom and co-workers found a 12.9 percent incidence of full recovery,[65] in comparison to only 7 percent found by Adler and Patterson.[1] It is impossible to state early which cases will recover or even to what degree. Therefore, a planned physical therapy program should be started 5 days after birth to give all patients every chance for recovery. The surgeon should not defer treatment with the expectation that spontaneous rehabilitation will occur.

Four times or more each day all joints of the infant's extremity should be placed through a full range of motion, and all muscles exercised. Perseverance is essential for the prevention of contractures. Such a program may later obviate surgical correction procedures (Fig. 9-11). It is apparent that in the beginning the patient must be supervised by the surgeon or therapist in order to carry out the repetitive exercises correctly.

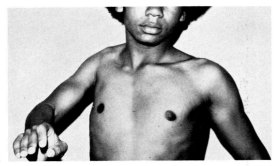

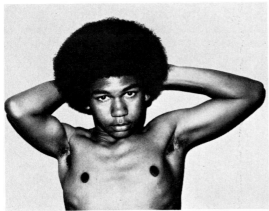

FIG. 9-11. A 16-year-old boy with severe Erb's palsy. A, His ability to actively abduct the arm is limited by the severe paralysis and atrophy of the deltoid. B, Note the excellent external rotation of the arm as evidenced by the patient's ability to place his hands behind his head. A lifelong daily exercise program was started at end of the first week of life. His upper extremity function was excellent even though the humerus was shortened.

Tying the arm of the infant to the bed sheet, bracing, and casting of the extremity in 90 degrees of abduction in as much external rotation as possible have been recommended as means of preventing contractures. There is a great danger in overimmobilizing the extremity because abduction-external rotation contractures may follow. Although Sever stressed bracing in 1916,[49] he withdrew this recommendation in 1925 in a report of 1100 patients, stating that excessive bracing hinders recovery.[51] The best conservative treatment revolves about repetitive nonviolent physical therapy by the parent and supportive passive bracing. When an effective program is carried out, surgery can be avoided in a majority of patients. In any event, the child should be watched for evidence of conversion of the internal rotation-adduction contracture at the shoulder to one of internal rotation-abduction from overtreatment.[38]

Later Treatment

After 3 or 4 years of age the child is old enough to undergo a complete assessment of his functional impairment. Previous examination records should be studied to determine the degree of progression of any functional loss. New x-ray films of the joints should be taken to further evaluate any deformities. Moreover, after 4 years of age the child is able to cooperate, especially in the postoperative period.

Surgical treatment of birth trauma is directed toward (1) releasing capsule and tendon contractures, (2) removing the action of deforming muscles and reinforcing partially or completely paralyzed muscles, and (3) altering abnormal bone contour or incongruent articular surfaces when they interfere with reasonable function or cause intractable pain. If contracture, incongruous glenohumeral articular surfaces, or dislocation is evident, tendon transfer alone obviously will not improve function. A careful analysis of the problem about the shoulder will enable the surgeon to select the most effective operations. Moreover, surgical management described in this section can be applied to help those patients who have permanent deformities resulting from brachial plexus lesions.

Not all patients with contractures or bone abnormalities require surgery. Many seem to function comfortably for long periods. Wickstrom and associates have shown that patients with internal rotation contractures and weak abduction at the shoulder have difficulty in moving the hand to the mouth or to other parts of the head.[65] Internal rotation contracture of more than 20 degrees requires forward flexion of the head and tilt toward the affected side, in addition to abduction and flexion of the shoulder to facilitate hand movement to the mouth. If the internal rotation contracture is more

Table 9-3. *Operations to Improve Function After Birth Trauma*

Shoulder Lesion	Author and Year	Operation
Joint contracture	Fairbank, 1913	Anterior capsule and subscapularis tendon release (Fig. 9-12A)
	Sever, 1916	Subscapularis and pectoralis major tendon release (joint capsule left intact) (Fig. 9-12B)
	L'Episcopo, 1934	Sever's operation plus teres major transfer to lateral humerus
	L'Episcopo, 1939	Sever's operation of teres major and latissimus dorsi transfer to lateral humerus (Fig. 9-13)
	Zachary, 1947	L'Episcopo's modification of teres major and latissimus dorsi transfer (Fig. 9-14)
Subluxation of humeral head	Fairbank, 1913	Fairbank's operation, and open reduction of joint and wire fixation
Paralyzed posterior deltoid	Moore, 1935	Transfer of anterior deltoid to restore paralyzed posterior deltoid
Internal rotation contracture	Rogers, 1916	Derotation osteotomy of humerus
Multiple muscle paralyses at shoulder joint	Steindler, 1919	Glenohumeral arthrodesis
Intractable painful arthritis	Post-Haskell, 1973 (see Chapter 10, Part B)	Total shoulder replacement (exceptional case)

than 45 degrees and there is moderate limitation of shoulder abduction, it may be possible to bring the hand to the mouth. Based upon the amount of disability of the patient, the surgeon may decide whether operation is necessary. Of course, any functional impairment of the elbow, wrist, or hand must be considered.

SURGICAL PROCEDURES TO IMPROVE LOST FUNCTION AT SHOULDER

Table 9-3 summarizes those operations found useful in the surgical treatment of birth palsies.

Fairbank's Release Operation

In 1913, Fairbank described his operation for shoulder joint contracture after birth palsy[17] (Fig. 9-12A). An incision is made over the deltopectoral groove from beneath the clavicle to a level just below the upper edge of the pectoralis major tendon. The deltoid and pectoralis major muscles are retracted. The patient's arm is externally rotated. If necessary, a 1.3-cm. incision is made in the flat, superior tendon of the pectoralis major in order to better define surrounding structures such as the anterior humeral circumflex vessels. The biceps groove is identified. A small transverse opening is made in the soft tissues above the anterior circumflex artery and below the subscapularis tendon near its insertion (Fig. 9-12A). A blunt curved dissector is pushed upward beneath the adherent capsule and subscapularis tendon. The capsule should be completely divided above, and care taken to avoid injury to the long head of the biceps in its groove. In elderly patients, it may be necessary to divide a tight coracohumeral ligament, supraspinatus tendon, and even a deformed coracoid process.

AFTERCARE. Although a plaster shoulder spica was originally recommended to maintain the arm in full external rotation and the forearm supinated with the elbow at the side for a 3-month period, it is more prudent to start gentle massage and motion exercises at the end of 2 or 3 weeks, and maintain the extremity in a splint for at least 3 months in abduction and external rotation during rest periods. Reduction of the subluxated humeral head is recom-

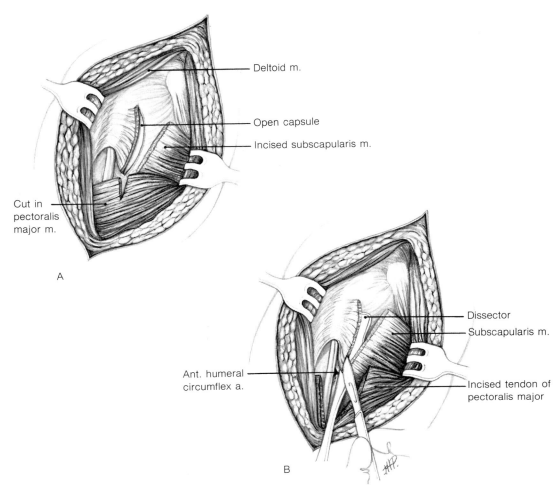

FIG. 9-12. A, Fairbank's operation. B, Sever's operation. (See text for discussion.)

mended before performing soft-tissue procedures.

Sever's Release Operation

Sever modified Fairbank's operation by dividing the pectoralis major and the subscapularis tendons, and thus he avoided opening the joint capsule in hope of preventing adhesions between the capsule and joint cartilage[49,50,52] (Fig. 9-12B). If the coracobrachialis and short head of the biceps are tight, they are also divided to allow external rotation and abduction. The surgical approach is the same as that used for the Fairbank operation.

The Fairbank and the Sever operations are worthwhile if they are performed before there is marked incongruity of the glenohumeral joint surfaces. The surgeon should have no preconceived notion as to which operation will be performed, but should release all tight, deforming structures.

AFTERCARE. A plaster shoulder spica is worn with the arm abducted, elevated, and externally rotated, and the hand supinated for 2 weeks. Thereafter, massage and motion exercises are supervised for at least several months and as long as 6 to 8 months, four times each week. The extremity should be supported in a splint for a minimum of 3 months in abduction and external rotation when not being exercised.

L'Episcopo's Operations to Restore Muscle Balance

Muscle transfer operations should be performed early, at 3 or 4 years of age, when maximum return of function has occurred. These should increase external rotation and prevent contracture and joint changes whenever possible. In 1934, L'Episcopo used Sever's operation to release contracted structures.[30] He believed that older children developed internal rotation contractures that resulted from a loss of muscle balance between the internal and external rotators at the shoulder. His operation is designed to restore balance between these two opposing groups of muscles by transferring the tendon of the contracted teres major, which changes it from an internal to an external rotator (Fig. 9-13).

The operation is performed in conjunction with Sever's operation. The patient is placed on his side and the shoulder and extremity are draped free. In the anterior

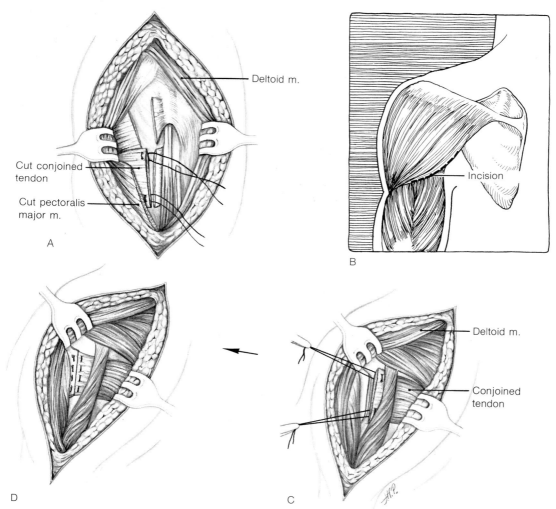

FIG. 9-13. L'Episcopo's operation (1939). A, Release of tight anterior structures. Conjoined tendon (latissimus dorsi and teres major) is cut close to its insertion. B, A posterior incision is made along posterior deltoid edge. C, The conjoined tendon is brought anterior to the long head of the triceps and, D, sutured into an osteoperiosteal flap in the humerus. (Modified from L'Episcopo, J. B.: Tendon transplantation in obstetrical paralysis. Am. J. Surg., 25:122–125, 1934.)

part of the operation the shoulder is tilted backward, and then toward the prone position for the actual muscle transfer. After release of all contracted anterior structures (Fig. 9-13A), a 10-cm.-long incision is made parallel with the posterior border of the deltoid (Fig. 9-13B). The deltoid, long head of the triceps, and teres major are identified. The long head of the triceps is retracted laterally to expose the tendon of the teres major and the humerus. The axillary nerve and posterior humeral circumflex artery must be protected. The teres major tendon is cut close to its insertion, and the long head of the triceps is laterally retracted to expose the posterolateral humerus and upper part of the origin of the lateral head of the triceps. An osteoperiosteal flap is raised in the shaft as close as possible to the short head of the triceps. The cut tendon of the teres major is buried and sutured beneath the flap (Fig. 9-13C and D). The wound is closed in layers.

In 1939, L'Episcopo reported on his operation of transferring not only the teres major but the latissimus dorsi as well.[31] He stated that if the capsule is contracted he performed Fairbank's operation. In his later operation, L'Episcopo used the same anterior and posterior incisions described previously, but divided the tendons of the latissimus dorsi and teres major through the anterior approach (Fig. 9-13A). The cut tendons were then passed posteriorly and sutured beneath a thin osteoperiosteal flap just above or at the origin of the lateral head of the triceps (Fig. 9-13D).

AFTERCARE. The extremity is placed in a plaster of Paris cast for 6 weeks with the arm abducted and externally rotated, and the forearm supinated. Thereafter, the cast is used as a removable splint for another 6 weeks, and gentle passive and active exercises are initially performed thrice weekly and increased progressively for at least 6 months.

Zachary's Modification of Teres Major and Latissimus Dorsi Transfers

Zachary modified L'Episcopo's method.[69] He recommended it for those patients with weak or paralyzed external rotators secondary to brachial plexus injuries.

In the first part of the operation, the patient's arm is abducted and internally rotated behind the back (Fig. 9-14A). With the Henry approach to the posterior humerus (Fig. 9-15), the long and lateral heads of the triceps are separated, and the teres major is identified at its insertion. The teres major tendon is cut and transplanted to the lateral humerus by passing the tendon through a slit in the origin of the lateral head of the triceps when the arm is externally rotated and abduction avoided (Fig. 9-14B). Similarly, the cut tendon of the latissimus dorsi is transplanted with the teres major.

AFTERCARE. The extremity is held in external rotation in a plaster shoulder spica for 5 weeks. After 4 weeks the extremity is removed from the cast periodically and gentle passive and active exercises are given, but abduction and internal rotation are always avoided.

Open Reduction of Posterior Dislocation

Fairbank recommended early open reduction of posterior dislocation of the shoulder, wherein the tight anterior joint structures are opened and the humeral head is reduced.[17] If an elongated coracoid process blocks reduction, this bone is also divided. A smooth pin is placed through the humeral head into the glenoid neck for 4 weeks. It is cut short beneath the skin, and its end bent to prevent migration. It is removed at the end of 4 weeks.

Moore's Transfer of Anterior Deltoid to Restore Paralyzed Posterior Deltoid Function

Moore reported his method of transferring the strong anterior deltoid to replace a paralyzed deltoid in patients with birth palsy.[39] By correcting muscle balance, internal rotation contracture may be prevented.

The patient is placed on the unaffected side with the extremity draped free. A semicircular incision is made transversely about

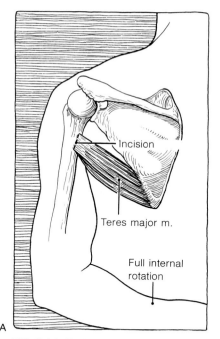

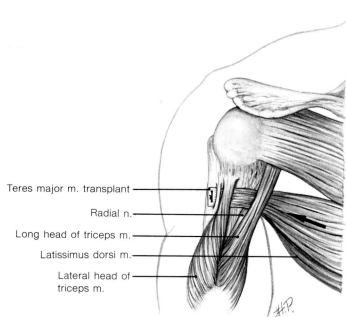

FIG. 9-14. Zachary's operation. A, With the extremity in internal rotation behind the back the teres major tendon insertion is transected. B, The cut teres major tendon is transferred to the lateral humerus. The cut tendon of the latissimus dorsi is similarly transferred with the teres. (Redrawn from Zachary, R. B.: Transplantation of teres major and latissimus dorsi for loss of external rotation at shoulder. Lancet, 2:757–758, 1947.)

the shoulder, extending from the middle of the spine of the scapula to just medial, beyond the acromioclavicular joint. When necessary, the anterior incision is continued inferiorly for 2.5 or 5.0 cm. The skin flap is dissected laterally.

A raw bed in the spine of the scapula is prepared for the transplanted deltoid. The patient's arm is at the place where the ridge of the spine spreads out to the acromion for 3.8 cm.

The lateral edge of the acromion with its attached muscle is cut. In children it is cartilaginous and easily cut with a knife or an osteotome. The deltoid muscle fibers are separated downward on either side of the cut acromial corners to a point halfway toward its insertion. The nerve supply must not be impaired.

If the subscapularis is tight it is divided. The arm is abducted and externally rotated, and the prepared muscle flap is attached to the spine.

AFTERCARE. The arm is immobilized in a plaster shoulder spica for 6 weeks. Thereaf-

ter, it is bivalved and the lower portion worn as a splint. The elbow is actively raised from the splint for 2 weeks. At the end of 8 weeks gentle motion exercises of the shoulder are permitted. At the end of a total of 10 weeks postoperatively the cast is discarded. The arm is in an abducted position. Gradually, the transplanted muscle adapts to a new length. During this time an abduction brace should be worn.

Rogers's Osteotomy of Humerus to Correct Internal Rotation Contractures[45]

Rogers described the use of osteotomy of the humerus just below the deltoid insertion to correct internal rotation contractures.[45] The operation improves the appearance of the extremity but does not rid the patient of the actual joint contracture, as do some of the release operations.

The humerus is approached through an incision in the deltopectoral groove. An osteotomy is made 5 cm. distal to the gleno-

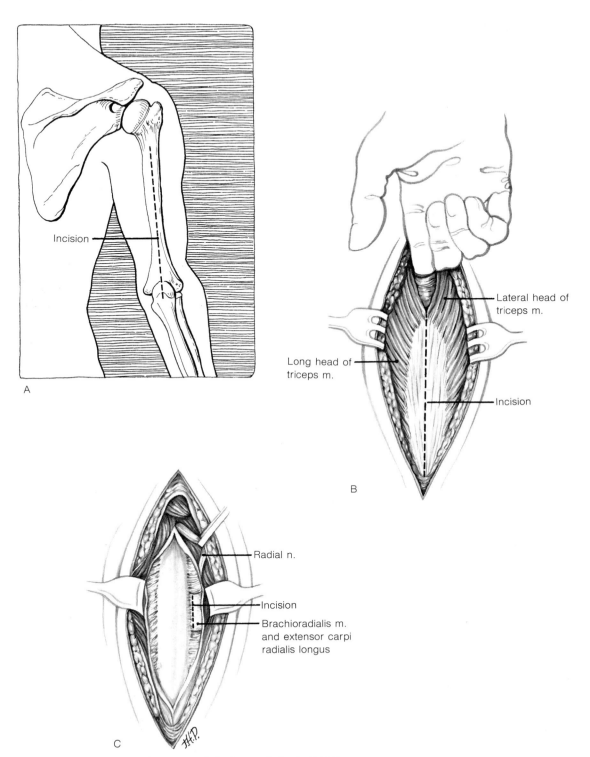

FIG. 9-15. Henry's posterior approach to the posterior humerus.

humeral joint. Under direct vision the distal fragment is externally rotated the desired amount (Fig. 9-16). In order to hold the bone fragments, temporary fixation of the fragments can be effected using the Roger-Anderson fixation technique for 4 to 6 weeks or until enough callus is present to prevent movement.

AFTERCARE. With the arm abducted, the elbow flexed, and the forearm supinated a plaster shoulder spica is worn for 8 weeks.

Arthrodesis

Arthrodesis of the glenohumeral joint should be considered in a teenage patient with severe contractures, who has poor shoulder muscle function.[18,57,60] The patients must meet the prerequisites for this operation (see Chapter 11, Arthrodesis).

Total Shoulder Replacement

In exceptional cases, elderly patients with excellent hand function may have an intractably painful shoulder joint secondary to arthritis, and may be candidates for total shoulder replacement. One such untreated patient had a nonfunctioning rotator cuff and an excellent serratus anterior and trapezius (Fig. 9-17). While total joint replacement relieved his pain, long-term results are not available to determine whether this method is worthwhile (see Chapter 10, Part B).

CONTRACTURE SECONDARY TO STROKE

Shoulder contracture following stroke is common. The condition is most often observed in adults past middle age and there-

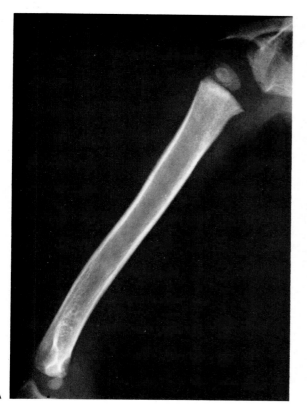
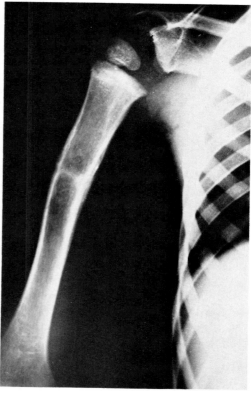

A

B

FIG. 9-16. A, A 4-year-old child with Erb's palsy developed an internal rotation-abduction contraction. The arm was hypoplastic. B, An osteotomy of the humerus was performed and excellent results were obtained. Roger Anderson temporary fixation was used.

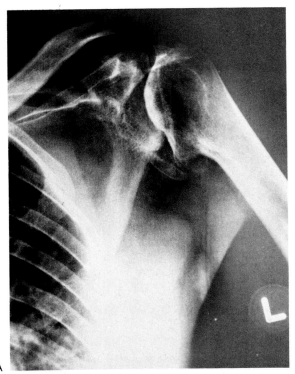 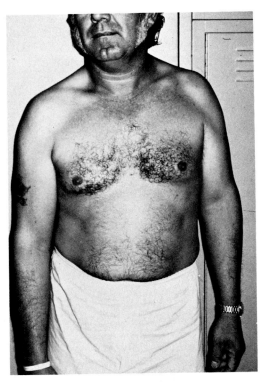

A   B

FIG. 9-17. A, A 53-year-old man had a severely deformed glenohumeral joint secondary to Erb's palsy. Note the deformity of the shaft. B, Total shoulder replacement relieved his pain and improved motion. At 2 years postoperatively, the result was very satisfactory.

fore associated with degenerative lesions about the shoulder joint. Moreover, spastic contracture of muscles and painful subluxation are often present (Fig. 9-18).

Early in the acute phase it is possible to minimize and even prevent subluxation in the less severe cases by supporting the shoulder with a sling to prevent overstretching of the muscles, and by having the patient perform frequent motion exercises until the time that the shoulder rotator muscles and deltoid function effectively.

When painful symptoms persist, and joint contracture results, it is occasionally beneficial to release the responsible tight internal rotators and adductor structures surgically, if the hand is functional. This procedure is relatively easy particularly in the young patient. I have not found this necessary in the elderly patient.

CONTRACTURE SECONDARY TO CEREBRAL PALSY

Experience has shown that it is extremely rare for contracture of the shoulder joint or for spastic muscles secondary to cerebral palsy to cause enough disability to require surgical correction.[37] If the patient does need such treatment for adduction-internal rotation contracture of the shoulder, the reader is referred to the section in this chapter that reviews methods described for the treatment of birth palsy contractures.

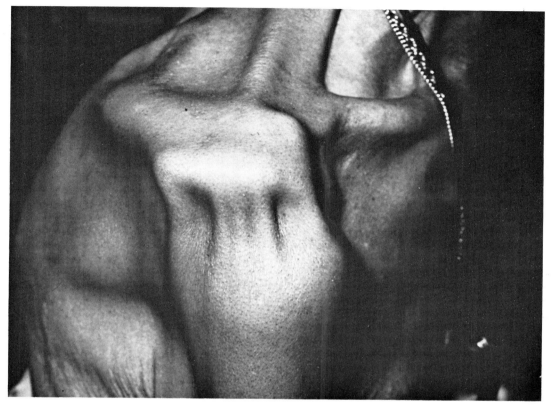

FIG. 9-18. A 70-year-old man developed a stroke and 10 weeks later complained of shoulder pain. There was full passive joint motion. When the extremity was unsupported, note the obvious joint subluxation and stretched deltoid. Pain subsided when the elbow was supported by a sling. A gentle motion exercise program was started.

REFERENCES

1. Adler, J. B., and Patterson, R. L.: Erb's palsy long-term results of treatment in eighty-eight cases. J. Bone Joint Surg., 49-A:1052–1064, 1967.
2. Babbitt, D. P., and Cassidy, R. H.: Obstetrical paralysis and dislocation of the shoulder in infancy. J. Bone Joint Surg., 50-A:1447–1452, 1968.
3. Bateman, J. E.: The Shoulder and Environs. St. Louis, C. V. Mosby Co., 1955.
4. Bateman, J. E.: Trauma to the Nerves in Limbs. Philadelphia, W. B. Saunders Co., 1962.
5. Brockway, A.: An operation to improve abduction power of the shoulder in poliomyelitis. J. Bone Joint Surg., 21:451–455, 1939.
6. Brunnstrom, S.: Muscle testing around the shoulder girdle. A study of the function of shoulder-blade fixators in seventeen cases of shoulder paralysis. J. Bone Joint Surg., 23:263–272, 1941.
7. Bunts, F. E.: Nerve injuries about the shoulder joint. Trans. Am. Surg. Assn., 21:520–526, 1903.
8. Chaves, J. P.: Pectoralis minor transplant for paralysis of the serratus anterior. J. Bone Joint Surg., 33-B:228–230, 1951.
9. D'Aubigne, R. M.: Treatment of residual paralysis after injuries of the main nerves (superior extremity). Proc. R. Soc. Med., 42:1831, 1949.
10. Davidson, W. D.: Traumatic deltoid paralysis treated by muscle transplantation. J.A.M.A., 106:2237, 1936.
11. Dehne, E., and Hall, R. M.: Active shoulder motion in complete deltoid paralysis. J. Bone Joint Surg., 41-A:745–748, 1959.
12. Dewar, F. P., and Harris, R. I.: Restoration of function of the shoulder following paralysis of the trapezius by fascial sling fixation and transplantation of the levator scapulae. Ann. Surg., 132:1111–1115, 1950.
13. Dickson, F. D.: Fascial transplants in paralytic and other conditions. J. Bone Joint Surg., 19:405–412, 1937.
14. Duchenne, G. B. A.: De l'Electrisation Localisee et de son Application a la Pathologie et a la Therapeutique, ed. 3, pp. 357–362. Paris, Balliere, 1872.
15. Durman, D. C.: An operation for paralysis of the

serratus anterior. J. Bone Joint Surg., 27:380–382, 1945.

16. Erb, W. H.: Ueber ein Eigenthumliche Localization von Lahmungen im Plexus Brachialis. Verhanl. d. Naturhist. Med. Ver Heidelberg, n. F.2:130–137, 1874.

17. Fairbank, H. A. T.: Birth palsy: Subluxation of shoulder joint in infants and young children. Lancet, 1:1217–1223, 1913.

18. Frankel, M. E., Goldner, J. L., and Stelling, F. H.: Partial shoulder girdle paralysis: Surgical management. South. Med. J., 62:1502–1508, 1969.

19. Haas, S. L.: Treatment of permanent paralysis of deltoid muscle. J.A.M.A., 104:99–103, 1935.

20. Hansson, K. G.: Serratus Magnus-Paralysis. Arch. Phys. Med., 29:156–161, 1948.

21. Harmon, R. H.: Anterior transplantation of the posterior deltoid for shoulder palsy and dislocation in poliomyelitis. Surg. Gynecol. Obstet., 84:117–120, 1947.

22. Harmon, R. H.: Surgical reconstruction of the paralytic shoulder by multiple muscle transplantations. J. Bone Joint Surg., 32-A:583–595, 1950.

23. Hass, J.: Muskelplastik bei Serratuslahmung. Zeitschr. f. Orthop. Chir., 55:617–622, 1931.

24. Herzmark, M. H.: Traumatic paralysis of the serratus anterior relieved by transplantation of the rhomboidei. J. Bone Joint Surg., 33-A:235–238, 1951.

25. Hildebrandt, J.: Ueber eine neue Methode der Muskeltransplantation. Arch. Klin. Chir., 78:75–84, 1906.

26. Horwitz, M. T., and Tocantins, L. M.: An anatomical study of the role of the long thoracic nerve and the related scapular bursae in the pathogenesis of local paralysis of the serratus anterior muscle. Anat. Rec., 71:375–385, 1938.

27. Horwitz, M. T., and Tocantins, L. M.: Isolated paralysis of the serratus anterior (magnus) muscle. J. Bone Joint Surg., 20:720–725, 1938.

28. Johnson, J. T. H., and Kendall, H. O.: Isolated paralysis of the serratus anterior muscle. J. Bone Joint Surg., 37-A:567–574, 1955.

29. Klumpke, A.: Contribution à l'etude des paralysies radiculaires du plexus brachial. Paralysies radiculaires totales. Paralysies radiculaires inferieures. De la participation des filets sympathiques oculo-pupillaires dans ces paralysies. Rev. Med., 5:591–616, 739–790, 1885.

30. L'Episcopo, J. B.: Tendon transplantation in obstetrical paralysis. Am. J. Surg., 25:122–125, 1934.

31. L'Episcopo, J. B.: Restoration of muscle balance in the treatment of obstetrical paralysis. N.Y. State J. Med., 39:357–363, 1939.

32. Lewis, D. D.: Trapezius transplantation in the treatment of deltoid paralysis. J.A.M.A., 55:2211–2213, 1910.

33. Liebolt, F. L., and Furey, J. G.: Obstetrical paralysis with dislocation of the shoulder. A case report. J. Bone Joint. Surg., 35-A:227–230, 1953.

34. Lowman, C. L.: The relationship of the abdominal muscles to paralytic scoliosis. J. Bone Joint Surg., 14:763–772, 1932.

35. Mayer, L.: Transplantation of trapezius for paralysis of abductors of Arm. J. Bone Joint Surg., 9:412–420, 1927.

36. Mayer, L.: Operative reconstruction of the paralyzed upper extremity. J. Bone Joint Surg., 21:377–383, 1939.

37. McCue, F. C., and Honner, R.: Deformities of upper limb in cerebral palsy; Their surgical management. South. Med. J., 63:355–359, 1970.

38. Milgram, J. E.: Discussion of L'Episcopo's presentation.[31]

39. Moore, B. H.: A new operation to relieve paralysis of the deltoid muscle. J.A.M.A., 99:2182, 1932.

40. Ober, F. R.: An operation to relieve paralysis of the deltoid muscle. J.A.M.A., 99:2182, 1932.

41. Osterhaus, K.: Obstetrical paralysis: A preliminary report of 2 cases. N.Y. Med. J., 88:887–891, 1908.

42. Pollock, L. J.: Accessory muscle movements in deltoid paralysis. J.A.M.A., 79:526–528, 1922.

43. Rapp, I. H.: Serratus anterior paralysis treated by transplantation of the pectoralis minor. J. Bone Joint Surg., 36-A:852–854, 1954.

44. Riedel, G.: Zur Frage de Muskeltransplantation bei Deltoideslahmung. Ergebn. d. Chir. u. Orthop., 21:489–542, 1928.

45. Rogers, M. H.: An operation for the correction of the deformity due to "obstetrical paralysis." Boston Med. Surg. J., 174:163, 1916.

46. Saha, A. K.: Surgery of the paralyzed and flail shoulder. Acta Orthop. Scand. (Suppl.), 97:5–90, 1967.

47. Scaglietti, O.: The obstetrical shoulder trauma. Surg. Gynecol. Obstet., 66:868–877, 1938.

48. Schottstaedt, E. R., Larsen, L. J., and Bost, F. C.: The surgical reconstruction of the upper extremity paralyzed by poliomyelitis. J. Bone Joint Surg., 40-A:633–643, 1958.

49. Sever, J. W.: Obstetric paralysis. Its etiology, pathology, clinical aspects and treatment, with a report of four hundred and seventy cases. Am. J. Dis. Child., 12:541–578, 1916.

50. Sever, J. W.: The results of a new operation for obstetrical paralysis. Am. J. Orthop. Surg., 16:248–257, 1918.

51. Sever, J. W.: Obstetric paralysis: Report of eleven hundred cases. J.A.M.A., 85:1862–1865, 1925.

52. Sever, J. W.: Obstetrical paralysis. Surg. Gynecol. Obstet., 44:547–549, 1927.

53. Smellie, W.: Collection of Preternatural Cases and Observations in Midwifery, Compleating the Design of Illustrating His First Volume on That Subject, Vol. III, pp. 504–505. London, 1764.

54. Smith, J. F., and Christensen, H. H.: Deltoid paralysis following shoulder injuries. Surg. Gynecol. Obstet., 41:451–453, 1925.

55. Spira, E.: The treatment of dropped shoulder. A new operative technique. J. Bone Joint Surg., 30-A:229–233, 1948.

56. Staples, O. S., and Watkins, A. L.: Full active ab-

duction in traumatic paralysis of the deltoid. J. Bone Joint Surg., 25:85–89, 1943.

57. Steindler, A.: Operative treatment of paralytic conditions of the upper extremity. J. Bone Joint Surg., 1:608–619, 1919.

58. Steindler, A.: Tendon transplantation in the upper extremity. Am. J. Surg., 44:26–271, 1939.

59. Steindler, A.: Orthopedic Operations. Springfield, Ill., Charles C Thomas, 1940.

60. Steindler, A.: The Traumatic Deformities and Disabilities of the Upper Extremity. Springfield, Ill., Charles C Thomas, 1946.

61. Steindler, A.: Reconstruction of the poliomyelitic upper extremity. Bull. Hosp. Joint Dis., 15:21–26, 1954.

62. Taylor, A. S.: Results from the surgical treatment of brachial birth palsy. J.A.M.A., 48:96–104, 1907.

63. Tubby, A. H.: A case illustrating the operative treatment of paralysis of the serratus magnus muscle by muscle grafting. Br. Med. J., 2:1159–1160, 1904.

64. Whitman, A.: Congenital elevation of the scapula and paralysis of serratus magnus muscle. J.A.M.A., 99:1332–1334, 1932.

65. Wickstrom, J., Haslam, E. T., and Hutchinson, R. H.: The surgical management of residual deformities of the shoulder following birth injuries of the brachial plexus. J. Bone Joint Surg., 37-A:27–36, 1955.

66. Wolf, J.: The conservative treatment of serratus palsy. J. Bone Joint Surg., 23:959–961, 1941.

67. Wolman, B.: Erb's palsy. Arch. Dis. Child., 23:129–130, 1948.

68. Wright, W. G.: Muscle training in the treatment of infantile paralysis. Boston Med. Surg. J., 163:567–574, 1912.

69. Zachary, R. B.: Transplantation of teres major and latissimus dorsi for loss of external rotation at shoulder. Lancet, 2:757–758, 1947.

10

Part A: Shoulder Arthroplasty

MELVIN POST

No joint in the human body is more difficult to salvage than the glenohumeral joint. Its unusual anatomic relationships, marked dependence on muscle integrity, and great vulnerability to trauma create problems that make successful reconstruction formidable. Still, it is worthwhile attempting to achieve a painless, functioning glenohumeral joint in order to permit the hand to be placed in a wide variety of positions that otherwise would not be possible. Although shoulder joint arthrodesis, resection, and prosthetic replacement of the humeral head have a place in the armamentarium of the orthopaedic surgeon, each has a serious drawback. Arthrodesis significantly limits movement of the shoulder and drastically curtails hand placement. Humeral head resection diminishes strength and motion function of the shoulder joint because the fulcrum is usually lost. Moreover, patients often continue to complain of localized discomfort. Prosthetic replacement of the humeral head may give good results, providing the shoulder girdle muscles, especially the rotator cuff muscles, are intact.

This chapter will consider (1) resection arthroplasty of the humeral head, (2) autogenous fibular graft replacement of the proximal humerus, (3) prosthetic replacement of the humeral head, and (4) total shoulder replacement. Whatever procedure he selects for his patient, the surgeon must base his judgment on careful preoperative analysis of the actual functioning anatomy of the upper extremity, predetermining what goals can be attained by surgical intervention, particularly as they relate to hand function.

RESECTION ARTHROPLASTY OF THE HUMERAL HEAD

Jones added immeasurably to our knowledge of shoulder joint physiology. He demonstrated that after humeral head resection a stable shoulder could be obtained by transplanting the rotator cuff muscles into the proximal humerus.[9] He was among the first who stated that the shoulder girdle must be in a fixed position and stabilized through muscle action on the scapula in order to allow the arm to be elevated. Stabilization of the scapula and clavicle is effected by the actions of the subclavius and pectoralis minor anteriorly, the trapezius and rhomboids posteriorly, and the serratus anterior muscle acting on the vertebral border of the scapula. Working synchronously these muscles fix the scapula. Although they are of primary importance, other muscles such as the short biceps and coracobrachialis attaching to the coracoid process can act as secondary stabilizers.

Once the scapula is stabilized the proximal humerus must be fixed within the shallow glenoid before the arm can be actively raised. This is accomplished by the subscapularis in front, and the supraspinatus, infraspinatus, and teres minor behind. These "short rotator" muscles are not small, nor are they unimportant, as was once erroneously believed. Their combined weight was shown by Jones to be greater than that of the deltoid.[9] Acting together, all the shoulder muscles permit prodigious work demands to be met. Thus, any injury or operation that disrupts the integrity of the joint or weakens muscle action impairs the function of the arm and the whole extremity.

Indications

In the past, humeral head resection was performed for resectable tumor, localized infection of the proximal humerus, severe crush injury, 4-part fractures and severe fracture-dislocations of the humeral head with obvious attendant loss of the blood supply to the fragments. In recent years improved surgical techniques and replacement procedures have greatly narrowed the indications for resection arthroplasty. The

procedure has its greatest worth in eliminating local infection in the proximal humerus (Fig. 10-1), and to a lesser degree is used for tumor removal (Fig. 10-2).

Prerequisites

The lesion should be localized to the proximal humerus and a functioning rotator cuff must be available for reattachment to the humeral shaft. The rest of the shoulder girdle musculature should be normal. Even when these conditions are met the patient may have limited motion and a varying degree of discomfort. Failure to meet these requirements will lead to a poor result.

Operation

The patient is placed in a semireclining position with the torso elevated 30 degrees by a sandbag placed behind the shoulder blade. The knees should be flexed slightly and the lower extremities wrapped with Ace

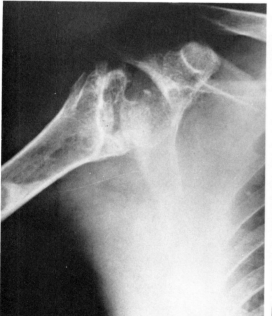
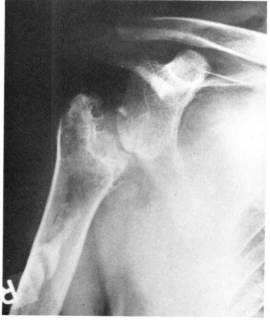

A

B

FIG. 10-1. A 34-year-old man had surgical treatment for a fracture of the proximal humerus. He developed a severe infection and had a subsequent humeral head resection and reattachment of the rotator cuff structures with fair results. The patient had poor active abduction and great discomfort. Note the development of irregular bone spurs on the film in both, A, abducted and, B, resting positions.

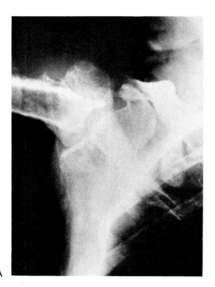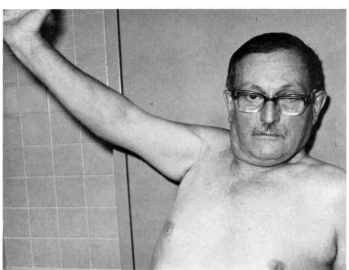

A   B

FIG. 10-2. A, Roentgenogram in the abducted position of a 55-year-old man who had a humeral head resection years before for tumor. Note the bone spur formation. B, This view of the patient demonstrates active abduction to 90 degrees. The patient complained of pain and stiffness that were not serious enough to warrant another surgical procedure.

bandages. The extremity is draped free and sterile sheets with wings are placed across a tilted half screen. The patient's head is isolated from the shoulder with a special U-shaped Vi-Drape in order to allow an assistant to stand above it and to the side. Endotracheal anesthesia should be employed. The chest wall must not be used as a "convenient table" for resting instruments.

The upper portion of the Henry approach can be utilized (Figs. 10-2 and 10-3A). A 12.5-cm. curvilinear incision is started over the superolateral acromion, then continued medially toward the acromioclavicular joint and lateral clavicle, and gently curved downward in the direction of the deltopectoral groove on the lateral side of the coracoid tip.

The cephalic vein is identified, its lateral muscle branches tied and cut, and the vein retracted medially. It is permissible to ligate the vein. The deltopectoral groove is followed proximally toward the clavicle. The deltoid is cautiously elevated from its clavicular origin with a millimeter of osteoperiosteal cuff. From previous operation, enough scar has formed so that repair sutures will hold if the muscle is transected

1.5 cm. beneath the clavicle. In heavy individuals it may be necessary to continue the elevation of the deltoid from the anterior acromion. When the muscle has been elevated, a plexus of veins normally is seen leaving the deep surface of the upper medial deltoid. These must be ligated and cut before complete lateral retraction of the muscle can be effected. The muscle must be kept moist with saline solution and gently retracted at its superior part. Pressure by the retractor blades at the undersurface of the middle of the belly must be avoided in order not to injure branches of the axillary nerve as they enter the muscle.

The subscapularis and its underlying capsule are now seen. In severe acute fracture the capsule is opened first by transecting the tendon of the subscapularis at the medial lip of the bicipital groove. Any bony fragments are carefully removed by sharp dissection but the tendon mass of the rotator cuff muscles is left. The proximal shaft is rounded by removing all sharp edges of bone. It may be necessary to transect the long head of the biceps and reattach it either to the tip of the coracoid or in its groove below.

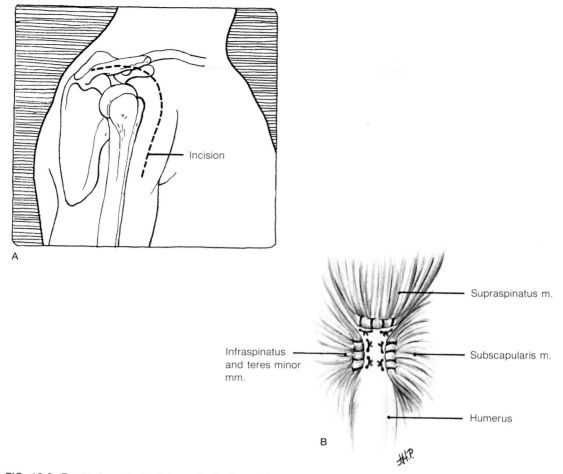

FIG. 10-3. Reattachment of rotator cuff. A, Dotted line indicates incision for anterior Henry approach to the shoulder. B, Jones's method for reattaching rotator cuff structures to the proximal humerus. The tendons of each of the muscles must be identified and directly attached to the shaft for best results (see text for discussion).

Traction is placed on the infraspinatus-teres minor, supraspinatus, and subscapularis tendons. An area on the lateral upper humeral shaft is marked as the site of attachment for these structures (Fig. 10-3B). It is important to define these structures. Merely attaching a large mass of capsule to the shaft haphazardly can preclude a successful result (see Fig. 10-1). The patient must be able to bring his arm to the side of the body without excessive tension on the muscles or the site of rotator cuff reattachment. Small slots are made in the cortex and heavy nonabsorbable sutures placed through drill holes and tendons. These are tied after the surrounding surface cortex is scarified. The wound is flushed with saline solution. The deltoid muscle flap is reattached to the clavicle with heavy nonabsorbable or synthetic suture placed through several drill holes in the clavicle.

Aftercare

The extremity is immobilized for 25 days in Velpeau position, and thereafter, gentle passive and pendulum motion exercises are started. After several more days active exercises are begun and gradually increased. It takes at least 6 months to achieve an optimum result.

In recent years my preference for this

operation has been limited more to the patient with severe localized infection. Even when a benign tumor is resectable some soft-tissue cuff about the proximal humerus is ordinarily removed in order to avoid entering the lesion. In this event, too much rotator cuff tissue and/or bone may be removed, precluding proper reattachment of the rotator muscles.

AUTOGENOUS FIBULAR GRAFT REPLACEMENT

Resection of the proximal humerus and replacement by a fibular graft is rarely indicated. This procedure has been used successfully for resectable tumor of the proximal humerus and distal radius.

In 1910, Rovsing reported a case of fibula transplantation used to fill a bony defect in the shoulder joint.[15] Albee reported three additional cases in 1921, wherein he not only transplanted the fibula to the humerus but preserved the surrounding muscles and reattached them to the transplant.[1] In 1926, Hammond described another case of transplant for painful shoulder that had previously been operated upon for an old fracture-dislocation of the proximal humerus.[5] Over the years, many similar but unreported procedures have undoubtedly been performed. Enneking and Roy have ingeniously utilized a fibular autograft for a resectable tumor of the proximal humerus, the fibular head coincidentally showing a benign exostosis approximating the shape of a humeral head (see Fig. 21-2B).

Although autogenous fibular grafts do unite with the remaining humeral shaft, functional results are ordinarily less than desirable. The result of this procedure, like that of total shoulder replacement for resectable tumor, is certainly better than a flail upper extremity. This operation has merit for carefully selected cases requiring extensive resection of the proximal humerus.

Indications

The operation should be reserved for resectable tumor of the proximal humerus when it is unlikely that humeral head resection and reattachment of the rotator muscles to the shaft will rid the patient of the lesion. In certain cases of traumatic loss of the proximal humerus or those requiring extensive resection of the proximal humerus, this method may be considered.

Operation

The patient is placed in a semireclining position, as described for humeral head resection. The Henry approach is utilized (Figs. 10-4 and 10-10A). After retraction of the deltoid muscle, the anterior circumflex humeral vessels are ligated and other smaller branches cauterized. Structures such as the short rotator muscles and pectoralis major are freed from the shaft extraperiosteally, and as much soft tissue is left attached to the bone as is necessary to ensure that tumor tissue is not left behind. The axillary nerve must be protected. If at all feasible as much of the deltoid insertion as possible should be preserved. The humerus is transected by power saw, and the diseased proximal shaft and head are removed. Care must be taken not to strip the periosteal tissue from the remaining bone.

A second surgical team may remove a fibular graft through a longitudinal incision. As much length is taken as is needed to fill the humeral gap. The peroneal nerve as well as all its branches must be isolated and protected. When the various muscles have been stripped from the fibular shaft and the bone has been transected below, the biceps tendon insertion and fibular collateral ligament above are transected close to their attachments. These structures are then sutured to the surrounding muscles and the wound is closed.

In the meantime, the distal part of the bone graft is shaped as needed to fit the medullary canal of the humerus. The outer fibular cortex should be scarified, preferably with a sharp rongeur. Care should be exercised not to break the graft. The graft should be secure and fit snugly, but not be unduly forced, into the humeral medullary canal. In some cases, it has been suggested that added strength in the graft may be

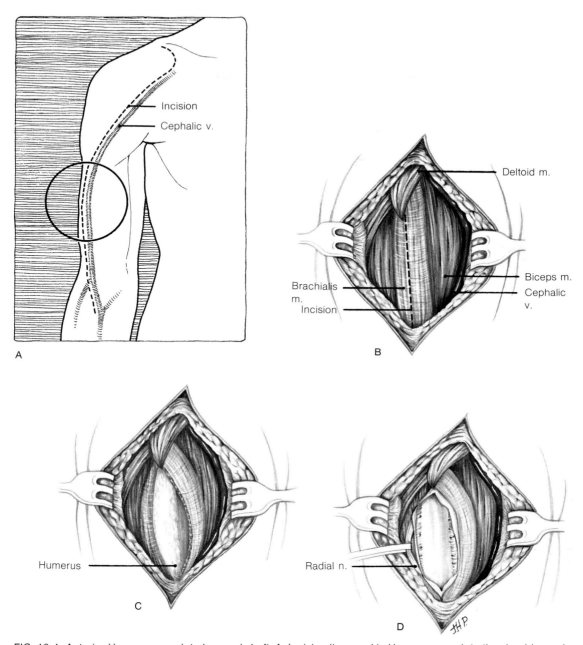

FIG. 10-4. Anterior Henry approach to humeral shaft. A, Incision line used in Henry approach to the shoulder and shaft. B to D, Surgical approach to the shaft structures within circle, for example, is shown (see text for discussion). This technique is ideal for performing an osteotomy of the humeral shaft at any level.

obtained by passing a heavy Steinmann pin or rod downward through the fibular intramedullary canal into the humeral canal. The tendons of the various muscles groups are then reattached to the graft through small drill holes in the bone. If necessary, stability of the graft can be enhanced with a Nicola biceps tendon transfer. The new "head" should be positioned so that it does not rest opposite the superior portion of the glenoid, but rather at its middle.

The wound is closed and Hemovac suction instituted for 24 hours. Postoperative blood loss is usually less than 75 ml.

Aftercare

The extremity must be protected in a plaster of Paris spica cast for at least 3 or more months until the graft appears to be healed both clinically and by roentgenographic examination. Gentle elbow and shoulder exercises are then started. Vigorous active exercises should not be allowed until consolidation is complete. Even then, gentle active exercises should be prescribed.

PROSTHETIC REPLACEMENT OF THE HUMERAL HEAD

When the proximal humerus alone is irreparably damaged, prosthetic replacement of the humeral head may be considered as an alternative method for preserving shoulder function. The surgeon not only must consider the bony abnormality but must be quite certain that the short rotator muscles are functioning in order to achieve a good result. At times this may be difficult to determine, such as when a low threshold of pain precludes adequate testing of muscle strength. Failure to obtain a stable fulcrum will almost certainly lead to a poor result. Neer is of the opinion that the prosthetic head should provide a gliding rather than a fixed fulcrum, which should result in leverage and simultaneously allow a loose fit of the metal head on its glenoid.[11] It has been my experience from having examined patients with such prosthetic replacements of the humeral head that seemingly well-performed operations for correct indications and good follow-up care have nevertheless led to poor results (Fig. 10-5).

Neer has employed four stem sizes: small, medium, large, and extra large. The latter is used when needed for the enlarged humeral canal in osteoporotic elderly bone. A series of holes are positioned beneath the dome of the metal head on the stem which allows for bone ingrowth. Haraldsson described a prosthesis used to replace the humeral head and the upper portion of humerus when involved with a destructive tumor.[6] In his operation a series of perforations were placed in the stem in order to permit the

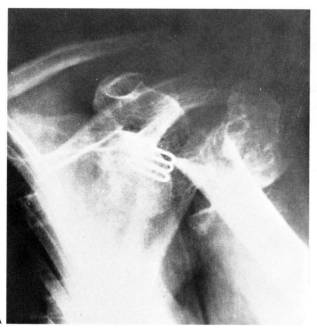
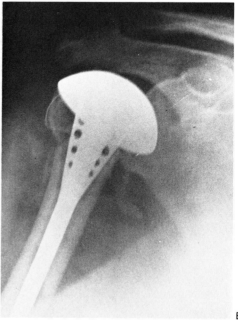

A

B

FIG. 10-5. A, A 65-year-old woman sustained a highly comminuted humeral head-surgical neck fracture-dislocation. B, It was correctly treated with a Neer hemiarthroplasty. The metal dome was stable. The patient was referred when she continued to have severe pain and stiffness in the shoulder.

muscles, preferably antagonists, to be sutured to one another to provide a permanent muscle-sling fixation.

Indications

Humeral head prosthetic replacement can be considered for acute fracture-dislocations or 4-part fractures of the humeral head in which the blood supply of the bone fragments is almost certainly lost. Fracture-dislocations with a 50 percent impression defect and split humeral head fractures are additional indications.[10]

According to Neer, best results are achieved with humeral head replacement for patients with symptomatic osteoarthritis.[12] The procedure may be considered for other reasons such as painful osteonecrosis, cartilage necrosis, or other degenerative conditions of the humeral head.

It should be remembered that mere loss of shoulder motion without severe pain is not an indication for this type of procedure or for total shoulder replacement. Moreover, when considering prosthetic replacement of the humeral head the shoulder girdle musculature including the short rotators should be strong. Therefore, this operation should not be considered for the severely painful, destroyed rheumatoid shoulder, because almost always there is atrophied muscle that will not permit enough of a stable fulcrum in the usual case. Nevertheless, hemiarthroplasty has occasionally been used with fair success. Clayton and Ferlic employed the Neer prosthesis in seven patients with symptomatic rheumatoid shoulders.[3] Neer reported one case.[12]

Contraindications

Prosthetic replacement of the humeral head should not be used (1) when the short rotators and other important muscles are nonfunctioning,[2] (2) when there is infection, and (3) when there is no hope of reattaching a functioning rotator cuff because of fracture or degenerative lesions of the humeral head. It should not be performed with the mistaken notion that a reattached severely weakened rotator cuff will somehow restore strength in these muscles. It is particularly contraindicated in the advanced symptomatic rheumatoid shoulder with an attenuated rotator cuff.

This operation is not recommended for traumatic conditions listed previously except in the acute phase, because in the chronic phase there is much scarring and atrophy about the rotator cuff that will ultimately give a poor result. This procedure like others is most worthwhile if the surgeon employs it for the appropriate case.

Operation

The patient is placed in a semireclining position with a sandbag or roll behind the involved shoulder. A 12.5- or 15.0-cm. curvilinear incision is made over the acromion and deltopectoral groove (see Fig. 10-10A to C). The deltoid is elevated from the clavicle and laterally reflected. If needed, it may also be elevated from the anterior acromion in order to facilitate additional exposure. The fascia is incised longitudinally and lateral to the coracoid. Neer recommends excision of the coracoacromial ligament, although this may not be needed all the time.[11] The subscapularis insertion is transected and the tendon elevated from its capsule by sharp dissection. Any movable attached fragments are excised from the tendon.

In acute fracture the bone fragments are excised. When the head is intact, as in osteoarthritis, a power saw is used to resect the humeral head, and care is taken to protect the region of the axillary nerve. Relatively little humeral head need be resected to make room for the dome of the prosthesis. However, osteophytes should be removed. The Neer prosthesis that best fits snugly into the humeral canal is selected. The revised Neer prosthesis has a 44.5-mm.-diameter head and three stem diameters (6.6, 9.5, and 12.9 mm.).[11] A drill of appropriate size is used to ream the humeral canal. The head is placed in the desired degree of retroversion via a triangular opening in the canal.

This is best estimated by placing the extremity in anatomic position and flexing the elbow 90 degrees during the placement. Although Neer first recommended 25 degrees of retroversion, he now employs 35 to 40 degrees of retroversion, because he believes this is important for the stability of the joint.[13]

Bechtol believes that for his shoulder prosthesis as much as 45 degrees of retroversion is needed for best results.[2]

When driven into the canal the edge of the dome should be parallel to the cut surface of the neck. In the event that the tuberosities are intact, it may be necessary to resect some additional bone so that the prosthetic head will not be displaced upward. Its surface must glide on the glenoid while the arm is passively abducted. The rotator cuff tendon and any attached bone fragments to be reduced are tied to the shaft anatomically, if possible, through small drill holes. Heavy nonabsorbable suture may be placed through one of the stem holes and tied circumferentially. The surgeon should strive to restore the anatomic continuity of the surrounding structures. The distal portion of the long head of the biceps is sutured in its groove and the excess tendon removed. The capsule is not closed, but the subscapularis tendon is repaired with the patient's arm in neutral position. If the tendon is contracted, it should be lengthened.

The deltoid is reattached to the clavicle as described for humeral head resection, and the wound closed. Hemovac drainage is maintained for 24 hours.

Aftercare

The extremity is maintained in Velpeau position. Neer recommends abduction and slight external rotation for posterior fracture-dislocation.[11] After 2 or 3 days, when postoperative pain has subsided, gentle passive exercises are instituted. Extremes of motion are avoided until after 3 weeks when the soft tissues have healed. Thereafter, active exercises are gradually increased. It usually takes months to achieve a good result, especially in those patients whose muscles were initially weak. In a cooperative patient a shoulder with long-standing preexisting disease may require at least a year or even longer to gain an optimum result.

Part B:
Total Shoulder Replacement

MELVIN POST
SAUL S. HASKELL

Total shoulder replacement is an experimental salvage procedure designed to rid the patient of pain and restore function when other operations will not serve the needs of the patient. Ten or more centers have designed or are now implanting total shoulder joints.

Lettin and Scales reported two cases of total shoulder joint replacement employing the Stanmore prosthesis.[8] Fenlin described his method of total shoulder with a large ball and a fixed fulcrum design.[4] Neer has used a revised prosthesis with enlarged head and short neck along with a polyethylene glenoid that avoids a fixed fulcrum and still permits resurfacing of the diseased glenoid.[12] Similarly, Bechtol performs a hemiarthroplasty and also resurfaces the glenoid, giving a nonhinged joint replacement.[2] Reeves and associates have stated the conditions needed for successful joint replacement and have implanted total shoulders of their own design.[14] Preliminary reports and still unanswered questions about which total shoulder design is best center around (1) whether the artificial joint should have a fixed fulcrum or be gliding and nonhinged, (2) whether the head should be large or small,[4] (3) whether the head should be fixed into the scapula or humerus,[7] and (4) what are the best methods for anchoring the scapular component. This section relates our personal experience with one particular fixed fulcrum design.

Prerequisites

A good range of active shoulder motion is possible with shoulder joint replacement provided the surrounding soft tissues allow such motion. All soft-tissue contractures must first be released, preferably at the time of joint replacement. Failure to release contracted tissues will give a corresponding limitation of joint motion. Because the upper extremity must work against gravity, the stronger the shoulder girdle musculature the better will be the result. Accordingly, it is essential to carefully examine the patient, taking into account the age, job requirements, and the expectations of the patient. The surgeon and patient must determine together what are the goals of the procedure, the chance of relieving the patient's pain and significantly increasing hand function. In a patient who desires a "normal" shoulder, the surgeon should not suggest that postoperative total shoulder function will ever equal the extraordinary strength, endurance, and wide range of synchronous movements of the uninjured glenohumeral joint no matter how excellent the result.

When the shoulder girdle musculature,

particularly the rotator cuff muscles, is severely damaged, a stable fulcrum is required for best results. The controversy over whether the fulcrum should be fixed or gliding (wandering) has not been resolved, except that it is virtually impossible in the severely damaged joint with its permanently weakened short rotator muscles to provide the delicately balanced stable fulcrum required for a successful replacement. It appears that fixed fulcrum prostheses give the best chance for solving the dilemma of the permanently damaged glenohumeral joint with nonfunctioning rotator cuff muscles.

Minimum requirements for successful joint replacement are (1) an intact glenoid and scapular neck, (2) functioning muscles to stabilize the scapula (serratus anterior and trapezius), and (3) a functioning deltoid that can elevate the arm against gravity, except in certain select cases in which a lesser goal is acceptable. The last condition is essential if the arm is to be actively elevated. However, if elimination of pain alone is expected, as in "flail shoulder" secondary to irreparable massive rotator cuff tear, for example, then total joint replacement is worthwhile even with a weakened deltoid. Many patients with sedentary jobs prefer a movable joint allowing a wider range of hand positions to arthrodesis that diminishes hand placement.

Evolution of Prosthetic Design and Insertion

A variety of shoulder prostheses have been designed including snap fits, non-dislocatable hinged joints, and reversed ball in the glenoid models. Snap fit designs fail to give control over the congruity of artificial joint surfaces. Non-dislocatable designs will break away from the glenoid vault, and the ball in the glenoid vault has the inherent characteristic of weakening the bone structure leading to failure. Therefore, the best design appears to be one in which the integrity of the glenoid vault is preserved as much as possible, and a controlled dislocation of a fixed fulcrum prosthesis allowed

before the glenoid component pulls from the glenoid. A total shoulder joint replacement must not be based purely on engineering principles, but more importantly also must take into account the living tissues, especially the bone tissue and what it is capable of tolerating.

When the glenohumeral joint is severely damaged and function of the short rotator muscles is lost, the insertion of a total shoulder prosthesis should (1) provide a fixed fulcrum, (2) allow lateral rotation, abduction, and a stable 360-degree arc of movement for full overhead motion of the arm, and (3) dislocate with excessive force before the scapular neck will fracture or the anchored metal glenoid pull away from the bone. Planned dislocation of the metal humeral head from its socket is easier to achieve with a small humeral head than with a large ball.

The first series of 24 cases of total shoulder replacement, inserted from June 1973 to July 1975, employed a 15-mm.-diameter metal humeral head that fit within two polyethylene halves that made a perfect sphere of similar diameter and had a peripheral lip diameter slightly smaller than the humeral head (Fig. 10-6). The assembled parts fit precisely within the metal glenoid (Fig. 10-7). A self-locking metal ring first placed about the humeral neck portion is tightened

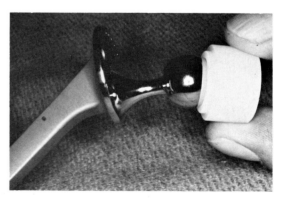

FIG. 10-6. Humeral component used in series I cases with 4-mm. neck, 15-mm.-diameter head, and plastic halves in which the head diameter is larger than the peripheral diameter of the fitted plastic pieces. The plastic pieces fit about the head, preventing easy dislocation when all the parts are assembled.

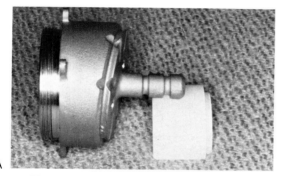

A

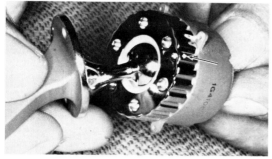

B

FIG. 10-7. A, A side view of the truncated metal glenoid with its central post resting on one plastic half of series I model. B, The assembled components. Note the anteriorly projecting eyelets through which a 20-gauge wire is first inserted. The wire is then inserted into the small hole on the locking ring (arrow).

about the metal glenoid. A fixed fulcrum is achieved by the apparatus which gives maximum protection to the fragile scapula.

Early cases had rectangularly shaped metal glenoids inserted. Truncated metal glenoids with a 10.5-degree angle of declination are now utilized (Fig. 10-7A), because it was discovered on cine studies that the metal humeral neck component, set at 145 degrees to the metal shaft, impinged slightly on the inferior plastic lip periphery when the arm is at the side. Merely changing the angle of the humeral neck to the face of the metal glenoid by 10.5 degrees lessened the abutment of the neck against the plastic lip, and is also less likely to cause polyethylene "flow." This obviously decreases the danger of dislocation of the head if the extremity should drop suddenly and forcefully to the side of the body. In addition, it may diminish the possibility of eventual metal fatigue and fracture at the neck. The change was

accomplished without significantly decreasing overhead motion. Even less chance of impingement can be achieved by decreasing the neck-shaft angle to 135 degrees, but there is a corresponding decrease in overhead motion. In the patient with weakened muscles and perhaps intrinsic muscle contractures who cannot possibly attain complete overhead motion, this extreme motion is superfluous. Thus, slight varus position of the metal neck may be desirable in some patients.

As in the normal shoulder joint, impingement in the region of the greater tuberosity and lateral collar of the prosthesis occurs at the lateral acromion during abduction. This is obviated if care is taken to position the metal glenoid centrally on the glenoid hollow, and the patient is instructed to externally rotate the arm during abduction. When adequate external rotation is prevented, complete overhead motion is lost in the artificial joint.

The first 24 total shoulders were constructed of stainless steel. The dimensions and calculated yield strengths at the neck of the humeral component are:

Neck diameter	4 mm.
Humeral head diameter	15 mm.
Calculated yield strength	824 lb.

Six complications were related to breakage of the humeral neck component (see under Complications). In order to lessen breakage, the newer series of total shoulder replacements are made of harder cast chromecobalt. The dimensions and calculated yield strengths of the thickened neck portion are:

Neck diameters	6.3 mm.	8 mm.
Humeral head diameters	22.0 mm.	22 mm.
Calculated yield strengths	3191 lb.	4970 lb.

In order to accommodate the heavier neck part the humeral head diameter was increased to 22 mm., and the outside diameter of the metal glenoid was correspondingly increased from 32 mm. to 35 mm. The plastic pieces also were slightly increased in size to accommodate the new head. Thus, the use of harder metal and greater neck strength should lessen the possibility of breakage from metal fatigue. In fact, since January 1976, not one series II neck component has broken in 26 cases.

Methods of Anchoring the Metal Glenoid Component

PRINCIPLE. The flat, membranous scapula contains few regions with a significant mass of cancellous bone for attaching a metal glenoid component. The cancellous vault is covered by a paper-thin cortical bone layer, and extends laterally from the scapular neck to the glenoid face, upward to the coronoid, and as an extension downward in pencillike fashion inside a thickened ridge along the axillary border of the scapula (Fig. 10-8). The volume and integrity of cancellous bone determine how a metal component can be affixed to the scapula.

The scapular neck region can be used to receive an artificial glenoid, or a spherical humeral head may be implanted directly into the scapula. The principle is to achieve a stable fulcrum for the upper humerus during abduction. Because pathologic conditions often destroy this stability, it is necessary to fix the fulcrum. However, this adds greater stress on the components and bone. Therefore, a safety feature has been employed by allowing the artificial humeral head to dislocate from its glenoid component with undue force, especially torque, before the scapula or the metal glenoid attachment is damaged.

Coronal sections of the scapula show that the largest volume of cancellous bone resides in the neck region. The cancellous bone in this region resembles a sieve throughout its mass (Fig. 10-8). The described design depends upon the protection of the cancellous vault and its overlying cortical cover. The integrity of the bone permits easy and adequate fixation of the metal glenoid component to the scapula. A weakened cancellous vault caused by severe osteoporosis, tumor, or surgical excavation decreases the strength of the bone and its attachment between the metal glenoid and the scapula.

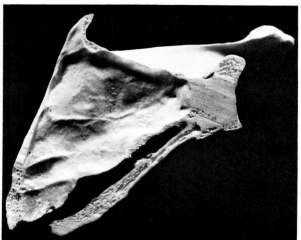

A   B

FIG. 10-8. A, A coronal section of a scapula shows the extent of the cancellous vault and the thinness of its cortical cover. B, A coronal section of the glenoid vault after it was injected with soft methyl methacrylate. Note the homogeneous dispersion of cement.

The attachment of the glenoid component can be accomplished with (1) screws alone, (2) helicoil suspension, or (3) a combination of screws, central metal glenoid post, and methyl methacrylate. Screw fixation alone is unreliable, whereas the helicoil system without the use of methyl methacrylate shows promise. In the latter system, $\frac{1}{4}$-in.-diameter short-length helicoils inserted into dry scapula bone can each withstand straight pulling forces of up to 80 pounds. Presently, the use of bone cement and heavy duty screws allows the strongest bond between the metal glenoid and scapula. The use of metal glenoid prongs has been avoided because it has been shown in vitro that implantation of such a system makes it impossible to remove the metal glenoid without destroying the glenoid.

TECHNIQUE. The glenoid face is carefully denuded of its cartilage with a sharp curette, but the subchondral cortical bone is left intact. A tapered 10.5-degree jig is used to drill a $\frac{1}{4}$-in.-diameter central hole 2 cm. deep (Fig. 10-9). With the drill bit in place, eccentric $\frac{1}{8}$-in. parallel drill holes are made 2.8 cm. deep into the scapular neck. In order to avoid rotation of the jig and ensure precise placement of the holes in the scapula, anterior and posterior short sharp prongs have been placed on the jig face. The diameter between these projection points is exactly the same as the diameter between the eccentric $\frac{1}{8}$-in. holes. The jig is first rotated into the transverse plane and $\frac{5}{64}$-in. diameter holes are drilled only through the glenoid cortex anteriorly and posteriorly on the midsection of the glenoid face utilizing the rotated eccentric holes. The jig is then oriented in the vertical direction, thus aligning the jig holes longitudinally. The pointed jig projections are pressed into the transverse holes to obviate the possibility of jig movement while drilling the glenoid. During the drilling all drill bits are left in place so as to be certain the jig does not move and the holes are parallel. Each hole is cautiously counterbeveled at several depths with a needle tip curette while care is taken not to break the walls between the holes.

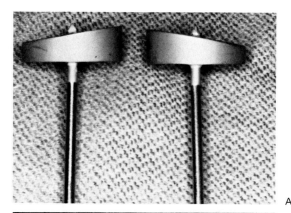

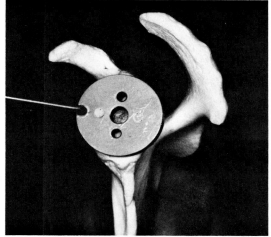

FIG. 10-9. A, Lateral views of the right and left glenoid guides with their anterior and posterior prongs. B, Correct alignment of the guide on its glenoid. The wider portion is positioned posteriorly. This permits three parallel holes to be made in the vault.

A 6-ml. disposable syringe is used to load each hole with methyl methacrylate in the "hairy" stage. During this process, cement extruding through the other holes when the first hole is filled demonstrates dispersion of the cement throughout the cancellous system. The cement is forced into the bone via one hole while the other two are covered with a finger (Fig. 10-8B). The glenoid central post and back plate are loaded with cement. The glenoid threads are protected with a plastic ring protector. A glenoid guide permits the glenoid component to be aligned with the scapular holes in a precise position after the metal central post is placed through the central hole. No effort is made to cover the sides of the metal glenoid with cement since this does not add to the holding power and may block tightening of the glenoid ring. While the cement is still soft heavy duty screws, $1\frac{1}{4}$- and $1\frac{1}{8}$-in. long, respectively, are placed through the superior and inferior holes of the back plate into the scapular neck. The screw heads must be below the inside surface of the back plate. They must be tight and care should be taken not to strip the threads made in the cancellous bone by the screw threads. The screws must be of the same chrome-cobalt metal as the metal glenoid.

Instead of removing cancellous bone from its vault, it is utilized and strengthened by filling its pores with cement. Thus, it is left intact to continue its scaffoldlike support of the overlying thin cortical bone. Whether the bone trabeculae remain viable is unknown but unlikely. When the metal glenoid is solidly fixed in place, the normal shoulder contour is preserved unless severe shoulder girdle atrophy already exists. In a very thin person the loss of contour is magnified.

Insertion of Humeral Component

PRINCIPLE. A small-sized humeral head is easier to dislocate with excessive force than a large diameter head. The small diameter head has been used in order to protect the metal glenoid-scapula attachment to bone. The newer series 22-mm.-diameter head also dislocates with excessive force.

TECHNIQUE. The patient's arm is held in anatomic position while the proximal humerus is cut at a 45-degree incline from the superolateral to the inferomedial shaft. The angle of the blade is retroverted 20 to 25 degrees to coincide with the position in which the humeral component is to be retroverted. The medial end of the cut bone should lie opposite the inferior edge of the glenoid or slightly below it (Fig. 10-10D and E). The angle of retroversion will vary in some cases. For instance, certain patients desire more internal rotation than others, and in this event the surgeon should aim for a bit more retroversion than usual. The periosteum and soft tissues should not be stripped from the shaft. With the metal glenoid and trial humeral component temporarily in place, the center of the ball must not lie above the center of the metal glenoid when the patient's arm rests at the side. Only enough of an opening in the humeral canal is made to accept the metal stem, and no larger. When this has been accomplished, the medullary canal is filled with methyl methacrylate and the humeral component inserted into the desired position.

BIOMECHANICS. In vitro studies show that the smallest straight pulling force required to dislocate the cemented metallic glenoid from the scapula is 121 pounds. Early model total shoulder joints allowed the metal humeral head to dislocate from its plastic cup at an average of 186 pounds of straight pulling force and to torque out at 55 inch-pounds. Series I cases (24 cases) now contain plastic cups that permit dislocation of the metal head from the cup at an average straight pulling force of 250 pounds and a torque of 116 inch-pounds. This increase was achieved by slightly thickening and lengthening the plastic lip edge. Beyond this point there is danger that the scapular neck will fracture with this particular design. It is for this reason that this total shoulder has been designed to dislocate. The larger diameter head component (series II) requires 285 pounds of straight pulling force to dislocate and has approximately the same torque values as have the series I components.

Consecutive mechanical testing using the same plastic cup under the same conditions in vitro proved that it requires significantly less force to redislocate the head, indicating that the polyethylene compresses and deforms. If a revision is needed, only a new plastic cup and locking ring should be used. Because the torquing force is the one that will usually cause dislocation, it must not exceed the critical value of 116 inch-pounds, nor must a pulling force of 121 pounds be surpassed in order to protect the metal glenoid-bone attachment. However, even this last figure may be revised upward in view of more recent laboratory data.

Of course, from these studies it is not possible to define actual in vivo conditions nor to base any conclusions of actual forces upon extrapolation of in vitro data until an instrumented total shoulder has been inserted.

Operation

The patient is placed in a semireclining position with a sandbag beneath the scapula. The extremity is draped free. An incision is started at the superolateral acromion, curved inward over the outer third of the clavicle, and then downward over the coracoid and along the deltopectoral groove for 7.5 to 10 cm. (Fig. 10-10A). Acute angles should be avoided in order to obviate skin slough.

The deltoid with a millimeter of osteoperiosteal cuff is elevated from its clavicular and anterior acromial origin (Fig. 10-10B). For revisions the deltoid may be incised 1.5 cm. beneath the clavicle because enough scar is usually present to hold the new sutures. The deltoid is cautiously retracted to avoid injury to the axillary nerve. After the subscapularis tendon is incised and retracted, the capsule is opened via a cruciate incision (Fig. 10-10C). The long head of the biceps is transected in its groove. Thereafter, the diseased humeral head with an appropriate amount of shaft is resected, a trial humeral prosthesis and power saw being used to obtain a correct angle (Fig. 10-10D and E). If the tendons of the rotator muscles are to be reattached later, they are tagged with sutures. In this procedure this is not ordinarily necessary as these structures are often nonfunctioning.

The glenoid is next prepared by first excising the labrum, articular cartilage, and any protruding osteophytes. If necessary, the anterior capsule and any hypertrophied synovium are resected. With a tapered hand reamer the intramedullary canal is opened only enough to receive the humeral stem.

After the glenoid and humeral intramedullary canal are prepared as described, the metal glenoid and humeral components are temporarily fitted in situ for correct posi-

tion, and thereafter cemented in place with the humeral component in 20- to 25-degrees retroversion. Before permanently cementing the components into place, the threads on the ring and glenoid should be tested for flaws, as any defects will prevent tightening that cannot be remedied later. The plastic glenoid thread protector is used to protect the threads.

The metal ring is placed about the humeral neck. The plastic halves are placed about the metal neck and the assembled parts are reduced into the metal glenoid by utilizing a clamp holder for the plastic halves. The ring is tightened with a special wrench. A number 20-gauge wire is placed through one of the holes spaced along the ring edge and one of the protruding anterior glenoid eyelets. It has been found easier to place the wire through the anterior eyelet before cementing the glenoid component. The wire is twisted. If the follow-up roentgenograms show unbroken wire, the surgeon can be certain the ring is secure. Loosening of the ring has not been encountered.

When closing the wound several small holes are drilled vertically through the clavicle and acromion and heavy synthetic or nonabsorbable suture is used to reattach the deltoid muscle. If the rotator muscles are to be reattached, wire or nonabsorbable suture is placed through the holes of the humeral collar before it is cemented in place and later used as the retaining suture for the rotator cuff. If the rotator muscles are not functioning they are not reattached. If there is a good functional pectoralis major acting as an internal rotator, the subscapularis is not reattached. The long head of the biceps is sutured distally into its groove and the excess proximal portion resected.

The range of motion is tested and recorded. Hemovac drainage is instituted for 24 hours.

Aftercare

The extremity is held in an immobilizer in internal rotation. Passive motion exercises are initiated, usually on the second or third

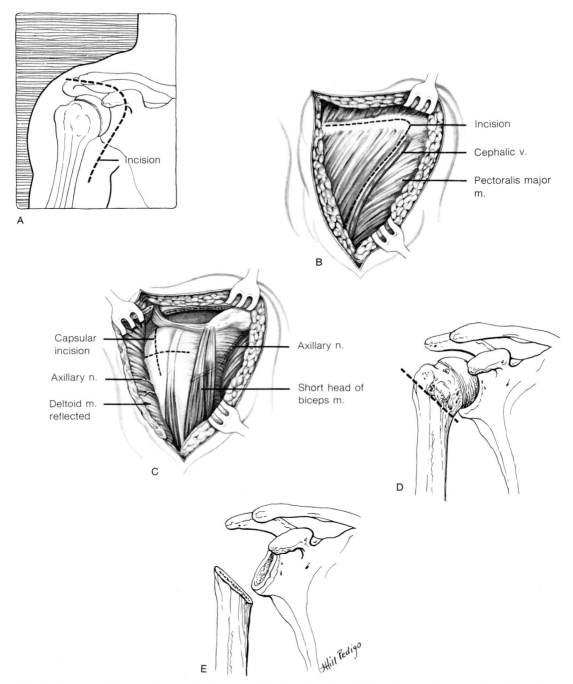

FIG. 10-10. A and B, Anterior surgical approach to the shoulder utilizing the proximal portion of the Henry technique. C, A cruciate cut is made in the capsule to isolate the humeral head. D and E, The line of osteotomy at the proximal humerus is shown along with the position of the cut shaft to its glenoid face when the arm is in anatomic position. Care must be taken to protect the axillary nerve when the deltoid is functioning.

postoperative day when acute pain has subsided, and not until 25 days later are gentle active motion exercises allowed when soft-tissue healing is adequate. In the beginning the joint acts like a frozen shoulder, and tends to cause discomfort during activity, but this disappears after several months. Frequent daily passive stretching exercises in forward flexion, abduction, external rotation, and internal rotation behind the back are instituted and increased as much as tolerated. Circumduction and pendulum exercises are not recommended.

The patient should forever avoid violent extremes of motion exercises, jerking movements as in pulling on a tight girdle, heavy lifting, or pulling with the operated extremity. Rifle hunting, pushups, and sports like skiing are contraindicated.

Nevertheless, the patients often disregard this advice and unfortunately play tennis or golf, or practice pushups in some cases. They also have an enormously high accident rate, about one third averaging three or more serious accidents a year postoperatively.

In order to gain optimum overhead motion the patient should be taught to first externally rotate the arm slightly. Finally, before operation the patient should be advised as to what motion and strength as a result of the procedure can be expected over a period time. Future results must never be overestimated.

Standardization of Examination Analysis

It is important for the results of any treatment to be standardized and objectively compared. Thus, a detailed analysis sheet is used to evaluate preoperative and postoperative data (Fig. 10-11). Joint motions are charted on diagramed cards.

The greatest emphasis is placed on the parameter of pain. Thus, this factor accounts for 75 percent of the rating scale. To rank improved range of motion and persistent pain equal, for example, will falsely skew the results. Whenever possible, the same physician should reexamine the patient.

Indications

Indications for total shoulder replacement include (1) the arthritides (Fig. 10-12), (2) osteonecrosis and cartilage necrosis of the humeral head, (3) severe humeral head fracture (Fig. 10-13), (4) resectable tumor of the proximal humerus (Fig. 10-14), (5) symptomatic old unreduced dislocation (Fig. 10-15), and (6) severe capsular insufficiency (Fig. 10-16).

The term "capsular insufficiency" is defined as a functional loss of stabilizing muscles that fix the humeral head in its glenoid. It may be caused by a loss of voluntary rotator muscle control relating to massive rotator cuff tear, nonunion of fractured bone (Fig. 10-17), or resection of the humeral head leading to a flail shoulder of non-neurologic origin (Fig. 10-16).

Intractable pain and nonfunctioning rotator cuffs should be the main reason for total shoulder replacement of this design for all the indications listed, with the exception of asymptomatic resectable tumor. This procedure is reserved for those patients who are likely to obtain poor results with other worthwhile operations. It is strictly salvage in nature. Each case must be individually studied. The fact that a total shoulder reconstruction can be performed in a particular case may not be the best procedure. For example, a young male laborer who must stress his upper extremity while working would obviously fare better with an arthrodesis.

Contraindications

Contraindications to total shoulder surgery include (1) previous infection, (2) paralyzed or flail shoulder due to neurologic deficit, (3) loss of scapular bone mass, and (4) psychiatric disorders.

In this grouping flail shoulder can be caused by poliomyelitis or brachial plexus injury wherein not only joint but scapular control is lost. Loss of scapular bone mass may result from tumor or bone demineralization so severe that there is no possibility of solidly affixing the metal glenoid compo-

MICHAEL REESE HOSPITAL AND MEDICAL CENTER
DEPARTMENT OF ORTHOPAEDIC SURGERY
ANALYSIS OF SHOULDER FUNCTION

NAME: _____   SEX: _____ UNIT # _____

DATE: _____   AGE: _____   SHOULDER: R _____ L _____ *(Dominance)

OPERATIONS & DATES: (1) _____

(2) _____

(3) _____

(4) _____

PREVIOUS INFECTION: _____   PSYCHIATRIC DISORDERS: _____

AGE GROUP: ( ) 25–35 ( ) 36–45 ( ) 46–55 ( ) 56–65 ( ) above 66

DIAGNOSIS: ( ) Fresh Fx. ( ) Old Fx. Head ( ) Non-union Fx.
( ) Malunion ( ) Osteonecrosis ( ) O.A. ( ) R.A. ( ) Tumor
( ) Capsular Insuff. ( ) Cartilage Necrosis ( ) Fx. Disl. ( ) Other

MUSCLE STRENGTH GRADE: Deltoid_____   Trapezius_____   Serratus Ant._____
Int. Rot. _____   Ext. Rot. _____   Extensors_____
Forward Flexors_____

I. PAIN   Points

A—None   75
B—Slight, occasional, activity not limited.   60–74
C—Mild, uses aspirin. No effect with light activity   45–59
   but moderate pain with moderate activity.
D—Moderate pain, tolerable, uses codeine, etc., curtails   30–44
   activities
E—Marked pain, serious limitations to total disability   0–29

II. FUNCTION   Active   Passive   Points

A—Full overhead motion, Int. Rot. behind   25
   back and in front
B—Forward flexion and abduction to 135°,   15–24
   reaches without difficulty
C—Abduction, forward flexion to 90° Dif-   11–14
   ficulty in raising arm actively.
D—Active abduct, forward flexion to 45° with   8–10
   difficulty
E—Can't raise arm at all; except ability to   0–7
   forward flex to 30° with great difficulty

points × 0.5 = _____

CAN PATIENT

1. Reach with hand behind head?_____

2. Reach behind back?_____

3. Touch opposite shoulder?_____

4. Perform toilet care with involved arm?_____

FIG. 10-11. Analysis sheet for shoulder function used at Michael Reese Medical Center.

5. Eating? _____

6. Combing hair? _____

7. Sleeping on side? _____

8. Dressing? _____

III. MOTION	Active	Passive	Points	Range
A—Backward Extension				
(0–25°)			1	
(25–50°)			2	
B—Forward Flexion				
(0–60°)			2	
(60–120°)			4	
(120–180°)			6	
C—Abduction				
(0–60°)			3	
(60–120°)			5	
(120–180°)			7	
D—Adduction				
(0–25°)			2	
(25–50°)			3	
(50–75°)			4	
E—Int. Rotation				
(0–30°)			2	
(30–60°)			3	
(60–80°)			4	
F—Ext. Rotation				
(0–30°)			1	
(30–65°)			2	

points $\times$ 0.5 = _____

COOPERATION

1. Excellent ( )
2. Good ( )
3. Average ( )
4. Fair ( )
5. Poor ( )

PATIENT RESPONSE

1. Enthusiastic ( )
2. Very Satisfied ( )
3. Satisfied ( )
4. Dissatisfied ( )
5. Failure ( )

COMPLICATIONS

1. Fx. Implant Device ( )
2. Dislocation of Implant ( )
3. Infection:
   (a) superficial ( )
   (b) deep ( )
4. Loosening of Implant
   (a) from humerus ( )
   (b) from glenoid ( )
5. Post-op. Injury to Shoulder
   (a) Fx. glenoid-scapula ( )
   (b) Fx. humerus ( )
6. Myositis Ossificans ( )
7. Soft Tissue Contracture ( )
8. Pulm, Embolus ( )
9. Blood Transfusion Reaction ( )
10. Hepatitis ( )
11. Wound Healing ( )
12. Allergy ( )
13. Other ( )

X-RAY

1. Implant Position
   (a) humeral   ( ) normal   ( ) altered   ( ) dislocation
   (b) glenoid   ( ) normal   ( ) altered   ( ) dislocation
2. Implant Loosening
   (a) humeral   ( ) normal   ( ) altered   ( ) dislocation
   (b) glenoid   ( ) normal   ( ) altered   ( ) dislocation
3. Fracture Implant   ( ) stem   ( ) neck
4. Lucent Lines   ( ) normal   ( ) abnormal

SIGNIFICANT INVOLVEMENT   R_____   L_____

    Elbow   _____   _____

    Wrist   _____   _____

    Hand   _____   _____

(TOTAL POINTS I, II, III = _____)

_____

Examiner

FIG. 10-11. Continued.

nent. Although a markedly weakened deltoid is a relative contraindication to replacement surgery, satisfactory results can be achieved in select cases if the patient understands that active overhead motion will not be gained. Rather, he may be able to comfortably but passively place his hand in a variety of positions after a successful replacement. In every patient, the stabilizing scapular muscles should be strong. For best results it is essential to have the complete cooperation of the patient. Accordingly, patients with known psychiatric disorders or senility are not good candidates for surgery. It is an unfortunate fact that the same patients who have been so pleased with their joints are the ones who have abused them and incurred complications. Finally, patients with Charcot joints resulting from syringomyelia or other causes should be excluded from this procedure.

Results

In June 1973, the first total shoulder replacement of this design was inserted. Over the next 25 months, 24 reconstructions of the smaller head (series I) were performed at Michael Reese Medical Center. The patients ranged in age from 27 to 77 years (average age, 53 years). These patients represented the very worst cases of symptomatic pathologic conditions of the shoulder selected for surgery from a far larger group of referred patients. All patients with the exception of one with a highly comminuted "split head" treated primarily with total joint replacement had had prior treatment that failed. Each had intractable pain and loss of function except for one patient with asymptomatic recurrent giant cell tumor of the proximal third of the humerus (see Fig. 10-14). The various conditions for which total joint replacements were performed were:

Osteoarthritis	3
Rheumatoid arthritis	1
Osteonecrosis	6
Capsular insufficiency	5
Recurrent giant cell tumor	1
Severe fracture	8
	24

Only one patient with acute humeral head fracture had a functioning rotator cuff. In the patient with resectable tumor, the rotator cuff was widely resected in order to avoid leaving any tumor tissue behind. Experience has shown that the rotator cuff

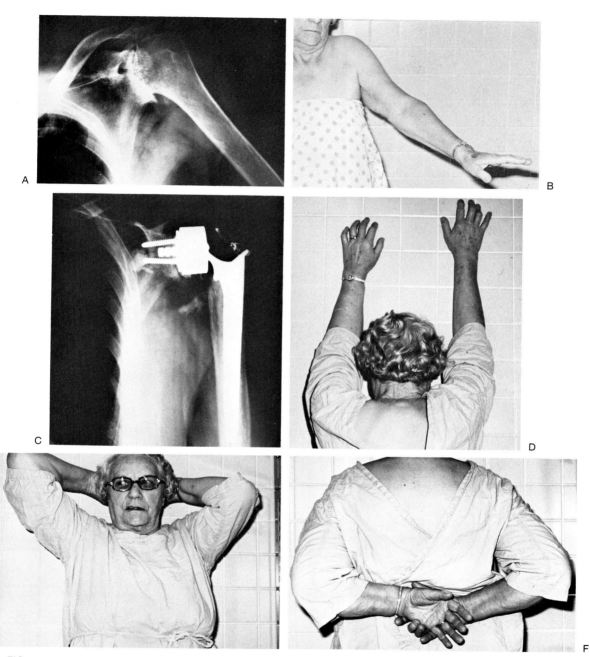

FIG. 10-12. A, A 69-year-old woman who had stiffness and severe pain in the left shoulder secondary to osteoarthritis underwent total shoulder replacement. B, Note the extent of preoperative abduction. C, Anteroposterior film shows the joint replacement. D to F, Three months after total replacement, she was able to move her arm without experiencing pain. At one year postoperatively, motion had increased beyond what is demonstrated. She maintained her own house, including vacuuming carpets. Two years postoperatively, the 4-mm. humeral neck broke necessitating revision. The result was very satisfactory.

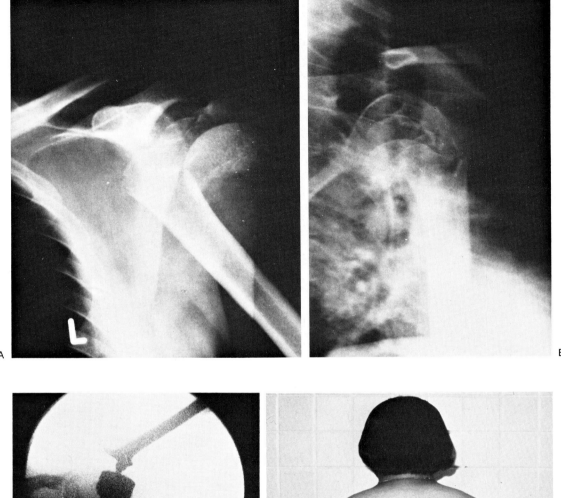

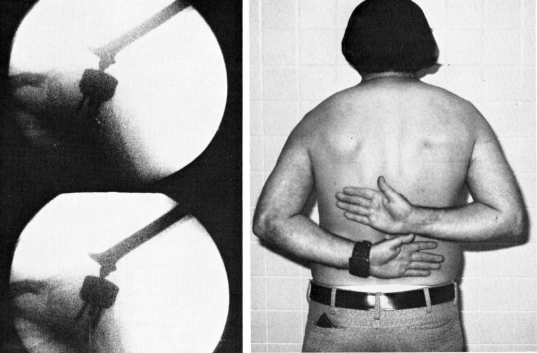

FIG. 10-13. See legend on facing page.

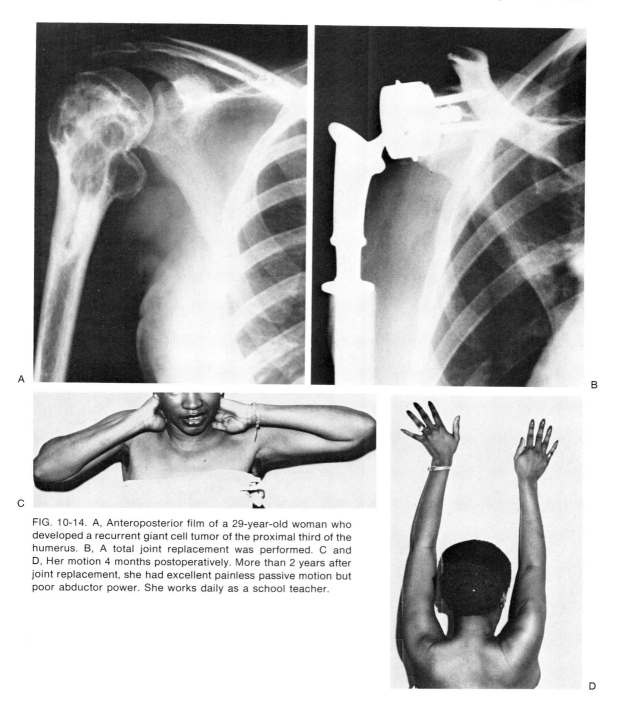

FIG. 10-14. A, Anteroposterior film of a 29-year-old woman who developed a recurrent giant cell tumor of the proximal third of the humerus. B, A total joint replacement was performed. C and D, Her motion 4 months postoperatively. More than 2 years after joint replacement, she had excellent painless passive motion but poor abductor power. She works daily as a school teacher.

FIG. 10-13. A, Left anteroposterior and, B, transthoracic lateral roentgenograms of a 37-year-old man who sustained a highly comminuted anterior fracture-dislocation of the humeral head and brachial plexus injury in a motorcycle accident. When seen 2 months after the accident he was in severe pain. C, Cine study of his joint replacement 3 months postoperatively. At 6 months postoperatively, he had almost full motion and had returned to work delivering heavy sewing machines. The rotator cuff was severely scarred and nonfunctioning. D, His motion is shown at 3 months postoperatively, before additional improvement. The result was excellent.

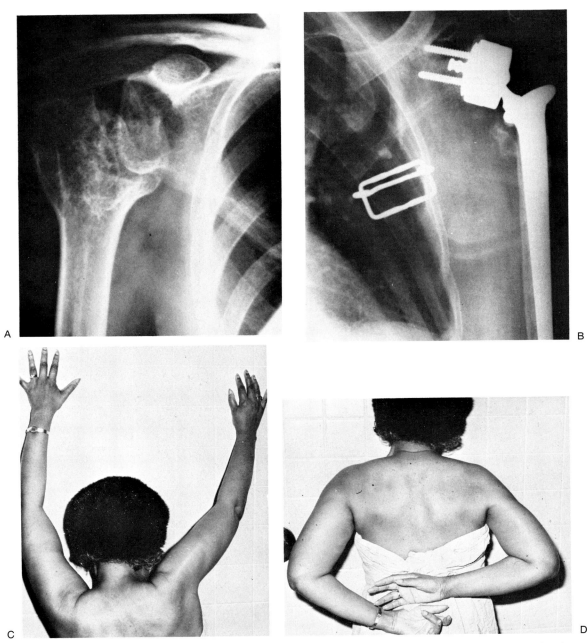

A

B

C

D

FIG. 10-15. A, A 53-year-old woman who had sustained a right posterior fracture-dislocation 6 years previously. Pain had become persistently severe. B, Anteroposterior roentgenogram of a rectangular series I total shoulder implant 3 months after the patient had dislocated her first total shoulder joint when her arm suddenly dropped. C and D, Two years later there was good painless, passive motion. Deltoid power was poor. With excessive use of the extremity there was occasional discomfort. The result was satisfactory.

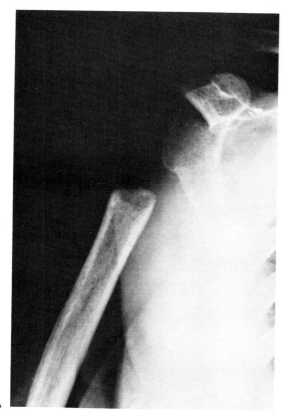
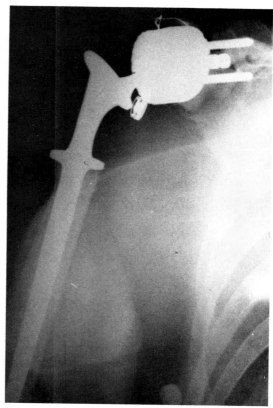

A

B

FIG. 10-16. A 44-year-old woman sustained a fracture of the right surgical neck and developed a nonunion following conservative treatment. An open reduction was performed. Over a 1-year period, osteonecrosis of the proximal fragment developed and was associated with severe pain. A, The proximal fragment was removed, but pain was severe and the shoulder was flail. B, A total joint replacement was performed with good results. There was no active abduction, but her severe pain was alleviated and the extremity became functional.

muscles are often nonfunctioning and irrevocably damaged when shoulder joint disease is chronic. Therefore, the surgeon should not hope for recovery of these short rotator muscles when they have not functioned for an extended period of time prior to reconstruction.

Many of the patients operated upon demonstrated multiple overlapping pathologic lesions that related to the symptoms of pain and loss of function, including nonunion and malunion of fractures of the proximal humerus, severe degenerative changes of the humeral head, cartilage necrosis, and osteonecrosis from which painful ankylosis and weak shoulder musculature often ensued.

Results improved with the passage of time after joint replacement. Usually 6 months were required for a maximum increase in joint motion. The original pain was almost immediately relieved in most of the cases, but here too, a time lapse of 4 to 6 months was needed before optimum pain relief was achieved. Decrease in pain was directly proportional to the motion regained postoperatively, and to the effort expended by the patient to follow through with his exercise program. Those patients with good musculature about the shoulder girdle obtained better results than those with weak musculature. Similarly, those patients who had fewer surgical procedures before replacement had better results. Interestingly, even those patients with weak muscles regained motion and strength that were not

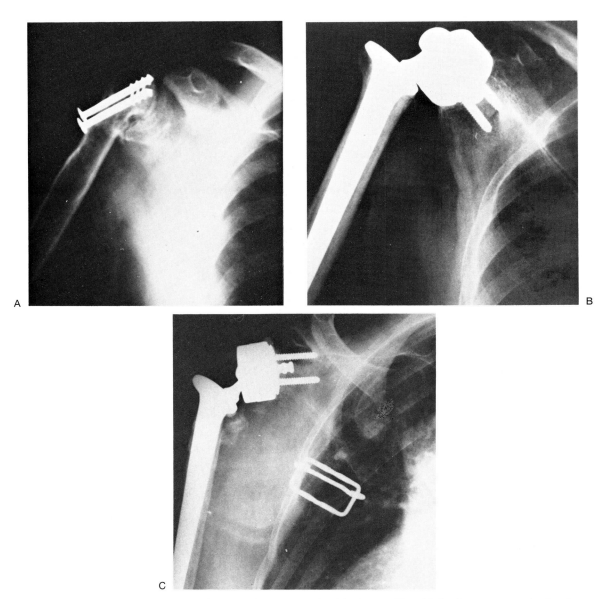

FIG. 10-17. A, A 62-year-old woman developed osteonecrosis of the humeral head following an open reduction for severe fracture. Pain and stiffness were severe. B, Three months after total shoulder replacement, the joint dislocated when the extremity dropped from the overhead position. C, A revision was performed with excellent results. There was excellent passive but poor active motion.

expected. This included patients who had previous multiple shoulder operations and were considered hopeless by their referring surgeons. This improvement probably followed because stable pivoting of the arm at the scapula permits primary muscles and some of the accessory shoulder muscles to exert residual function. Ordinarily, with a strong deltoid the forces on the glenohumeral articulation are compressive with the arm in abduction, whereas a weak deltoid will allow distraction at the articulation, a condition that can best be termed "the hanging subluxed joint." This fact, of course, explains why a fixed fulcrum joint can still produce a good result in a patient with a markedly weakened or even no deltoid strength.

Data in the first 24 cases indicate 77 percent overall improvement. The patients rated their shoulders satisfactory to excellent, and were more enthusiastic about results than was the surgeon. A minimum period of as long as 6 months must elapse before a good result is achieved. The patients appear to lose their previous pain, but may have some muscular discomfort while performing motion stretching exercises.

Each case should be compared with preoperative findings and not with the normal shoulder joint. In a patient with poor preoperative motion, weak muscles, and much pain, who achieves a good passive range of painless motion, the result is rated good (see Fig. 10-15). In a patient with painful shoulder and limited overhead motion with good muscles, who obtains excellent, painless active motion, the result will be excellent (see Fig. 10-13). The difference between what is considered a satisfactory or an excellent result depends upon a comparison with the preoperative data base. It is not merely a numerical rating obtained from an analysis sheet. Consider the patient with resectable tumor of the proximal humerus who had full function before replacement, but demonstrated relatively poor postoperative active abduction (see Fig. 10-14). Rated numerically, the result would be classed as very poor; it was rated good because the patient accomplished her goal of painless, passive overhead motion, even though the numerical rating value was negative.

Series II (8-mm.-diameter humeral necks), started in January 1976, included patients with varying pathologic conditions:

Chronic posterior fracture-dislocation	2
Idiopathic osteonecrosis (bilateral)	1
Capsular insufficiency	4
Osteoarthritis	8
Traumatic arthritis	2
Steroid osteonecrosis	2
Steroid osteonecrosis (renal disease)	1
Rheumatoid arthritis	4
Failed Bechtol total shoulder	1
Radiation necrosis	1

One elderly patient had two revisions for humeral head dislocations following severe states of inebriation. He is considered a failure. Notably, at each operation the metal glenoid component was found to be sound. The other patients show satisfactory to excellent results in the first postoperative year.

Management of Complications

The complications in the first 24 cases (series I) were:

Dislocations	3
Broken neck stems	6
Prosthesis removed (trauma)	1

The first two patients with low torque plastic pieces sustained dislocations several months after joint replacement when their arms dropped suddenly while reaching overhead (see Fig. 10-17). Both patients received later model, higher torque plastic inserts and experienced no subsequent complications. Another patient fell down a flight of steps 3 months after shoulder joint replacement and severely fractured the scapula and ipsilateral hip. She required an Austin-Moore hip prosthesis and removal of the prosthetic shoulder joint, but until then had had an excellent result. Thereafter, the arm had poor active abduction mainly because she lost the fulcrum. One other patient with a truncated cup slipped in a bathtub 8 months after joint reconstruction and dislocated the prosthetic joint when her extended arm caught on the tub edge (Fig. 10-18). The plastic pieces were easily replaced. Two other patients fractured the metal necks, one 15 months and the other 8 months, after initial joint replacement. The first patient had hunted and used a high powered rifle and shotgun (Fig. 10-19). New metal stems, plastic pieces, and metal glenoid rings were inserted in each case. The glenoids were solidly attached to their scapulae. Loosening of the metal glenoid thus far has not been seen in more than 4 years.

When the neck fractures, a $\frac{1}{8}$-in.-diameter carbon tip drill bit is employed to make a hole in the head, and the hole is tapped so

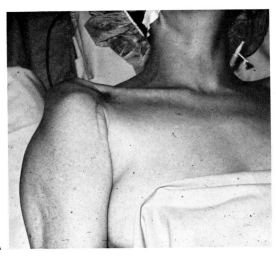
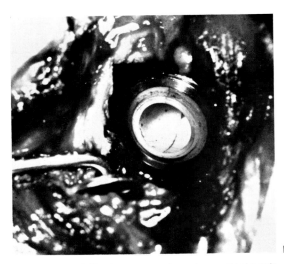

A   B

FIG. 10-18. A 45-year-old woman underwent total shoulder replacement following a nonunion of a surgical neck fracture. There was severe deltoid weakness anteriorly. A, Eight months postoperatively, the patient slipped in a bathtub and dislocated the artificial joint. B, At revision operation, the plastic halves and metal glenoid are shown after removal of the locking ring. A new humeral component, plastic pieces, and ring were inserted with good results. Two years later the patient had a Harmon transfer of the functioning posterior deltoid anteriorly.

that a screw can be inserted for removal of the head and cup by gentle traction, if needed. Another method to remove the fractured proximal humeral piece is to grasp the peripheral plastic lip with a towel clip and apply traction. No attempt should be made to grasp the broken ends because scratching of the fractured metal surfaces interferes with laboratory analysis. The metal intramedullary portion is easily removed by using a metal punch and mallet in the longitudinal direction. A new humeral stem is implanted with methyl methacrylate. If a change in the angle of retroversion is desired, the cement in the humeral canal is removed with osteotomes and a cortical window, if necessary. Drilling out the cement from its canal is not recommended because the shaft may fracture, especially in osteoporotic bone. It is not always necessary to open the cortex below in order to gut the intramedullary canal.

Finally, one patient in whom a total acromionectomy had previously been performed developed a transient painful tenalgia crepitans over the acromioclavicular joint region which in time cleared without treatment.

For some unexplained reason this total group of patients had a high incidence of accidents including falls. Fortunately, in consideration of the gravity of the accidents, there were no additional complications.

Conversion of Previous Arthroplasty to Fixed Fulcrum Total Shoulder

When pain and poor shoulder function persist following a nonhinged total joint replacement, a fixed fulcrum total shoulder replacement can still be accomplished with good results if the scapular vault is preserved. Consider the situation in which a nonhinged total replacement has failed. If the plastic glenoid articular component is already firmly attached to the glenoid, it should be left undisturbed for fear of damaging the glenoid vault. The plastic glenoid can be used as the interface between the new metal glenoid and scapula (Fig. 10-20).

Comments

It is true that patients do well with the procedures other than total joint reconstruction described in this chapter. How-

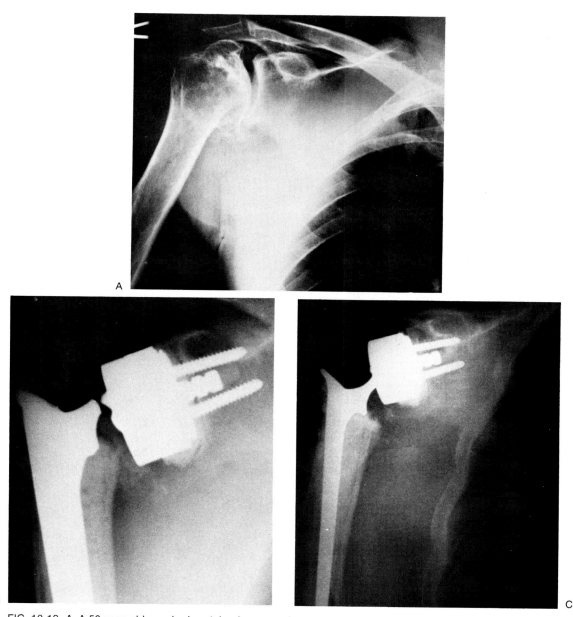

FIG. 10-19. A, A 50-year-old man had sustained a severe fracture of the humeral head years previously. Pain and stiffness of his shoulder increased. There was considerable deltoid atrophy. B, After series I total shoulder replacement, he had improved motion and pain relief. Fifteen months postoperatively, he went deer hunting and broke the neck portion of the prosthesis, shown on this x-ray film. C, The revised total joint replacement.

ever, experience has shown that hemiar-throplasty will not guarantee good results when there is disease of both articular surfaces of the glenohumeral joint, or even of the proximal humerus alone when there is a nonfunctioning rotator cuff. Many patients exhibit significant glenoid articular patho-logic changes that can cause pain. Again, for unexplained reasons, large numbers of examined patients with shoulder joints destroyed by rheumatoid disease have minimal complaints of pain and usually do well with conservative treatment, in comparison to patients with painful joints affected by a

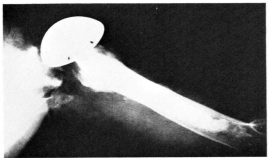

A

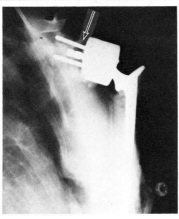

B

FIG. 10-20. A modified axillary view shows a Bechtol total shoulder replacement in a 64-year-old woman who had undergone several previous operations, including a failed Neer hemiarthroplasty and a Bechtol hemiarthroplasty, for severe fracture of the humeral head. Note the severe anteversion of the prosthetic head and its subluxation from its unseen plastic glenoid component. The deltoid power was poor and the rotator cuff did not function. B, Anteroposterior view of a series II fixed fulcrum total shoulder that was inserted and produced satisfactory results. The arrow points to the region of the plastic Bechtol glenoid component that was left in situ and used as an interface between the new metal glenoid component and the remaining glenoid vault. The bone was severely osteoporotic.

lesser degree of osteoarthritis. If the short rotator muscles do not have adequate function or cannot be reattached even when normal, then the patient will require a prosthesis of the fixed fulcrum design.

A fixed fulcrum prosthesis does not require functioning rotator cuff muscles, al-

though desirable, to obtain a good result. In many of the patients, the deltoid was markedly weakened for a variety of reasons, and following reconstruction deltoid function improved (Fig. 10-21). The results were rated satisfactory to excellent by the patients because not only was there pain relief, but their extremities became more functional. Even with poor active abduction but good passive overhead motion, patients can comfortably place their hands in a greater number of positions not previously possible, adding to their function. Thus, although a poor deltoid is generally considered a contraindication to surgery, in certain select cases it is not an absolute contraindication if the patient and surgeon understand that although active abduction may be poor, pain may be relieved and passive motion improved.

With an old massive tear of the rotator cuff, marked superior subluxation of the shaft may result because of the upward pull of the unopposed deltoid. In this case, resection of 2.5 cm. or more of proximal humerus may be needed in order to fit the components correctly. Ordinarily, this will not compromise function if the deltoid is functioning and there are no surrounding contractures.

Patients with spastic muscles and contracted soft tissues are not considered good candidates for replacement. If contracted structures cannot first be released, results will be less than optimum. However, in patients having had extensive radiation for breast carcinoma, for example, in whom shoulder replacement is needed, pain relief is dramatic even if overhead motion is compromised by the impossibility of freeing all contracted tissues.

It remains to be seen whether or not this shoulder design will endure under long-term use. Most certainly, improved prosthetic joints will evolve, which may increase the indications for the use of total shoulder prostheses.

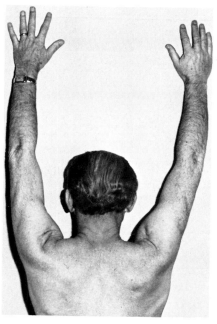
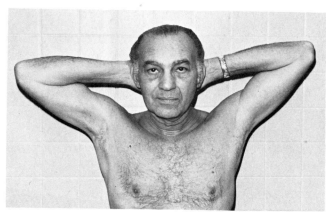

A

B

FIG. 10-21. A and B, A 67-year-old man had a series II fixed fulcrum total shoulder replacement for capsular insufficiency in which the rotator cuff did not function. He previously had had a calcium deposit removed surgically. Note the extent of his motion, particularly on the operated upon right side, 8 months following surgery. Now, 16 months postoperatively, he has a satisfactory result except for an occasional muscular ache in the lateral right arm during excessive activity.

REFERENCES

1. Albee, F. H.: Restoration of shoulder function in cases of lost head and upper portion of humerus. Surg. Gynecol. Obstet., 32:1–19, 1921.
2. Bechtol, C. D.: Personal communication, 1976.
3. Clayton, M. L., and Ferlic, D. C.: Surgery of the shoulder in rheumatoid arthritis. Clin. Orthop., 106:166–174, 1975.
4. Fenlin, J. M., Jr.: Total glenohumeral joint replacement, Orthop. Clin. North Am., 6:565–583, 1975.
5. Hammond, R.: Transplantation of the fibula to replace bony defect in the shoulder joint. J. Bone Joint Surg., 8:627–635, 1926.
6. Haraldsson, S.: Reconstruction of proximal humerus by muscle-sling prosthesis. Acta Orthop. Scand., 40:225–233, 1969.
7. Kölbel, R., and Friedebold, G.: Schultergelenkersatz. Z. Orthop., 113:452–454, 1975.
8. Lettin, A. W. F., and Scales, J. T.: Total replacement of the shoulder joint. Proc. R. Med. Soc., 65:373–374, 1972.

9. Jones, L.: The shoulder joint—Observations on the anatomy and physiology. Surg. Gynecol. Obstet., 75:433–444, 1942.
10. Neer, C. S.: Articular replacement for humeral head. J. Bone Joint Surg., 37-A:215–228, 1955.
11. Neer, C. S.: Prosthetic replacement of the humeral head: Indications and operative technique. Surg. Clin. North Am., 43:1581–1597, 1963.
12. Neer, C. S.: Replacement arthroplasty for glenohumeral osteoarthritis. J. Bone Joint Surg., 56-A:1–13, 1974.
13. Neer, C. S.: Personal communication, 1975.
14. Reeves, B., Jobbins, B., and Flowers, M.: Biomechanical Problems in the Development of a Total Shoulder Endoprosthesis. In Proceedings of the British Orthopaedic Society. J. Bone Joint Surg., 54-B:193, 1972.
15. Rovsing, T.: Erfaringer og Overvejelser Over Lungekirurgi, Hospitalstidende, Kobenh., LIII: 436–440, 1910.

11

Arthrodesis of the Shoulder

MELVIN POST

With the near disappearance of tuberculosis and poliomyelitis the need for shoulder arthrodesis has greatly diminished in the Western World. Newer techniques of shoulder arthroplasty and improved management of shoulder disorders have also narrowed the reasons for this operation. Patients are often dissatisfied with the results of fusion, frequently complaining of the limited positions for hand placement.

This chapter reviews the various essential factors that must be considered if the best results are to be attained with shoulder arthrodesis.

Indications

Shoulder arthrodesis remains a worthwhile procedure in properly selected cases. With successful fusion the patient can raise the hand to the mouth and head, grasp objects in front of him, and forcefully push and pull. It is recommended for (1) low-grade infections of the shoulder such as tuberculosis in the hope of preventing disease progression, and to provide a stable, painless shoulder joint, and (2) specific paralytic conditions, usually poliomyelitis flail shoulder (Fig. 11-1), irreversible brachial plexus damage (Fig. 11-2), or other disorders causing paralysis of the glenohumeral muscles associated with severe loss of function.

In the past, shoulder arthrodesis was performed for failed treatment of massive rotator cuff tears or degenerative conditions caused by trauma, and is still occasionally done for intractable painful arthritis of the glenohumeral joint from any cause[3] (Fig. 11-3). However, total shoulder joint replacement now may offer a better way of

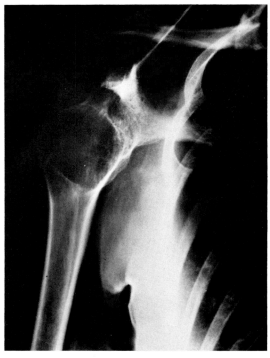

FIG. 11-1. Poliomyelitis patient with flail shoulder, including weak shoulder stabilizers, had had fusion at 10 years of age. Abduction position was excessive. Now in adulthood, the scapula wings markedly when the arm is at the side.

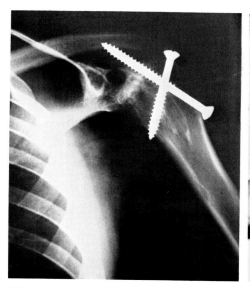 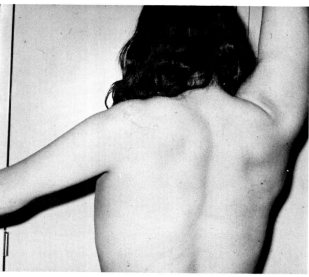

A   B

FIG. 11-2. A 16-year-old boy had sustained a severe left brachial plexus injury with irreparable loss of motor control of the shoulder joint after a traumatic shoulder dislocation. A, Roentgenogram shows solid Moseley-type fusion. At 18 years of age, the patient had painless scapulothoracic motion but was unhappy over the "stiffness." B, The extreme of passive overhead motion corresponds to the amount of scapular rotation.

managing some of these problems. The needs of each patient must be assessed. Because far fewer shoulder arthrodeses are now done, arthrodesis should not be dismissed as a method of treatment if it can best solve a problem and afford a functional extremity.

Prerequisites

Before undertaking shoulder arthrodesis, it is important for the patient to have a stable scapula for control of upper extremity movement. The normal glenohumeral fulcrum is transferred to the scapulothoracic region. Thus, the muscles that insert into the scapula must be strong. There should be good strength in the trapezius and serratus anterior muscles. As a general rule, when the patient lacks this strength arthrodesis should not be performed. In some patients, serratus anterior strength may be deficient but still permit a satisfactory result if arm abduction is not excessive and the trapezius remains strong. This is particularly true when other functioning muscles, such as the levator scapulae and rhomboids, that attach to the scapula help

stabilize the shoulder blade. Moreover, a good range of scapulothoracic motion must be demonstrated preoperatively. At operation, adduction contractures must be corrected.

Timing of Procedure

Shoulder fusion can be successfully performed in children who have reached 10 years of age because ossification of the humeral epiphysis is usually complete by then.[11] The years between 12 and 15 are best for joint fusion,[5] because enough cancellous bone is present in the humeral head and operation can be done without interfering with growth of the arm (Table 11-1). The procedure can be performed in a patient as young as 8 years if indicated. It has been reported to have been performed in children as young as 6 years. Early fusion should be discouraged because of possible epiphyseal injury and growth disturbance after fusion, the tendency for change of the angle at the fusion site with growth, and the chance that there will be failure of fusion.[16] Nevertheless, Barr and associates showed that arthrodesis done before the age of 12

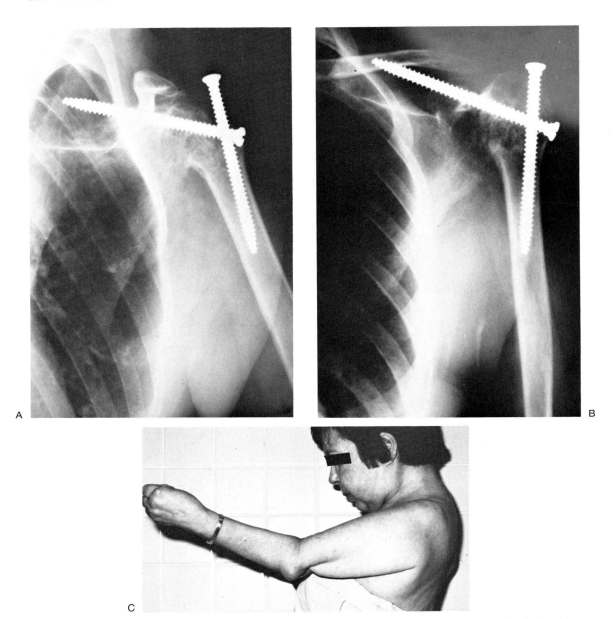

FIG. 11-3. A, Patient with rheumatoid arthritis had a Moseley-type fusion for a severely painful left shoulder. B, Slightly different view shows no true arthrodesis. In any event the shoulder was painless. C, Movement of the left upper extremity. The patient was happy with the result.

years allowed a better range of motion of the shoulder girdle than in the older age groups.[2]

Optimum Position for Arthrodesis

The final position of shoulder fusion (1) must permit the hand to reach the face, head, and midline of the body in front and behind, (2) must permit lifting, pulling, and pushing, (3) must allow comfort of the extremity with the arm at the side, and (4) should permit the scapula to lie flat against the chest wall.

In 1942, the Research Committee of the American Orthopaedic Association reported

Table 11-1. *Recommended Positions for Shoulder Arthrodesis*

Author	Year	Abduction (Degrees)	Forward Flexion (Degrees)	External Rotation (Degrees)	Internal Rotation (Degrees)	Minimum Age for Fusion (Years)	Best Age for Fusion (Years)
Gill	1931	45 or less (measured from vertebral border of scapula)				10	
Brett	1933	70 (adult)	20			8	12–15
Barr and associates	1942	70–90 (arm from side of body)	15–25	25–30		6	12.5 (average)
May	1962	65	60	40			After 10
Charnley and Houston	1964	45 (clinical position to side of body)	45		45		
Rowe	1974	15 to 20 (arm from side of body)	25 to 30		45 to 50		
Beltran and associates	1975	50	20		25		

on their study of 102 fusions in 101 patients.[2] The report dealt only with patients of infantile paralysis who ranged in age from 6 to 30 years. In a large majority of cases, results were less than excellent and the most frequent reason was some error in postoperative position. This fact related to the difficulty in controlling postoperative movement of the scapula. The Committee concluded that the best position for fusion occurred when abduction of the arm in relation to the trunk was 70 to 90 degrees (or 45 to 50 degrees when measured from the vertebral border of the scapula), forward flexion from the plane of the scapula was 15 to 25 degrees, and tilting upward of the flexed forearm was 25 to 30 degrees above the horizontal position (external rotation) (Fig. 11-4). Most cases in this report dealt with children afflicted with poliomyelitis, many of whom lost 10 to 20 degrees of abduction. In adults, this loss does not occur when internal rotation is used.

Care must be exercised to avoid excessive flexion or else winging of the scapula will result. When serratus anterior strength is deficient the angle of fusion in abduction should not be over 30 degrees in relation to the vertebral border of the scapula. The curve of the chest wall as well as the strength of the muscles must be considered when deciding the position of flexion. Moreover, excessive rotation and abduction will lead to a poor functional and cosmetic result.

The best functional position for shoulder fusion has been studied by numerous investigators over the years. Table 11-1 summarizes opinions of some of these authors. It is obvious that there is no standard position. However, Rowe stated that poor results are obtained with excessive abduction and forward flexion of the arm.[15] It appears that Rowe is correct in making this statement (Fig. 11-5). He concluded that lifting and elevation of the hand to the face are achieved more efficiently when there is no humeral abduction. This is primarily accomplished by elbow flexion of 135 degrees started with the arm in neutral at the side of the body and supplemented by scapula rotation (30 degrees of forward flexion of the shoulder). He believes that the only reason for more humeral abduction is the presence of strong scapulothoracic muscles and weak elbow flexors. In this instance, flexing the elbow to permit the hand to reach the mouth is more easily achieved by the hori-

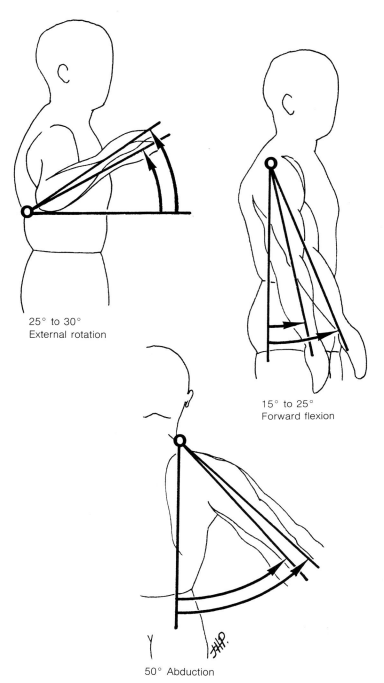

25° to 30°
External rotation

15° to 25°
Forward flexion

50° Abduction

FIG. 11-4. Barr Committee recommendation for optimum arthrodesis of the shoulder. Abduction angle is measured from vertebral border of the scapula. (Modified from the Report of the Research Committee of American Orthopaedic Association: J. Bone Joint Surg., 24:699, 1942.)

zontal position of the forearm. After shoulder fusion, hand placement at any point depends primarily upon the relative movements of abduction, rotation, and flexion of the fused shoulder.

METHODS OF FUSION

Successful shoulder fusion requires effective contact between cancellous bone of the humeral head and glenoid, and ade-

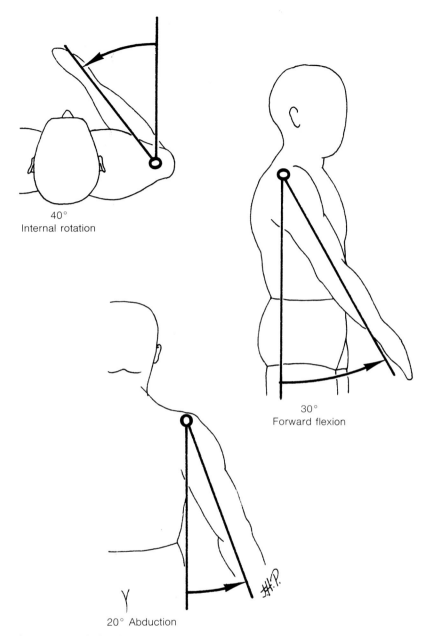

40°
Internal rotation

30°
Forward flexion

20° Abduction

FIG. 11-5. Rowe's recommendation for optimum arthrodesis of the shoulder. Abduction angle is measured from the side of the body. (Modified from Rowe, C. R.: Re-evaluation of the position of the arm in arthrodesis of the shoulder in an adult. J. Bone Joint Surg., 56-A:919, 1974.)

quate postoperative immobilization. Fortunately, both the humeral head and vault of the scapular neck have abundant cancellous bone. Unfortunately, the small area of the glenoid face and the difficulty of maintaining a desired position between humeral head and scapula make fusion of the gleno-

humeral joint technically more difficult than fusion of other joints in the body.

Since Albert's attempt to perform shoulder fusion in 1881, various techniques have been devised to accomplish shoulder fusion.[1] They may be classified into (1) intra-articular,[7] (2) extra-articular,[6,14,19] (3) combined intra-articular and extra-artic-ular,[5,10–13,17,18] and (4) compression ar-throdeses.[4,8,9]

Intra-articular Method

The method of intra-articular fusion alone without supplementation by screw fixation and cancellous bone grafting is in-adequate. Combined intra-articular and extra-articular methods appear to give the best results. The surgeon should select the method that fits the needs of the patient considering the anatomy that is present at the time of fusion. He should not rely on clinical evaluation and patient comfort alone to determine true arthrodesis as de-termined by roentgenologic study (Fig. 11-4). Barr and associates showed that re-gardless of whether or not fusion actually occurs, the joint becomes stable within 5 months of operation. Even with nonunion, fibrous union is usually sufficient to main-tain joint position.

Carroll reported on 15 cases of intra-articular fusion in which he used a wire loop for fixation which still allowed a change in the position postoperatively.[7]

Extra-articular Methods

Various extra-articular methods for shoulder fusion have been reported. One popular operation is the Brittain, in which a posterior approach is used and an arrow-shaped tibial graft is placed between the humerus and axillary border of the scapula. However, Saha reported difficulty in ob-taining rigid fixation and stated the results were far from satisfactory.[16]

Putti's Technique

Putti described his method of sliding a section of scapular spine and acromion across the posterosuperior joint into a raw defect of the humerus made by raising an osteoperiosteal flap (Fig. 11-6C).[14] The pa-tient is placed on the unaffected side and an incision is made along the surface of the entire spine of the scapula to the acromion.

The incision is directed downward to the deltoid insertion. The spine is exposed by subperiosteal dissection and detached from its base. An osteotomy is performed on the posterior portion of the acromion and this portion forms the distal part of the autoge-nous graft. The deltoid muscle is split so as to expose the capsule and proximal 5 cm. of humeral shaft. If the axillary nerve is cut, it does not matter because a functioning del-toid muscle is not needed after shoulder fusion. A bone flap measuring about 3.8 by 1.9 cm. is raised on the lateral humerus. The shoulder is abducted the desired amount, and the bone graft inserted beneath the bone flap.

AFTERCARE.   The extremity is placed in a plaster shoulder spica cast. At 8 to 12 weeks distal extremity joint motion is started. However, support is continued until fusion is complete.

Watson-Jones's Technique

In 1933, Watson-Jones reported on his extra-articular method for shoulder joint fusion.[19] He recommended it primarily for tuberculosis of the humeral head in which the upper end of the humerus was so exten-sively involved there was little hope of good bone being available for arthrodesis. In his method the acromion and lateral clavicle are angled downward and implanted in the region of the greater tuberosity without en-croaching on the diseased area. With recent advances in the chemotherapy of tubercu-losis this procedure is no longer commonly required.

The technique employs a straight incision over the point of the shoulder, centering over the acromial tip (Fig. 11-6A and B). The incision is extended upward midway be-tween the clavicle and scapular spine, and downward for a total of 12.5 or 15.0 cm. Flap dissection permits exposure of the whole outer surface of the upper 7.5 cm. of humerus, the outer third of the clavicle, the acromioclavicular joint, and the outer third of the spine of the scapula. After the deltoid is separated subperiosteally from the clavi-cle, acromion and scapula, both surfaces of

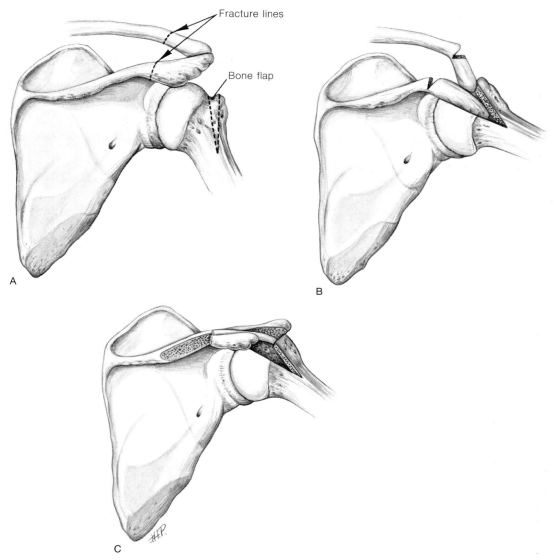

FIG. 11-6. Techniques of extra-articular arthrodesis. A and B, Watson-Jones's technique. C, Putti's method.

the acromion are taken back to raw cancellous bone.

A broad bone flap, 2.5 cm. wide and 2.5 cm. long, is raised from the outer surface of the humerus and is gently levered outward with an osteotome so it is not fractured at its base. The clavicle is partly fractured 5 cm. from its lateral end, and the scapular spine is similarly broken at a distance from its end that is in register with the clavicular fracture. With the patient's arm in the desired position of abduction, the whole acromioclavicular mass is angulated downward, hinged at the breakage points, and wedged beneath the raised humeral bone flap. Fixation is secured by a few strong sutures. Autogenous bone may be added if needed.

AFTERCARE. Following wound closure the extremity is placed in a plaster spica. After 4 months the plaster cast is removed and the extremity kept immobilized on an abduction frame in which the patient may practice abduction exercises. When the scapular muscles are sufficiently developed to enable the limb to be held in active abduction against gravity the frame is gradually discarded.

Combined Intra-articular and Extra-articular Methods

Good results can be achieved with intra-articular fusion when supplemented with extra-articular methods. It appears that internal fixation and postoperative external immobilization for an adequate time contribute to true arthrodesis. The following methods have been successfully employed by various authors.

Gill's Technique

In 1931, Gill presented his intra-articular, extra-articular method for achieving glenohumeral fusion (Fig. 11-7C). To date, it has remained popular among orthopaedic surgeons even though a lesser abduction angle than suggested by Gill is not easily achieved with this method. In this technique the capsule is opened and freely excised over the superior portion of the joint from its attachment to the edge of the glenoid fossa within 2.5 cm. of its humeral insertion. The soft tissues beneath the undersurface of the acromion are excised with the capsule. The tendon of the long head of the biceps may be spared and left attached to its glenoid origin. The inferior and superior surfaces of the acromion are denuded but the elevated proximal superior periosteal base is left intact.

The articular cartilage of the glenoid is removed along with the underlying paper-thin glenoid cortex. Similarly, cartilage and subchondral bone are removed from the medial anterior part of the humeral head so that cancellous bone will contact the glenoid. A wedge of bone is removed from the outer and anterior portion of the humerus, thus creating a cleft beneath the raw acromion. When the patient's arm is abducted to the desired degree, the acromion fits into the cleft to a depth of about 1.3 cm. The remaining capsule is then sutured to the

periosteum left over the superior aspect of the acromion. The extremity is placed in a plaster of Paris spica cast made prior to operation. This method can be modified by using internal fixation with two long wood screws. The screws should be placed across the head into the glenoid and base of the scapular spine and across the superior acromion into the humeral intramedullary canal.

Schulz later in 1931 described a similar method for fusing the shoulder.[17]

Brett's Technique

Brett believed optimistically that the introduction of bone grafts would secure solid fixation of the fusion site and solve the problem of nonunion.[5] After the humeral head and glenoid face are made raw, a tibial cortical graft, large enough to fit snugly, is passed through a $\frac{3}{8}$-in. hole just below the greater tuberosity and then through the glenoid into the spine of the scapula. The acromion is taken back to raw bone after it is denuded of soft tissue and broken in greenstick fashion, so that a broad raw bone surface can be fixed to the humeral head. The capsule is sutured down on the humerus for additional stability.

May's Technique

May described his technique of dissecting the soft tissues subperiosteally from the distal clavicle, the acromion, and scapular spine via the strap incision of Henry[12] (see Fig. 10-10A and B). Following dislocation of the long head of the biceps from its groove, the undersurface of the acromion is denuded to bleeding raw bone. The glenoid cartilage is removed and also cut back to bleeding raw bone with curved gouges. A partial osteotomy of the acromion is performed near its base, and the clavicle likewise divided at the junction of its middle and distal thirds. The distal portion of each bone is angled downward to contact the denuded humeral head (Fig. 11-7B). With the patient's arm held in the desired position the humeral head and glenoid are

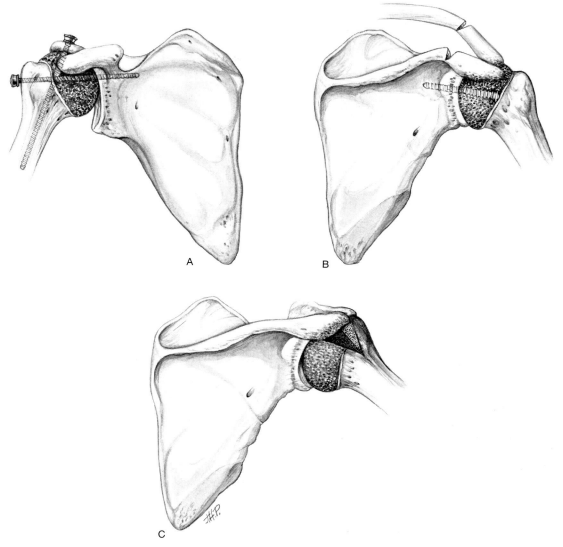

FIG. 11-7. Techniques of combined intra-articular and extra-articular arthrodesis. A, Moseley's technique. (Redrawn from Moseley, H. F.: Arthrodesis of the shoulder in the adult. Clin. Orthop., 20:158, 1961.) B, May's method. (Redrawn from May, V. R., Jr.: Shoulder fusion. A review of fourteen cases. J. Bone Joint Surg., 44-A:66, 1962.) C, Gill's technique. (Redrawn from Gill, A. B.: A new operation for arthrodesis of the shoulder. J. Bone Joint Surg., 13:287, 1931.)

shaped to produce a snug fit. A large wood screw is then placed through the head into the glenoid and spine of the scapula. Then the angled acromion and clavicle are fitted into a mortised groove in the humeral head. If necessary, multiple bone chips from the ilium may be used. Finally, the capsule is sutured down snugly and the wound closed.

AFTERCARE. After any of the combined methods of fusion, the extremity is placed into a well-padded, previously made shoulder spica which is changed at 10 days to a new shoulder spica cast. Thereafter, the patient should be seen periodically to be sure the cast fits well and that the patient is comfortable. Aftercare is continued as described for extra-articular arthrodesis.

Davis and Cottrell's Technique

Davis and Cottrell believe in their method of fusion performed with the patient sitting upright. (1) The glenohumeral joint is temporarily and preoperatively fixed with small Steinmann pins so that the optimum position for function is established by trial and error. (2) Immobilization in a shoulder spica is accomplished preoperatively and a window is made in the spica cast through which the operation is performed. (3) Rigid internal fixation is achieved with screws. (4) An intra-articular muscle-pedicle, cancellous bone graft fashioned from the acromion is then placed as a bridge across the denuded superior joint space. The downward angulation of the acromion allows fusion between these bones and the humeral head with the arm held in less abduction, as suggested by Rowe.[15]

Moseley's Technique

Finally, the method of Moseley appears to have merit.[13] In this operation a horseshoe-shaped incision is made over the acromion and the lateral flap reflected halfway down the deltoid muscle. Enough of the deltoid is detached from the acromion, the scapular spine, and the clavicle to expose the humeral head. Exposure may be increased by vertically splitting the deltoid. The rotator cuff is completely detached from its insertion, the intra-articular biceps tendon resected, and its distal end sutured in its bicipital groove. The inferior surface of the acromion is denuded to raw bone, and the humeral head and glenoid face are similarly denuded to raw cancellous bone. A long nail or screw is driven through the upper humerus below the greater tuberosity at the surgical neck level and through the glenoid, after the humeral head is superiorly displaced, to contact the raw acromion (Fig. 11-7A). A second nail or screw is driven downward through the acromion into the humeral intramedullary canal, thus securing the fixation.

Movements are checked to be certain the patient's arm can be brought to the side,

and the hand to the mouth and top of the head. Thereafter, the soft tissues are closed.

AFTERCARE. A plaster of Paris spica is applied at the time of surgery or the next day. Immobilization is continued as described for extra-articular arthrodesis.

Compression Methods

Charnley and Houston's Technique

Charnley first reported his method of applying compression to the shoulder in order to obtain glenohumeral arthrodesis in 1951.[8] In another report, Charnley and Houston described the same method used in 19 additional patients, 13 of whom had tuberculosis.[9] The technique originally required transfixion by two Steinmann pins, which restricted adjustment of the final position, but the latter report offered latitude for adjustment of the final fixed position.

The joint is exposed by a saber-cut incision made over the lateral acromion. The joint is cleared of debris, the upper half of the glenoid is denuded of its articular cartilage, and the undersurface is curetted to bare bone. The articular cartilage of the humeral head is removed and the arm of the patient held in the desired position for arthrodesis. A pedicle graft is raised from the site of the greater tuberosity, judging the direction of the osteotome from the lateral acromion. Some bone is now resected from the superior surface of the humeral head so that it lies flush against acromion when it is displaced upward (Fig. 11-8).

A 25-cm.-long, 4-mm.-diameter nail for the scapula is inserted first into the base of the acromion and then into the glenoid vault. A second nail is inserted perpendicular to the axis of the humerus.

AFTERCARE. After wound closure a plaster spica is applied but the compression pins are left free from the plaster. Although Charnley and Houston describe a compression clamp, it is possible to utilize Roger-Anderson fixation for similar compression. The extremity is immobilized in a plaster spica for an average of 4.8 weeks at which

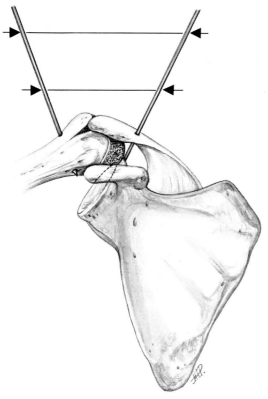

FIG. 11-8. Charnley's compression arthrodesis. Direction of arrows shows points of compression applied by cross rods. (Redrawn from Charnley, J. and Houston, J. K.: Compression arthrodesis of the shoulder. J. Bone Joint Surg., 46-B:617, 1964.)

time the pins are removed, and the arm again is supported for an additional average period of 5.3 weeks. A disadvantage of this method is the possibility of developing pin tract infection.

Beltran and Associates' Technique

Beltran and co-workers reported their operation of compression arthrodesis in 11 patients with various problems.[4] In this method, stability of the superiorly displaced, denuded humeral head against the raw undersurface of the acromion and glenoid is maintained by means of a compres-

sion screw introduced through the humeral head and glenoid and with a screw and washer through the upper surface of the humeral head (Fig. 11-9). Further stability is achieved by means of a fibular bone graft inserted beneath the compression device.

Two days before operation the extremity is placed in a plaster shoulder spica and the position verified by x-ray films. The day before operation a large window is removed from the spica cast leaving the anterior aspect of the shoulder, the anterolateral arm, the forearm, and the hand uncovered. The operation is performed with the patient in the semireclining position. An anterior approach is used. The clavicular origin of the deltoid is detached, and the coracoid is cut and later reattached. Once the humeral head, undersurface of acromion and glenoid are gouged to raw bone, and the desired position for arthrodesis is determined, a hole is made through the humeral head and glenoid with a reamer. The tip of the compression screw is directed perpendicularly toward the center of the glenoid vault. During this time a second team removes a 10-cm.-long pencil-shaped graft. A second parallel hole is made 2.5 cm. below the first. The screw is aimed toward the infraglenoid tubercle. The graft is gently tapped into place. Lastly, a screw with washer is placed through the acromion into the humeral head.

The shoulder spica cast is next completed and maintained for 2 weeks, at which time it is removed and the unsupported use of the shoulder allowed.

Immobilization

Regardless of the method used to obtain fusion, adequate postoperative external immobilization is required for a long enough period to achieve solid fusion. Most surgeons recommend 3 to 5 months of immobilization in a plaster spica. Table 11-2 lists some average times in plaster spica casts and the results of such treatment.

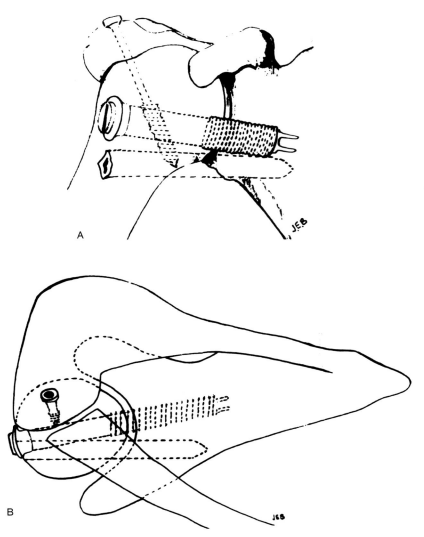

FIG. 11-9. Beltran's method for compression fusion of the shoulder. A, Anterior view of arthrodesis showing compression screw, bone graft at level of infraglenoid tubercle, and vertical screw crossing the acromion into the humeral head. B, Superior view shows the three elements that give stabilization at fusion site. (From Beltran, J. E., Trilla, J. C., and Barjau, R. B.: A simplified compression arthrodesis of the shoulder. J. Bone Joint Surg., 57-A:538–539, 1975.)

Table 11-2. *Lengths of Time and Results of Immobilization*

Author	Shoulders (Number)	Average Time in Plaster Spica (Weeks)	Nonunion Rate (Percent)
Barr and associates	102	15.2	22*
Davis and Cottrell	10	11.3	0
May	14	12	0
Charnley and Houston	19	9.1	5.3
Beltran and associates	11	2	18†

*Multiple methods.
†Union equivocal by x-ray examination in two cases.

REFERENCES

1. Albert, E.: Chirurgische Mittheilungen. Zentralbl. Chir., 8:776, 1881.
2. Barr, J. S., Freiberg, J. A., Colonna, P. C., and Pemberton, P. A.: A survey of end results on stabilization of the paralytic shoulder. J. Bone Joint Surg., 24:699–707, 1942.
3. Barton, N. J.: Arthrodesis of the shoulder for degenerative conditions. J. Bone Joint Surg., 54-A:1759–1764, 1972.
4. Beltran, J. E., Trilla, J. C., and Barjau, R.: A simplified compression arthrodesis of the shoulder. J. Bone Joint Surg., 57-A:538–541, 1975.
5. Brett, A. L.: A new method of arthrodesis of the shoulder joint, incorporating the control of the scapula. J. Bone Joint Surg., 15:969–977, 1933.
6. Brittain, H. A.: Architectural principles in arthrodesis. Edinburgh, E. and S. Livingstone, 1942.
7. Carroll, R. E.: Wire loop in arthrodesis of the shoulder. Clin. Orthop. 9:185–189, 1957.
8. Charnley, J.: Compression arthrodesis of the ankle and shoulder. J. Bone Joint Surg., 33-B:180–191, 1951.
9. Charnley, J., and Houston, J. K.: Compression arthrodesis of the shoulder. J. Bone Joint Surg., 46-B:614–620, 1964.
10. Davis, J. B., and Cottrell, G. W.: A technique for shoulder arthrodesis. J. Bone Joint Surg., 44-A:657–661, 1962.
11. Gill, A. B.: A new operation for arthrodesis of the shoulder. J. Bone Joint Surg., 13:287–295, 1931.
12. May, V. R., Jr.: Shoulder fusion. A review of fourteen cases. J. Bone Joint Surg., 44-A:65–76, 1962.
13. Moseley, H. F.: Arthrodesis of the shoulder in the adult. Clin. Orthop. 20:156–162, 1961.
14. Putti, V.: Arthrodesis for tuberculosis of the knee and of the shoulder. Chir. Organi Mov., 18:217, 1933.
15. Rowe, C. R.: Re-evaluation of the position of the arm in arthrodesis of the shoulder in the adult. J. Bone Joint Surg., 56-A:913–922, 1974.
16. Saha, A. K.: Surgery of the paralysed and flail shoulder. Acta Orthop. Scand. (Suppl.), 97:5–90, 1967.
17. Schulz, O. E.: Arthrodesis acromio-humeralis osteoplastica. J. Bone Joint Surg., 13:722–724, 1931.
18. Steindler, A.: Orthopedic Operations: Indications, Technique and End Results. Springfield, Ill., Charles C Thomas, 1940.
19. Watson-Jones, R.: Extra-articular arthrodesis of the shoulder. J. Bone Joint Surg., 15:862–871, 1933.

12

Arthritis of the Shoulder

MICHAEL H. ELLMAN

The shoulder is susceptible to any of the degenerative, metabolic, or inflammatory processes that affect other diarthrodial (synovial) joints. The majority of patients with shoulder pain do not have arthritis but periarticular disease of the shoulder with inflammation of the tendons, bursae, or other musculotendinous components of the shoulder capsule. Approximately 5 to 10 percent of patients with shoulder pain has arthritis that may be part of a polyarticular disease such as rheumatoid arthritis or ankylosing spondylitis, or it may be a monoarticular arthritis as seen with septic arthritis. Patients with monoarticular shoulder disease present diagnostic difficulties, because the list of possible diagnoses may include most of the disorders causing arthritis. Establishing a rheumatologic diagnosis requires integration of laboratory data including synovianalysis, appropriate roentgenograms, a thorough history, and physical examination. Remember that shoulder pain may be referred from the cervical spine or other extra-articular sites, such as the heart, aorta, and abdominal viscera, that are affected by disease.

There are many different forms of arthritis, and a comprehensive classification that could include 60 to 100 types is beyond the scope of this chapter. A limited outline of the more common arthritides involving the shoulder will help the physician to organize a differential diagnosis of shoulder arthritis and evaluate the patient.

I. Disorders primarily affecting the appendicular skeleton
 A. Rheumatoid arthritis
 B. Systemic lupus erythematosus and other "collagen" disorders
 C. Gout
 D. Pseudogout
 E. Infectious arthritis
 F. Tumors
 G. Miscellaneous disorders: rheumatic fever, hypothyroidism, hemochromatosis, sarcoid, hemophilic arthritis, etc.
II. Disorders primarily affecting the axial skeleton
 A. Ankylosing spondylitis
 B. Spondylitis of inflammatory bowel disease
III. Disorders frequently affecting both the axial and appendicular skeleton
 A. Osteoarthritis
 B. Juvenile rheumatoid arthritis
 C. Psoriatic arthritis
 D. Reiter's syndrome
IV. Miscellaneous disorders with frequent shoulder involvement
 A. Shoulder-hand syndrome
 B. Osteonecrosis
 C. Polymyalgia rheumatica
 D. Neuropathic joint disease (Charcot's arthropathy)
 E. Amyloidosis

These specific disorders are discussed later in the chapter. Finally, an outline of anti-inflammatory therapy is included to assist the physician in the initial treatment of shoulder arthritis.

SHOULDER ASPIRATION AND SYNOVIANALYSIS

Shoulder effusion is uncommon in most of the arthritides, but when present the fluid should be aspirated and carefully examined. Demonstration of sodium urate crystals in the synovial fluid, for example, can establish a diagnosis of gouty arthritis and no further diagnostic studies are needed. Effusion of the shoulder from any cause usually produces anterior bulging of the shoulder capsule. To obtain synovial fluid for diagnosis, I prefer to aspirate the joint with an 18- or a 20-gauge needle, inserting the needle at the point of maximal shoulder swelling, after cleansing the skin with alcohol or other topical antiseptic. Ethyl chloride sprayed at the site of insertion of the needle usually suffices for anesthesia. An 18-gauge needle is used for aspiration when thick, purulent synovial fluid is anticipated. Joint fluid must be treated as a precious commodity so that maximal diagnostic information is obtained.

Listed in Table 12-1 are the laboratory procedures available at most institutions for analyzing synovial fluid. Clear synovial fluid of normal viscosity generally requires no special laboratory testing, although occasionally the spun sediment will reveal calcium pyrophosphate crystals diagnostic of pseudogout. All inflammatory shoulder fluid should be cultured for microorganisms.

Synovial fluid has generally been classified into several categories reflecting the degree of synovial inflammation:

Group I. Transparent or nearly transparent joint fluid (white blood cells < 2000 mm.[3])
    A. Osteoarthritis
    B. Trauma
    C. Systemic lupus erythematosus
    D. Hypothyroidism
    E. Sarcoid
    F. Shoulder-hand syndrome
Group II. Slightly cloudy or cloudy synovial fluid (white blood cells usually > 2000 mm.[3])
    A. Rheumatoid arthritis
    B. Rheumatic fever
    C. Gout, pseudogout
    D. Reiter's syndrome

Table 12-1. *Laboratory Procedures for Synovial Fluid Analysis*

Test	Instructions

Synovianalysis:
  color of fluid
  white blood cell count
  differential count
  mucin clot
  viscosity
  polarized light microscopy
	Collect in tube or syringe with heparin. Inflammatory joint fluid contains fibrinogen and other clotting factors and will clot.

Microbiology:
  Gram stain
  bacterial culture
  culture for fungi and mycobacteria
	Sterile tube required. For suspect gonococcal arthritis, fluid should be placed on chocolate agar plates at time of aspiration.

Biochemistry I:
  total protein
  total hemolytic complement
	Plain tubes. These tests need not be performed routinely. See text for discussion of complement determination.

Biochemistry II: glucose determination	Tubes with sodium fluoride and potassium oxalate. Requires simultaneous blood glucose determination.

E. Ankylosing spondylitis
F. Psoriatic arthritis
G. Juvenile rheumatoid arthritis
H. Other inflammatory arthritides

Group III. Cloudy synovial fluid (white blood cells usually $> 50,000$ mm.^{3})
    A. Infectious arthritis
    B. Some cases of gout

Group IV. Hemorrhagic synovial fluid
    A. Trauma
    B. Bleeding disorders, especially deficiencies of factor VIII or factor IX
    C. Tumors

There is a great deal of overlap between disorders, but the classification is simple and is generally accepted by most rheumatologists and orthopaedic surgeons. It provides initial baseline information for the formulation of a differential diagnosis.

A number of rheumatic disorders can be diagnosed by an astute clinician simply by examining the joint fluid under the light microscope. Lupus erythematosus (LE) cells are occasionally seen in synovial fluid of patients with systemic lupus erythematosus. The presence of fat or bone marrow cells suggests a fracture communicating between the joint and the bone marrow cavity. Dark blue or brown inclusions in synovial fluid macrophages have been seen in ochronosis. Sickled red blood cells are diagnostic of sickle cell anemia or sickle trait. The crystal-induced arthropathies, gout and pseudogout, may be diagnosed definitively with the light microscope plus additional polarizing discs.

The polarizing light microscope is a standard microscope with a rotating stage and two polarizing discs, one above and one below the microscope stage. The polarizing discs will transmit only light waves that vibrate parallel to their axes. The two discs are placed perpendicular to each other, allowing no light transmission. The microscope stage viewed through the eyepiece appears black. Most crystals and crystalline material are birefringent, the property of being able to resolve polarized light into perpendicular planes. Sodium urate and calcium pyrophosphate (pseudogout) crystals present in joint fluid resolve transmitted light so that they appear white on a black background (Fig. 12-1).

The addition of a crystalline color compensator placed between the microscope stage and the upper polarizing disc will allow differentiation between sodium urate and calcium pyrophosphate crystals. The

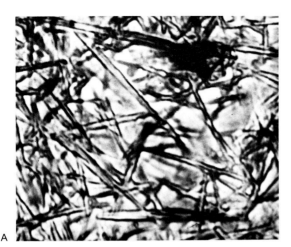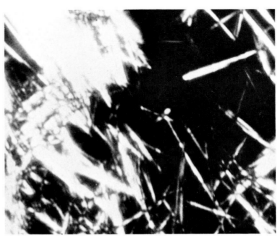

A   B

FIG. 12-1. A, Sodium urate crystals from a tophaceous deposit seen under the phase-contrast light microscope. Original magnification 440×. B, The same material seen with the polarized light microscope. The sodium urate crystals appear white on a black background.

color compensator differentially slows transmitted light so that the light components are out of phase, cancelling some light frequencies. The light reaching the eyepiece will now be perceived as having color. With a first-order red plate color compensator plus the polarizing discs, sodium urate crystals will appear yellow and calcium pyrophosphate crystals blue when they lie parallel to the slow axis of vibration of the color compensator. The technique for identifying these crystals is called compensated polarized light microscopy. Sodium urate crystals are always needle shaped; calcium pyrophosphate crystals may be needle shaped but are usually rhomboid (Fig. 12-2). The crystals are usually intracellular, having been phagocytosed by polymorphonuclear leukocytes.

Knowledge of the composition and derivation of normal synovial fluid is essential for the understanding and interpretation of synovial fluid content in disease states. Synovial fluid is a dialysate of plasma with the addition of hyaluronic acid (in the form of sodium hyaluronate), a nonsulfated polysaccharide composed of equimolar amounts of D-glucuronic acid and N-acetyl D-glucosamine. The synthesis of the hyaluronic acid occurs locally by the synovial tissue. The two monosaccharide components of hyaluronic acid are polymerized to form a long chain, high molecular weight, randomly coiled structure complexed with synovial fluid proteins. This hyaluronate-protein complex imparts to synovial fluid much of its unique characteristics, including its ability to exclude large molecules, its high viscosity, and its non-Newtonian flow properties.

Normal synovial fluid is clear and colorless and practically acellular. It contains approximately 3.5 mg. of hyaluronate/gram of synovial fluid and less than 2.0 gm. percent of total protein. Small molecules such as glucose, uric acid, urea, sodium, and potassium are in concentrations similar to that of plasma.

The appearance and clarity of joint fluid and knowledge of the white blood cell count allow classification of the fluid into

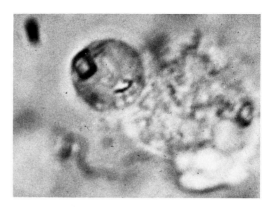

FIG. 12-2. A rhomboid-shaped calcium pyrophosphate crystal has been phagocytosed by a polymorphonuclear leukocyte. Phase-contrast light microscope original magnification 440×.

noninflammatory, inflammatory, possibly infectious, and hemorrhagic categories that are helpful in formulating an initial diagnostic impression (see outline, p. 239). The differential white blood cell count also provides important information. Most chronic inflammatory arthritides are characterized by a predominance of polymorphonuclear leukocytes. Systemic lupus erythematosus is an exception and usually has a predominance of lymphocytes. Serial synovial fluid white blood cell counts are helpful in monitoring the success of antibiotic treatment in septic arthritis.

The mucin clot test and estimation of the joint fluid viscosity are measurements of the integrity of the high molecular weight hyaluronate-protein complex. Inflammatory arthritides are associated with joint fluid with low viscosity and a poor mucin clot test. The former may be tested by simply placing a drop of synovial fluid between the thumb and forefinger and separating the digits. Normal joint fluid will string out for an inch or more. Addition of a drop or two of normal synovial fluid into 5 percent acetic acid (mucin clot test) will produce a tight ropey mass consisting of protein and hyaluronate. Synovial fluid from inflammatory joints will produce friable and shredded fragments of clot in the mucin clot test, and will not string out when placed between the thumb and forefinger. The quality of the mucin clot and viscosity of the joint fluid reflect the degree of polymerization of the hyaluronic acid and protein. A poor mucin clot and low viscosity may reflect disruption of this complex by inflammatory cells with release of their lysosomal enzymes, or synthesis of smaller hyaluronic acid molecules by inflamed synovial tissue. The results of the tests are rough estimates of the degree of joint inflammation. Occasionally group I (noninflammatory) joint fluid will have low viscosity and a poor mucin clot because of the dilution of hyaluronic acid by plasma dialysate.

Inflammatory joint fluid should be Gram stained and cultured whenever the possibility of infectious arthritis exists. Gonococcal arthritis is now the most common pyogenic arthritis in adults. This organism is difficult to culture, but serial aspirations and plating of the joint fluid on optimal media (usually chocolate agar plates) at the bedside will increase the percentage of positive results of cultures.

Protein analysis of synovial fluid is occasionally helpful to the clinician. Normal noninflammatory joint fluid has low quantities of high molecular weight proteins. In inflammatory arthritis, the synovial fluid protein concentration increases from values approximating 20 percent of plasma protein content to 75 percent or greater. As the synovial fluid protein increases in inflammatory states, it begins to qualitatively and quantitatively mirror the pattern of plasma protein.

The synovial fluid glucose level compared with simultaneous measurement of the serum glucose is frequently helpful when infectious arthritis is suspected. Synovial fluid glucose values in joint infections are usually less than half of serum levels and are often barely detectable. In noninfectious, inflammatory arthritis, the synovial fluid glucose may be 20 to 30 mg. percent lower than serum glucose. In noninflammatory joint fluid, there is little or no difference between serum and synovial fluid glucose values. Synovial fluid and serum complement determination will be discussed later in more detail.

LABORATORY AIDS IN RHEUMATOLOGY

Correct interpretation of laboratory tests in rheumatology will help the clinician diagnose and assess the activity of arthritis when this information is correlated with the history, physical examination, roentgenograms, and the routine baseline laboratory data. Only the more common and readily available rheumatologic tests are described. For an in-depth discussion on laboratory tests and their interpretation, the reader is referred to *Laboratory Diagnostic Procedures in the Rheumatic Diseases.*[6]

ERYTHROCYTE SEDIMENTATION RATE. The sedimentation rate is a useful screening test that positively correlates with the degree of inflammation. It is also a helpful discriminator between the inflammatory and noninflammatory arthritides. For example, noninflammatory disorders such as osteoarthritis, psychosomatic rheumatism, and shoulder pain secondary to cervical spine radiculopathy are usually associated with normal sedimentation rates. Patients with systemic inflammatory arthritis such as rheumatoid arthritis and ankylosing spondylitis ordinarily have high sedimentation rates, and the activity of the disease and the response to therapy can frequently be gauged by the level of this test. Diseases with primary vascular inflammation, namely, systemic lupus erythematosus, polyarteritis nodosum, and polymyalgia rheumatica, are associated with very high sedimentation rates.

The sedimentation of erythrocytes in blood is defined by Stokes' law, relating the rate of fall of a particle in a liquid to twice the square of its radius. The red cells indirectly increase their radii by stacking one on top of another, forming rouleaux. Asymmetric large molecules in plasma such as fibrinogen, alpha globulin, and gamma globulin promote rouleau formation which increases the sedimentation rate. Fibrinogen is the most asymmetric protein molecule in normal plasma and is usually the chief determinant of the sedimentation rate. Erythrocytes that are unable to stack because of abnormal or nonuniform shapes will settle slowly even in the presence of inflammatory states. Patients with sickle cell anemia or congenital spherocytosis or patients with diseases associated with anisocytosis or poikilocytosis are examples of those whose erythrocytes are unable to stack and will have low sedimentation rates. Patients with acute hepatitis or congestion of the liver also have low sedimentation rates because of low fibrinogen levels.

The Westergren sedimentation rate was introduced into laboratory medicine in 1926 and has several advantages over other methods. The blood is diluted with sodium citrate diminishing the whole blood viscosity. The wide-bore glass tube used in this test also reduces the resistance to gravity at the interface of the glass and the erythrocytes. Westergren sedimentation rate values increase slightly with age of the patient and higher values are seen in women than in men. Women over the age of 70 may have values as high as 50 mm./hour without overt evidence of inflammation.[9]

URIC ACID MEASUREMENT. Measurement of serum uric acid is almost always obtained when evaluating patients with acute arthritis. The value of this test depends on proper interpretation of the analytic method employed and knowledge of its normal range. Serum is saturated with urate at levels approximating 6.8 mg. percent. Crystallization of monosodium urate from serum occurs above this level with predilection for deposition on cartilage and in synovium. The mean serum urate in adult men is 5.1 mg. percent, with an upper limit of approximately 7 mg. percent (two standard deviations from the mean). Serum urate levels in women are about 1 mg. percent less than those in men. Current autoanalysis colorimetric methods for uric acid determinations tend to overestimate true urate by an average of 0.4 mg. percent. Uric acid determination using the enzyme uricase, an enzyme specific for converting uric acid to the nonpurine compound allantoin, is the most accurate method for determining uric acid. This procedure should be used when careful metabolic studies are needed. However, an assay with partial uricase digestion combined with a colorimetric method provides a reliable and accurate value for most requirements.

The prevalence of gouty arthritis is associated with the degree and duration of hyperuricemia. In the study by Hall and associates, 27.5 percent of men with uric acid values between 8.0 and 8.9 mg. percent and 90 percent of men with uric acid levels greater than 9.0 mg. percent developed gouty arthritis.[10]

Several commonly used medications increase uric acid levels such as salicylates in doses less than 3 gm./day, and thiazide, ethacrynic acid, and furosemide diuretics. Ethanol ingestion increases serum uric acid by decreasing urate secretion. Large doses of salicylates, probenecid, sulfinpyrazone, allopurinol, and phenylbutazone lower serum urate.

Disorders that are associated with hyperuricemia include hypothyroidism, advanced renal disease, lead nephropathy, and hematologic malignancies especially polycythemia vera, multiple myeloma, and chronic myelogenous leukemia, and chronic hemolytic anemias such as sickle cell anemia. Hyperuricemia in childhood is almost always secondary to hematologic malignancies, Down's syndrome, renal failure, type 1 glycogen storage disease, or the Lesch-Nyhan syndrome. Hypouricemia is marked in patients with xanthinuria and in patients with excessive renal excretion of urate such as those with Wilson's disease, adult Fanconi's syndrome, and isolated renal tubular abnormalities of urate resorption.

RHEUMATOID FACTOR. Most patients with rheumatoid arthritis have an IgM antibody in their serum directed against IgG. This antibody is called rheumatoid factor and is present in approximately 70 percent of patients with rheumatoid arthritis.

Rheumatoid factors are observed in many chronic illnesses and are even present in normal subjects. In one review, in which human gamma globulin-coated latex particles (latex fixation test) were used, 24 percent of normal persons over the age of 60 had positive results of agglutination tests.[2]

Patients with rheumatoid arthritis who have high titers of rheumatoid factor frequently have severe arthritis and more of the extra-articular manifestations of the disease including vasculitis, nodules, and pulmonary involvement. There is little evidence, however, that rheumatoid factor is involved in the pathogenesis of rheumatoid arthritis. Infusion of rheumatoid factor into normal subjects or into those with rheumatoid arthritis does not cause arthritis in the former or worsen the arthritis in the latter.

The ideal laboratory test for diagnosing rheumatoid arthritis would combine high sensitivity with high specificity. No such test exists. Rheumatoid factor, as detected by incubating the patient's serum with sheep red blood cells coated with antisheep rabbit IgG, has an estimated 70 to 90 percent specificity for rheumatoid arthritis but is not a sensitive test. The commonly employed latex fixation (rheumatoid factor) test is more sensitive but less specific than the sheep red blood cell test.

The demonstration of rheumatoid factor is helpful to the clinician, because this factor is usually not present in diseases that mimic rheumatoid arthritis such as ankylosing spondylitis, juvenile rheumatoid arthritis, and psoriatic arthritis. Rheumatoid arthritis is primarily diagnosed by the clinical parameters of the disease. The absence of rheumatoid factor should not deter one from diagnosing rheumatoid arthritis if the clinical patterns diagnostic of this disease are present.

ANTINUCLEAR ANTIBODIES. The antinuclear antibody (ANA) test has replaced the LE cell preparation as a screening test for systemic lupus erythematosus (SLE). The ANA test is extremely sensitive for diagnosing SLE. Rarely is the result of the test negative during active disease. Positive results of tests are common in diseases other than SLE especially chronic inflammatory disorders. A variety of collagen vascular diseases such as scleroderma, rheumatoid arthritis, and Sjögren's syndrome produce a high incidence of positive results of the ANA test. The high degree of sensitivity makes the ANA a good screening test in patients with arthritis possibly secondary to SLE. A negative result usually excludes SLE.

The usual ANA tests are performed by standard indirect immunofluorescent technique using sections of rat liver as the nuclear antigen source. The patient's serum is incubated with slides containing rat liver slices. Antinuclear antibodies present in serum will combine with nuclei (nuclear antigens) present in the rat liver. The antigen-antibody complex (rat liver nuclei plus antinuclear antibody in patient's serum) can be detected using a fluorescent microscope after incubation with a fluorescein-tagged antibody specific for human gamma globulin.

There are four well-recognized nuclear immunofluorescent patterns. The homogeneous pattern (the entire nucleus is fluorescent) is produced by antibody to nucleoprotein and is commonly seen in SLE and drug-induced SLE. The shaggy pattern, also called peripheral, marginal, or rim pattern (the rim of the nucleus is fluorescent), is produced by antibody to DNA and is almost always specific for SLE. A speckled pattern of nuclear staining is seen in some cases of SLE, all cases of mixed connective tissue disease, and frequently in scleroderma. A fourth pattern of fluorescence, nucleolar (fluorescent staining only of the nucleoli), is seen in some patients with scleroderma.

COMPLEMENT DETERMINATION. The complement system comprises a group of serum proteins, interacting with antigen-antibody complexes and biologic membranes, that are important in mediating many of the phenomena normally associated with acute inflammation. Activation of this system results in a number of biologic effects including cytolysis, release of anaphylotoxins (substances that contract smooth muscles and alter capillary permeability), release of leukocyte chemotactic factors, and enhancement of phagocytosis. Complement is activated and consumed in several disorders associated with arthritis, including systemic lupus erythematosus, mixed cryoglobulinemia, serum sickness, and infectious hepatitis associated with Australia antigenemia. A small percentage of patients with severe, destructive and long-standing rheumatoid arthritis having high titers of rheumatoid factor also have low serum complement. A distinctive feature of rheumatoid factor-positive (seropositive) rheumatoid arthritis is the finding of low synovial fluid complement in the presence of high or normal serum complement (Fig. 12-3). The entry of complement proteins into the articular cavity in rheumatoid arthritis is normal, but many of the individual complement components can be detected in synovial fluid white blood cells, on cartilage, or in the synovial membrane indicating that complement is activated locally. This consumption of complement, probably by attaching to antigen-antibody complexes, may play a significant role in mediating the severe articular inflammatory process seen in rheumatoid arthritis.

Most laboratories estimate serum complement by measuring C3, the third component of the complement system and the component normally present in the highest concentration. Radial immunodiffusion assay is generally employed, and values are interpreted in relation to standard immunodiffusion plates. Most data collected on synovial fluid complement are based on a total hemolytic complement assay. This system measures the lysis of 50 percent of sensitized sheep red blood cells incubated with synovial fluid or serum containing complement. Normally, the complement level in synovial fluid is directly correlated with the synovial fluid protein concentration (Fig. 12-3). This measurement of synovial fluid complement is occasionally helpful in diagnosing rheumatoid arthritis in patients with an atypical pattern of disease.

HISTOCOMPATIBILITY (HLA) SEROTYPING. With the advent of organ transplantation it became apparent that acceptance or rejection of a donor graft by a host is dependent, in part, on certain inherited genetically determined antigens detected on the surface of nucleated cells. This important histocompatibility determinant in man resides on the sixth chromosome and is called the histocompatibility locus antigen (HLA) system. There are four recognizable loci on this complex (A to D), each locus with two alleles, one inherited from each parent. Three of the loci can be detected by lymphocyte cytotoxic techniques employing monospecific antiserum to the antigens. In 1973, several groups of investigators found that a specific B-locus antigen, HLA B27, was associated with ankylosing spondylitis.[3,16] Eight to nine percent of the Caucasian pop-

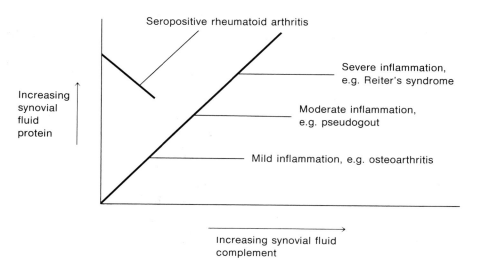

FIG. 12-3. Synovial fluid total hemolytic complement. Synovial fluid complement levels normally are directly related to the synovial fluid protein level. Patients with rheumatoid factor-positive rheumatoid arthritis have low synovial fluid complement in spite of high synovial fluid protein concentrations.

Table 12-2. *Diseases Associated with HLA B27*

Disease	Positivity of HLA B27 (Approximate Percent)
Ankylosing spondylitis	90
Reiter's syndrome	80
Spondylitis and inflammatory bowel disease	70
Psoriasis with spondylitis	35
Control patients (Caucasian population)	9

ulation carries the HLA B27 genetic marker, whereas greater than 90 percent of patients with ankylosing spondylitis are HLA B27-positive (Table 12-2). This HLA serotyping confirmed the strong hereditary basis of ankylosing spondylitis and has been an important diagnostic tool in confirming early ankylosing spondylitis. It has been estimated that up to 20 percent of asymptomatic subjects with HLA B27 has subclinical evidence of ankylosing spondylitis.[4] The spondylitis associated with inflammatory bowel disease, psoriatic arthritis, and Reiter's syndrome also has an increased association with the HLA B27 serotype (Table 12-2).

The causal role of the HLA system in the diseases mentioned is not known. A plausible explanation that correlates with extensive animal studies states that the HLA genes are closely linked to other genes responsible for disease susceptibility and that the HLA B27 gene in man serves as a marker for this gene(s). In mice there is close linkage of the histocompatibility system with genes controlling immune responses.

COMMON ARTHRITIDES WITH SHOULDER INVOLVEMENT

RHEUMATOID ARTHRITIS. Rheumatoid arthritis is a clinical disorder characterized by symmetric and generally progressive involvement of the small joints of the hands with eventual involvement of most other joints. Distal interphalangeal joint and spine involvement occur late in the disease. It is uncommon for shoulder involvement to be the initial and it is never the sole manifestation of rheumatoid arthritis. The involvement is usually bilateral, but often more severe on the dominant side. At times, shoulder pain is very severe especially at nighttime, contrasting with other involved joints that are more painful and stiff in the morning. The shoulder symptoms frequently do not correlate well with the general severity and activity of the rheumatoid arthritis. There are no diagnostic changes in the shoulder on roentgenograms. Marginal erosions, periarticular osteoporosis, and cystic changes in the subchondral bone are frequently noted. However, these changes can be seen in other inflammatory arthritides (Fig. 12-4). The roentgenographic finding of inferior erosions of the distal clavicle and erosions of the humeral head suggests the presence of systemic or polyarticular disease rather than of a monoarticular arthritis. When shoulder pain or effusion is

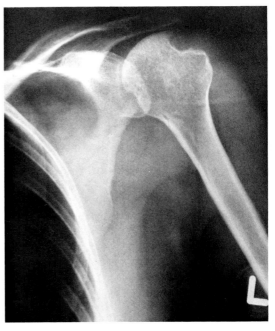

FIG. 12-4. A roentgenogram of the shoulder of a young woman with severe rheumatoid arthritis. There are extensive erosions of the humeral head on the medial and lateral aspects.

out of proportion to the general severity of the rheumatoid disease, septic arthritis must be considered, and appropriate cultures of the aspirated joint fluid are mandatory.

The treatment of the rheumatoid shoulder is generally that of the basic management of rheumatoid arthritis. It encompasses anti-inflammatory medication, adequate rest, and a supervised physical therapy program. Salicylates remain the mainstay of drug treatment and are effective to some degree in all patients with rheumatoid arthritis. Chrysotherapy has withstood the test of time and is the second-line choice of therapy in patients not adequately responding to salicylates. The antimalarials are effective drugs in reducing the inflammation in rheumatoid arthritis and several drugs newly introduced into rheumatology (D-penicillamine, azathioprine, and cyclophosphamide) are beneficial in selected patients. The occasional use of intra-articular steroids is effective in the treatment of shoulder symptoms as adjunctive therapy to the basic drug management and physical therapy. Although few untoward effects have been observed, aseptic technique is essential and repeated injections may adversely alter cartilage metabolism. Intra-articular therapy is especially effective when the disease is generally inactive except for the shoulder. Active shoulder range of motion exercises should be initiated early in the disease in order to prevent loss of shoulder motion. Although vigorous physical therapy to the shoulder is recommended, excessive force must be avoided.

SYSTEMIC LUPUS ERYTHEMATOSUS AND OTHER COLLAGEN DISEASES. Inflammatory arthritis is common in the collagen-vascular diseases (systemic lupus erythematosus, scleroderma, polymyositis, polyarteritis nodosum). Arthritis is the most frequent clinical manifestation of systemic lupus erythematosus and is common in the other collagen-vascular diseases, although destructive changes are unusual. Shoulder involvement causing significant inflammation and effusion is rare. However, osteonecrosis of the humeral head is not infrequent in systemic lupus erythematosus and will be discussed later.

GOUT. Gout is an inflammatory arthritis initiated by the interaction of sodium urate crystals with polymorphonuclear leukocytes. When serum is supersaturated with urate there is deposition of sodium urate crystals in connective tissue, especially cartilage and synovium. These crystals may break free during trauma or stress or other poorly defined inciting factors and are phagocytosed by leukocytes. The polymorphonuclear leukocyte is unable to digest the phagocytosed urate crystal, leading to cell rupture and release of proteolytic enzymes and other cell contents into the joint fluid. Chemotactic factors are released, attracting more cells to the area and resulting in further phagocytosis of crystals, rupture of cells, release of more chemotactic factor and more enzymes, which produce a cyclic pattern of inflammation that may ultimately destroy cartilage and soft tissue.

Shoulder involvement in gout is much less common than involvement of other joints such as the first metatarsophalangeal joint, wrists, and knees. Podagra (involvement of the metatarsophalangeal joint of the first toe) is the initial manifestation of gouty arthritis in approximately 50 percent of cases. The shoulder is rarely the first joint to be involved, but patients with polyarticular gout and patients with long-standing, untreated hyperuricemia with tophaceous deposits may have shoulder involvement. As in other gouty joints there is exquisite pain accompanied by warmth, tenderness, and swelling. With the polarized light microscope, aspirated joint fluid reveals the typical sodium urate crystals within polymorphonuclear leukocytes. The detection of urate crystals is specific for gout, and conversely their absence makes gouty arthritis unlikely. Systemic treatment with colchicine or anti-inflammatory drugs such as indomethacin or phenylbutazone is always indicated when gouty arthritis is diagnosed. Colchicine, although occasionally effective in sarcoid arthritis and pseudogout, is almost specific for gout. Aspirin is less effective and, when used in doses less than approximately 3 gm./day, elevates serum uric acid by blocking urate secretion in the kidney. Intra-articular steroids instilled into the shoulder joint provide effective relief of pain. Once the acute attack is terminated, long-term therapy to lower the plasma urate should be undertaken if basal serum urate levels are greater than 8.0 to 8.5 mg. percent. Probenecid, in doses of 0.5 to 1.5 gm./day, effectively lowers serum uric acid by suppressing resorption of renal tubular urate. The drug is not consistently effective in patients also taking salicylates or diuretics. Allopurinol inhibits xanthine oxidase, the enzyme that converts purine degradation products to uric acid. The drug decreases both serum and urine urate and is the drug of choice in patients with gouty arthritis and renal disease. Patients with tophaceous gout and those with hyperuricemia secondary to malignancies with tissue breakdown or excessive purine synthesis should also be treated with allopurinol. The usual dose range of allopurinol is 100 to 600 mg./day, 300 mg. daily being the average dose.

PSEUDOGOUT. Pseudogout is a common arthritic disorder of the elderly. It has been generally recognized as a disease entity only since 1961. The hallmark of pseudogout is deposition of calcium pyrophosphate dihydrate crystals on cartilage, producing the characteristic linear, stippled, and punctate calcifications observed on roentgenograms (chondrocalcinosis) (Fig. 12-5). The knees and wrists are the most common sites of chondrocalcinosis. The calcium pyrophosphate crystals present in the synovial fluid of pseudogout patients are quite distinctive when seen under a polarized light microscope. The interaction of calcium pyrophosphate crystals with polymorphonuclear leukocytes initiates inflammation similar to the inflammatory response observed with true gout. The arthritis in pseudogout may be quite severe and similar to gout, thus the name pseudogout. It may be mild, often similar to the symptoms of osteoarthritis. The crystals may even be present in joints without causing symptoms. The knees, wrists, and hips are more commonly in-

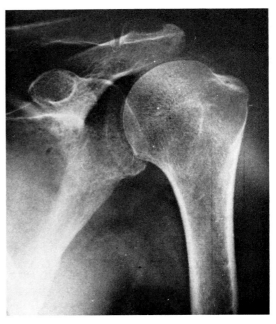

FIG. 12-5. There is a thin rim of calcification (chondrocalcinosis) surrounding the humeral head. The linear, stippled calcification is almost specific for calcium pyrophosphate crystal deposition. This patient also had similar calcifications in the cartilage of the knees and wrists.

volved than the shoulder. In patients with multiple joint involvement, it is not unusual to find chondrocalcinosis of the shoulder. The shoulder may occasionally be the joint initially involved in pseudogout. The acutely involved shoulder is warm and swollen, and the inflammatory synovial fluid has many leukocytes containing intracellular calcium pyrophosphate crystals. Like gout, failure to demonstrate these crystals usually makes the diagnosis of pseudogout untenable. Thorough aspiration of the joint often suffices as satisfactory treatment. Most anti-inflammatory medications such as aspirin, indomethacin, and phenylbutazone, and intra-articular corticosteroids also provide effective therapy. There are several metabolic disorders associated with pseudogout and these should be looked for in every newly diagnosed patient. Hyperparathyroidism may be present in as many as 7 percent of patients, and there is an increased incidence of pseudogout in patients with hemochromatosis, Wilson's disease, and true gout.

INFECTIOUS ARTHRITIS. See Chapters 6 and 7.

TUMORS. Primary tumors of the shoulder are uncommon but should be considered in the differential diagnosis of patients with monoarticular arthritis. Joint pain and synovial thickening with hemorrhagic joint fluid in the absence of trauma or bleeding disorders are clues to the presence of tumor or tumorlike lesions (Table 12-3). Tumors metastatic to joints are more common than primary malignant joint tumors. We have occasionally seen patients with multiple myeloma and lytic lesions involving the humeral head appear initially because of shoulder pain. Cytologic examination of joint fluid may provide valuable information to the physician. Figure 12-6 demonstrates the histologic findings of synovial chondromatosis of the shoulder in a patient with shoulder pain and swelling.

ARTHRITIS ASSOCIATED WITH MISCELLANEOUS MEDICAL DISORDERS. Almost any of the medical disorders associated with arthritis can involve the shoulder. Viral illnesses such as viral hepatitis, rubella, mumps, and infectious mononucleosis may have a significant arthritic component.

Several metabolic disorders are associated with arthritis. Hypothyroidism may be manifest by joint stiffness and effusion. Occasionally, gout and pseudogout are associated with hypothyroidism. Hemochromatosis is also associated with pseudogout and with a distinctive pattern of degenerative

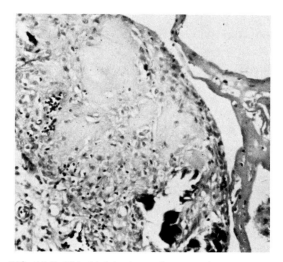

FIG. 12-6. This histologic section reveals an area of metaplastic cartilage formation within synovial connective tissue in a patient with synovial chondromatosis. Notice the remnants of calcified tissue. Hematoxylin and eosin. Original magnification 220×.

arthritis. There is usually involvement of the second and third metacarpophalangeal joints and knees, but shoulder arthritis is not uncommon.

The shoulder is involved in approximately 7 to 8 percent of patients with rheumatic fever and arthritis.[8] The arthritis is migratory, often very painful, and usually part of a polyarticular presentation. The joint fluid is inflammatory and, like other joint involvement in rheumatic fever, improves dramatically with administration of salicylate.

In one survey of 157 patients with hemo-

Table 12-3. *Primary Tumors or Tumorlike Lesions of the Shoulder*

Lesion	Distinguishing Features
Synovial (osteo)chondromatosis	Roentgenographic demonstration of intra-articular loose bodies. Histologic features of metaplastic formation of cartilage developing within synovial connective tissue.
Pigmented villonodular synovitis	Hemorrhagic joint fluid and characteristic synovial histologic appearance of appreciable vascularity and conspicuous hemosiderin deposition.
Hemangioma	Hemorrhagic joint fluid, reduction in size of joint with elevation of affected limb; hemangiomas elsewhere and characteristic pathologic changes.
Synovial sarcoma	Malignancy uncommonly involving the shoulder, usually para-articular, highly pleomorphic; tumor may produce hyaluronate and structurally may be caricature of synovial tissue.

philia A and B, 21 patients (13.4 percent) had shoulder involvement and 7 patients had bilateral disease.[1] Shoulder arthritis was rare in children; the majority of patients were over 20 years of age. There is significant synovial hypertrophy in hemophilic arthritis, and hemosiderin deposition is found throughout all layers of the synovium and within the cartilage. The arthritis is often associated with significant cartilage and joint destruction probably mediated by release of lysosomal enzymes, including cathepsin D, from the synovial cells. Treatment is similar to that for knee and other joints involved in hemophilia: blood factor replacement, immobilization, and analgesics. Orthopaedic surgical treatment of hemophilic patients including joint replacement has recently become possible with the use of factor-replacement therapy.[15]

SARCOID. Sixteen to twenty-five percent of patients with sarcoid has arthritis. Approximately one fourth of the patients with arthritis will have shoulder involvement.[17] There are two major forms of sarcoid arthritis: an acute and transient arthritis associated with erythema nodosum and hilar adenopathy, which usually only involves the ankles, but may involve the shoulder when multiple joints are affected; and a more persistent or chronic arthritis associated with granulomas in the synovium. The arthritis is usually not destructive and it spares the axial skeletal. It usually involves the hands, knees, and ankles and occasionally the shoulder.

ANKYLOSING SPONDYLITIS. Shoulder involvement in ankylosing spondylitis is quite common. It may be present in up to 25 percent of patients and it contributes significantly to the morbidity of the disease.[7] Shoulder involvement, however, is almost never an isolated finding. There is a marked male predominance in this disease ranging between 4 to 1 and 15 to 1. The signs and symptoms of ankylosing spondylitis include back stiffness and immobility, especially in the morning, decreased range of motion of the cervical and lumbosacral spine, and frequent peripheral joint arthritis. Occasionally, aortitis and iritis are extra-articular

manifestations. Typical sacroiliac and spine changes on roentgenograms, mild anemia, elevated erythrocyte sedimentation rate, and the frequent presence of the HLA B27 serotype are the usual laboratory and radiologic findings. Erosive changes of the shoulder are common radiologic features but are not specific for ankylosing spondylitis.

Satisfactory treatment of pain and stiffness is usually accomplished with indomethacin or high dose salicylate therapy. Occasionally, long-term phenylbutazone therapy is required, although this necessitates frequent monitoring of the leukocyte count. Persistent shoulder pain may be treated with intra-articular steroids. Early and repetitious physical therapy will help maintain the functional range of shoulder motion.

SPONDYLITIS AND INFLAMMATORY BOWEL DISEASE. Spondylitis occurs in approximately 5 percent of patients with inflammatory bowel disease (ulcerative colitis, regional enteritis, and granulomatous colitis). The disease is clinically indistinguishable from primary ankylosing spondylitis but male predominance is not as striking. The shoulder is the most common peripheral joint involved, 33 percent of patients in one series.[13] There is little correlation between the extent and activity of the bowel involvement with the spondylitis. Occasionally, the spondylitis may even antedate the diagnosis of inflammatory bowel disease. Medical or surgical amelioration of the bowel disease does not seem to alter the course of the spondylitis. Treatment is similar to that of primary ankylosing spondylitis.

OSTEOARTHRITIS. Primary osteoarthritis uncommonly involves the shoulder. When this disease affects large joints there is a predilection for knees and hips. Osteoarthritis of the cervical spine with radiculopathy may cause referred pain to the shoulder that mimics primary shoulder arthritis. Patients with prior injuries to the shoulders and those placing unusual long-term stresses on the shoulder may develop secondary osteoarthritic changes. Shoulder pain in these patients may be due to degenerative changes of the glenohumeral joint but is frequently due to inflammation of the musculotendinous structures of the surrounding region. Changes of osteoarthritis on roentgenograms reveal new bone formation (osteophytes) and joint space narrowing with subchondral sclerosis (see Fig. 10-12). These findings are uncommon in inflammatory arthritis. Osteoporosis is not evident on roentgenograms unless there is long-standing disuse. Conservative treatment including mild anti-inflammatory medications, range of motion exercises, and avoidance of overuse usually provides adequate pain relief.

JUVENILE RHEUMATOID ARTHRITIS (JRA). Shoulder involvement is present in approximately 25 percent of patients with juvenile rheumatoid arthritis. Knees, ankles, wrists, and the cervical spine are more often the initial and more severely involved joints. Approximately 20 percent of patients with juvenile rheumatoid arthritis appear with an acute febrile illness that may precede the actual arthritis often for a considerable period of time. In approximately half the patients the disease is polyarticular in onset, four or more joints being involved. The remainder of the patients have mono- or oligo-articular arthritis with less than four joints affected. There is a distinctive rash that helps establish the diagnosis of juvenile rheumatoid arthritis. It is an erythematous, usually macular, rarely pruritic rash, chiefly limited to the trunks and limbs and frequently appearing only in the late afternoon or early evening during a febrile episode. The radiologic picture of juvenile rheumatoid arthritis distinguishes it from adult rheumatoid arthritis. In juvenile rheumatoid arthritis, the findings are relatively late destruction of cartilage, peripheral joint ankylosis, early involvement of the cervical spine and temporomandibular joint, and frequent periosteal new bone formation. Shoulder involvement producing erosive changes, however, may be similar to other inflammatory arthritides. If juvenile rheumatoid arthritis starts prior to bone maturation, there may be underdevelopment of the joint (Fig. 12-7).

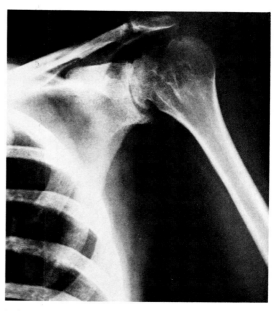

FIG. 12-7. This roentgenogram of a patient with long-standing juvenile rheumatoid arthritis demonstrates erosive changes of the humeral head, joint space narrowing, and osteophyte formation at the inferior margin of the joint. The underdeveloped humeral head and shaft distinguish it from adult onset inflammatory arthritis.

Physical therapy, rest, and salicylates usually provide adequate treatment for shoulder involvement. Intra-articular steroids are seldom used in children because of the potential deleterious effect on cartilage metabolism. Systemic therapy with parenteral gold may reduce joint inflammation in patients who have an inadequate response to high doses of salicylates.

PSORIATIC ARTHRITIS. Psoriatic arthritis is a distinctive form of arthritis present in approximately 7 percent of patients with psoriasis. Shoulder involvement occurs in up to 30 percent of patients with psoriatic arthritis, although the shoulder is not usually the first joint affected. Patients with psoriatic arthritis plus spondylitis may have an even higher incidence of shoulder disease. It is generally a mild inflammatory disease almost always involving the hands, usually in an asymmetric pattern. Distal interphalangeal joint involvement is common and it may be associated with fingernail changes such as pitting, ridging, discoloration, and thickening of the nail plate. The disease differs from rheumatoid arthritis in that it has asymmetric joint involvement, frequent early sacroiliac and spine involvement, absence of rheumatoid factor, frequent lack of systemic manifestations, and distinctive roentgenographic features. The latter features include osteolysis of the phalanges, periosteal new bone formation, erosions and widening of the distal interphalangeal joints, and ankylosis of the interphalangeal joints. Erosions may be present on the superior margin of the humeral head. However, there are no specific changes in the shoulders visible on radiograms. Psoriatic arthritis usually responds well to intermittent or long-term anti-inflammatory therapy such as high dose salicylates, indomethacin, or ibuprofen. Occasionally phenylbutazone therapy is required. Intra-articular corticosteroids for shoulder involvement unresponsive to oral anti-inflammatory medications frequently benefit the patient.

REITER'S SYNDROME. Reiter's syndrome is an acute inflammatory arthritis, primarily occurring in sexually active males and usually preceded by urethritis or dysentery. Conjunctivitis, balanitis circinata, painless superficial ulcers of the tongue and buccal mucosa and skin lesions—keratoderma blennorrhagica—are commonly associated with the arthritis. Shoulder involvement is common although it is an unusual site for initial presentation. Fingers and toes often have sausage-shaped soft-tissue swelling, and peripheral joints frequently have periosteal new bone formation visible on roentgenograms. These changes are similar to those seen in psoriatic arthritis. The erythrocyte sedimentation rate is often very elevated. There is a high association between Reiter's syndrome and the presence of the HLA B27 serotype (see Table 12-2). The symptoms of Reiter's syndrome are usually acute and short-lived but occasionally may become chronic or run an intermittent course. The disease usually responds to anti-inflammatory medications such as salicylates, indomethacin, and phenylbutazone.

The occasional use of intra-articular corticosteroids for shoulder involvement unresponsive to oral anti-inflammatory therapy is effective in relieving symptoms.

SHOULDER-HAND SYNDROME (THE REFLEX SYMPATHETIC DYSTROPHY SYNDROME). See Chapter 14.

OSTEONECROSIS. Osteonecrosis (avascular or aseptic necrosis) is a painful, destructive arthropathy thought to be caused by interruption of vascular supply to the bone. The humeral and femoral heads are the two most common sites of disease, humeral head involvement being one half to one tenth as common as that of the femoral head. The latter is a common cause of chronic hip disease. Although the incidence of osteonecrosis of the humeral head is unknown, it is not an uncommon cause of severe or chronic shoulder pain and disability. In most cases of osteonecrosis, there is no known underlying cause, but there are a large number of diseases etiologically associated with it. Hypercorticism, usually iatrogenic, has been implicated causally with increasing frequency. Patients receiving corticosteroids for treatment of systemic lupus erythematosus and rheumatoid arthritis seem especially at risk, as do patients receiving corticosteroids after renal transplantation. Sickle cell anemia patients, especially those with SC hemoglobinopathy have a high incidence of osteonecrosis. As many as 17 percent of patients with SS hemoglobin may develop shoulder osteonecrosis[5] (see Fig. 14-21). It is even more common in patients with SC hemoglobin; as many as 31 percent of patients may have shoulder involvement.[5] The putative role of corticosteroids in systemic lupus erythematosus is unknown but osteonecrosis may occur in patients never receiving corticosteroids. Alcoholism, caisson disease, Gaucher's disease, radiation therapy, and trauma are all associated with osteonecrosis. Sodium urate crystals have been found in a number of synovial specimens obtained at operation from patients with osteonecrosis implicating gout as a possible frequent etiologic cause.

In patients with caisson disease, nitrogen

bubble embolization and, in alcoholics with cirrhosis or fatty infiltration of the liver, fat embolization to the end arteries of the long bones are the likely causes of the bone necrosis. In systemic lupus erythematosus and rheumatoid arthritis without steroid use, vasculitis of the end arteries has been the suggested mechanism of disease. Infiltration of the bone and blood vessels by the glucocerebroside-containing cells in Gaucher's disease is usually found when osteonecrosis occurs. Vascular impairment, trauma, and reduced ability of bone to remodel may all play an etiologic role in producing osteonecrosis.

Roentgenogram findings of osteonecrosis are quite specific. In early stages of the disease, spotty or streaky sclerotic foci near areas of resorption and infarction are common (see Fig. 5-35). More advanced states of osteonecrosis will reveal sequestration and disintegration of bone.

Medical management of osteonecrosis is usually limited to analgesic therapy and mild anti-inflammatory medications along with joint immobilization. Patients with SS and SC hemoglobinopathy may have humeral head involvement and minimal symptoms. The disease in these patients is occasionally diagnosed during routine chest x-ray examination. In patients with severe or unremitting shoulder pain, prosthetic replacement of the humeral head may provide considerable relief of pain.

POLYMYALGIA RHEUMATICA. Polymyalgia rheumatica is a common disease entity of the elderly. It is characterized by protean symptoms including pain and stiffness of the shoulder and hip girdle, prominent morning stiffness, depression, weight loss, headache, and fatigue. A markedly elevated erythrocyte sedimentation rate, often greater than 100 mm./hour, is almost a prerequisite for diagnosis. There is a definite articular component to the disease, shoulder synovitis being most common. This may be demonstrated with radioisotopic joint scans showing increased shoulder uptake of the radionuclide. Results of physical examination are often surprisingly normal in patients in spite of a myriad of symptoms,

although modest limitation of shoulder motion may occur. Vascular bruits over large blood vessels and tenderness over the temporal arteries may also be present. The disease should be suspected in any elderly patient with shoulder girdle pain and constitutional symptoms of an ill-defined nature associated with an elevated sedimentation rate. Rheumatoid arthritis, other collagen diseases especially systemic lupus erythematosus and polymyositis, and neoplasms have to be excluded. Temporal artery biopsy specimens may reveal giant cell infiltration of the vessel wall in a patchy distribution. Sudden irreversible blindness may occur in untreated patients as a result of the vasculitis. Treatment with oral corticosteroids provides effective therapy and an unusually prompt amelioration of symptoms, usually within 48 hours.

NEUROPATHIC JOINT DISEASE (CHARCOT'S ARTHROPATHY). Neuropathic joint disease is a progressive arthropathy leading to gross destruction of the joint. It is a complication of a number of neurologic diseases that interfere with sensory innervation of the joint. Tabes dorsalis, diabetic neuropathy, and syringomyelia are frequently associated with neuropathic joint disease. The former two disorders are unusual causes of upper extremity joint disease, whereas in cervical syringomyelia upper extremity joint destruction occurs in approximately 25 percent of patients. The shoulder is the most frequently involved joint, followed by the elbow, cervical spine, and the wrist. There are often large effusions in the shoulder with markedly inflammatory joint fluid with white blood cell counts as high as 50,000/mm.[3] (Fig. 12-8). The disease is monoarticular in approximately 85 percent of the cases and is characterized by joint effusion, hypermobility, and relatively minimal pain. The complete absence of pain with shoulder involvement is unusual. Roentgenograms reveal progressive joint destruction with fragmentation and disintegration of the articular surfaces (Fig. 12-9). In spite of the extensive destruction, there is often surprisingly good joint function. Hypertrophic changes and loose joint bodies

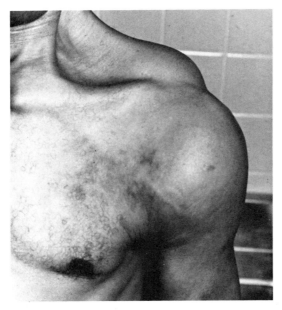

FIG. 12-8. Massive soft-tissue swelling of the shoulder in a patient with cervical syringomyelia and neuropathic joint disease. This picture corresponds temporally with Figure 12-9B.

are common initial findings. Treatment of the involved shoulder is unsatisfactory. Immobilization or restriction of use will reduce the swelling and discomfort. Intra-articular steroids have produced little pain relief, in our experience, and may hasten the progression of the disease.

AMYLOIDOSIS. Amyloidosis frequently involves the shoulder. Although almost any joint can be involved with amyloid, there is predilection for large joints, especially the shoulder. There is often striking fullness of the shoulder because of the extensive amyloid infiltration of the periarticular and synovial tissue that is sometimes called the "shoulder pad" sign. A noninflammatory joint effusion with few white blood cells and a normal mucin clot is common. Subcutaneous nodules in the absence of rheumatoid factor are considered a distinguishing feature of amyloidosis. Carpal tunnel syndrome is common because of amyloid infiltration in the subcutaneous tissue of the

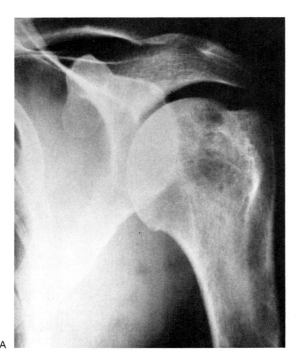

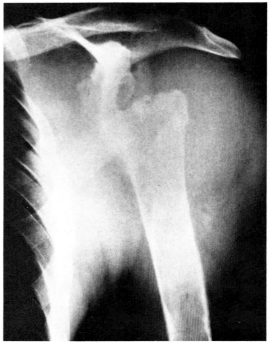

A

B

FIG. 12-9. A, Shoulder roentgenogram of the patient shown in Figure 12-8 at the onset of shoulder involvement. The patient had cervical syringomyelia with arthritic involvement of his cervical spine and contralateral elbow. B, Two years later, there is marked soft-tissue swelling and total destruction of the humeral head.

volar area of the wrist. Most patients with amyloid articular involvement have multiple myeloma as the underlying disease process.

PRINCIPLES OF TREATMENT

Systemic anti-inflammatory therapy is indicated in all patients with serious inflammatory arthritis involving the shoulder. In most patients, shoulder involvement is part of a polyarticular disease and therapy is directed toward reduction of inflammation and maintenance of function of all the joints. Except for local corticosteroid instillation into the shoulder, there is no specific oral or parenteral anti-inflammatory medication specific for shoulder arthritis. This section includes an outline of the commonly used anti-inflammatory medicines in rheumatology and indications for corticosteroid injection of the shoulder. Discussion of certain drugs, such as cyclophosphamide, azathioprine and D-penicillamine, that have extensive side effects and are limited to selected patients with rheumatoid arthritis and several other joint and vascular diseases is beyond the scope of this chapter. Readers are referred to several reviews on the treatment of inflammatory arthritis.[11,14] Drug therapy in rheumatology is not an exact science and herein is my preference for the treatment of shoulder arthritis (Table 12-4).

ASPIRIN. Salicylate therapy is the mainstay of most anti-inflammatory programs. The drug has successfully withstood the test of time regarding efficacy and safety. It is the drug of choice for most inflammatory arthritides. Its major drawback is the high doses required to achieve adequate anti-inflammatory activity. In most adults, 10 to 16 5-gr. tablets daily, administered in divided doses, are required to achieve therapeutic serum levels of 20 to 25 mg. percent. Reduction of inflammation occurs gradually after the initiation of aspirin even at these doses. Tinnitus and reversible hearing loss occur at higher salicylate levels. Upper gastrointestinal intolerance (nausea, vomiting, and epigastric discomfort) is a com-

mon side effect but is usually alleviated when the aspirin is administered with food or antacids or with the substitution of enteric-coated aspirin tablets that do not dissolve in the stomach. There is a slight increased incidence of benign gastric ulcers and of major upper gastrointestinal bleeding not due to duodenal ulcers in patients regularly taking aspirin. These two disease associations with aspirin, although statistically significant, are low in incidence when one considers the extensive use of aspirin and its high degree of effectiveness.[12] Aspirin significantly prolongs the bleeding time but this usually has little clinical significance. In young children, toxic levels of salicylate can produce systemic alkalosis followed by life-threatening acidosis. Salicylate levels should be frequently monitored in children, and signs of salicylism should be searched for in children receiving high dose aspirin therapy.

Aspirin sensitivity is an uncommon complication characterized by angioedema, rarely anaphylactic shock, bronchial asthma, rhinitis, urticaria, and nasal polyps. The symptoms may start suddenly and require epinephrine and/or aminophylline therapy, and occasionally corticosteroids. More often, symptoms of aspirin sensitivity will include a history of poorly controlled asthma or recurrent nasal polyps often requiring surgery. Indomethacin and some of the newer, mild anti-inflammatory medications such as ibuprofen have caused similar intolerance.

The mechanism of the anti-inflammatory effects of aspirin is not known. Aspirin, like many of the other anti-inflammatory drugs, suppresses prostaglandin synthesis.

CHRYSOTHERAPY. Gold therapy has been used in the treatment of rheumatoid arthritis since 1927. It has been proved effective in rheumatoid arthritis in many large and well-controlled studies and is the treatment of choice in patients with rheumatoid and juvenile rheumatoid arthritis not adequately responding to aspirin alone. The drug has also been used with sporadic success in psoriatic arthritis. Chrysotherapy should not be used in patients with mini-

Table 12-4. *Drugs Frequently Used for Inflammation of the Shoulder in Adults**

Drug	Dose	Indication	Common Side Effects
Aspirin 5-gr. tablets	Children: 80–100 mg./kg./day Adults: 10–16 tablets/day (Therapeutic serum level of approximately 20–25 percent)	Drug of choice for rheumatoid arthritis and rheumatic fever. Effective in most inflammatory arthritides. Should not be used in gouty arthritis. Doses less than 3 gm./day will raise uric acid levels.	Dose-related tinnitus; angioedema; asthma; gastrointestinal intolerance and bleeding
Chrysotherapy	Gold sodium thiomalate or gold thioglucose, 50 mg. IM weekly after test doses	Effective in rheumatoid arthritis, juvenile rheumatoid arthritis, and occasionally useful in psoriatic arthritis	Rash, proteinuria, and leukopenia, usually dose related
Colchicine 0.6-mg. tablets	Acute attacks: 0.6 mg. hourly until relief or toxicity. No more than 6 to 8 tablets/24 hours Maintenance therapy: 0.6 mg. twice daily	Considered specific therapy for acute gouty arthritis but often effective in pseudogout; most effective when used early in a gouty attack; provides adequate therapy for prevention of gouty arthritis	Abdominal cramping; diarrhea; nausea; vomiting
Ibuprofen 400-mg. tablets Naproxen 250-mg. tablets	Ibuprofen: 1200 to 2400 mg./day Naproxen: 500 mg./day in divided doses	Mild anti-inflammatory and analgesic drugs; moderately effective in most arthritides; good alternative drugs for patients intolerant to aspirin	Mild gastrointestinal intolerance; headache
Indomethacin 25-mg. capsules	50 to 150 mg. daily in divided doses	Consistently effective in gout and pseudogout; effective in ankylosing spondylitis, Reiter's syndrome, psoriatic arthritis and periarticular shoulder pain	Headache and upper gastrointestinal intolerance
Phenylbutazone 100-mg. tablets	100 to 400 mg. daily in divided doses	Consistently effective in gout and pseudogout; effective in ankylosing spondylitis, Reiter's syndrome and psoriatic arthritis (because of fatalities with agranulocytosis the drug should not be used before trial of other medication)	Sodium retention causing edema; upper gastrointestinal intolerance; agranulocytosis; aplastic anemia
Prednisone 5- and 20-mg. tablets	Dose depends on specific disease treated	Drug of choice for shoulder-hand syndrome and polymyalgia rheumatica; most effective anti-inflammatory drug	Gastrointestinal intolerance; salt retention; capillary fragility; osteoporosis; many others

* Consult textbook of pharmacology for complete listing of side effects and indications

mally active disease or in patients with only few involved joints. Gold is not recommended if the diagnosis is uncertain or if only the shoulder joints are active in a polyarticular disease. Side effects of chrysotherapy are frequent but most often are not major. Cessation of gold therapy is usually adequate treatment for most of the side effects. Rash is common and is usually preceded by pruritus. Rarely, the rash may progress to exfoliative dermatitis that requires hospitalization and corticosteroid therapy. Leukopenia and thrombocytopenia occur infrequently but require cessation of therapy. Proteinuria and nephritis occur in approximately 1 to 3 percent of patients. Eosinophilia precedes many of the toxic gold reactions, especially the leukopenia and rash. Corticosteroids will hasten recovery from most of the toxic effects of gold.

COLCHICINE. Colchicine is effective in the treatment of gouty arthritis. It is occasionally effective in pseudogout attacks and has been reported to be effective in the treatment of the acute arthritis occurring with sarcoidosis. It is the drug of choice for maintenance therapy in gout by preventing attacks of arthritis. In patients with possible gouty arthritis of the shoulder, optimal diagnostic evaluation requires aspiration of the joint and demonstration of sodium urate crystals in the synovial fluid by a polarizing light microscope. If significant effusion is not present, or appropriate laboratory facilities with a polarizing microscope are not available, then a trial of colchicine is indicated. Marked improvement within 24 to 36 hours and the demonstration of hyperuricemia constitute an acceptable method for diagnosing gout.

Maintenance therapy of gout, in order to prevent attacks, usually requires 0.6 mg. of colchicine twice daily. For the treatment of acute gouty arthritis, colchicine, 0.5 to 0.6 mg., is administered hourly for 6 hours until relief or gastrointestinal toxicity intervenes. The drug is most effective when started early in the gouty attack. Colchicine is excreted by the small intestine, and significant gastrointestinal cramping and diarrhea with marked fluid loss may occur.

These symptoms may be very serious in the elderly patient and in patients with renal insufficiency and electrolyte imbalance.

IBUPROFEN AND NAPROXEN. These drugs, newly introduced into rheumatology, have demonstrable anti-inflammatory and analgesic effects in patients with inflammatory joint disease. Both drugs are often the equal of high dose aspirin therapy in rheumatoid arthritis and osteoarthritis. Occult gastrointestinal blood loss and the frequency of upper gastrointestinal symptoms are less common than with aspirin. Major side effects are uncommon, although blurred vision, skin rash, and nausea and vomiting occur.

The role of these drugs as anti-inflammatory therapy in rheumatology is not clear. They are effective and relatively safe for shoulder arthritis but are expensive and no more effective than high dose aspirin therapy in patients with rheumatoid arthritis or osteoarthritis. Combination therapy with ibuprofen or naproxen and aspirin has provided additive anti-inflammatory effect in some patients with rheumatoid arthritis.

Patients with gastrointestinal distress or true allergic symptoms from aspirin frequently can tolerate ibuprofen or naproxen. We have used these drugs in patients with acute gouty arthritis who are unable to tolerate colchicine, indomethacin, or phenylbutazone. Both drugs are primarily excreted by the kidney and should be used in caution in patients with renal insufficiency.

INDOMETHACIN. Indomethacin has been used in the United States as an anti-rheumatic drug since 1965. The drug has anti-inflammatory, antipyretic, and mild analgesic effects. It is effective in the treatment of acute gouty arthritis and pseudogout, and in the management of most patients with ankylosing spondylitis, Reiter's syndrome, and psoriatic arthritis. The drug is helpful in acute periarticular pain of the shoulder secondary to inflammation of the musculotendinous structures. Indomethacin is not as consistently effective as aspirin in rheumatoid arthritis, juvenile rheumatoid arthritis, and osteoarthritis and should not be used routinely for these disorders.

Indomethacin is administered in doses of 25 mg. three to five times daily. Side effects include gastrointestinal intolerance, headache, and light-headedness. The headache is frequently frontal in location and often occurs on awakening. Gastrointestinal distress is minimized when the medication is taken with food or antacids. The drug should not be used in patients with, or with a past history of, ulcer disease. The drug is mainly excreted by the kidneys. Indomethacin inhibits prostaglandin synthetase activity but its exact mode of action as an anti-inflammatory drug is not known.

PHENYLBUTAZONE. Phenylbutazone is an effective anti-inflammatory drug for the treatment of gout, pseudogout, Reiter's syndrome, ankylosing spondylitis, and psoriatic arthritis. It is less effective than aspirin and should not be used routinely in most patients with rheumatoid arthritis, juvenile rheumatoid arthritis, and osteoarthritis. The side effects of phenylbutazone may be serious but are uncommon when the drug is used for short treatment periods, as in the treatment of acute gout. Nevertheless, the side effects of phenylbutazone limit the use of this drug in the treatment of uncomplicated arthritis. Upper gastrointestinal distress and salt retention are the most common adverse effects. The drug prolongs the prothrombin time in patients taking oral anticoagulants. Hematologic abnormalities include agranulocytosis and aplastic anemia that may not be reversible with cessation of therapy. Fatalities have been reported secondary to these hematologic complications. Patients with ankylosing spondylitis, psoriatic arthritis, or Reiter's syndrome unresponsive to indomethacin, aspirin, and the newer anti-inflammatory drugs may have a trial of phenylbutazone if they are cognizant of the potential complications. Frequent white blood cell determinations are performed in these patients in an attempt to monitor possible hematologic toxicity.

CORTICOSTEROIDS. The corticosteroid drugs are effective anti-inflammatory agents. The drugs have numerous, serious adverse effects and thus should not be used routinely in uncomplicated arthritis. The corticosteroids should not be prescribed in undiagnosed shoulder arthritis and should never be used when there is a possibility of septic arthritis. The drug is the treatment of choice for shoulder-hand syndrome, administered in doses of 20 to 40 mg. of prednisone daily for 10 to 14 days, followed by slow tapering of the dose. In shoulder-hand syndrome and in other arthritides requiring the use of steroids, there is frequent exacerbation of arthritis when the drug is withdrawn quickly. Corticosteroids effectively treat the vasculitis in patients with polymyalgia rheumatica, preventing eye and other major organ damage. The shoulder girdle pain and shoulder synovitis seen in polymyalgia rheumatica often respond to milder anti-inflammatory drugs but corticosteroids are the drugs of choice. Corticosteroids are frequently lifesaving in systemic lupus erythematosus, the vasculitis of rheumatoid arthritis, the heart involvement in rheumatic fever, and other forms of vasculitis and muscle inflammation. Small doses of corticosteroids (5 mg. of prednisone or its equivalent) are frequently used in reducing the morning stiffness in rheumatoid arthritis. Short courses of high dose corticosteroids are occasionally useful in relieving acute shoulder pain in patients with polyarticular disease, such as rheumatoid arthritis or psoriatic arthritis.

The adverse effects of corticosteroids are legion, and include psychiatric disturbances, osteoporosis, edema, increased susceptibility to infection, cataracts, glaucoma, gastrointestinal ulceration, and many others.

Intra-articular Corticosteroids. Intra-articular corticosteroids are effective in the treatment of inflammatory arthritis of the shoulder. The medication quickly reduces inflammation, alleviates pain, diminishes effusion, and allows joint function to return toward normal. Intra-articular corticosteroids are ideally used in a patient with polyarticular disease responding well to systemic anti-inflammatory therapy except for one or two persistently inflamed joints. In the shoulder, pain relief can be dramatic, allowing use of the joint and greatly assisting rehabilitative efforts.

Intra-articular corticosteroid treatment provides only temporary improvement but may be repeated at widely spaced periodic intervals. It is not effective in patients with degenerative, noninflammatory arthritis, and it should not be used when the diagnosis of the shoulder pain is unclear. It is contraindicated in septic arthritis.

Most rheumatologists believe that the judicious use of intra-articular corticosteroids is safe. The medication reduces inflammatory effusion and decreases the temperature of the inflamed joint, markedly reducing the proteolytic and collagenolytic effects of the lysosomal enzymes present in inflammatory joint fluid. Intra-articular corticosteroids also have deleterious effects on cartilage metabolism, limiting their frequent use.

Hydrocortisone and synthetic water-soluble corticosteroids are rapidly absorbed from joint fluid to produce high serum levels. Corticosteroids in the form of their water-insoluble salts or esters are the drugs of choice for intra-articular use. They have long-acting effects in the reduction of joint inflammation and have few systemic adverse reactions. Prednisolone tertiary butylacetate and triamcinolone hexacetonide are two examples of long-acting intra-articular preparations that are metabolized locally by synovial tissue and produce a relatively long anti-inflammatory effect.

Intra-articular corticosteroid injection is accomplished by injecting 20 to 40 mg. of prednisolone tertiary butylacetate or triamcinolone hexacetonide into the glenoid fossa just medial to the head of the humerus and below the tip of the coracoid process with a 20-gauge needle. Alternatively, injection of corticosteroids into the bulge of the humeral head just short of the periosteum with the needle placed between the periosteum and synovium will allow easy instillation into the shoulder. The corticosteroid crystals are the size of sodium urate crystals and can produce short-lived inflammation following injection. Immobilization and cold applications provide adequate treatment for this side effect.

REFERENCES

1. Ahlberg, A.: Hemophilia in Sweden. VII. Incidence, treatment and prophylaxis of arthropathy and other musculoskeletal manifestations of hemophilia A and B. Acta Orthop. Scand. (Suppl.), 77, 1965.
2. Bartfeld, H.: Distribution of rheumatoid factor activity in non-rheumatoid states. Ann. N.Y. Acad. Sci., 168:30–38, 1969.
3. Brewerton, D. A., Hart, F. D., Nicholls, A., Caffrey, M., James, D. C. O., and Sturrock, R. D.: Ankylosing spondylitis and HLA-27. Lancet, 1:904–907, 1973.
4. Calin, A., and Fries, J. F.: Striking prevalence of ankylosing spondylitis in "healthy" W27 positive males and females. N. Engl. J. Med., 293:835–839, 1975.
5. Chung, S. M. K., and Ralston, E. L.: Necrosis of the humeral head associated with sickle cell anemia and its genetic variants. Clin. Orthop., 80:105–107, 1971.
6. Cohen, A. S.: Laboratory Diagnostic Procedures in the Rheumatic Diseases, 2nd ed. Boston, Little, Brown & Co., 1975.
7. Dilsen, N., McEwen, C., Popple, M., Gersh, W. J., DiTata, D., and Carmel, P.: A comparative roentgenologic study of rheumatoid arthritis and rheumatoid (ankylosing) spondylitis. Arthritis Rheum., 5:341–368, 1962.
8. Feinstein, A. R., and Spagnuolo, M.: The clinical patterns of acute rheumatic fever: A reappraisal. Medicine, 41:279–305, 1962.
9. Gilbertsen, V. A.: Erythrocyte sedimentation rates in older patients. Postgrad. Med., 38:A44–A52, 1965.
10. Hall, A. P., Barry, P. E., Dawber, T. R., and McNamara, P. M.: Epidemiology of gout and hyperuricemia. Am. J. Med., 42:27–37, 1967.
11. Hollander, J. L., and McCarty, D. J., Jr.: Arthritis and Allied Conditions: A Textbook of Rheumatology, 8th ed. Philadelphia, Lea & Febiger, 1972.
12. Levy, M.: Aspirin use in patients with major upper gastrointestinal bleeding and peptic ulcer disease. N. Engl. J. Med., 290:1158–1162, 1974.
13. McEwen, C.: Arthritis accompanying ulcerative colitis. Clin. Orthop., 57:9–17, 1968.
14. Pearson, C., and Dick, W. C. (Eds.): Current Management of Rheumatoid Arthritis in Clinics of Rheumatic Diseases, Volume 1. Philadelphia, W. B. Saunders Co., 1975.
15. Post, M., and Telfer, M. C.: Surgery in hemophilic patients. J. Bone Joint Surg., 57A:1136–1145, 1975.
16. Schlosstein, L., Terasaki, P. I., Bluestone, R., and Pearson, C. M.: High association of an HLA antigen, W27, with ankylosing spondylitis. N. Engl. J. Med., 288:704–706, 1973.
17. Spilberg, I., Siltzbach, L. E., and McEwen, C.: The arthritis of sarcoidosis. Arthritis Rheum., 12:126–137, 1969.

13

Orthopaedic Management of the Arthritic Shoulder

MELVIN POST

It is paradoxical that a variety of disease states commonly cause such painful, disabling arthritis of the multiple joints that comprise the shoulder girdle, and yet are often excluded from the needed attention that most other similarly affected joints in the body receive. One reason is the fact that conservative and operative treatments for the shoulder arthritides have not given the gratifying results seen after such therapy for other joints. Another factor may be that such disease states as osteoarthritis, rheumatoid, and even hemophilic arthritis disable multiple other joints so severely that often the shoulder region is overlooked. It is true, for example, that the patient who is afflicted with rheumatoid arthritis of the shoulder seldom has complaints that warrant major surgery in comparison to other patients with painful joints from different disorders. But when observed these rheumatoid patients require effective multidisciplinary care, and occasionally require definitive treatment of severe shoulder arthritis. Similarly, each case of shoulder arthritis, regardless of cause, must be assessed as to which type of treatment is warranted for the individual.

The surgeon who undertakes the responsibility for managing the symptomatic arthritides should not have a pessimistic attitude. Moreover, the disease process must be understood, as well as those principles of treatment that can give successful results (see Chapter 12).

ANATOMY

The surgeon who realizes that arthritic disease can adversely affect the acromioclavicular, sternoclavicular, and glenohumeral joints, as well as the surrounding soft tissues, correctly understands that a defect in any of these structures alters the smooth function of the shoulder. Although the scapulothoracic articulation is not a true joint, its muscles must remain strong for normal shoulder function. It can compensate for a loss of glenohumeral joint function. Likewise, painful arthritic involvement of the acromioclavicular and sternoclavicular joints can compromise the normal movement of the upper extremity.

MANAGEMENT OF DISEASE STATES

It seems clear that (1) all the joints should be evaluated before starting treatment so that the type of disease can be established, (2) it be determined whether a proliferative synovitis, localized bursitis, or tendinitis is present, and (3) the extent to which damaged articular cartilage and arthritis exists be ascertained. Following this evaluation treatment priorities can be stated. In our medical center, treatment is rendered in a multidisciplinary setting whenever possible. This obviates multiple visits to multiple specialists by the patient.

Closed Treatment

As long as the patient is maintained in a comfortable, controlled state by conservative measures, open methods are avoided. Treatment of diverse conditions such as rheumatoid and hemophilic arthritis requires the "control and suppression of the inflammatory synovial process."[5] Yet, each condition needs far different methods of closed treatment. In the former, the inflammatory response is controlled with salicylates and other drugs, whereas aspirin is absolutely forbidden in the hemophilic patient. Rather, it is important to distinguish an inflamed hemophilic joint from one that is swollen following hemorrhage, for example.

In general, the occasional local intraarticular injection of steroid into the glenohumeral and clavicular joints, into an inflamed shoulder bursa, or into a bicipital tendon sheath may provide relief of pain. Failed treatment of bicipital tendinitis or bursitis may occasionally portend an arthritic state.

It is worthwhile giving the patient a physical therapy program, and using the modalities of heat and massage. It is essential to instruct the patient in the performance of shoulder exercises early in order to prevent contractures of the capsule and muscles about the shoulder, and to preserve the normal gliding movement of the tissues.[6] Violent exercises that can injure tissues are not recommended. Codman exercises that stress circumduction, external rotation, and forward flexion motion are favored.[2] It is important to know when to start an exercise program. Obviously, during an acute stage of glenohumeral synovitis or bursitis the patient is unlikely to perform exercises until there is adequate pain relief.

Open Treatment

When closed treatment methods fail or a disease process advances causing attendant symptoms surgical methods are indicated.

Bursectomy

Frequently repeated local steroid injections into bursae and the bicipital sheath are contraindicated because this therapy eventually leads to chronic irritation and fluid production on rare occasions. More commonly fibrosis and contracture will result. In any event, when pain from bursitis persists, especially when a thick-walled bursa continues to produce fluid, a bursectomy should be performed.

The bursal sac is excised through a saber-cut incision, as is used for rotator cuff repairs (see Chapter 15). The excision should not be attempted through a small incision because it may be impossible to excise the entire bursa through a limited surgical approach. Early postoperative exercises are recommended.

Synovectomy

Despite the large volume of the shoulder capsule, synovectomy is not ordinarily employed as an early definitive procedure, even in the patient with severe rheumatoid arthritis.[4] It is performed when a proliferative synovitis exists, or as a necessary part of an arthroplastic procedure. In this event, the bicipital tendon and its sheath are usually involved in the inflammatory process. In this case, I resect the intracapsular portion of the tendon and reattach the distal long head of the biceps to the humerus below.

When a persistent synovitis and associated pain are present, synovectomy can be accomplished through an anterior approach such as is used in shoulder dislocation repair or total shoulder replacement. After synovectomy the capsule is closed tightly. Early postoperative motion exercises avoiding gravity are recommended.

Resection Arthroplasty

The acromioclavicular joint is frequently affected in shoulder disease, whereas the sternoclavicular joint is rarely involved by arthritis. However, when each is involved by rheumatoid or osteoarthritis and fails to respond to conservative treatment, resection of the inner or outer ends of the clavicle (lateral to the coracoclavicular ligament) combined with synovectomy gives good results.

Arthroplasty

When the painful arthritic glenohumeral joint is disabling, shoulder arthroplasty can be rewarding. A hemiarthroplasty com-

bined with synovectomy, when needed, gives good results if the surrounding shoulder musculature, particularly the external rotators, is strong.[1] Humeral head resection may relieve pain but often fails to give satisfactory motion. Shoulder arthrodesis also relieves pain but curtails motion. When other joints are affected this procedure may create problems (Fig. 13-1). On the other hand, hemiarthroplasty performed in the presence of weak or nonfunctioning external rotator muscles may give pain relief but poor function (Fig. 13-2). Even the use of a spacer in such shoulders does not increase active motion.

Four- to eighteen-month follow-ups of two patients with fixed fulcrum total shoulder replacements for severe rheumatoid arthritis and destroyed rotator cuffs show good early results (Fig. 13-3). For the osteoarthritic shoulder, total joint replacement

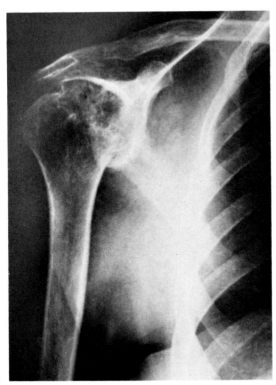 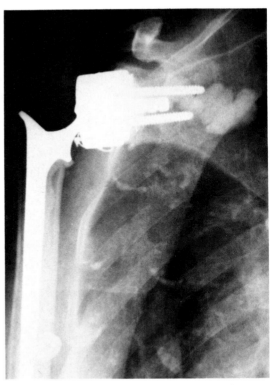

A   B

FIG. 13-1. A 50-year-old woman who had multiple joint involvement from rheumatoid arthritis had previously undergone left shoulder arthrodesis with good relief of pain. A, The right arthritic shoulder was now severely painful. The rotator cuff was markedly attenuated and nonfunctioning. B, A fixed fulcrum total shoulder replacement relieved her pain and gave the patient satisfactory passive overhead motion.

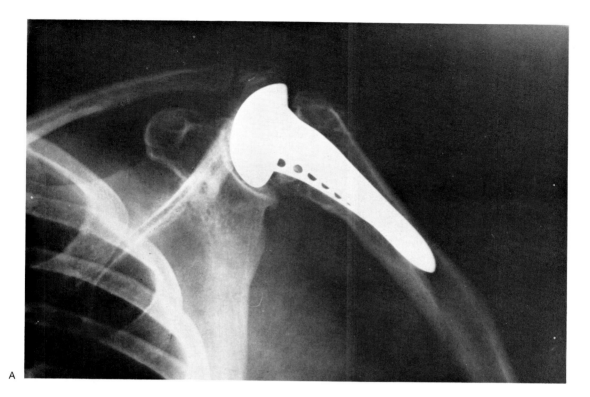

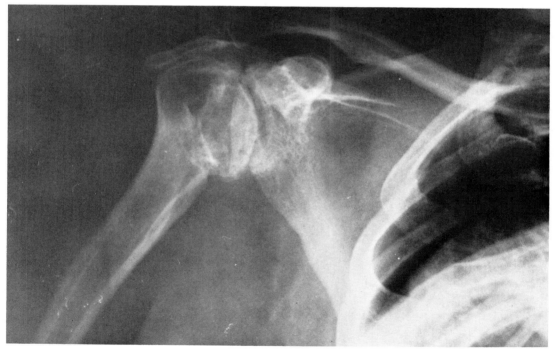

FIG. 13-2. A, A 28-year-old woman with severe rheumatoid arthritis had a Neer hemiarthroplasty of the left shoulder. There was good pain relief but the shoulder was stiff. The rotator cuff was nonfunctioning. B, The right shoulder is now severely disabled with a nonfunctioning rotator cuff. In this case, a fixed fulcrum total shoulder replacement is indicated.

also works well (Fig. 13-4) (see Chapter 10, Part B).

Glenoidectomy

In an attempt to relieve pain and restore shoulder function, Gariépy[3] and Wainwright[7] each showed their results of glenoidectomy at the Sixth Combined Meeting of the Orthopaedic Associations of the English Speaking World in 1976. Gariépy stated that removing a 7- to 8-mm. slice of glenoid through an anterior approach gave good pain relief in 12 rheumatoid shoulders. He stated that the prerequisites of this operation require (1) the humeral head not be too deformed, (2) the systemic disease not be too severe, (3) adequate musculature, and (4) postoperative supervision.[3] However,

the postoperative motion was not impressive. Wainwright performed a similar glenoidectomy through a posterior approach in nine patients with generalized arthritis, and his results equaled those of Gariépy.[7]

The procedure leaves the rotator cuff untouched, and therefore assumes that it is functioning and continues to do so, a fact that may not be true. The further statement by Gariépy that this procedure does not preclude future implant arthroplasty is true only for hemiarthroplasty, but is not true for a fixed fulcrum total shoulder replacement. For such an implant to remain fixed to the glenoid mandates that the whole cancellous glenoid vault be intact. Therefore, if total joint replacement is contemplated at any future time, I do not recommend glenoidectomy which serves to weaken the vault.

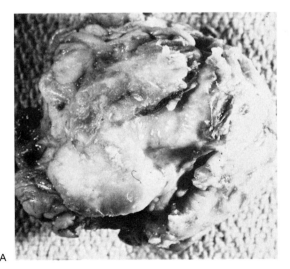

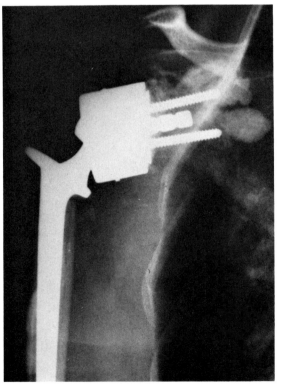

A   B

FIG. 13-3. A, A 48-year-old woman with severe rheumatoid arthritis had intractable right shoulder pain markedly decreasing hand function. Note the destructive changes in the humeral head, including the erosion on the medial side of the anatomic neck, following total shoulder replacement. B, Anteroposterior view shows total shoulder replacement. The rotator cuff could not be identified at operation.

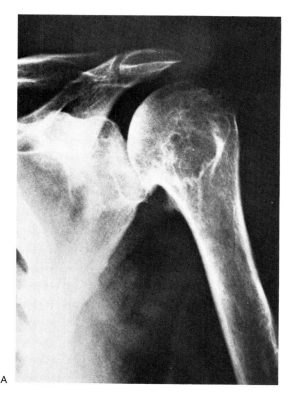
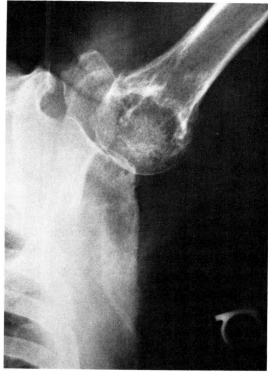

A

B

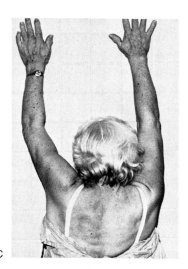
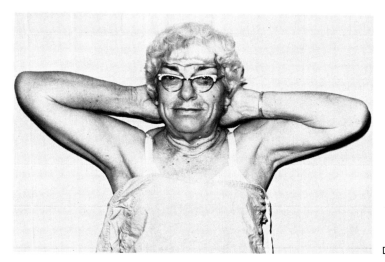

C

D

FIG. 13-4. A 63-year-old woman had severe left shoulder pain. Anteroposterior views in the, A, neutral and, B, overhead positions show osteoarthritic changes and inferior subluxation of humeral head. A nonfunctioning rotator cuff was present. A total joint replacement (series I) was performed. C and D, Multiple views show the extent of painless shoulder motion 19 months after surgery. The result so far is excellent.

REFERENCES

1. Clayton, M. L.: Personal communication, 1975.
2. Clayton, M. L., and Ferlic, D. C.: Surgery of the shoulder in rheumatoid arthritis. A report of nineteen patients. Clin. Orthop., 106:166–174, 1975.
3. Gariépy, R.: Glenoidectomy in the Repair of the Rheumatoid Shoulder. Paper read at the Sixth Combined Meeting of the Orthopaedic Associations of the English Speaking World, September 15, 1976, London.
4. Linscheid, R. L.: Surgery for rheumatoid arthritis—Timing and techniques: The upper extremity. J. Bone Joint Surg., 50-A:605–613, 1968.
5. Sbarbaro, J. L.: The rheumatoid shoulder. Orthop. Clin. North Am., 6:593–596, 1975.
6. Swanson, A. B.: Flexible Implant Resection Arthroplasty in the Hand and Extremities. St. Louis, C. V. Mosby Co., 1973.
7. Wainwright, D.: Audiovisual Presentation on Glenoidectomy—A Method of Treating the Painful Shoulder. Sixth Combined Meeting of the Orthopaedic Associations of the English Speaking World, September 15, 1976, London.

14

Miscellaneous Painful Shoulder Conditions

MELVIN POST

Of all complaints of pain afflicting man shoulder pain stands near the top of the list as to both frequency and disability. The shoulder seems to serve as the focal point for a variety of pain stimuli that may be local or referred. No other region demands a more thorough understanding of the anatomy or a greater clinical acumen when assessing pain.

Too many painful conditions about the shoulder are merely ascribed to a general category such as "fibrositis" and treated ineffectively for a prolonged time. The physician must strive to establish the etiology and the location of the disease process early, because failure to do so may lead to unnecessary muscle atrophy, restricted motion, and more pain. Every effort must be made to determine the organic nature of the pain, whether local or referred, even to decide what effect emotion has on this experience, and to prescribe appropriate treatment.

ANATOMY

The first systematic study of the nerve supply of the shoulder joint was described by Rüdinger in 1857, who showed it to be derived from the axillary and suprascapular nerves.[18] Gardner found that the nerve supply of human fetal shoulder joints arises from the axillary, suprascapular, and lateral anterior thoracic nerves, from the posterior cord, from the sympathetic ganglia, and possibly from the radial nerve.[7]

An articular branch of the axillary nerve enters the inferior region of the capsule and then ramifies, extending laterally to the bicipital sulcus, and superiorly to the anterior and posterior capsule. Recurrent branches of the radial nerve may reach both the bicipital sulcus and inferior capsule.

The suprascapular nerve gives an upper branch to the periosteum of the coracoid process, the coracoacromial ligament, and superior capsule. A lower branch of this nerve supplies the posteroinferior region of the capsule. It also supplies the scapula as well as the shoulder joint in the infraspinatus fossa.[8]

The posterior cord supplies an articular branch mainly to the anterior capsule. Gardner found that it anastomoses with the bicipital branch of the axillary nerve, and also with sympathetic fibers, and very occasionally with a twig from the lateral anterior thoracic nerve.[7] A branch from the latter nerve supplies the acromioclavicular joint. During its course, it gives a twig to the anterosuperior capsule. Thus, like the blood supply to this area, the shoulder joint region contains a rich nerve supply. It is easy to see how the surgeon may be misled into wrongly diagnosing a painful shoulder when the nerve supply overlaps so closely.

267

Some commonly and not so commonly encountered painful shoulder conditions are:

I. Musculoskeletal disorders
  A. Glenohumeral synovitis
  B. Calcific tendinitis
  C. Bicipital tendinitis and rupture
  D. Biceps tendon subluxation
  E. Muscle ruptures (pectoralis major and triceps)
  F. Frozen shoulder
  G. Glenohumeral and acromioclavicular arthritis
  H. Scapulothoracic disorders

II. Entrapment and neuritic syndromes
  A. Paralytic brachial neuritis
  B. Supraclavicular nerve entrapment
  C. Carpal tunnel syndrome
  D. Compression syndromes secondary to bone lesions

III. Neurovascular compression syndromes
  A. Scalene anticus syndrome
  B. Axillary venous thrombosis compression syndrome
  C. Costoclavicular syndrome
  D. Brachiocephalic vascular syndrome
  E. Subclavian steal syndrome
  F. Sympathetic disorders (shoulder-hand syndrome)

IV. Storage diseases
  A. Alkaptonuria
  B. Gaucher's disease

V. Arthropathies
  A. Sickle cell disease
  B. S-C disease
  C. S-thalassemia
  D. S-A disease
  E. Decompression sickness
  F. Hemophilia

VI. Unusual causes of shoulder pain
  A. Tietze's syndrome
  B. Friedrich's disease
  C. Sternoclavicular hyperostosis

MUSCULOSKELETAL DISORDERS

Acute Synovitis of Glenohumeral Joint

Synovitis of the shoulder joint is uncommon when compared to the frequency of the condition in other joints such as the knee joint. The causes for shoulder joint synovitis are the same as those for other joints, namely, most often the arthritides, trauma, and infections. The inflamed synovium may produce a considerable volume of synovial fluid and is symptomatic of the disease state.

The joint is swollen and movements are painful. Often, the humeral head may subluxate inferiorly not only because of the effusion but also as a result of the lost tone in the shoulder girdle muscles.

The diagnosis may be established by aspirating the joint and examining the synovial fluid. An attempt should be made to obtain a specific diagnosis (see Chapter 12 on Rheumatology). Treatment varies with the cause of this condition. However, immobilization of the extremity remains the cornerstone of treatment. When the joint inflammation subsides an effective rehabilitation program to restore joint motion and muscle strength is necessary for best results.

Calcific Tendinitis

Calcific tendinitis, subdeltoid bursitis, and subacromial bursitis are terms that represent a progression of a disease process that can cause excruciating pain. The condition is most often observed in people over 30 years of age, and seldom in young adults.[17]

PATHOLOGY AND PATHOGENESIS. The subacromial bursa lies beneath the superior portion of the deltoid muscle and extends upward beneath the acromion. It separates the greater tuberosity of the humerus from the deltoid muscle and acromion (see Fig. 15-2A). The subdeltoid bursa is a large one between the deep surfaces of the deltoid and the joint capsule (see Fig. 15-2A). Both bursae are frequently continuous and serve to decrease friction when the humerus moves beneath the acromion. The walls of the bursae are usually loose and collapsed. In any event, the inner walls are well lubricated by a thin layer of bursal fluid.

In most cases, bursal inflammation starts as a result of pathologic changes in the underlying tendon.[2,5] Pedersen and Key found that in patients suffering from calcific subdeltoid bursitis the basic process was degeneration of the tendon or muscle in the rotator cuff.[16] Calcified deposits may lie dormant in the tendon for years.[20] The calcium salts deposit in the necrotic collagen tissue. This material becomes enclosed, forming a granuloma that eventually becomes visible on roentgenograms. Subsequently, the calcific mass, composed of calcium salts, produces a swelling much like a boil. Its core is white with a turgid zone about the center. Until this point is reached there are few or no symptoms. Then all at once the slightest event such as turning in bed, according to Codman,[6] causes tension in the tendon and leads to rupture of a few superficial fibers, allowing the calcified particles to discharge into the bursa (Fig. 14-1).

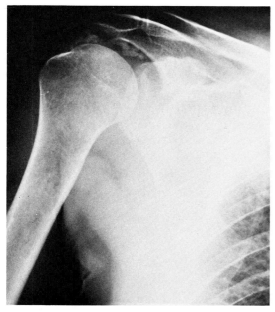

FIG. 14-1. A 55-year-old man merely raised his arm above his head and developed excruciating pain in the right shoulder. An anteroposterior roentgenogram showed an extensive calcification of the subacromial bursa. The anterolateral aspect of the shoulder joint was swollen and exquisitely tender. He was treated with aspiration of the semiliquid calcific mass through an 18-gauge needle and intra-articular injection of steroid. He had immediate relief of pain. The following day motion exercises were started. Symptoms have not recurred after several years.

Thus, an acute bursitis is produced. Increased fluid is produced and mixes with the calcified particles. The walls of the bursa become distended. Fibrin formation traps the specks of calcium. After the calcified particles are forced into the bursa and enmeshed in fibrin they are rapidly eliminated by the action of leukocytes.

Codman stated that perforation into the bursa was nature's way of clearing the calcium particles and mitigating the symptoms without treatment.[6] However, when the inflammation of the bursa is intense a "frozen shoulder" may result. The defect in the base of the bursa is nearly always present over the critical zone. Codman believed that varying degrees of supraspinatus rupture are the basis of almost all the lesions noted in this area.[6]

Within the bursa, synovial villi are commonly present. Codman also reported finding cordlike bands of fibrous consistency, like the bands found in the olecranon bursa at operation.[6] Adhesions form between the inflamed walls of the bursa often acting as one mechanism for producing a frozen shoulder.

On attempting to aspirate a soft calcific mass during an acute attack of bursitis, not uncommonly several milliliters of slightly yellow clear fluid may first be obtained. It was Codman's contention that in this case the supraspinatus is ruptured and permits a free communication between the joint and bursa.[6]

DIAGNOSIS. Calcific tendinitis is most often seen in middle-age adults, although I have treated an increasing number of patients in their twenties. There does not appear to be any correlation of pain and injury, or use of the arm. Why some persons are more prone than others to accumulation of calcium deposits in the supraspinatus tendon is still a mystery.

In the acute phase the patient holds the shoulder at the side absolutely still. He complains of severe ache in the shoulder especially at night. The level of the pain may range from a dull ache to excruciating unbearable pain. Often, the patient may complain that the pain is over the lateral aspect of the deltoid distally rather than at the point from where it originates at the joint. Any attempt to abduct or rotate the arm increases pain. If the arm is elevated the scapula may rotate while the glenohumeral joint is fixed. Occasionally, in a thin person swelling is seen over the site of the calcium deposit. This spot may be exquisitely tender, or the tenderness may be diffuse over the region. Most often the patient resists any movement, but when the arm is gently abducted the point of tenderness may disappear beneath the acromion (Dawbarn's sign).

When a history of injury is obtained, 1 to 3 days usually elapse before the pain of the bursitis attack intensifies. In these instances, the patient often states he has used much local heat as therapy in the vain hope of relieving his suffering.

Multiple roentgenograms of the arm should be taken in order to disclose a calcium deposit (Fig. 14-2).[4,5] In my experience, even a small calcium deposit detected on the roentgenogram may cause substantial degrees of pain. Even though most attacks of shoulder bursitis are subacromial or subdeltoid, it is important for the surgeon to know the locations of multiple other bursae about the shoulder which may be the source of pain when inflamed. In early disease states the shoulder may appear normal on roentgenograms. Later, sclerosis of the tuberosities, eburnation, spicules, small detached particles of bone, or cystic bone changes may appear (Fig. 14-3). I no longer employ local injection of anesthetics for diagnosis. Rather, I rely more on the history and examination, reserving the injection of local anesthetic and steroid for treatment.

TREATMENT. When the symptoms of true bursitis are mild to moderate the condition may be treated conservatively. The extremity is rested in a sling for several days, and analgesics are taken for pain. I do not recommend using local heat in the very acute

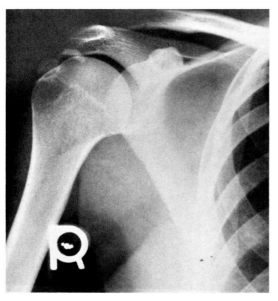
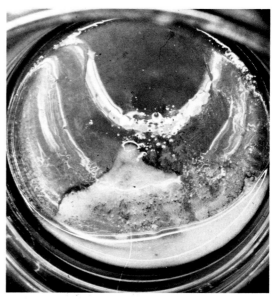

A   B

FIG. 14-2. A 28-year-old woman complained of excruciating pain during a 24-hour period after having lifted her infant. A, An anteroposterior film reveals a calcification in the subacromial bursa overlying the supraspinatus tendon. Note the sclerosis of the greater tuberosity, indicating that the disease process had been present for some time. When the head of the humerus disappeared beneath the acromion the pain lessened. B, A large amount of calcium salt was obtained after the bursa was irrigated with 40 ml. of 0.5 percent local anesthetic. When the fluid was decanted, whitish calcium salts appeared to be toothpastelike in consistency. The aspiration process was repeated 48 hours later because of an exacerbation of severe pain. During this aspiration, 2 cc. of straw-colored bursal fluid were obtained along with additional calcium salts.

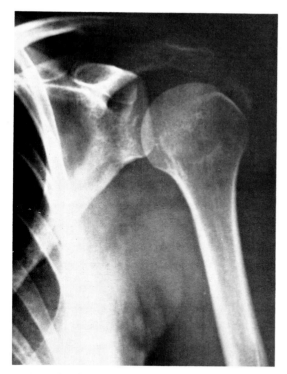

FIG. 14-3. A middle-age adult complained of moderate shoulder pain for 1 week. Note the calcification in the subdeltoid bursa and the sclerosis of the greater tuberosity. Relief was obtained through the intra-articular injection of local steroid even though a minimum amount of calcium salts was obtained during attempted aspiration.

phase as this often intensifies the pain. Instead, I advise the patient to use cold packs to the shoulder for relief of pain. After the acute phase is over and gentle motion exercises are begun, gradually increasing activity over 4 to 6 weeks, a mild amount of local heat can be employed if the patient desires. Although I prescribe short courses of oral anti-inflammatory drugs in many cases, I believe the occasional well-placed injection of steroid is more effective.

Injection Therapy. When severe pain cannot be controlled by simple measures, then injection of local anesthetic and intra-articular preparations of steroids into the inflamed site is useful.[57] This form of treatment may abort an attack of subdeltoid bursitis, in a high percentage of cases, that otherwise would have disabled the patient over an extended period of time.

While the location of calcium deposit on roentgenograms is desirable more reliance should be placed on a careful examination of the patient and the most painful, tender spot selected for injection.[13,15] While the patient is recumbent and the shoulder raised on a roll behind the shoulder blade, the skin is surgically prepared and draped. A sterile injection kit is used for injection. A wheal is raised with a 25-gauge needle using 1 percent local anesthetic. A long 18-gauge needle is inserted into the tender site, and the local anesthetic is slowly infiltrated as the needle is advanced. When the calcium mass is penetrated there is sudden, momentary intense pain if the calcium mass is under tension. At this point a definite resistance is felt. One or two milliliters of anesthetic are injected and the plunger of the syringe is released or pulled back. Often a cloudy white fluid is seen, indicating calcium particles in the anesthetic irrigating fluid. The material may be as thick as toothpaste and homogeneous, or appear as amorphouslike small clumps (Fig. 14-2B). If two needles are simultaneously used for irrigation, saline solution may be employed to wash the bursa. Although much calcium material may be obtained, I have never been able to totally evacuate the entire calcium mass as evidenced by roentgenograms. Nevertheless, in most cases there are dramatic relief of pain and early recovery from the disability.

Before withdrawing the needle steroid is injected into the bursa. The patient is advised not to use local heat for the first 24 to 36 hours following injection or needle irrigation, as this merely increases the hyperemia in the bursal wall. Rather, cold applications are recommended. Occasionally, pain does not abate and the treatment is repeated within a few days. I have found an increased incidence of the collection of clear straw-colored bursal fluid in the aspirate of such cases and even the accumulation of additional calcium material not obtainable during the first treatment. In these cases, it is likely that the bursa connects with the joint through ruptured supraspinatus fibers. This treatment is safe if aseptic principles are scrupulously followed. In many thousands of injections into bursae and joints at Michael Reese Medical Center over the years, there has been only one case of infection resulting from such treatment.

I do not believe it matters whether the arm is held abducted or at the side after injection as long as early motion exercises are started, which is a chief goal of such treatment. I prefer to place the shoulder through a complete range of motion under the protection of the local anesthetic. As the local anesthetic dissipates, pain often increases for 24 to 36 hours. Usually, motion exercises may be started in earnest the next day. The patient must be impressed with the importance of this part of the treatment in order to avoid a frozen shoulder that will only prolong treatment.[12]

Surgical Management. Rarely, when the simpler forms of treatment fail to relieve pain, the mass of calcified material should be excised.[3,11] In this event the calcified deposits may be found to be multiple, varying in size from a pinhead to much larger. They may be buried in the supraspinatus tendon, even replacing the tendon fibers, or appear as a tense boil impinging on the overlying inflamed bursal wall. Fluid within the bursa itself may appear cloudy with whitish calcium material.

The patient is placed in a semireclining position with a sandbag behind the back, and the involved extremity surgically prepared and draped free. The rotator cuff is exposed by a saber-cut incision, as is used for the exploration of the rotator cuff. A 5-cm. vertical incision may be used alternatively, starting at the acromial edge, if extreme care is taken not to split the deltoid fibers more than 3.8 cm. distally in order not to injure the branches of the axillary nerve.

The bursa is opened. The arm may be rotated to further inspect the rotator cuff structures. All calcium deposits are removed from the bursal floor and supraspinatus tendon. Thereafter, only the edges of the deltoid fascia are sutured, followed by skin closure. The arm is placed in 20 degrees of abduction for a few days and gentle motion exercises are then started. Sling immobilization is terminated as soon as the pain permits. Pain relief is dramatic.

Complete Acromionectomy. It is seldom necessary to perform total acromionectomy when treating painful shoulders. Armstrong reported on 95 acromial excisions used for painful shoulders resulting from periarthritis, "frozen shoulder," or a supraspinatus lesion, when it was thought a mechanical impingement was present and conservative treatment had failed.[1] Armstrong stated that persistent, prolonged disabling pain often requires such an operation.[1] He also believed that true limitation of shoulder movement and a doubtful diagnosis were contraindications to this procedure. Hammond agreed with this viewpoint.[9,10] He emphasized that there must be a complete active or passive range of motion. Surgery should not be performed when shoulder motion is limited by adhesive capsulitis since the condition can be made worse.[1] First, motion should be restored if such surgery is contemplated for pain relief.

The statement that complete excision of the acromion does not cause untoward effects is not always true. I have found significant loss of deltoid power in such cases subsequently referred for shoulder arthroplasty because of progression of the disease state. It is true that new bone can form in the reattachment of the deltoid to raw bone, but it does not follow that complete acromionectomy is needed to provide relief of symptoms.

Partial Anterior Acromionectomy. Partial anterior acromionectomy, advocated by Neer, is recommended for patients with evidence of chronic bursitis who may have partial tears of the supraspinatus tendon and are thought to have pain resulting from mechanical impingement of the irritated supraspinatus area beneath the anterior acromial edge.[14] Experience has shown that Neer is correct when he advises removal of the anterior edge and the undersurface of the acromion in this situation.[14] If adhesions or spurs are discovered at operation and are likely to cause impingement on the rotator cuff they are removed. (For details of the surgical procedure, see Chapter 15 on

Rotator Cuff Injuries.) In these instances, the attached coracoacromial ligament is also removed. It is unnecessary to perform lateral or total acromionectomy in most patients, since the pathologic lesion most often resides beneath the anterior lip of the acromion. Moreover, total acromionectomy is disabling because more often than not the deltoid is weakened when it loses its normal fulcrum. Some of these patients later require extensive shoulder arthroplasties and it would be better if the acromion has not been removed.

Paraglenoid Osteotomy of Scapula. Stamm and Crabbe recommended paraglenoid osteotomy through the neck of the glenoid as an alternative method for treating intractable painful shoulder conditions caused by bursitis.[19] The rationale for this operation revolves around the downward displacement of the glenoid and humerus so that there is no longer any friction between the humerus and the acromion. The technique is essentially the same as that described for recurrent posterior shoulder dislocations, except that the osteotomy is directed obliquely so that the glenoid can be levered downward. I have no experience with this operation for relief of shoulder pain, but it is apparent that it should be used only in highly selected cases.

Bicipital Tendinitis and Ruptures

A common cause of shoulder pain is disease of the long head of the biceps tendon. Too many surgeons tend to dismiss this painful condition as one that will automatically abate with "tincture of time." Unfortunately for many patients this is not true. As long as the biceps tendon and its investment sheath are involved in a disease process, the resulting pain prevents normal shoulder function.

ANATOMY. The long head of the biceps resides within the capsule and yet is not within the synovial cavity, although it is covered by the synovium. When the glenohumeral joint is fixed the biceps muscle provides three functions: (1) flexes the forearm on the arm, (2) aids in supinating the

forearm if the radius is pronated, and (3) elevates the arm forward and brings it into a medial position. If the forearm is fixed, the biceps elevates the shoulder, and acts on the arm, flexing it on the forearm.[32]

The biceps muscle is innervated by a branch of the musculocutaneous nerve, supplying both the long and short heads after the branch divides.

PATHOLOGY AND PATHOGENESIS. In 1928, Meyer called attention to the supratubercular ridge, a bony ridge on the lesser tuberosity.[42] He described the widening, flattening, and fibrillation of the articular portion of the biceps tendon, and its attrition and fraying of the intra-articular and intertubercular portions, reporting complete tears in some cases. That these changes and eventual rupture may be the result of tenosynovitis was suggested by Ewald in 1927.[30] Codman doubted that such a lesion existed.[6] Gilcreest stated that there was a "common bicipital syndrome" wherein wear and tear of the tendon caused subsequent rupture and dislocation of the tendon.[32] He stated that in older persons degenerative changes occur, the muscles lose their normal elasticity, and eventual tearing of some muscle fibers results. The long head of the biceps also undergoes continual attrition, which may not be painful but finally causes rupture.

Lippmann believed that bicipital tendinitis was the basic lesion in the causation of frozen shoulder.[40] He showed that the biceps tendon does not move passively in its groove when the biceps is contracted. Rather, motion of the shoulder entails movement of the humeral head along the long head. There is minimal excursion of the tendon during internal rotation of the arm and maximal excursion during external rotation.

Waugh and associates reported on 50 cases of rupture of the long head of the biceps and believed that many cases are unrecognized and untreated.[50] Hitchcock and Bechtol stated that lesions of the long head of the biceps were a common cause of shoulder pain and disability.[33] They believed that a shallow bicipital groove was a contributing cause to dislocation of the tendon. They supported Meyer's contention that the supratubercular ridge helped to prevent dislocation of the tendon.[42] They concluded that a shallow or flat bicipital groove permitted easy dislocation of the tendon. It was also shown that during motion, if the tendon of the long head of the biceps was involved by adhesions, the limited excursion of this structure transmitted a pull on the sensitive surrounding tissues, including the periosteum and fasciae. Thus, pain production may be due largely to stretching of these adhesions during motion. It is this fact that led Hitchcock and Bechtol to suggest resection of the long head of the biceps tendon and fixation of its distal portion in the raw bed of its groove.[33]

Crenshaw and Kilgore, in a series of surgically treated cases, showed that in the acute stage of bicipital tendinitis there were capillary dilatation, edema of the tendon and synovium, and cellular infiltration of these structures, the end result being the formation of adhesions between the tendon and its sheath.[27]

In the chronic phase the biceps tendon becomes frayed, narrowed, and fibrosed, which results in the formation of dense adhesions between the tendon and its sheath. Any surgeon who has once operated upon such a case cannot doubt these pathologic changes, or the existence of this entity as a cause of shoulder pain.

DIAGNOSIS. The chief complaint of the patient is pain over the anterior shoulder. The onset of pain may be acute or insidious. In young adults, a history of excessive use of the shoulder such as in playing tennis is often given as a cause of the pain. Often, the patient cannot precisely isolate his discomfort and may lay the hand over the whole front of the shoulder. The one constant feature in pinpointing the diagnosis is mild to severe tenderness along the intertubercular groove. Absence of tenderness suggests that another diagnosis is likely.

Occasionally, full overhead motion may be limited in the shoulder joint of such patients. In the vast majority, there is a normal range of shoulder motion. Codman

showed that peritendinitis of the long head of the biceps may be associated with other lesions, such as supraspinatus rupture.[6]

Three signs are often associated with this condition.[50] The tests are described in Chapter 2 on Diagnosis. They are (1) Yergason's supination sign, in which a positive response indicates wear and tear of the long head of the biceps or synovitis of its sheath; (2) Ludington's sign, in which a positive result indicates rupture; and (3) Heuter's sign, in which flexion of the pronated forearm is more energetic when the biceps is tense than when the forearm is supinated. Contraction of the biceps in pronation causes a movement of supination immediately afterward. This sign is absent with biceps tendon disruption. Lippmann described still another test that causes sharp pain when the examiner's finger moves the biceps tendon from side to side in its groove.[40] Crenshaw and Kilgore described a useful test, called Speed's test.[27] The patient anteriorly elevates the shoulder against resistance while extending the elbow and supinating the forearm. A positive response occurs when pain is limited to the bicipital groove. These tests are not pathognomonic but suggest a disease state in the region of the bicipital groove.

MANAGEMENT. Most cases can be treated conservatively by resting the extremity in a sling and using analgesics as required for pain relief. Although I have employed local steroid injections in the more resistant cases, I am less than convinced that there is a consistent, lasting effect from such treatment. In fact, one wonders whether multiple steroid injections may be deleterious considering the marked changes noted in patients receiving such injection therapy. In any event, one or two steroid injections may prove useful in some patients.

In the occasional case of chronic bicipital tenosynovitis that is resistant to all conservative measures, over 4 to 6 months of pain relief can be achieved with surgical treatment. Especially if a frozen shoulder results or is impending, little hope for relief of pain is possible so long as the causative factors remain uncorrected.

The goal of surgical treatment is to eliminate the movement of the biceps tendon-tendon sheath structures in the bicipital groove, and to release any adherence of the tendon to the surrounding structures. Gilcreest described a method of attaching a distal ruptured end to the short head of the biceps or to the coracoid process.[32] Lippmann sutured the tendon to the lesser tuberosity.[40] DePalma[28] and DePalma and Callery[29] described an operation wherein they cut the tendon near its origin and remove it from its sheath and groove, and suture it to the coracoid process or to the short biceps. Suture of the biceps to the short head of the biceps (Fig. 14-4), or the method of Hitchcock and Bechtol[33] work well in providing pain relief. In the latter operation, after the proximal portion is resected, the long head of the biceps tendon is sutured to the floor of the raw intertubercular groove.

The aforementioned operations may be accomplished in the following manner. After draping of the extremity as in a shoulder repair for dislocation, a curvilinear incision is made over the deltopectoral groove.

The deltoid and pectoral muscles are separated and the tendinous cuff is inspected.

The capsule and transverse humeral ligament are incised over the long biceps tendon, thereby allowing visualization of the biceps tendon in its groove (Fig. 14-4A). Abduction of the extremity will disclose whether the tendon moves freely in its groove or is adherent.

For the transfer of the damaged tendon to the short biceps tendon, a $\frac{1}{4}$-in. incision is made in the capsule superiorly, near the origin of the long head of the biceps, and the tendon severed. It is withdrawn from its sheath and either sutured to the scarified surface of the short head of the biceps under slight tension, or woven through a slit in this structure and then sutured to itself and excess tendon is excised (Fig. 14-4B).

In the Hitchcock-Bechtol method, the floor of the groove is made raw using a $\frac{1}{4}$-in. curved gouge. The distal tendon is roughened and attached beneath a raised osteoperiosteal flap using heavy suture. The proximal intra-articular portion of the tendon is resected.

The shoulder is placed through a com-

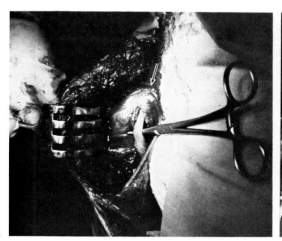 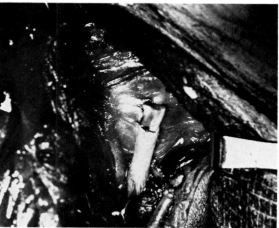

A   B

FIG. 14-4. A 30-year-old woman failed to respond to multiple local injections of steroid for bicipital tendinitis over a 2-year period. A, At operation, the long head of the biceps tendon was visualized in its groove after incision of the transverse humeral ligament. Note the frayed tendon surface overlying the hemostat. A small $\frac{1}{4}$-in. incision was made in the superior capsule near the glenoid rim (arrow). The biceps tendon was transected at its glenoid origin and the tendon withdrawn below. Multiple adhesions were found between the tendon and its groove. The long head of the biceps was transferred to the coracoid region. B, The scarified tendon is shown sutured in place to the base of the coracoid and the surrounding soft tissues (or it may be woven, under slight tension, through a slit made in the short head of the biceps). After completion of the repair, excess tendon is removed.

plete range of motion before closure in either operation. The wound is closed.

Aftercare includes rest of the extremity in a sling for 10 to 14 days and then the initiation of gentle passive motion exercises. After 3 to 4 weeks, active motion exercises are allowed and gradually increased. It is not unusual for the patient to have some difficulty in attaining complete overhead motion until 6 to 8 weeks postoperatively. Violent exercises should be avoided for 6 weeks.

Either operation provides for pain relief and does not appear to weaken the shoulder.

Rupture of Biceps Muscle or its Tendon

The biceps ruptures commonly in comparison to similar structures in the body. The pathologic alterations leading to rupture in elderly adults have been described under the section on Bicipital Tendinitis.

Ruptures of muscles or their tendons are the result of muscle action. In the older adult a less forceful contraction is needed to rupture the long head of the biceps, for example, than in the younger adult patient. In the former case, degenerative pathologic changes in the tendon permit relatively easy rupture (Fig. 14-5). In fact, there may be no history or only a slight history of trauma, whereas in the younger patient a history of acute trauma is often elicited (Fig. 14-6).[34] Such a history may include the lifting of very heavy objects.[47] The sudden contracture of the biceps muscle against an asynchronous movement may cause such a tendon rupture.

In the elderly patient, long-standing attrition of the tendon may lead to elongation of the tendon and eventual complete rupture. The distal end may reattach spontaneously in its groove or to the transverse humeral ligament. Occasionally, the intrascapular portion of the long head of the biceps may disappear completely or fuse with its joint capsule.

The biceps brachii may rupture at any place along its course, depending on the force and mechanism of injury. Since there is greater wear on the flattened long tendon portion as it passes over the articular surface of the head, it is understandable why proximal rupture occurs much more frequently than distal rupture, although the latter is by no means as rare as once was believed.[23,31,50]

DIAGNOSIS. Most patients report a sudden "snap" that occurs in the act of lifting light to heavy objects. Occasionally, the older patient cannot recall any history of injury. In any event, the patient may feel mild to considerable pain over the muscle structure and bunching up of the muscle with attempted contraction, and observe ecchymosis (Figs. 14-5 and 14-6). The patient may complain of some weakness in the arm, although he may be more disturbed merely by his inability to contract the muscle.

Bunching of the muscle belly is the most common finding. If the long head of the biceps is ruptured, the bunching of the muscle is distal, whereas rupture of the distal biceps brachii tendon causes the contracted belly of the biceps muscle to appear high above the crease of the elbow (Fig. 14-7). In the latter case, occasionally the distal biceps tendon is intact and biceps brachii muscle fibers are torn and pulled upward.

MANAGEMENT. Treatment of the rupture depends on the site and degree of rupture, preexisting disease, the age and occupation of the patient, and his future requirements. For example, in the elderly patient who is retired, surgical correction is not necessary, but a rupture in a younger or middle-age laborer often requires repair in order to restore needed strength of the arm. Good judgment and discussion of the condition with the patient are needed for the treatment that is selected for the individual.

If the tear is incomplete or conservative treatment is recommended by the surgeon, the extremity should be immobilized in a sling for 2 or 3 weeks with the elbow flexed about 90 degrees in the acute case. After 3 weeks, gentle exercises are begun.

If surgery is selected as the best method

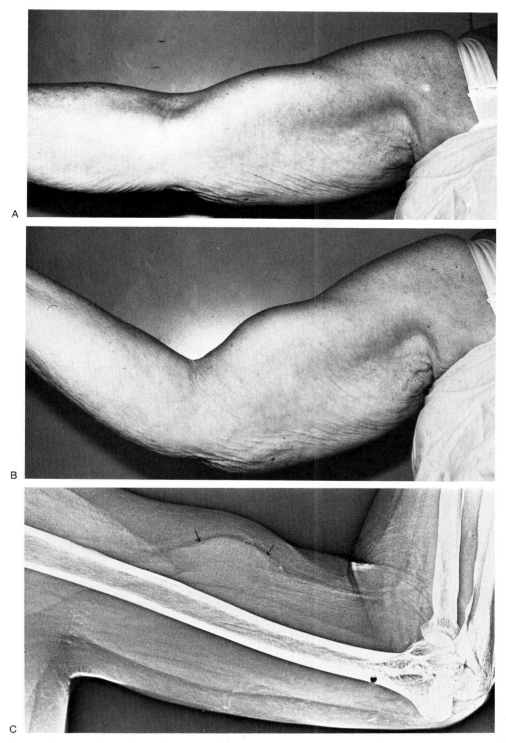

FIG. 14-5. A 65-year-old woman tore the proximal portion of the long head of the biceps tendon after lifting a 10-pound object. A, Note the relatively normal looking contour of the biceps muscle with the arm extended. B, With slight flexion, notice the bunching up of the muscle belly distally. C, Xeroradiogram shows the bunching of the muscle belly distally and the proximal depression in the soft tissue on the anterior aspect of the injured arm.

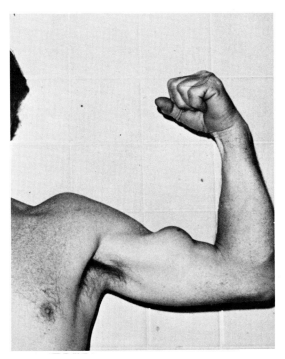

FIG. 14-6. A 48-year-old man tore the proximal long head of the biceps tendon of the left arm while wrestling. Note the bunching of the muscle belly distally in the left arm. The patient refused surgical treatment because there was good residual strength and little functional impairment.

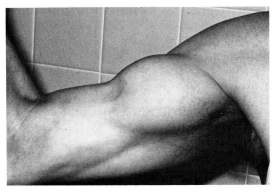

FIG. 14-7. A young man tore his distal biceps tendon while lifting a heavy object. During extension of the arm, there was a relatively normal-appearing outline of the biceps contour. Forty-eight hours after injury, however, note the proximal bunching of the biceps muscle belly during flexion. Ecchymosis was seen in the cubital fossa. The patient had a desk job and few symptoms. He refused surgical repair.

for treating a rupture of the long head of the biceps, I prefer to suture the distal end to the scarified short head of the biceps near its insertion into the coracoid process, passing it through a slit in the short tendon. If rupture occurs in the middle of the tendon, the fresh edges can be overlapped and sutured together providing the tissue is not greatly degenerated. In the very rare event that the biceps brachii function is destroyed, the method of Clark, transplanting a portion of the pectoralis major, may be used to restore function if such function is desirable.[25]

Wagner[49] and Friedmann[31] reported on their techniques for reinserting a ruptured tendon of the distal biceps. In Friedmann's method a hole is made in the region of the radial tuberosity, and the tendon pulled into the medullary canal of the radius by wires placed through holes drilled in the distal cortex.[31] He uses the pullout wire technique and reported good results in 13 cases. However, the reader must be careful not to injure the surrounding neurovascular structures when attempting a repair of the torn distal biceps tendon.

Boyd and Anderson reported on their method of reinserting the distal biceps tendon into the radial tuberosity.[24] In their operation a curvilinear incision is made over the cubital fossa. The torn distal end of the biceps is located. With blunt dissection the original tunnel between the ulna and radius is located. After flexing the patient's elbow an incision is made on the posterolateral elbow. The muscles attached to the lateral olecranon are elevated and retracted laterally along the plane of the interosseous membrane, thereby exposing the head and neck of the radius. Care is taken to avoid injury to the motor branch of the radial nerve.

The patient's forearm is pronated to allow visualization of the radial tuberosity. A trapdoor is made in the tuberosity and two drill holes are made at the base of the hinge. Heavy suture placed through the severed tendon is passed through the radius and ulna and out the second incision. The heavy suture is threaded through the holes in the base of the trapdoor. The elbow is flexed, and the tendon placed into the trapdoor and held with a forceps as the heavy suture is tied. Reinforcing sutures are placed in the surrounding tissues.

The elbow is immobilized in a plaster of Paris splint in 110 degrees of flexion in moderate supination. At 2 weeks postoperatively, a new splint is applied for 4 additional weeks. Thereafter, motion exercises are gradually increased.

Subluxation of Biceps Tendon

Subluxation or dislocation of the long head of the biceps from its groove is not as common in the young adult as in the older patient. O'Donohue reported 10 cases of subluxating biceps tendon, 8 of the cases occurring during sport activity.[43] In the younger patients degenerative change is not the chief reason for this condition. Meyer reported three factors in normal joints, and possibly six factors in all, that favor dislocation.[42] He cited the supratubercular ridge, and the anterior wall of the sulcus formed by the lesser tuberosity that normally acts as a trochlea for the tendon in the usual position of medial rotation. The other factors that favor dislocation include the normal course of the intracapsular portion of the tendon and its relation to the humeral head, the much greater width of the proximal portion of the tendon, the possibility that the capsular attachment may be weakened by intracapsular bursae, and possible restriction of the capsular attachment to the anatomic neck in the region proximal to the lesser tuberosity. He was not impressed with the ability of the transverse humeral ligament to retain the tendon in its groove.

In a classic paper, Abbott and Saunders reviewed the literature and described the function of the long head of the biceps. They showed that at the start of abduction the humeral head glides upward on the long head of the biceps, and then downward with further abduction.[21] They described the functional synchronization of the shoulder muscles and believed that the long

head of the biceps mechanically guides and redirects the humeral head in its backward and downward path so that glenohumeral motion is harmonious.

Hitchcock and Bechtol described the variation in the angle of the medial wall of the bicipital groove as ranging from 90 to 15 degrees.[33] Seventy percent of the cases had a 60- to 75-degree angle. As the angle decreases toward 15 degrees and the groove becomes shallow, there is a tendency for the bicipital tendon to slip medially over the lesser tuberosity.

DIAGNOSIS. There may be a history of a definite and severe wrenching injury, followed by a disability. A young patient often complains that there is a painful snap in his shoulder, especially when throwing an object. The tendon may snap over the lesser tuberosity as the arm is positioned in external rotation, and snap back into its groove in the neutral position.[21,38] O'Donohue believes that it may even snap over the greater tuberosity as the arm moves into medial rotation in exceptional cases.[43] There may be acute swelling over the anterior aspect of the shoulder, and there is tenderness over the long head of the biceps. The condition tends to worsen and tenderness increase along the groove. An older person tends to accept his disability to a greater degree as he is more willing to curtail his activity and accept his disability unless pain increases. Limitation of motion and loss of strength in forward flexion and abduction are characteristic.

Crenshaw described a test to disclose this condition.[26] The patient holds a 5-pound weight in each hand, and brings the extended arms overhead, holding them in extreme external rotation. As the examiner places his fingers on the long head of the biceps, the patient lowers the arm to the side in the coronal plane. As the arm reaches 110 to 90 degrees, there may be an audible snap that is associated with a sharp pain.

The longitudinal axial roentgen view of the intertubercular groove may show an abnormal shallow groove.

MANAGEMENT. Reduction of the tendon

into its groove is often accomplished by medial rotation of the humerus with the arm at the side.

If symptoms are disabling and there is subluxation or dislocation of the tendon from its groove, then especially in the young adult patient surgery is indicated.

The method described by Hitchcock and Bechtol, resecting the intra-articular portion above the bicipital groove, is recommended in such cases.[33] When there is doubt that the tendon will remain in the groove, the long head of the biceps can be transferred to the short head of the biceps, as previously described for bicipital tendinitis, although this is seldom necessary.

Aftercare includes Velpeau immobilization for 10 to 14 days and a sling for an additional week, after which gentle motion exercises are started and gradually increased.

Rupture of Pectoralis Major Tendon

Rupture of the pectoralis major is rare to the extent that not a single case of this condition has been observed at Michael Reese Medical Center in more than 20 years. Pulaski and Chandlee reviewed the literature on 17 patients up to 1941 and reported a case of their own.[46] Since then scattered reports have appeared in the literature.[36] Kawashima and co-workers reported two cases and reviewed the literature.[35]

The condition has been reported only in males involved in accidents, the causes ranging from a crush injury of the chest wall to a sudden pull force on the involved upper extremity. In their case report and review of the literature, Park and Espiniella showed that the most common cause of pectoralis major rupture was due to heavy lifting with incoordination of muscle action.[44] Pectoralis major rupture has been reported in infants and in the elderly, the greatest peak occurring in the 20- to 30-year period of life.

PATHOLOGY AND PATHOGENESIS. Among 26 cases reviewed by Kawashima and associates, rupture occurred in 6 cases at the tendinous insertion, 9 cases at the mid-muscular portion, 5 cases at the musculo-tendinous junction, and 6 cases at the muscular origin.[35]

Marmor and co-workers stated that the pectoralis major was not needed for normal shoulder function, but was necessary for athletic performance or other strenuous activity.[41] McEntire and associates showed that partial to total ruptures of the pectoralis major may occur.[37]

DIAGNOSIS. The most common symptom is a sudden, sharp pain in the arm and shoulder as the injury occurs. Occasionally, the patient describes a snapping sensation in the shoulder. Commonly, swelling and ecchymosis result over the site of rupture. If the swelling is not massive a groove or depression may be palpated. With attempted contraction pain is increased and there is weakness in adduction and internal rotation of the arm. A visible bulge of torn muscle may be seen during contraction. If the diagnosis is in doubt, the normal pectoralis shadow will not be visible on a xeroradiogram.

TREATMENT. Park and Espiniella reviewed 10 cases treated surgically with 80 percent excellent and 10 percent good results and compared them with 21 other cases treated conservatively with only 17 percent excellent and 58 percent good results.[44]

If the rupture is significant and is likely to cause disability then surgical repair should be considered. However, if the patient is elderly and a poor risk it is unlikely that surgical treatment will enhance his well-being in future years. Lindenbaum reported a successful operative repair of an avulsed pectoralis major insertion performed in a 25-year-old man 6 months after the initial injury when the patient complained of excessive weakness that prevented him from participating in professional football.[39] Therefore, the treatment selected for each patient must be carefully considered and individualized. It is important to distinguish the site of rupture. McEntire and associates recommended early surgical repair for distal tendon injuries, and conservative therapy for rupture of the muscle belly, based upon the experience of 11 injuries.[37] In their cases proximal muscle injury responded well to conservative therapy.

If surgical repair is performed, 6 weeks of immobilization in a plaster spica cast is recommended to ensure healing, followed by gentle active exercises for an additional 4 to 6 weeks before full activity is permitted.

Rupture of the Triceps

Rupture of the triceps brachii is more uncommon than pectoralis rupture, as evidenced by the paucity of reports in the literature.[22,48]

Preston and Adicoff reported a single case of rupture of the triceps tendon and both quadriceps, presumably owing to weakening of the tendons by deposits of calcium in a patient who had hyperparathyroidism.[45] The triceps was not repaired as it caused little disability.

Searfoss, Tripi, and Bowers found only two reported cases and added a case of their own.[48] Anderson and LeCocq stated that excessive force against the resistance of the contracted triceps muscle results in olecranon fracture rather than in tendon rupture.[22]

When rupture occurs, a depression or sulcus may be palpated or seen in the tri-

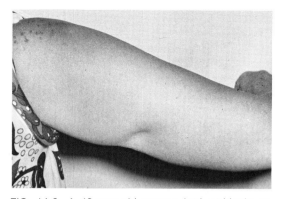

FIG. 14-8. A 48-year-old woman had suddenly extended her right arm against an immovable object and felt discomfort. She had sustained a partial tear of the triceps muscle. Two years later, note the dimpling effect in the posteromedial aspect of the midarm. She was asymptomatic except for slight loss of extension power.

ceps contour (Fig. 14-8). With complete rupture of the triceps tendon, active extension is lost.

If there is a complete tear of the triceps tendon surgical repair is indicated in order to restore active extension motion. In this case, an average of 5 weeks in an extension splint is recommended. The degree of extension should be less than complete, but not flexed so as to cause any traction on the suture line of the repaired rupture.

Adhesive Capsulitis

One of the most common and disabling painful disorders of the shoulder, described as early as 1882 by Putnam,[71] and yet least understood, is adhesive capsulitis (frozen shoulder). It accounts for more cases than that of bicipital tendinitis, and affects females slightly more than males. Usually, the condition is observed starting in middle age, but is occasionally seen in the early thirties because this disorder has varied causes leading to the aftermath termed "frozen shoulder."

Duplay was the first to discriminate between the all inclusive category of "arthritis" and the more specific "humeroscapular periarthritis."[58] This condition is equivalent to what is now called frozen shoulder. King and Holmes,[61] Codman,[53] Meyer,[66] and others[67,68] further refined this condition. For example, Meyer noted that disease of the long head of the biceps could be a cause of this disorder, describing the pathology of degeneration in cadavers.[66] However, although it was Codman who clearly described the clinical picture of frozen shoulder, he was unclear as to its pathology.[54] Pasteur described the syndrome "tenobursitis," which he believed caused frozen shoulder.[70] He first equated bicipital tenosynovitis with frozen shoulder. In 1943, Lippmann reported that adhesive tenosynovitis caused frozen shoulder, and believed that the basic pathologic lesion was a tenosynovitis of the long head of the biceps.[63]

DePalma reported that muscular inactivity was the cause of frozen shoulder, stating that anything that hindered scapulohumeral movement favored muscular inactivity.[56] He stressed that bicipital tenosynovitis was the most common factor. Neviaser found in surgically explored shoulders that the capsule adhered to the underlying humeral head and with manipulation the capsule could be stripped from the head, as well as torn at the reflected fold.[67] Although Neviaser reported little or no hemorrhage with manipulation,[67] this is not always the case in my experience. Kopell and Thompson reasoned that the pain originated in a compressive neuropathy of the suprascapular nerve.[62] I have not been able to confirm this view over the years.

McLaughlin,[64,65] and others,[52,54,55,60] reviewed the chief causes of frozen shoulder, including a variety of painful neck conditions, apical lung tumor invading the brachial plexus (see Fig. 5-25), cardiac conditions, pulmonary tuberculosis, disorders of the extremity, especially those relating to the shoulder, and even Colles' fracture. He listed a variety of other conditions which included shoulder joint infection, calcific deposits of the tendons about the shoulder, neoplasms, trauma, metabolic disorders such as gout, and other causes. McLaughlin's basic premise was that a shoulder that moves through a normal range of motion even a few times each day will not become frozen. Therefore, he believed that the immediate cause of every frozen shoulder is prolonged dependency. One can attest to the veracity of this statement by recalling such disparate experiences as the patient with a radical mastectomy who often develops frozen shoulder because of her fear in mobilizing the ipsilateral extremity, or the rare case of scleroderma (Fig. 14-9).[132]

MECHANISM. From the belief that limitation of shoulder motion, due to intrinsic or extrinsic factors, is the main determinant in causing frozen shoulder, it appears that inflammation of portions of the capsule or of the biceps mechanism evokes an abnormal change in these tissues. The soft tissues are saturated with a serofibrinous exudate that produces adhesions. A change in the collagen and an accumulation of serofibrinous fluid over large surface areas and in the

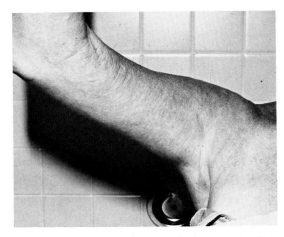

FIG. 14-9. A 54-year-old woman had a long-standing history of scleroderma. She showed classic evidence of a frozen shoulder. Note the limited overhead motion that was associated with considerable pain. The skin showed typical changes associated with this condition including coarsening and edema. There were no soft-tissue changes about the joint. In a similar case of scleroderma there are extensive soft-tissue calcifications (see Fig. 5-48).

recess of the capsule predispose to stiffness. That bicipital tenosynovitis is often related to frozen shoulder is borne out by the findings in those cases that are occasionally operated upon for relief of pain.

Reeves reported arthrographic changes in frozen shoulder cases, wherein there is a diminution of joint volume.[73] This occurred at pressures rising to 1000 mm. Hg without the dye filling the subscapular bursa, the bicipital tendon sheath, or the inferior recess of the capsule. However, with resolution of the disease process it was again possible to fill the joint with serial intra-articular injections. Reeves observed that manipulation in abduction caused a rupture of the inferior capsule and rupture of the subscapularis tendon in external rotation.[73]

DIAGNOSIS. It is easy to establish the diagnosis. The patient typically complains of a mild ache in the affected shoulder. The pain often starts in the outer part of the upper arm and may even radiate upward or downward, especially while the patient attempts overhead motion of the extremity. In the beginning the discomfort may be so mild that the patient may defer medical

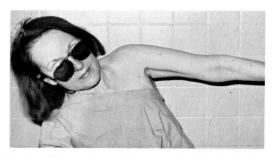

FIG. 14-10. A 40-year-old woman had had adhesive capsulitis over a 2-year period which failed to respond to conservative treatment. Note the marked limitation of shoulder motion. The patient had voluntarily fixed the scapula and had to tilt the body in order to gain any abduction motion. Pain was severe. She refused manipulation under anesthesia. Eventually pain decreased but normal motion was markedly decreased.

treatment. In some of these cases the problem may vanish. Although some surgeons believe it is a self-limiting condition this is not always the case (Fig. 14-10). The pain may persist for months to years and then cease, or progress until the patient is totally disabled with pain. The patient cannot pinpoint one painful area and describes the whole shoulder as being painful. Generally, as the pain increases the normal range of motion decreases. At times it may be difficult to assess the problem because there may also be superimposition of pain from the neck or back of the shoulder.

The patient may become fatigued with pain and even emotionally depressed. Lippmann has pointed out that most patients are well before 10 months have elapsed,[63] although I have seen the condition persist for up to 3 years despite treatment. I agree with the observation that the condition does not usually recur in the same shoulder if the cause is eliminated. Although pain may subside, a significant number of patients are often left with some degree of permanent loss of the normal range of glenohumeral motion. Nevertheless, uncomplicated cases recover promptly.[5]

It is generally true that the patient who has a prolonged, severe illness will have a larger amount of residual pain and stiffness of the affected shoulder. The range of shoulder motion should be carefully recorded and the scapular motion observed. Ordinarily, it is common to note tenderness over the bicipital groove. Tenderness over other parts of the joint is not often observed.

The sine qua non of frozen shoulder is the definite limitation of shoulder motion. During the acute phase the patient will resist passive overhead motion testing, complaining of increased pain. In the chronic or late stage of the disorder there is more freedom of motion and virtually no pain when the involved joint is moved within its constricted arc of motion. Attempted motion beyond this point will elicit a painful response.

TREATMENT. Ideal treatment for frozen shoulder is not yet at hand. It varies with the degree and duration of the pain, the loss of shoulder function, and even with the inciting factor. Many cases can be treated conservatively on an outpatient basis providing the patient is cooperative. In any event, a careful examination should determine the reason for the condition, so that treatment may be directed not only to the amelioration of the pain but also to the elimination of the causative factor.

In the early acute phase, analgesics are given for the pain. The patient should be encouraged to gently place the shoulder through a full range of motion. The surgeon should not merely instruct the patient to perform these exercises, but demonstrate the detail of the desired movement. This is best accomplished in recumbency, and the extremity is allowed to gradually move overhead in a slow, repetitive fashion. The patient may hold a lightly weighted piece of dowel with both hands while doing this exercise. Motion exercises in internal rotation behind the back, lateral arm elevation, and external rotation are also practiced. In addition, a bulky, soft pillow should be placed in the axillary region to keep the arm abducted during sleep periods. Heat applications are not recommended as the average patient tends to overuse this modality of therapy.

As the pain subsides in the acute phase, it is even more important to encourage movement through as full an arc of motion as possible. Such methods as holding a length of dowel or exercising with a pulley device are good ways to achieve an increased range of shoulder motion if they are practiced often and effectively each day. It is not possible to state a period of time that is needed to continue these exercises. Rather, the surgeon should use good clinical judgment to decide such things as how much the patient should exercise, and the type of exercise and its duration. As a general rule, I encourage the patient to exercise until the pain ceases and maximum active shoulder motion results without exacerbation of pain. At no time in the early stage of the disease is manipulation or force used to regain motion. In an occasional case in which there is one point that is exceptionally tender, as in the biceps sulcus, local anesthetic and intra-articular steroid injection can be given to ease the discomfort. It should not be given with the specious argument that local steroid injection will lessen the formation or "dissolve" adhesions. Occasionally, oral anti-inflammatory drugs help to lessen the discomfort and indirectly improve motion.

In the chronic phase, especially when an outpatient therapy exercise program has failed to restore shoulder motion and the pain is intractable, a more vigorous treatment plan is needed.[59,69] Manipulation under anesthesia was first advocated by Putnam in 1882.[71] The patient is admitted to the hospital when it is determined that further conservative treatment on an outpatient basis is fruitless. The general medical condition should be known, as well as the degree of radiolucency of the bone in the elderly patient. I have seen more than a rare iatrogenic fracture of the humerus occur from overzealous manipulation.

Manipulation of the shoulder joint under general anesthesia should be discussed with the patient before the procedure is performed. Its purpose is to tear the adhesions that restrict motion. In so doing the capsular structures may also be stretched and torn. This cannot be avoided and may result in local joint hemorrhage, swelling, and ecchymosis. Furthermore, this method does not obviate the need for an effective, immediate physical therapy program postmanipulation.

During manipulation the arm should be supported by the surgeon throughout the procedure and not merely jerked or pulled through a range of motion. The joint should be gently but firmly stretched through a full range of motion that should include overhead motion, abduction, and internal and external rotation, and should be compared to the opposite normal shoulder if the patient states both shoulder joints had normal motion. As the adhesions are torn a snap is usually felt or heard. In most cases it is not necessary to repeat this manipulation if motion exercises are started by the next morning. Analgesics should be given freely for severe pain that may follow. In some patients, like those who have had radical mastectomy, the hand and rest of the extremity may swell dramatically. In this event the swelling may be controlled with an elastic sleeve.

Andrén and Lundberg described their method of treating chronic frozen shoulder by distending the joint capsule with dye until there is resistance, and repeating the procedure several times.[51] The patient moves the arm several times and as larger fluid volumes are required saline solution is used. Stein reviewed 21 patients who underwent infiltration brisement and claimed good results.[74] I have no experience with either method.

Other treatment methods such as ultrasound and x-ray treatment have no merit in the care of frozen shoulder in my opinion.[72]

Occasionally, surgical treatment is required to remove the offending cause of frozen shoulder, such as a calcific deposit or a bicipital tenosynovitis, that is recalcitrant to conservative treatment.

Glenohumeral and Acromioclavicular Arthritis

The exact location of the shoulder pain often will allow the surgeon to take prompt corrective measures in helping the patient.

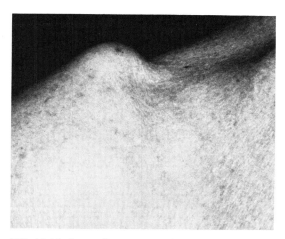

FIG. 14-11. A ganglion was noted in an elderly woman who had slight discomfort over the acromioclavicular joint. The cyst itself could be transilluminated. It was associated with arthritis of the joint. The patient was treated by aspiration of the cyst contents and injection of steroid into the joint. Symptoms were not so severe that surgery was required.

Arthritic conditions of the glenohumeral joint are covered elsewhere in this text. Merely ascribing a diagnosis such as arthritis of the acromioclavicular joint will not alleviate a painful joint. At times resection of the lateral end of the clavicle may be necessary for best results. When a ganglion forms it is not always necessary to resect the lesion unless the pain is disabling or cosmetically unappealing (Fig. 14-11). More often such lesions may not cause symptoms. Such arthritic lesions may be suspected early when the normal acromioclavicular interval of 1 to 3 mm. is narrowed. If pain results from degenerative changes in this joint, its limited mobility may interfere with normal arm movement.

Scapulothoracic Disorders— Snapping Scapula[75-79]

Movement of the anterior surface of the scapula over the convexity of the posterior and posterolateral chest wall may occasionally produce a slight friction as a result of normal muscle action but has no pathologic significance. Occasionally, a patient may complain of a snap during scapulothoracic movement which may be pathologic, as in the case of an osteochondroma interfering with the normal articulation. An audible snap is usually pathologic and may be painful.

Any abnormality in the scapulothoracic articulation may cause pain during movement. If the pain is intractable and conservative treatment fails, surgical treatment is indicated if the cause can be determined. This may require resection of an osteochondroma or resection of a portion of the scapula that is incongruent with its opposing rib cage articulation, for example.

In less severe cases degeneration in the soft tissues of the scapulothoracic articulation may cause a grating that may produce pain of a less severe nature. Most of these cases can be treated conservatively.

ENTRAPMENT AND NEURITIC SYNDROMES

Compression upon a nerve or artery may occur at various places in the upper extremity; namely, at the thoracic outlet, the suprascapular notch, the arm, and the wrist, all of which may cause pain in shoulder. The site of compression or the nerves involved in neuritic disorders can be determined by a careful examination in most instances.

Paralytic Brachial Neuritis

Paralytic brachial neuritis was described by Spillane in 1943.[116] It is characterized by a spontaneous onset of severe shoulder pain followed by severe weakness and atrophy in the affected muscles as the pain subsides.[84] It is often missed because surgeons may not be familiar with this syndrome. Magee and DeJong reviewed 23 cases and found that occasionally both shoulders may be involved.[109]

Within hours or days after the onset of pain in the shoulder, weakness of the muscles of the shoulder girdle may ensue, and vary from very mild to severe. The paralysis may persist for weeks or months, with a tendency toward slow recovery. In some cases cutaneous sensory deficit may result. In these cases the motor and sensory loss seem to follow a peripheral nerve. This may add confusion to the diagnosis with the vain expectation that a viral disorder, such as herpes zoster, as sometimes occurs, may be the offending cause.

The sexes are equally affected. The age range varies from 8 to 64 years. However, most of the cases occur in patients in the third through the sixth decades of life. The results of the cerebrospinal fluid examination are normal. Recurrence is rare but has been noted. There seems to be no common denominator in the causation of the illness.

Diagnostic studies such as electromyography may be helpful in specifically localizing the lesion. When it is thought to be necessary roentgenograms of the cervical spine and myelography with examination of the cerebrospinal fluid will help the physician determine whether other conditions cause the problem.[98]

Paralytic brachial neuritis may be confused with poliomyelitis, but whereas poliomyelitis is seasonal, brachial neuritis occurs at any time. It may also be confused with the motor effects of herpes zoster which can be severe, and amyotrophic lateral sclerosis. In brachial neuritis the overall prognosis is good and there is a tendency toward recovery of shoulder function. During the recovery phase exercises should be prescribed to prevent shoulder stiffness or frozen shoulder.

Supraclavicular Nerve Entrapment

Gelberman, Verdeck, and Brodhead reported a case of compression of the middle branch of the supraclavicular nerve as it passed through an osseous tunnel in the clavicle of a teenager.[96] Pain occurred in the midclavicular region 1 month after a stretching injury to the neck. Surgical treatment, including resection of the entrapped nerve proximal and distal to the bony canal, resulted in cessation of the pain and persistent numbness over the anterior shoulder.

Carpal Tunnel Syndrome[103,112,117,119]

Compression of the median nerve at the wrist may produce pain radiating upward and to the shoulder region in as many as 15 percent of the cases. Care should be taken to differentiate this syndrome from cervical neuritis. Once the diagnosis of carpal tunnel syndrome is confirmed by electromyographic and nerve conduction velocity studies, release of the carpal ligament is indicated when conservative treatment fails. During operation, the nerve should be released proximally in the lower forearm as well as into the palm. Care should be exercised not to injure the palmar branch of the median nerve.

Compression Syndromes Related to the Supracondylar Process

A small bony spur, varying from 2 to 20 mm. in length, occasionally projects from the humerus 5 to 7 cm. proximal to the medial epicondyle and points obliquely downward and forward in a medial direction (Fig. 14-12).[99,101] It is present in 1 percent of the population and is often bilateral.[86] In some cases a fibrous band joins the tip of the process to the medial epicondyle. Through the foramen formed by the supracondylar spur and the fibrous band passes the median nerve. The pronator teres may have an anomalous origin from the spur.[86] Other bone lesions may cause similar symptoms (Fig. 14-13).

Attention may be called to the process when it is fractured or when it causes compression of the median nerve that may mimic carpal tunnel syndrome. Fragiadakis and Lamb reported a case of ulnar nerve compression related to a supracondyloid process.[93] When its presence is suspected it is easily palpated. When fracture occurs treatment is not indicated except for immobilization of the extremity until pain subsides. Rarely, median nerve compression occurs leading to symptoms. Compression of the nerve is caused by tightness of the nerve against the spur by the fibrous band. Should this condition arise the spur should

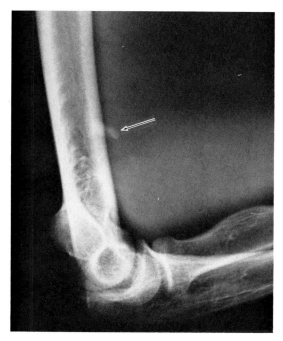

FIG. 14-12. A supracondylar process (arrow) was found in a 15-year-old boy who had symptoms of median nerve compression after a football injury. The process was resected and there was complete resolution of the symptoms.

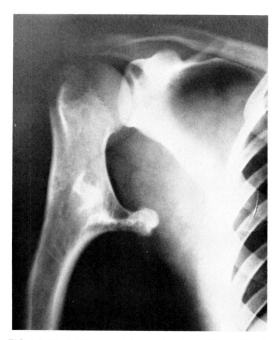

FIG. 14-13. A 32-year-old man developed hypesthesia in the median and ulnar nerve sensory distribution of the right upper extremity. An osteochondroma was resected which resulted in cure.

be removed thus freeing the neurovascular bundle.

Suprascapular Nerve Entrapment

The obscure and uncommon syndrome of suprascapular nerve entrapment can cause severe shoulder pain and disability, and is easily cured if only it is recognized. The condition was described by Kopell and Thompson in 1963.[102] However, it is often overlooked as a possible source of shoulder pain.

ANATOMY. The suprascapular nerve is derived from the upper trunk of the brachial plexus formed by the roots of C5 and C6 at a place known as Erb's point. The nerve passes downward, usually behind the brachial plexus, to the superior edge of the scapula and then through the suprascapular notch (see Fig. 14-14B). The roof of the notch is formed by the transverse scapular ligament. The notch is shaped like the letter "U" and may be deep and narrow or shallow and wide. Although the nerve may sometimes fit snugly in its notch, there is no clear evidence that a relationship exists between one particular-shaped suprascapular notch and entrapment symptoms of its nerve.

The suprascapular nerve reaches the posterior scapula after passing through the notch, supplies the supraspinatus muscle, and gives off articular branches to the glenohumeral and acromioclavicular joints.[102] Sensory and sympathetic fibers of the nerve innervate about two thirds of the shoulder capsule.[115] The nerve then turns around the lateral edge of the scapular spine to innervate the infraspinatus. There are no sensory endings on the skin for this nerve.

MECHANISM. Suprascapular nerve compression may result because of acute trauma such as fracture, a direct blow to the shoulder, encroachment of the suprascapular notch because of intrinsic or extrinsic reasons, or its cause may be unknown and is then termed idiopathic. Kopell and Thompson believe that certain extremes of scapular motion render the nerve taut, kinking it over the edge of the foramen.[102] They relate a number of ways in which abnormal scapular movements may produce a suprascapular neuropathy foremost of which may be a variety of trauma. Clein stated that transmitted forces, direct injuries, and traction are important in the causation, but that traction injury was most significant.[89]

DIAGNOSIS. The diagnosis of suprascapular nerve entrapment is made by exclusion and is based upon the abnormal findings from electrodiagnosis. The hallmark of suprascapular nerve entrapment is pain. The pain is deep and poorly delineated. Although the pain is usually localized to the posterior and lateral aspects of the shoulder, it may be referred down the arm, to the neck, or to the upper anterior chest wall. A patient characterized the pain as burning, aching, and "crushing," in one case I have attended.

In severe cases of neuropathy, atrophy and weakness of the supraspinatus and infraspinatus may be noted. Occasionally, certain scapular motions may be painful. In this event the patient may attempt to restrict shoulder motion. Adduction of the extended arm across the body tenses the nerve and so may increase pain. Thumb pressure over the region of the suprascapular notch may cause severe tenderness.

Local and systemic diseases such as diffuse peripheral neuropathy and cervical disc pathology must be excluded as causes of shoulder pain. This is important when one considers that pain from the C3-4 level is referred to the upper border of the trapezius and that pain from the C6-7 region, to the inferior angle of the scapula, for example. Additional confirmatory evidence may be gained by blocking the nerve as suggested by Rose and Kelly.[115] This may be achieved by using a 25-gauge spinal needle and 1 percent local anesthetic. The suprascapular notch is approached posteriorly and superiorly. Pain relief is dramatic but not long lasting. In one severe case, the patient had an associated "frozen shoulder" but after injection could move the shoulder with ease without fear of pain.

Definitive confirmation of the diagnosis rests with the electromyogram. It is not enough simply to order this test and expect the electromyographer to test for this condition. The surgeon must suspect the syndrome and be specific in ordering the study. Khalili has shown that an increased latency time is an indication of impaired conductibility.[100] When the suprascapular nerve is stimulated at the suprascapular space, the evoked potentials are picked up in the supraspinatus muscle by a single coaxial needle electrode. The conduction time from stimulating electrode to the pickup needle is measured and compared with the opposite side. The mean latency is thought to be 2.7 msec. with a range of 1.7 to 3.7 msec. A decrease in the amplitude or marked polyphasicity of evoked potentials is also significant. If significant neuropathic change is present, the findings vary from a reduction in the interference pattern to a severe degree of denervation in the supraspinatus and infraspinatus muscles.

Neuropathic lesions of other nerves such as the long thoracic must be differentiated.

TREATMENT. On occasion, a patient may obtain relief of pain by resting the extremity for a period of time.[87] However, when a patient fails to respond to treatment as expected, surgical release of the entrapped nerve at its notch is required. I do not believe that bone resection is indicated about the notch unless pressure phenomenon is caused by the callus of an associated fracture or a bone tumor, for example.

Clein reported on a posterior surgical approach to the suprascapular notch,[89] whereas Murray stated that the anterior surgical approach via a saber-cut incision was best for exposure because the posterior approach may cause scarring and additional postoperative pain in the area that is painful, and may produce injury to the anatomic structures on the dorsal and medial aspects of the scapula.[111]

Although either surgical approach is acceptable, in my personal experience I believe that the posterior approach is easier, safer, and not likely to cause muscle damage if good surgical technique is exercised. The patient may leave the hospital within several days after surgery. If the diagnosis is proved preoperatively, pain relief is likely to be dramatic and permanent.

Posterior Surgical Approach. The patient is placed in the prone position and the involved extremity draped free. A transverse incision is made $\frac{1}{4}$ in. above the scapular spine and parallel along its length (Fig. 14-14A). The trapezius muscle is elevated from the spine with a millimeter of bone, care being taken not to elevate the underlying supraspinatus. The trapezius is gently retracted upward (Fig. 14-14B). With the gloved index finger, the superior edge of the suprascapular notch is located by palpation. Blunt dissection is employed to free the supraspinatus from the posterosuperior edge of the scapula, and occasionally the surrounding tissues are dissected with a blunt-tip scissors. Care is taken to avoid injury to the easily identified suprascapular artery after the trapezius and supraspinatus are retracted upward and downward, respectively (Fig. 14-14C).

If doubt exists as to location of the suprascapular notch, a nerve stimulator is used and the contraction of the supraspinatus observed. Two straight nerve root retractors aid in gently retracting the suprascapular artery and isolating the transverse scapular ligament from its underlying nerve. The ligament is resected with a number 11 scalpel blade. No bone is removed unless there is definite evidence of bony encroachment upon the nerve, as in the case of a bone tumor or a mass of fracture callus.

The muscles are allowed to fall back into place. Several drill holes are made in the

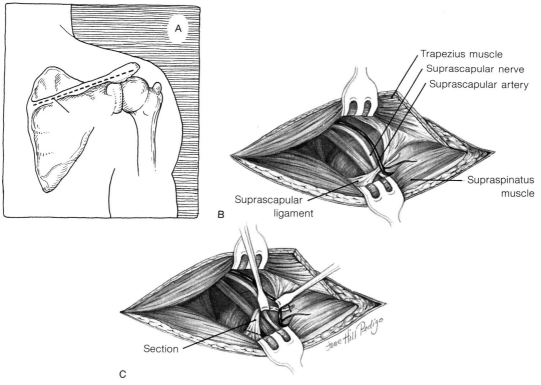

FIG. 14-14. Method of resecting the transverse scapular ligament. A, The dotted line indicates the skin incision overlying the scapular spine. B, After elevation of the trapezius from the scapular spine and upward retraction of the muscle, the supraspinatus notch and its transverse ligament are palpated. The supraspinatus muscle is then retracted downward to bring into view the suprascapular artery and nerve. C, With nerve root retractors the suprascapular artery and the transverse scapular ligament are isolated, permitting easy removal of the ligament with a number 11 scalpel blade.

scapular spine for reattachment of the trapezius. The overlying fascia and skin are closed. If muscle retraction is gentle one need not fear damage to the nerve supply to the surrounding muscle.

The extremity is immobilized in Velpeau position for 10 to 14 days, and thereafter, gentle passive motion exercises are started. After 3 weeks gentle active exercises are initiated.

NEUROVASCULAR COMPRESSION SYNDROMES

After Adson and Coffey described their method for relieving neurovascular symptoms in the upper extremity in 1927, in which they sectioned the scalene anticus attachment at its rib,[81] a plethora of papers followed that still leaves the budding surgeon confused and uncertain as to the best treatment for the patient with evidence of a compression syndrome. With each group of papers the pendulum seems to swing from the side of conservatism to radical surgical treatment, and back toward conservatism. Thirty years ago many cases of painful shoulder thought to be associated with scalene anticus syndrome obtained unsuccessful results from section of the muscle insertion. Clagett stated that 60 percent of patients with scalene anticus operations were not relieved.[88] In my experience this is probably true, undoubtedly because there were mistakes in the diagnosis, or there was an inexact understanding of the mechanism causing the symptoms.[94] Merely concluding that one of a variety of positive compression tests is present in a patient is not enough in evaluating such a case. For this reason the surgeon should be cautious in making such a diagnosis, particularly when surgical treatment is contemplated (Figs. 14-15 to 14-17) (see Chapter 2, Diagnosis).

MECHANISM. Adson and Coffey reviewed the anatomy of cervical rib and the relationship of the brachial plexus and subclavian vessels to this structure, and found that the anterior scalene produced compression of the subclavian artery and brachial plexus against the cervical rib.[81] In their highly

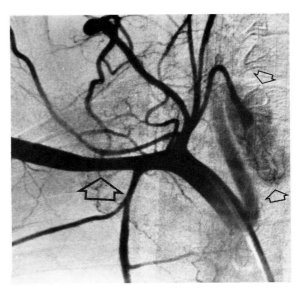

FIG. 14-15. An arteriogram shows the constricted portion of the subclavian artery (small arrows) secondary to invasion by a Pancoast tumor (large arrow). (Courtesy of Swamy, S., Segal, L., and Mouli, S. C.: Percutaneous Angiography, Springfield, Ill., Charles C Thomas, 1976. Reproduced with permission of the publisher.)

selected cases it was attractive to divide the muscle insertion rather than to perform a more formidable rib resection. Gradually, it became apparent that a better definition of the mechanism causing compression syndrome was needed. Falconer and Weddell, as well as others,[121] described the costoclavicular compression of the subclavian artery and vein and related it to the anterior scalene syndrome.[92] They showed that cure of the symptoms was effected by resecting the offending rib from beneath the artery, and pointed out that division of anterior scalene muscle alone may be ineffective[92] (Fig. 14-18). Adson eventually came to believe in this concept of rib removal in addition to scalenotomy when circumstances suggested this approach[80] (Fig. 14-19).

In 1947, Gage and Parnell showed that a number of anatomic factors predisposed to neurovascular and anterior scalene disorders in a moderately high percentage of persons.[95] The factors include (1) a relationship between the anterior scalene tendon and fifth to seventh cervical nerves; (2) the

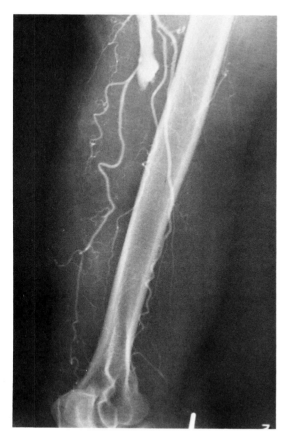

FIG. 14-16. An adult with a below the knee amputation had used crutches for many years, often leaning on the crutch pads in the axillary regions. He developed symptoms secondary to an occlusion of the axillary artery. At operation, an aneurysm was found and repaired. (Courtesy of Swamy, S., Segal, L., and Mouli, S. C.: Percutaneous Angiography. Springfield, Ill., Charles C Thomas, 1976. Reproduced with permission of the publisher.)

of determining by careful examination the exact sites of nerve compression. Williams believed that when no anatomic abnormality was found in a suspected scalene anterior syndrome, tension on the neurovascular bundle as it passed over the first rib could be relieved by resecting the rib.[120] Lishman and Russell believed that few cases of brachial neuropathy originated from the region of the thoracic outlet.[106] They stated that brachial neuropathic lesions can be situated along widely separated points of the nerves, and are often incorrectly attributed to thoracic outlet compression. As an example, Lotem and associates described radial nerve palsy in

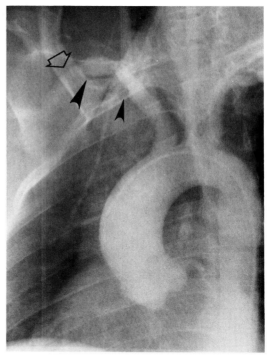

FIG. 14-17. An adult sustained a fracture of the right first rib which was associated with neurovascular compression symptoms of the upper extremity. An arteriogram shows the constricted portion of the subclavian artery (dark arrows) over the healing fractured first rib (outlined arrow). Collateral circulation to the hand was adequate and surgery was not performed in view of the patient's age (78 years) and poor medical condition. (Courtesy of Swamy, S., Segal, L., and Mouli, S. C.: Percutaneous Angiography. Springfield, Ill., Charles C Thomas, 1976. Reproduced with permission of the publisher.)

existence of a minor anterior scalene muscle in 60 percent of cases; (3) the passage of the fifth to seventh cervical nerves through the anterior scalene or between the minor and major anterior scalene; (4) the relative rigidity of the anterior and middle scalenes at their rib attachments; (5) the diminution in the triangle caused by the insertion of the minor scalene between the artery and brachial plexus; (6) the variation in the width of the anterior scalene; and (7) the anatomic relationship between the brachial plexus, subclavian artery, and the first rib. These authors also stressed the importance

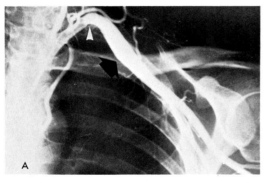

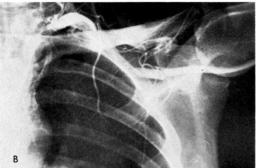

FIG. 14-18. A, A 24-year-old woman had neurovascular compression symptoms associated with a cervical rib. Note the relatively normal flow of dye in the subclavian and axillary arteries (white and black arrows). B, During hyperabduction of the involved extremity, note the occlusion of dye in the subclavian artery overlying the cervical rib. There was no adequate runoff of dye into the upper extremity. The cervical rib was removed, which resulted in cure. (Courtesy of Swamy, S., Segal, L., and Mouli, S. C.: Percutaneous Angiography. Springfield, Ill., Charles C Thomas, 1976. Reproduced with the permission of the publisher.)

tebral artery from the subclavian on the left side or distal to the carotid artery and proximal to the vertebral artery on the right side, and cause a demand for blood by the corresponding arm that is often greater than the collateral arterials can supply.[122] This creates a negative pressure in the subclavian artery and sucks blood from the vertebral artery which may produce diverse symptoms that include syncope, headache, and hemiparesis. Lain described the "military brace syndrome" wherein military personnel develop an Erb's palsy when they strongly retract and depress the shoulders, and displace the head backward for a prolonged time period.[105]

De Villiers reported 41 cases of first rib resections for thoracic outlet compressions in whom 8 patients had venous obstruction and in which angiography showed a tight thoracic outlet to be the underlying cause of venous thrombosis.[90]

DIAGNOSIS. In establishing the correct cause of a particular compression syndrome at the thoracic outlet, it is essential to correlate all symptoms with objective findings. Thus, neural, vascular, combined neurovascular, and sympathetic etiologic factors should be considered.[97,104] The surgeon should not rely on examination alone before resorting to surgical treatment. Clinical evidence of diminished circulation, for example, to the distal part of the extremity should be confirmed by arteriograms when definitive treatment is contemplated.

Scalene Anticus Syndrome

In scalene anticus syndrome, pain is the most common symptom.[80] Some of the findings include a pulsating mass above the clavicle and a bruit in the same area. Paresthesias and even anesthesia may be present. Vasomotor disturbance in which one hand is cooler, dusky, and associated with hyperhidrosis may be present. The pain may vary from a dull ache to very sharp. Exertional activity may increase the symptoms causing shoulder and arm pain. A careful inspection may reveal atrophy of muscles innervated by the brachial plexus.

three cases in which the nerve was compressed as it passed through the posterior compartment through a fibrous arch located just proximal to the deltoid insertion.[108]

Rosati and Lord categorized the various neurovascular compression disorders at the shoulder girdle in an excellent monograph that greatly clarifies these conditions and their treatment.[114] They reviewed the various etiologic factors and found that congenital and traumatic factors played a significant role. Other compressions of the subclavian artery occur near its origin just proximal to the origin of the ipsilateral ver-

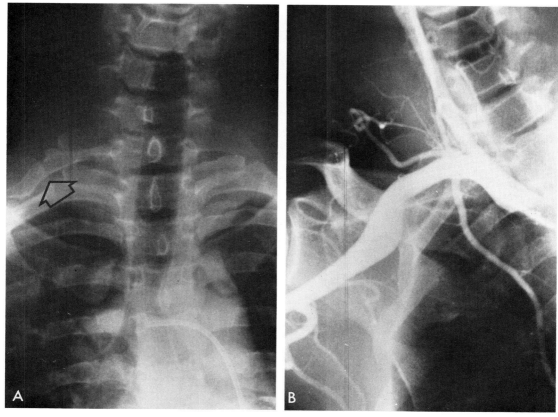

FIG 14-19. A, An adult had neurovascular compression symptoms in the right upper extremity associated with a cervical rib (arrow). B, An arteriogram shows a constriction in the subclavian artery at the cervical rib and poststenotic dilatation. At operation, a clot in the subclavian artery was found and removed along with the cervical rib, which resulted in cure. (Courtesy of Swamy, S., Segal, L., and Mouli, S. C.: Percutaneous Angiography. Springfield, Ill., Charles C Thomas, 1976. Reproduced with permission of the publisher.)

Vascular symptoms may predominate to the point where vasomotor symptoms as in a Raynaud's condition may appear. The anterior scalene syndrome may occur in the absence of a cervical rib. Results of the Adson test are positive (see Chapter 2, Diagnosis). Adson believed that a positive vascular response is a pathognomonic sign of a cervical rib or scalene anticus syndrome and indicates whether or not the volume of the pulse at the wrist has been altered.[80] I do not believe that the surgeon should place so much reliance on this test. Nevertheless, with a negative response, scalenotomy is contraindicated.

If other conditions such as discogenic, musculoskeletal disorders, neoplasms, neu-

ropathies, and shoulder-hand pain syndromes that follow coronary occlusion or cardiac surgery have been excluded as a cause of symptoms, the patient can be treated for this condition.[83,105,107,110,113]

Conservative treatment should be attempted first, correcting posture, resting the upper extremity, or even injecting the anterior scalene muscle with local anesthetic while care is taken to avoid injecting the phrenic nerve. Mild to moderate cases are best treated conservatively. However, when conservative treatment fails to relieve symptoms in more severe, proved cases, division of the scalene anterior tendon is indicated. In some cases partial or complete cervical rib resection is needed. In any

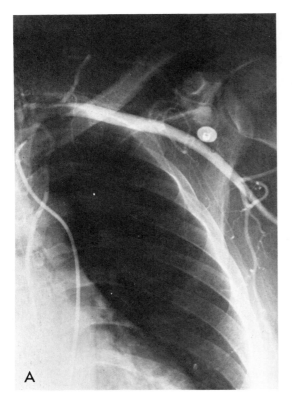
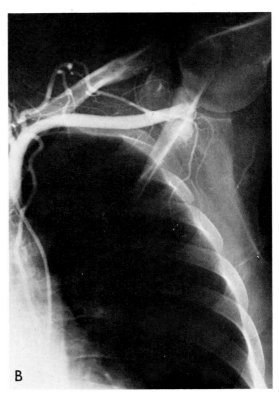

FIG. 14-20. A, An adult had an asymptomatic positive Adson sign. An arteriogram shows the normal flow of dye through the subclavian and axillary arteries with the extremity in neutral position. B, In hyperabduction, the axillary artery shows a complete block of the dye overlying the shoulder joint. The condition was noted bilaterally. However, the patient, in reality, had cervical neuritis that was successfully treated with conservative measures. (Courtesy of Swamy, S. Segal, L., and Mouli, S. C.: Percutaneous Angiography. Springfield, Ill., Charles C Thomas, 1976. Reproduced with permission of the publisher.)

event, such a case requires specialized consideration and treatment (Fig. 14-20).

Sympathetic Disorders (Shoulder-Hand Syndrome)[82,83,85,118,123]

Reflex sympathetic dystrophy can be one of the most disabling conditions acquired by man. Numerous names have been assigned to this entity, including causalgia, shoulder-hand syndrome, painful disability following coronary occlusion, reflex dystrophy, and Sudeck's atrophy. Evans has reviewed the pain mechanism and stated that a prolonged series of pain impulses start a vicious circle of reflexes that spread through a pool of many neuron connections upward, downward, and across the spinal cord.[91] A summation of these impulses constantly crosses the involved synapses in the central nervous system, including those of the sympathetic motor neuron cells in the lateral horn of the spinal cord controlling vasomotor tone and the sweat glands.

Shoulder-hand syndrome may ensue with the slightest trauma, even as little as a bruise or sprain. Steinbrocker described three phases in the clinical evolution of such cases.[118] In phase I, a painful shoulder disability is accompanied or followed by diffuse swelling, exquisite tenderness, and vasomotor changes in the hand and digits of the extremity. Spotty demineralization in the shoulder and hand may be present. This condition is bilateral in 20 percent of the cases. This phase lasts 3 to 6 months. Immediate treatment is necessary.

In phase II, pain in the shoulder subsides.

Some vasomotor changes may persist. The skin and muscles may become noticeably atrophic. The nails also may atrophy and the palmar fascia may thicken, resembling Dupuytren's contracture.[123] This phase also lasts 3 to 6 months. Treatment is imperative and the prognosis poor.

In phase III, trophic changes and atrophy progress. Irreversible flexion deformities of the fingers may result. The vasomotor changes are generally absent. Here, the prognosis is very poor.

The surgeon should not become pessimistic no matter how long the duration of symptoms. Steinbrocker stated that as long as any swelling, tenderness, or vasomotor changes persist, there remains a chance for at least some recovery.[118]

In treatment it is important to attain a state of general well-being for the affected patient. Vigorous surgical measures have not proved effective. Analgesics in adequate amounts should be given for the pain. Sedatives, other than phenobarbital, should be prescribed. Steinbrocker believes that this drug may act synergistically in some persons prone to reflex neuromuscular disorders.[118]

Local anesthetic injection at the shoulder or other tender points may be useful. Passive and active exercises to the shoulder and hand are desirable, along with moderate heat modalities.[82]

The most effective measures for relief of shoulder-hand syndrome are sympathetic block or systemic administration of corticosteroid in early cases. The results of surgical sympathectomy are varied. In two patients I have treated who received such treatment, the results were less than satisfactory.

STORAGE DISEASES

Alkaptonuria (Ochronosis)

Alkaptonuria is a rare disorder of amino acid metabolism characterized by the urinary excretion of breakdown products which appear black on oxidation.[130] The condition is inherited as a mendelian recessive trait affecting tyrosine and phenylala-

nine breakdown. The disease is due to the absence of the enzyme homogentisate oxygenase. Some patients with alkaptonuria develop ochronotic arthritis. Laskar and Sargison reviewed the literature and reported 4 cases.[130] Abe and associates reported on 13 cases in one family of whom 6 had bone and joint changes.[124]

Most cases of ochronosis occur after 40 years of age. Males are affected twice as often as females. When homogentisic acid accumulates in the body it forms brownblack pigment granules as a result of slow oxidation. If this accumulation is mild the person may be unaware that the condition exists. When it does occur ochronotic arthritis develops, the degree depending upon the severity of the alkaptonuria.

Gaucher's Disease

Gaucher's disease is a systemic storage disease of the reticuloendothelial system that affects many organs and tissues in the body. Two clinical forms occur: an acute infantile type, and a chronic adult type, the latter being most common and starting at any age. Three genetic forms have been described: (1) an infantile form transmitted as an autosomal recessive; (2) an adult form also transmitted as an autosomal recessive (most common); and (3) an adult type transmitted as an autosomal dominant.

Abnormal oval or spheroid cells in the liver, spleen, lymph nodes, and bone marrow become distended with a cerebroside which may exist in different forms such as kerasin. The disease probably relates to the absence of an enzyme responsible for the degradation of cerebrosides. These so-called Gaucher's cells cause severe destruction of the bone and other tissues.

With destruction of the bone there often are severe degenerative changes of the joint surfaces, including the shoulder, and pathologic fractures (see Figs. 5-44 and 5-45). Local pain may be severe. The chemical changes relate to elevations in the acid phosphatase without a concomitant increase in alkaline phosphatase. Examination of biopsy specimens will easily establish the diagnosis.

ARTHROPATHIES

Sickle Cell Disease

Sickle cell disease (SS) and to a lesser extent sickle cell trait (SA) affect bone, causing infarcts in the bone and osteonecrotic areas in the diaphysis and at the ends of the long bones.[133] The pathogenesis of the bone changes stems directly from the abnormal hemoglobin and the lowered oxygen tension that results. This causes increased viscosity and stasis of the red blood cells.

Sickle cell trait occurs in 8 percent of the American black population. These patients show a positive sickle preparation without anemia. Although bone changes in sickle cell anemia (SS) and in hemoglobin (SC) disease variant, and in hemoglobin S-thalassemia are well documented (Fig. 14-21, see also Fig. 5-39), bone necrosis is now known to occur to a lesser extent in sickle cell trait (SA). The greatest incidence of

bone infarction occurs first with the SC variant and next with sickle cell anemia (SS).

Two simultaneous but different bone changes occur. First, ischemia and infarction of the bone lead to an osteosclerosis and osteonecrosis which may be persistently painful (Figs. 14-21 and 14-22). Early bone and joint changes may be seen as early as 11 years of age and progress with time. As a reaction to the chronic hypoxia the marrow becomes hyperplastic, the marrow spaces widen, and the bone cortex thins.[133] Eventually, bone necrosis increases.

When evaluating a patient with hemoglobinopathy affecting bone, such a diagnosis should not be based on scanty clinical evidence. Other rare conditions may mimic these conditions. For example, Bosworth reported a case of a possible epiphysitis or localized osteomyelitis of the humeral head.[125]

The patient can be treated conservatively with analgesics early in the disease. In the severe case with complaints of intractable pain, surgical treatment consisting of hu-

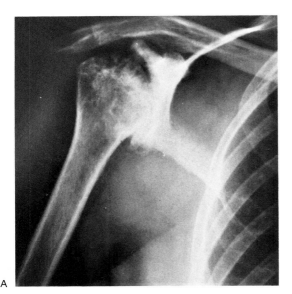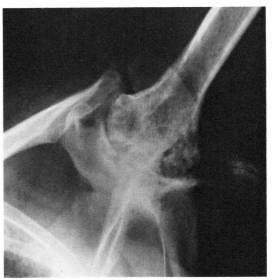

A   B

FIG. 14-21. A 24-year-old black woman had severe bilateral pain in the shoulders secondary to osteonecrosis resulting from sickle cell disease. A, The right side shows marked narrowing of the glenohumeral joint. Infarcts are seen within the humeral head and proximal diaphysis. B, The left humeral head has severe changes. The patient had excellent overhead motion although pain was severe.

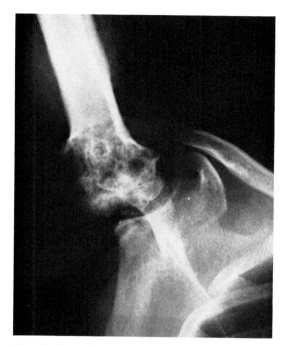

FIG. 14-22. A 45-year-old woman with hemoglobin S-C disease had severe pain in her right shoulder. Note the marked osteonecrosis within the humeral head and destruction of the articular surface. The patient had excellent overhead motion.

meral head resection and arthroplasty may be required. However, assurance cannot be given that such methods will relieve the pain, since other areas of bone infarction in the humerus and surrounding bone may also be associated with the pain. It is obvious then that surgical treatment should be selected for those patients whose pathologic lesion is primarily in the humeral head alone.

Steroid Osteonecrosis of Humeral Head

Numerous cases of humeral head osteonecrosis have been observed in those patients receiving steroids for hematologic or chronic renal problems. Dyreborg and Pilgaard reported three such cases in young men receiving steroids for aplastic anemia.[127] They found the femoral and humeral heads to be involved. The exact cause of the pathologic alteration is unexplained,

although several reasons have been offered.[127]

Osteonecrosis of the humeral head can occur in those patients who have received multiple local steroid injections into the glenohumeral joint. The pathologic condition of such humeral heads not only shows extensive cartilage destruction but true necrosis of the bone. Similarly, in patients receiving prolonged oral steroids osteonecrosis of the humeral head may occur. Occasionally, a patient may have received radiation treatment for cancer of the breast, for example. These cases may demonstrate radiation necrosis of the humeral head.

Early treatment mandates that administration of all steroids be stopped. However, the disease process often progresses, and if pain increases to an intolerable level arthroplasty is indicated in selected patients.

Decompression Sickness

Chronic bone disease is not uncommonly seen in those persons who work in compressed air. The cause of decompression sickness, known as the bends, has been understood for years. However, it has only recently been shown that significant bone changes occur even with a single exposure in those working in tunnels.[131] I have examined a number of such workers who had severe shoulder pain associated with varying degrees of osteonecrosis in the proximal humerus, often bilateral (Fig. 14-23). It could not always be demonstrated that symptoms arose only when an articular surface was involved. McCallum and associates described the classic roentgen features in a group of persons who worked in tunnels in Great Britain from 1958 to 1963.[131] The bone changes may show (1) a band of increased density in the region of the old epiphyseal line, (2) "bone islands," (3) "snow-cap" lesions, (4) small lakes in the medulla, (5) calcified lakes, and in my experience eventual collapse of the subchondral bone in the humeral head. Strangely, the humeral head is affected twice as often as the femur and apt to cause more pain.

When the humeral head is hopelessly

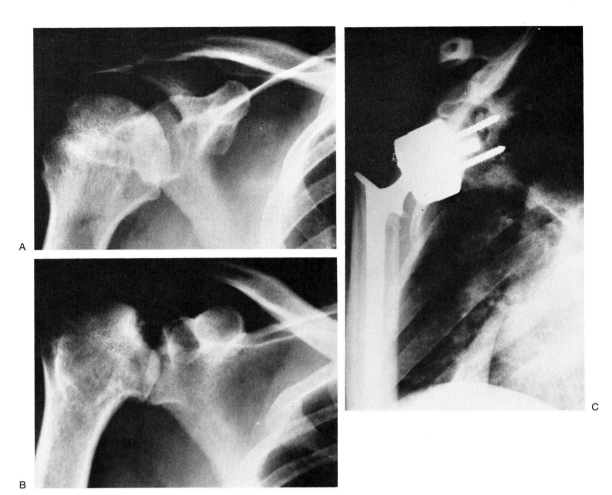

FIG. 14-23. A, A 47-year-old black man developed severe pain in the right shoulder. The history was questionable as to whether or not the patient had worked in a deep tunnel. However, a thorough medical evaluation failed to disclose any other reason for the severe osteonecrosis noted in the humeral head. B, Several months later the pain increased, and progressive, extensive changes in the humeral head were noted over the years. There were marked atrophy of the deltoid and a nonfunctioning rotator cuff. C, A total shoulder replacement was performed with good results. Although there was considerable pain relief and improvement in overhead motion, the patient still had some discomfort in the shoulder region during excessive activity.

damaged and pain is persistent, arthroplasty is indicated in selected individuals (Fig. 14-23C).

Hemophilic Arthropathy

Hemophilia includes two different bleeding disorders, each of which is transmitted by sex-linked recessive inheritance. Factor VIII (classic hemophilia) deficiency is clinically indistinguishable from factor IX deficiency.

Hemorrhages into the shoulder are rela-tively common but occur much less often than into the knee, for example. Early bleeding causes synovitis which often progresses in time. Bleeding into the humeral head and about the epiphyseal plate at first creates microcysts, which later coalesce and weaken the bone mass beneath the articular surface. Atrophy of muscles and soft-tissue contractures result, thereby establishing a vicious cycle that is often associated with considerable pain. The changes are classic (see Fig. 5-43).

Pain should never be treated with certain

anti-inflammatory drugs, or aspirin or aspirin-containing medications, as aspirin decreases platelet adhesiveness and increases bleeding. Bleeding should be treated with factor replacement therapy unless an inhibitor is present.[134] During an acute hemorrhage the upper extremity and shoulder girdle should be immobilized, and active gentle shoulder exercises started as soon as possible. Force must be avoided and manipulation is contraindicated. Painful glenohumeral inferior subluxation should not be manipulated since this is not a true dislocation. Rather, it results from the "piston effect" of a large volume of blood in the joint which cannot be aspirated. Rest, factor replacement, and gentle exercises usually lead to recovery in most instances. However, with progressive bleeding, overhead motion is gradually lost.

In the rare event that a pseudotumor forms, it must be eradicated early to save life and limb (see Fig. 22-10A).

UNUSUAL CAUSES

Tietze's Syndrome

Tietze's syndrome is a rare condition in which a painful nonsuppurative, benign swelling of the sternoclavicular or first to sixth sternochondral junctions occurs.[129] The condition is usually unilateral and both sexes are affected.

The left second sternocostochondral junction is affected in 35 percent of the cases, followed by the right second sternocostochondral junction in 30 percent of the cases. The cause is unknown.

Clinically, a sudden or gradual onset of anterior upper chest pain, associated with swelling of the affected costal cartilage, may result. Although the pain is intermittent and lasts from a few days to weeks, the swelling lasts for months to years. The course of the condition is characterized by exacerbations and remissions. Results of roentgen studies are normal except for occasional findings of calcium deposits in the affected cartilage. Blood chemistries are normal. The condition should be considered in the differential diagnosis of anterior chest pain and chest wall swelling. Buchmann reported 31 cases of sternoclavicular joint swelling, in which 21 were monoarticular, 4 with involvement of one or two other joints.[126] Eleven cases were probably related to systemic joint disease. Multiple other causes were discovered for the joint swelling including degenerative joint changes. Buchmann coined the term "sternoclavicular syndrome" for isolated sternoclavicular swelling.[126]

Treatment consists of local heat, analgesics, and local anesthetic injections. Unfortunately, more than one such case has had unnecessary radical resection for the mistaken diagnosis of malignant tumor.

Friedrich's Disease

Another unusual cause of swelling in the sternoclavicular joint is a condition associated with aseptic necrosis of the sternal end of the clavicle. Fischel and Bernstein reported one such case in which a 15-year-old boy was affected with swelling of the right sternoclavicular joint.[128] The diagnosis is based on radiologic findings of aseptic necrosis of the medial clavicle in which irregular punctate calcification of the involved area may be seen (see Fig. 5-28). Biopsy examination confirms the diagnosis. Radical treatment is not indicated (see Chapter 5, Radiologic Diagnosis).

REFERENCES

Bursitis and Calcific Tendinitis

1. Armstrong, J. R.: Excision of the acromion in treatment of the supraspinatus syndrome. Report of ninety-five excisions. J. Bone Joint Surg., 31-B:436–442, 1949.
2. Arner, O., Lindvall, N., and Rieger, A.: Calcific tendinitis of the shoulder joint. Acta Chir. Scand., 114:319–331, 1958.
3. Bartels, W. P.: The surgical treatment of acute subacromial bursitis. J. Bone Joint Surg., 22:120–121, 1940.
4. Bosworth, B. M.: Examination of the shoulder for calcium deposits. Technique of fluoroscopy and

spot-film roentgenography. J. Bone Joint Surg., 23:567–577, 1941.

5. Bosworth, B. M.: Calcium deposits in the shoulder and subacromial bursitis. A survey of 12,122 shoulders. J.A.M.A., 116:2 477–2482, 1941.

6. Codman, E. A.: The Shoulder; Rupture of the Supraspinatus Tendon and Other Lesions in or About the Subacromial Bursa. Boston, Thomas Todd Co., 1934.

7. Gardner, E.: The innervation of the shoulder joint. Anat. Rec., 102:1–17, 1948.

8. Goss, C. M. (Ed.): Gray's Anatomy, 29th Am. ed., Philadelphia, Lea & Febiger, 1974.

9. Hammond, G.: Complete acromionectomy in the treatment of chronic tendinitis of the shoulder. J. Bone Joint Surg., 44-A:494–504, 1962.

10. Hammond, G.: Complete acromionectomy in the treatment of chronic tendinitis of the shoulder. J. Bone Joint Surg., 53-A:173–180, 1971.

11. Heggö, O.: Tendinitis calcarea supraspinati. 14 Operated cases. Acta Orthop. Scand., 35:126–131, 1964.

12. Howard, L. G.: Neck and shoulder pain syndromes. Med. Clin. North Am., pp. 1289–1307, September, 1952.

13. Lowell, J. D.: Management of bursitis. N. Engl. J. Med., 269:798–800, 1963.

14. Neer, C. S., II.: Anterior acromioplasty for the chronic impingement syndrome in the shoulder. A preliminary report. J. Bone Joint Surg., 54-A:41–50, 1972.

15. Patterson, R. L., and Darrach, W.: Treatment of acute bursitis by needle irrigation. J. Bone Joint Surg., 19:993–1001, 1937.

16. Pedersen, H. E., and Key, J. A.: Pathology of calcareous tendinitis and subdeltoid bursitis. Arch. Surg., 62:50–63, 1951.

17. Rogers, M. H.: A study of one hundred cases of subdeltoid bursitis. J. Bone Joint Surg., 16:145–150, 1934.

18. Rüdinger, N.: Die Gelenknerven des Menschlichen Korpers. Erlangen, Verlag von Ferdinand Enke., 1857.

19. Stamm, T. T., and Crabbe, W. E.: Paraglenoid osteotomy of the scapula. Clin. Orthop., 88:39–45, 1972.

20. Wardle, E. N.: Calcification in the supraspinatus tendon. J. Bone Joint Surg., 17:789–791, 1935.

Bicipital Tendinitis, Subluxation of the Bicipital Tendon, and Rupture of Tendons About the Shoulder

21. Abbott, L. C., and Saunders, J. B. de C. M.: Acute traumatic dislocation of the tendon of the long head of the biceps brachii. A report of six cases with operative findings. Surgery, 6:817–840, 1939.

22. Anderson, K. J., and LeCocq, J. F.: Rupture of the triceps tendon. J. Bone Joint Surg., 39-A:444–446, 1957.

23. Biancheri, T. M.: Sulla rottura sottocutanea del bicipite brachiale. Chir. Organi Mov., IX:580–588, 1925.

24. Boyd, H. B., and Anderson, L. D.: A method for reinsertion of the distal biceps brachii tendon. J. Bone Joint Surg., 43-A:1041–1043, 1961.

25. Clark, J. M. P.: Reconstruction of biceps brachii by pectoral muscle transplantation. Br. J. Surg., 34:180–181, 1946.

26. Crenshaw, A. H. (Ed.): Campbell's Operative Orthopaedics, 5th ed. p. 1495. St. Louis, C. V. Mosby Co., 1971.

27. Crenshaw, A. H., and Kilgore, W. E.: Surgical treatment of bicipital tenosynovitis. J. Bone Joint Surg., 48-A:1496–1502, 1966.

28. DePalma, A. F.: The painful shoulder. Postgrad. Med., 21:368–376, 1957.

29. DePalma, A. F., and Callery, G. E.: Bicipital tenosynovitis. Clin. Orthop., 3:69–85, 1954.

30. Ewald, H.: Bizepsriss und Unfall. Munch. med. Wochanschr., 74:2214–2215, 1927.

31. Friedmann, E.: Rupture of the distal biceps brachii tendon. J.A.M.A., 184:182–184, 1963.

32. Gilcreest, E. L.: The common syndrome of rupture, dislocation and elongation of the long head of the biceps brachii. An analysis of one hundred cases. Surg. Gynecol. Obstet., 58:322–340, 1934.

33. Hitchcock, H. H., and Bechtol, C. O.: Painful shoulder. Observations on the role of the tendon of the long head of the biceps brachii in its causation. J. Bone Joint Surg., 30-A:263–273, 1948.

34. Kanter, P. J., and Callahan, J. J.: Spontaneous rupture of the biceps brachii. A case report. Orthop. Rev., 4:37–38, 1975.

35. Kawashima, M., Sato, M., Torisu, T., Himeno, R., and Iwabachi, A.: Rupture of the pectoralis major. Report of 2 cases. Clin. Orthop., 109:115–119, 1975.

36. Kingsley, D. M.: Rupture of the pectoralis major. Report of a case. J. Bone Joint Surg., 28:644–645, 1946.

37. McEntire, J. E., Hess, W. E., and Coleman, S. S.: Rupture of the pectoralis major muscle. A report of eleven injuries and review of fifty-six. J. Bone Joint Surg., 54-A:1040–1045, 1972.

38. Lieberman, H. S.: Traumatic subluxation of the long head of the biceps brachii. A case report. J. Bone Joint Surg., 22:425–428, 1940.

39. Lindenbaum, B. L.: Delayed repair of a ruptured pectoralis major muscle. Clin. Orthop., 109:120–121, 1975.

40. Lippmann, R. K.: Frozen shoulder; periarthritis; bicipital tenosynovitis. Arch. Surg., 47:283–296, 1943.

41. Marmor, L., Bechtol, C. D., and Hall, C. B.: Pectoralis major muscle. Function of sternal portion and mechanism of rupture of normal muscle: Case reports. J. Bone Joint Surg., 43-A:81–87, 1961.

42. Meyer, A. W.: Spontaneous dislocation and destruction of tendon of long head of biceps brachii. Fifty-nine instances. Arch. Surg., 17:493–506, 1928.

43. O'Donohue, D. H.: Subluxating biceps tendon in the athlete. J. Sports Med., 1:20–29, 1973.

44. Park, J. Y., and Espiniella, J. L.: Rupture of pectoralis major muscle. A case report and review of literature. J. Bone Joint Surg., 52-A:577–581, 1970.

45. Preston, F. S., and Adicoff, A.: Hyperparathyroidism with avulsion of three major tendons. Report of a case. N. Engl. J. Med., 266:968–971, 1962.

46. Pulaski, E. J., and Chandlee, B. H.: Ruptures of the pectoralis major muscle. Surgery, 10:309–312, 1941.

47. Rankin, J. O.: Rupture of the long head of the biceps brachii. J. Bone Joint Surg., 15:1003–1006, 1933.

48. Searfoss, R., Tripi, J., and Bowers, W.: Triceps brachii rupture: Case report. J. Trauma, 16:244–246, 1976.

49. Wagner, C. J.: Disinsertion of the biceps brachii. Am. J. Surg., 91:647–650, 1956.

50. Waugh, R. L., Hathcock, T. A., and Elliott, J. L.: Ruptures of muscles and tendons with particular reference to rupture (or elongation of long tendon) of biceps brachii with report of fifty cases. Surgery, 25:370–392, 1949.

Adhesive Capsulitis (Frozen Shoulder)

51. Andrén, L., and Lundberg, B. J.: Treatment of rigid shoulders by joint distention during arthrography. Acta Orthop. Scand., 36:45–53, 1965.

52. Braun, R. M., West, F., Mooney, V., Nickel, V. I., Roper, B., and Caldwell, C.: Surgical treatment of painful shoulder contracture in the stroke patient. J. Bone Joint Surg., 53-A:1307–1312, 1971.

53. Codman, E. A.: On stiff and painful shoulders: The anatomy of the subdeltoid subacromial bursa and its clinical importance: Subdeltoid bursitis. Boston Med. Surg. J., 154:613–620, 1906.

54. Codman, E. A.: The Shoulder; Rupture of the Supraspinatus Tendon and Other Lesions in or About the Subacromial Bursa. Boston, Thomas Todd Co., 1934.

55. Dee, P. E., Smith, R. G., Gullickson, M. J., and Ballinger, C. S.: The orthopaedist and apical lung carcinoma. J. Bone Joint Surg., 42-A:605–608, 1960.

56. DePalma, A. F.: Loss of scapulohumeral motion (frozen shoulder). Ann. Surg., 135:193–204, 1952.

57. DePalma, A. F., and Kruper, J. S.: Long-term study of shoulder joints afflicted with and treated for calcific tendinitis. Clin. Orthop., 20:61–72, 1961.

58. Duplay, S.: De La Periarthrite Scapulo-Humérale. Rev. Prat. d. Trav. de Med., 53:226–227, 1896; translated, M. Week 4:253–254, 1896; On Scapulo-Humeral Periarthritis.

59. Haggart, G. E., Dignam, R. J., and Sullivan, T. S.: Management of the "frozen" shoulder. J.A.M.A., 161:1219–1222, 1956.

60. Johnson, J. T. H.: Frozen-shoulder syndrome in patients with pulmonary tuberculosis. J. Bone Joint Surg., 41-A:877–882, 1959.

61. King, J. M., Jr., and Holmes, G. W.: Diagnosis and treatment of four hundred and fifty painful shoulders. J.A.M.A., 89:1956–1961, 1927.

62. Kopell, H. P., and Thompson, W. A. L.: Pain and the frozen shoulder. Surg. Gynecol. Obstet., 101:92–96, 1959.

63. Lippmann, R. K.: Frozen shoulder; periarthritis; bicipital tenosynovitis. Arch. Surg., 47:283–296, 1943.

64. McLaughlin, H. L.: On the "frozen shoulder." Bull. Hosp. Joint Dis., 12:383–393, 1951.

65. McLaughlin, H. L.: The "frozen shoulder." Clin. Orthop., 20:126–131, 1961.

66. Meyer, A. W.: Chronic functional lesions of the shoulder. Arch. Surg., 35:646–674, 1937.

67. Neviaser, J. S.: Adhesive capsulitis of the shoulder. A study of the pathological findings in periarthritis of the shoulder. J. Bone Joint Surg., 27:211–222, 1945.

68. Neviaser, J. S.: Adhesive Capsulitis of the Shoulder. Instructional Course Lectures of the American Academy of Orthopaedic Surgeons, 6:281–291, 1949.

69. Omer, G. E., and Thomas, S. R.: The management of chronic pain syndromes in the upper extremity. Clin. Orthop., 104:37–45, 1974.

70. Pasteur, F.: Les Algies del Épaule et al Physiotherapie. La Téno-bursite Bicipitale. J. Radiol. d'Électrol., 16:419–426, 1932.

71. Putnam, J. J.: The treatment of a form of painful periarthritis of the shoulder. Boston Med. Surg. J., 107:536–539, 1882.

72. Quin, C. E.: Humeroscapular periarthritis. Observations on the effects of x-ray therapy and ultrasonic therapy in cases of "frozen shoulder." Ann. Phys. Med., 10:64–69, 1969.

73. Reeves, B.: Arthrographic changes in frozen and post-traumatic stiff shoulders. Proc. R. Soc. Med., 59:827–830, 1966.

74. Stein, I.: Managing frozen shoulder syndrome. Orthop. Rev. 5:92, 1976.

Scapulothoracic Disorders

75. Michele, A. A.: Scapulocostal syndrome. N.Y. State J. Med., 55:2485–2493, 1955.

76. Michele, A., Davies, J. J., Krueger, F. J., and Lichtor, J. M., Scapulocostal syndrome (fatigue-postural paradox). N.Y. J. Med., 50:1353–1356, 1950.

77. Milch, H.: Snapping scapula. Clin. Orthop., 20:139–150, 1961.

78. Mosely, H. F.: Shoulder Lesions. London, E. & S. Livingston, Ltd., 1969.

79. Steindler, A.: Lectures on the Interpretation of Pain in Orthopaedic Practice. Springfield, Ill., Charles C Thomas, 1959.

Nerve Entrapment, Neuritis, Neurovascular Compression Syndromes, and Reflex Sympathetic Dystrophy

80. Adson, A. W.: Cervical ribs: Symptoms, differential diagnosis and indications for section of the insertion of the scalenus anticus muscle. J. Intern. Coll. Surg., 16:546–559, 1951.
81. Adson, A. W., and Coffey, J. R.: Cervical rib. A method of anterior approach for relief of symptoms by division of the scalenus anticus. Ann. Surg., 85:839–857, 1927.
82. Amick, L. D., Gilmer, W. J., and Sutton, F. D.: The holistic approach to the shoulder-hand syndrome. South. Med. J., 59:161–167, 1966.
83. Askey, J. M.: The syndrome of painful disability of the shoulder and hand complicating coronary occlusion. Am. Heart J., 22:1–12, 1941.
84. Bacevich, B. B.: Paralytic brachial neuritis. Case report. J. Bone Joint Surg., 58-A:262–263, 1976.
85. Baer, R. D.: Shoulder-hand syndrome: Its recognition and management. South. Med. J., 59:790–794, 1966.
86. Barnard, L. B., and McCoy, S. M.: The supracondyloid process of the humerus. J. Bone Joint Surg., 28:845–850, 1946.
87. Bateman, J. E.: Nerve injuries about the shoulder in sports. J. Bone Joint Surg., 49-A:785–792, 1967.
88. Claggett, O. T.: Research and prosearch (Presidential Address). J. Thorac. Cardiovasc. Surg., 44:153–166, 1962.
89. Clein, L. J.: Suprascapular entrapment neuropathy. J. Neurosurg., 43:337–342, 1975.
90. De Villiers, J. C.: A brachiocephalic vascular syndrome associated with cervical rib. Br. Med. J., 2:140–143, 1966.
91. Evans, J. A.: Reflex sympathetic dystrophy. Surg. Gynecol. Obstet., 82:36–43, 1946.
92. Falconer, M. A., and Weddell, G.: Costoclavicular compression of the subclavian artery and vein: Relation to the scalenus anticus syndrome. Lancet, 245:539–543, 1943.
93. Fragiadakis, E. G., and Lamb, D. W.: An unusual cause of ulnar nerve compression. Hand, 2:14–16, 1970.
94. Freiberg, J. A.: The scalenus anterior muscle in relation to shoulder and arm pain. J. Bone Joint Surg., 20:860–869, 1938.
95. Gage, M., and Parnell, H.: Scalenus anticus syndrome. Am. J. Surg., 73:252–268, 1947.
96. Gelberman, R. H., Verdeck, W. N., and Brodhead, W. T.: Supraclavicular nerve-entrapment syndrome. J. Bone Joint Surg., 57-A:119, 1975.
97. Glass, B. A.: The relationship of axillary venous thrombosis to the thoracic outlet compression syndrome. Ann. Thorac. Surg., 19:613–621, 1975.
98. Haymaker, W., and Woodhall, B.: Peripheral Nerve Injuries. Philadelphia, W. B. Saunders Co., 1962.
99. Kessel, L., and Rang, M.: Supracondylar spur of the humerus. J. Bone Joint Surg., 48-B:765–769, 1966.
100. Khalili, A. A.: Neuromuscular electrodiagnostic studies in entrapment neuropathy of the suprascapular nerve. Orthop. Rev., 3:27–28, 1974.
101. Kolb, L. W., and Moore, R. D.: Fractures of the humerus. Report of two cases. J. Bone Joint Surg., 49-A:532–534, 1967.
102. Kopell, H. P., and Thompson, W. A. L.: Peripheral Entrapment Neuropathies. Baltimore, Williams & Wilkins Co., 1963.
103. Kummel, B. M., and Zazanis, G. A.: Carpal tunnel syndrome: Shoulder pain as presenting complaint. Clin. Orthop., 92:227–230, 1973.
104. LaBan, M. M., Zemenick, G. A., and Meerschaert, J. R.: Neck and shoulder pain. Mich. Med., 74:549–550, 1975.
105. Lain, T. M.: The military brace syndrome. A report of 16 cases of Erb's palsy occurring in military cadets. J. Bone Joint Surg., 51-A:557–560, 1969.
106. Lishman, W. A., and Russell, W. R.: The brachial neuropathies. Lancet, 2:941–947, 1961.
107. Lorenze, E. J., III.: Painful shoulder syndrome following cardiac surgery. Arch. Phys. Med. Rehabil., 37:555–559, 1956.
108. Lotem, M., Fried, A., Levy, M., Solzi, P., Najenson, T., and Nathan, H.: Radial palsy following muscular effort. A nerve compression syndrome possibly related to a fibrous arch of the lateral head of the triceps. J. Bone Joint Surg., 53-B:500–506, 1971.
109. Magee, K. R., and DeJong, R. N.: Paralytic brachial neuritis. Discussion of clinical features with review of 23 cases. J.A.M.A., 174:1258–1262, 1960.
110. Michelsen, J. J., and Mixter, W. J.: Pain and disability of shoulder and arm due to herniation of the nucleus pulposus of cervical intervertebral disks. N. Engl. J. Med., 231:279–287, 1944.
111. Murray, J. W. G.: A surgical approach for entrapment neuropathy of the suprascapular nerve. Orthop. Rev., 3:33–35, 1975.
112. Posch, J. L., and Marcotte, D. R.: Carpal tunnel syndrome. An analysis of 1,201 cases. Orthop. Rev., 5:25–35, 1976.
113. Raaf, J. E.: Surgical treatment of patients with cervical disk lesions. J. Trauma, 9:327–338, 1969.
114. Rosati, L. M., and Lord, J. W.: Neurovascular Compression Syndromes of the Shoulder Girdle. New York, Grune & Stratton, 1961.
115. Rose, D. L., and Kelly, C. R.: Shoulder pain. Suprascapular nerve block in shoulder pain. J. Kans. Med. Soc., 70:135–136, 1969.
116. Spillane, J. D.: Localised neuritis of the shoulder girdle. A report of 46 cases in the MEF. Lancet, 2:532–535, 1943.
117. Spinner, M., and Spencer, P. S.: Nerve compression lesions of the upper extremity. A clinical and experimental review. Clin. Orthop., 104:46–67, 1974.

118. Steinbrocker, O.: The shoulder-hand syndrome: Present perspective. Arch. Phys. Med., 49:388–395, 1968.

119. Thompson, W. A. L., and Kopell, H. P.: Peripheral entrapment neuropathies of the upper extremity. N. Engl. J. Med., 260:1261–1265, 1959.

120. Williams, A. F.: The role of the first rib in the scalenus anterior syndrome. J. Bone Joint Surg., 34-B:200–203, 1952.

121. Winsor, T., and Brow, R.: Costoclavicular syndrome. Its diagnosis and treatment. J.A.M.A., 196:697–699, 1966.

122. Wright, I. S., and Cameron, D. J.: The subclavian steal and other shoulder girdle syndromes. Trans. Am. Clin. Climatol. Assoc., 76:13–25, 1964.

123. Wright, V.: The shoulder-hand syndrome. Rep. Rheum. Dis., 24:89–91, 1966.

Arthropathies, Osteochondritides, Osteonecrosis, and Miscellaneous Painful Conditions

124. Abe, Y., Oshima, N., Hataneka, R., Amako, T., and Hirohata, R.: Thirteen cases of alkaptonuria from one family tree with special reference to osteoarthrosis alkaptonuria. J. Bone Joint Surg., 42-A:817–831, 1960.

125. Bosworth, D. M.: An unusual shoulder lesion. J. Bone Joint Surg., 18:1078–1079, 1936.

126. Buchmann, M.: Swelling of the sternoclavicular joint. Acta Med. Orient., 17:65–72, 1958.

127. Dyreborg, E., and Pilgaard, S.: Osteonecrosis in three young men previously treated with steroid for aplastic anaemia. Acta Orthop. Scand., 45:199–205, 1974.

128. Fischel, R. E., and Bernstein, D.: Friedrich's disease. Br. J. Radiol., 48:318–319, 1975.

129. Frey, G. H.: Tietze's syndrome. A new entity in the differential diagnosis of anterior chest wall swelling. Arch. Surg., 73:951–954, 1956.

130. Laskar, F. H., and Sargison, H.: Ochronotic arthroplasty. A. Review with four case reports. J. Bone Joint Surg., 52-B:653–666, 1970.

131. McCallum, R. I., Walder, D. N., Barnes, R., Catto, M. E., Davidson, J. K., Fryer, D. I., Golding, F. C., and Paton, W. D. M.: Bone lesions in compressed air workers. With special reference to men on the Clyde Tunnels 1958 to 1963. J. Bone Joint Surg., 48-B:207–235, 1966.

132. Meszaros, W. T.: The regional manifestations of scleroderma. Radiology, 70:313–325, 1958.

133. Nachamié, B. A., and Dorfman, H. D.: Ischemic necrosis of bone in sickle cell trait. Mt. Sinai J. Med. N.Y., 41:527–536, 1974.

134. Post, M., and Telfer, M. C.: Surgery in hemophilic patients. J. Bone Joint Surg., 57-A:1136–1145, 1975.

15

Injuries to the Rotator Cuff

MELVIN POST

Codman, in 1911 and 1927, described one of the major causes of painful shoulder, namely, rupture of the supraspinatus tendon.[9,10] He first suggested air or opaque fluid arthrography of the shoulder joint, and recommended early operative repair for complete rupture in order to obtain satisfactory results.[10] Codman[11] discovered that Smith[64] in 1834 had made essential observations of "varying percentages of defects in the capsule of the shoulder joint at or about the region of the insertion of the supraspinatus tendon." Smith also found that the long biceps tendon could be involved, by becoming detached from the superior glenoid rim and forming a new attachment in its groove.[64]

Codman's brilliant work on the shoulder was the impetus for numerous articles in the following years that have helped to clarify the diagnosis, pathology, and treatment of this condition.[9-13] To this day Codman's writings have been proven to be remarkably advanced and accurate, with little changing except for the refinement in diagnosis and techniques of operative repair.

ANATOMY

The rotator cuff of the shoulder joint is composed of the short muscles of the shoulder whose muscular and tendinous fibers are closely applied to the fibrous capsule of the shoulder joint. The articular cartilage gradually changes to fibrocartilage

which blends with tendinous fibers at its attachment to the bone (Codman).[9-11] The anatomic structures comprising this region include the subscapularis, the smaller supraspinatus, and the larger infraspinatus-teres minor muscles. The tendons of these muscles cross the joint and blend or fuse with each other and the underlying capsule. They form a musculotendinous cuff about the joint and attach to both tuberosities of the humeral head along the upper two thirds of the anatomic neck. The long head of the biceps in its groove passes between the tuberosities beneath this attachment. Lewis[34] showed that in the stillborn the supraspinatus is fleshy up to its insertion via a short fibrous portion at its end part.[64]

The synovial membrane is reflected from the margin of the glenoid hollow over the labrum, lining the inner surface of the capsule and covering the inferior part and sides of the anatomic neck of the humerus (Fig. 15-1). The long biceps tendon passes within the capsule and is enclosed in a tubular sheath of synovium, which starts at the tendon's attachment at the superior glenoid rim, continues downward in its intertubercular groove, and ends at the level of the surgical neck (Fig. 15-1). Thus, the tendon traverses the joint but is not within the synovial cavity.

There are eight bursae associated with the shoulder joint.[25] However, during arthrography it is the subacromial bursa into which the radiopaque dye tends to leak

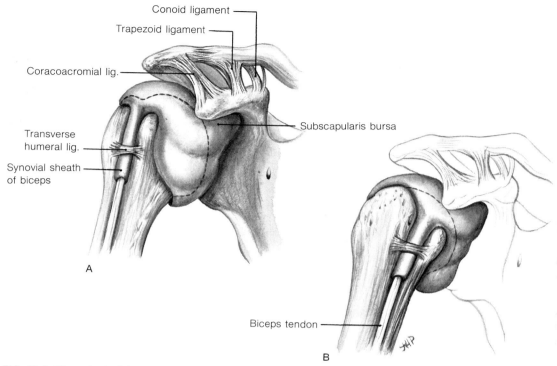

FIG. 15-1. The extent of the synovial membrane is shown with the humerus in, A, external rotation and, B, slight internal rotation. The dotted line indicates the outline of the humeral articular surface.

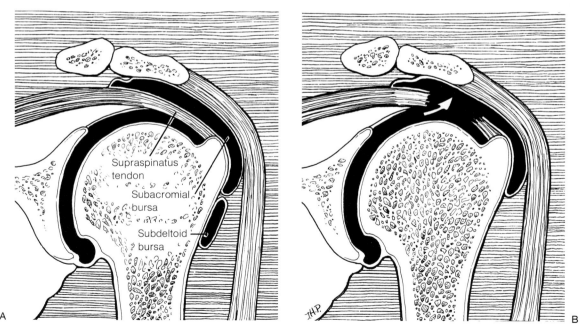

FIG. 15-2. A, Coronal section of the normal shoulder joint. Note the separation of the subacromial bursa from the glenohumeral joint by the supraspinatus tendon. B, When the rotator cuff is ruptured, the subacromial bursa and the joint communicate.

from a complete rotator cuff tear, and therefore is important anatomically (Fig. 15-2). It lies between the undersurface of the acromion and the joint capsule, usually extending under the coracoacromial ligament. It is often continuous with the subdeltoid bursa.

BLOOD SUPPLY OF THE ROTATOR CUFF

In 1939, Lindblom showed that there were areas of relative avascularity in the supraspinatus tendon close to its insertion, and a similar zone of avascularity in the long biceps tendon near its origin.[36] Subsequently, Laing described the arterial supply to the humerus and emphasized the importance of the anterolateral branch of the anterior humeral circumflex artery.[33] He noted that arterial branches perforate the head via the region of the rotator cuff attachment. Moseley and Goldie investigated the vascularity of the rotator cuff attempting to relate it to rupture and calcium deposition.[48] They reviewed a "critical portion" named by Codman 1 cm. medial to the attachment of the supraspinatus tendon and renamed it the "critical zone." They concluded that the morphologic distribution of arteries in the rotator cuff showed no evidence that the critical zone is significantly less vascularized than other areas of the tendinous cuff.[48] Also, they found the "critical zone" to be that region of anastomoses between the osseous and tendinous vessels, age not influencing this pattern.

Rothman and Parke described six arteries that provide the arterial supply to the rotator cuff.[60] They are the suprascapular, anterior humeral circumflex, and posterior circumflex humeral, contributing 100 percent of the time to the cuff, and in descending order of frequency the thoracoacromial, suprahumeral, and subscapular arteries. Rothman and Parke stated that the critical zone was hypovascularized in relation to the rest of the cuff and concluded that the region of hypovascularization in the supraspinatus and infraspinatus tendons was most prone to degenerative changes.[60] They

postulated that ischemia leads to the release of lysozymes which cause additional connective tissue destruction in the joints of patients, as in those of hemophilia and rheumatoid arthritis patients.

Rathbun and Macnab further elucidated the vascularity pattern of the critical zone and found a constant avascularity of this region.[58] They suggested the positions of the rotator cuff tendons predispose them to constant pressure from the humeral head, and tend to squeeze the blood supply out of the vessels when the arm is in the resting position of adduction and neutral rotation.

ROTATOR CUFF FUNCTION

Abduction of the arm is initiated by supraspinatus action and its activity continues throughout the entire range of abduction. Normal abduction capacity of the shoulder occurs because this important structure creates a fixed fulcrum by depressing the humeral head and holding it against the glenoid while the deltoid exerts its action. However, it was shown by Linge and Mulder that suprascapular nerve block only weakened abduction and did not limit it.[38] This is compatible with the findings in the injured patient that not only rotator cuff trauma but ensuing deltoid atrophy may result in loss of abduction strength, but not in a loss of abduction with elimination of supraspinatus action alone.[61]

CLASSIFICATION

Bosworth categorized rotator cuff lesions according to the pathologic anatomy.[4-6] Later, McLaughlin employed such a classification to treat patients with various ruptures of the rotator cuff.[40] The classification is:

I. Incomplete rupture
II. Complete rupture
   A. Pure transverse rupture
   B. Pure vertical or longitudinal tears
   C. Tear with retraction of the tendon edges
   D. Massive avulsion of the cuff

Incomplete tears do not involve the whole cuff thickness. Surface tears may cause irregularities and irritation of the bursal floor, or the tear may be present within the substance of the cuff and involve neither inner nor outer surfaces.

Complete tears of the cuff involve the whole thickness of the cuff which permits a direct communication between the subdeltoid or subacromial bursa and the joint cavity (Fig. 15-2). These lesions may be divided into four subtypes: pure transverse rupture, pure vertical or longitudinal tears, tear with retraction of tendon edges, and massive avulsion of the cuff.

The pure transverse lesion is uncommon,

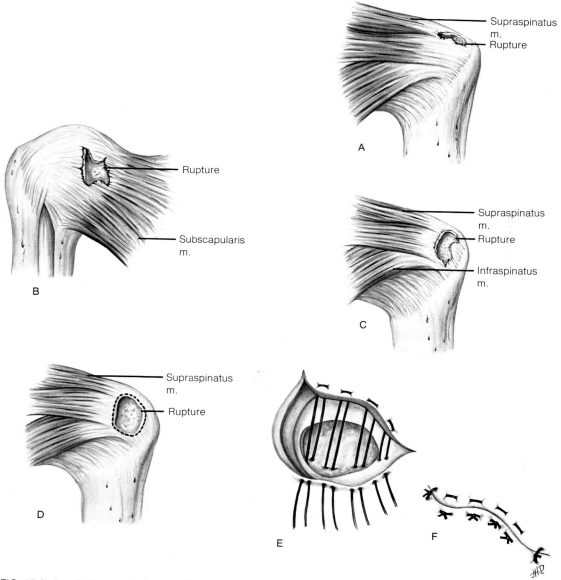

FIG. 15-3. A to C, Types of rotator cuff tears are shown from the front and back. D, In chronic rotator cuff tear, a rim of tissue should be resected to normal vascularized tissue, indicated by dotted line. The amount of resected tissue may be a small rim or a great deal more, if necessary to achieve a sound repair. E and F, One method of closure.

and is not ordinarily observed in the young person, according to McLaughlin.[40] It is seen in patients past 35 years of age who have rotator cuffs weakened by attrition. There is minimal retraction of the edges which makes direct end-to-end suture of freshened edges relatively easy.

Pure vertical or longitudinal tears are most often seen in young patients who have thick, strong cuffs. These ruptures may be found in the cuff portion between the subscapularis and supraspinatus, a region termed the coracocapsular ligament by Jones.[28] Smaller tears often heal spontaneously, but larger ones may require operative repair.

Tears with retraction of torn cuff edges are usually transverse (Fig. 15-3). Not only the cuff but the tendons may be avulsed from their insertion. These cuffs are often

subject to attrition which makes the tendinous tissue weak. The lesion tends to evolve and enlarge into the type in which there is retraction of torn transverse and longitudinal edges.

Massive cuff avulsions or complete avulsion and retraction of the external rotators occur with a longitudinal split separating the supraspinatus and subscapularis. The extent of the rupture is such that the humeral head may subluxate superiorly (Fig. 15-4).

PATHOLOGY AND PATHOGENESIS

Whether trauma or degeneration comes first before cuff rupture has been a subject of controversy for years. Codman and Akerson[13] and later Codman[11] believed that trauma was the more important of the two.

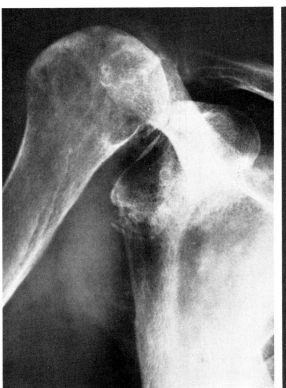
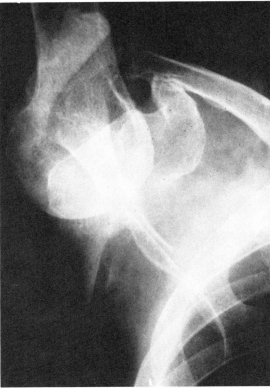

A
B

FIG. 15-4. A, A 66-year-old man had a chronic massive rotator cuff tear. Note the severe superior displacement of the humeral head and disappearance of the normal interval between the acromion and humeral head. B, On passive overhead movement, the humeral head subluxates inferiorly because of the lack of control of the rotator cuff structures.

Meyer considered the important factor to be attrition caused by degenerative changes.[44] Pettersson reported no tears in patients under 30 years of age who had habitual dislocation.[57] In the series of anteroinferior shoulder dislocations reported by Pettersson, 31 percent showed tendon rupture without intra-articular bone injury, the average age being 63 years in 99 cases.[57] He stated that spontaneous ruptures occurring in healthy joints result from degenerative changes due to age, and possibly chronic trauma without an actual history of injury. Spontaneous ruptures were not found in any patient under 55 years of age in 71 healthy joints studied arthrographically.

Keyes reported that age, prolonged use, and trauma were the main factors causing tears in the senile shoulder.[30] DePalma and associates described the changes in the shoulder joint that occur with age,[19] supporting Meyer's belief that attrition is an important factor in cuff tears.[45] Skinner agreed that ruptures are usually preceded by a long period of wear on the supraspinatus tendon.[63] The consensus of authors now is that the degenerated tendon will rupture when trauma is superimposed on the weakened rotator cuff.[6-17,19,24,30,40,46,53,54,57,63,68]

MICROSCOPIC AND CORRELATED PATHOLOGY. Codman[11] and Codman and Akerson[13] showed that the critical zone contained varying degrees of necrosis interspersed with large calcified areas of minute calcium specks, or no calcification at all of the necrotic fibers. Some or all of these fibers may rupture. The tendon attachment to bone may become irregular on its surface or be torn in spots. This area may thicken and show chronic inflammation in the tendon. The synovial reflection almost always changes with tears in the rim, and there may be thinning and loss of the articular cartilage in some cases.

Skinner described some of the structural disturbances occurring with rupture of the supraspinatus tendon including (1) fusion of the aponeurosis and joint capsule, (2) deposition of calcium in the aponeurotic sheet, (3) disappearance of the long head of the biceps, (4) rupture of the supraspinatus tendon, and (5) bony changes.[63] Once the portion of the supraspinatus tendon becomes thin, a fusion results between the aponeurosis and capsule so that during abduction there is little chance of pinching of the capsule, which might occur if a bursa formed between the joint capsule and the aponeurosis. Marked changes may occur in that portion of the greater tuberosity laid bare by retraction of the supraspinatus. Thus, the bony surface becomes rough, irregular, and pitted. In time, the area may become smooth again by rubbing on the undersurface of the acromion. Bosworth reported that a sharp exostosis at the tendinous attachment of the greater tuberosity may occur.[4] He also described two cases of osteochondritis, one in a 17-year-old patient. Both patients erroneously were thought to have classic symptoms of supraspinatus tear.

In 1943, Wilson and Duff described the pathology of rupture and degeneration of the supraspinatus tendon.[69] Wilson later concluded, from a series of experiments in rabbits, that the degeneration observed in the human supraspinatus tendon was caused by trauma during the life of the individual.[70] They believed that incomplete ruptures prevented communication with the subacromial bursa, and that at times the rent was within the substance of the tendon and affected neither surface.[69,70] Such partial tears may be inflamed, or may cause an adherence to the wall of the overlying bursa or even a pannus formation and irregularity over the cuff.

Cotton and Rideout studied 106 necropsy specimens, correlating the pathologic changes with radiologic findings.[14] Both shoulders were examined in each case and abnormalities were found in 68 shoulders. The diagnostic criteria of cuff tear in the 68 shoulders of 38 subjects included (1) cysts in 56 joints, (2) irregularity of the cortex of the greater tuberosity in 31 shoulders, (3) sclerosis of the greater tuberosity or of the groove between it and the articular surface in 27, (4) exaggeration of the groove between the greater tuberosity and the articular surface of the humeral head in 8, (5) narrowing of the acromiohumeral interval in 11, and (6) sclerosis of the humeral surface of the acromion in 9 shoulders. Cotton and Rideout found cuff tears in 35 of the 38 subjects, the average age of the subjects being 70.7 years, and concluded that changes on radiograms could not be correlated with the severity of tears or associated abnormalities except in complete rupture with superior subluxation of the humeral head. In addition, they found villous synovial proliferation in 14 cases, of which 5 had changes on histologic sections resembling pigmented villonodular synovitis.

The collagen bundles show a loss of normal wavy outlines and assume a homogeneous appearance.[70] The nuclei of the fibroblasts become a bit oval and deranged, followed later by a greater loss of normal tendon structure associated with a disappearance of discrete collagen strands. Early fibrillation results, and an increase in the blood vessels within the tendon structures is seen. Of 46 experimentally traumatized rabbit supraspinatus tendons, Wilson found that 86 percent showed a loss of the wavy configuration of the collagen bundles, which produces a homogeneous appearance.[70]

The natural conclusion of authors like Rathbun and Macnab of such studies suggests that these lesions require excision of the diseased, degenerated, avascular tendon in order to obtain a sound operative repair.[58]

DIAGNOSIS

Patients sustaining symptomatic rotator cuff tears are usually in their middle years of life.[24,57] Many are older than 50 years of age, and frequently give a history of recurrent attacks of shoulder pain, most often on the dominant side. Occasionally, the patient relates a history of acute trauma from a fall (Fig. 15-5). Usually, there is a history of chronic persistent or recurring attacks of pain without a specific history of injury. Often, the pain is worse during the night

and awakens the patient from a sound sleep.

Especially with trauma after an acute rupture, the patient experiences pain that increases hours later and has a feeling of weakness, and occasionally is unable to abduct the arm at all (Fig. 15-5A). In my experience, there is seldom a loss of active abduction except in those cases with massive avulsions of the rotator cuff or those patients with failed surgery for such tears. Occasionally, there is an associated adhesive capsulitis which causes limited overhead passive motion. Most patients retain the ability to abduct the arm against gravity (Fig. 15-6). However, abduction weakness is quite significant.

The shoulder is held adducted in the acute phase, and any attempt to move the extremity, especially to abduct it, increases the pain.

Dawbarn described a sign in which a tender point is present over the greater tuberosity.[15] Fracture, bursitis, and rupture of the supraspinatus show this sign, which is the disappearance of the tender point during full abduction when the painful spot is carried beneath the protective arch of the acromion. The presence of crepitus is not pathognomonic of a tear but if present should cause the surgeon to be aware of such a lesion. I agree wholeheartedly with Samilson and Binder that pain, weakness in shoulder elevation, and "popping" or grating are the three most common symptoms of full-thickness tears.[61]

In chronic, large tears the supraspinatus and infraspinatus may be atrophic, a condition easily detected if both shoulders are examined together.

In a patient with a tear whose abduction motion is restricted because of pain, it is sometimes worthwhile infiltrating local anesthetic because testing active abduction motions at this time will usually reveal weakness. In any event, I do not rely on clinical evaluation alone for diagnosis if surgery is contemplated, except when a single trauma has avulsed the rotator cuff tendon and a piece of attached bone is ob-

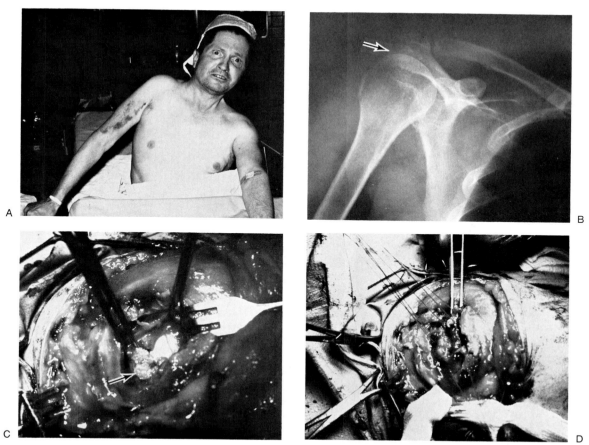

FIG. 15-5. After a fall, a 55-year-old man complained of severe shoulder pain and an inability to abduct his arm. A, Two weeks after injury, note the extent of ecchymosis of the axilla and arm and the inability of the patient to abduct the arm. B, The arrow points to an avulsed bone fragment. The lesion was surgically exposed through a saber-cut incision. C, The arrow points to avulsed cuff, the attached bone fragment, and the rotator cuff defect immediately beyond. D, The repair. A partial anterior acromionectomy was performed. The result was excellent.

served on routine roentgenograms (Fig. 15-5B).

Roentgen Diagnosis

Cotton and Rideout reported that rotator cuff tears are constantly related to cyst formation in the subcortical bone of the anatomic neck of the humerus, partial avulsion of the tendinous insertion of the cuff, loss of the marginal articular surface, or excessive grooving at this margin and "bridge formation."[14] They regard sclerosis of the greater tuberosity in the absence of other radiographic evidence as an unreliable sign.

Skinner suggested that the acromiohumeral interval was narrowed with tear.[63] Golding found the interval normally measures 7 to 13 mm.,[23] whereas Cotton and Rideout stated such reliance with a full-thickness tear was not warranted since one of their cases with a complete tear had a normal interval measurement.[14] They considered sclerosis of the inferior acromial surface to be a more reliable sign of acromial articulation[14] (Fig. 15-7). Weiner and Macnab[66] agreed with Golding,[23] and showed that the normal acromiohumeral interval was 7 to 14 mm., and that an interval of 5 mm. or less should be considered

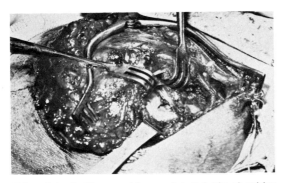

FIG. 15-6. A 45-year-old man injured his shoulder lifting a heavy weight. He had complained of shoulder pain and stiffness for 4 months. A rotator cuff tear was demonstrated by arthrograms. The retractors are beneath the anterior acromion and coracoacromial ligament. A small jagged rotator cuff tear is visible superiorly. An excellent result was achieved by partial anterior acromionectomy and repair.

compatible with a rotator cuff tear. I agree with the latter viewpoint.

Shoulder Arthrography

Shoulder arthrography is an excellent diagnostic tool for accurately determining ro-

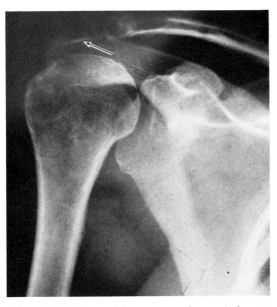

FIG. 15-7. A 55-year-old woman was known to have a rotator cuff tear. Note the decrease in the normal interval between the humeral head and acromion. The arrow points to sclerotic area at the inferior acromial surface.

tator cuff tears and differentiating other local pathologic lesions that may cause similar symptoms. It should be used in patients when any doubt exists as to the cause of shoulder pain.[50] Shoulder arthrograms give a visible record of demonstrable soft-tissue pathologic alterations involving the glenohumeral joint. Moreover, the procedure is simple to perform on an outpatient basis, and its accuracy approaches 95 percent at Michael Reese Medical Center.

In 1927, Codman first suggested this method, stating that he recommended injection of air or opaque fluid.[10] He attempted air injection but apparently had no success in interpreting the x-ray films. The worth of air contrast arthrography to study the inferior recess of the glenohumeral joint after dislocation was reported by Oberholzer in 1933.[54] Subsequently, Lindblom and Palmer[37] and Lindblom[35] performed a series of shoulder arthrograms in 1938 which proved the accuracy of this diagnostic method for rotator cuff tears. In 1957, Kernwein and associates reported their operative findings in 54 patients culled from a series of 96 patients with shoulder arthrograms.[29] A number of authors reported their findings in various pathologic lesions in the shoulder joint that are described later in this section.[31,51-53,59,67] This helped to establish the criteria for correct interpretation of various abnormal conditions in the shoulder joint that are important because physical findings are not pathognomonic.

INDICATIONS. Contrast arthrography is useful for confirming a diagnosis of full-thickness rotator cuff tear. It can be used to differentiate other lesions such as (1) recurrent shoulder dislocations, (2) bicipital lesions, (3) adhesive capsulitis, and (4) partial rupture of the rotator cuff. In this last group of lesions a false negative finding may result in view of the fact that large, deep tears may be missed.

TECHNIQUE. Before arthrograms are taken, routine films in the anteroposterior plane, with the patient's arm in varying degrees of internal and external rotation as desired, and axillary and lateral transthoracic planes should be obtained. A history should be elicited as to possible drug allergies, especially to iodine preparations. In this event, the test should be cancelled.

The patient, the physician performing the test, and personnel should wear surgical caps and masks. The physician should scrub his hands as in surgery. The skin about the patient's shoulder should be cleansed for 10 minutes as in any surgical preparation, and the patient should lie supine on the x-ray table in a room with an image intensifier.

The materials needed for performing the test are two 20-ml. Luer-Lok syringes, a 25-gauge needle with 1 percent procaine HCl (Novocain) to anesthetize the skin, a 20-gauge spinal needle to enter the joint, and a 15-in. length of sterile plastic tubing with an adapter that connects the syringe and needle.

The most common approach for insertion of the spinal needle is anterior. If this approach fails or there is some reason that one wishes to avoid the anterior surface of the shoulder, the posterior approach can be used. In the anterior approach a small skin wheal is raised about 1.3 cm. lateral to the coracoid tip. A spinal needle is directed posteriorly while the patient's arm is in anatomic position. The position of the point of the needle can be checked using a cine-fluoroscope. As the needle tip enters the space between the humeral head and the glenoid, the patient's arm can be internally rotated slowly, and the position of the needle tip again checked on the cine screen. As 4 to 5 ml. of 1 percent Novocain are injected into the joint via the plastic tubing, a definite reflux phenomenon occurs (fluid returns to the syringe). With massive rotator cuff tears this phenomenon may not occur. The first few milliliters should enter the joint easily. Failure to do so gives a clue that there is extravasation about the joint capsule. Now, 8 ml. of meglumine diatrizoate (Renografin-60) are injected with a fresh syringe. The dye can be observed entering the joint on the cine screen. During this injection period the patient will often complain of a sensation of fullness, but may cry out in pain if there is extravasation of the

dye. After injection, the needle is withdrawn and the wound covered with a Band-Aid. Following the arthrographic examination the patient may have soreness in the shoulder for a few days. If pain persists the patient should be examined. There has never been a case of any infected joint, including the shoulder, at Michael Reese Medical Center following countless arthrographic examinations.

In the seldom-used posterior approach, the patient is placed in the prone position with the arm in anatomic position, and the spinal needle tip is directed anteriorly into the space between the glenoid and humeral head. The injection technique is the same as that in the anterior approach.

NORMAL ARTHROGRAPHIC FINDINGS. The interpretation of the findings on an arthrogram depend upon a knowledge of the normal anatomy of the glenohumeral capsule, its synovial lining, and the surrounding bursae. The anatomy of the synovial membrane has been described in the beginning of this chapter (see Fig. 15-1). The synovial membrane and the capsule are normally loose. These structures form a recess or pouch inferiorly which is obliterated when the arm is abducted (see Fig. 15-10).

The synovial membrane, in addition to forming a covering for the long biceps tendon within the joint, is prolonged medially to form the subscapularis bursa, an extension of the capsule beneath the coracoid (Fig. 15-8). The bursa usually communi-

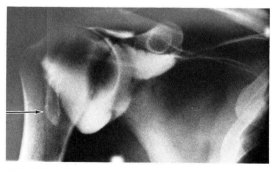

FIG. 15-8. Arthrogram of a normal arm in neutral position. The arrow points to the outline of the biceps sheath. Note the thin meniscus between the head of the humerus and the glenoid.

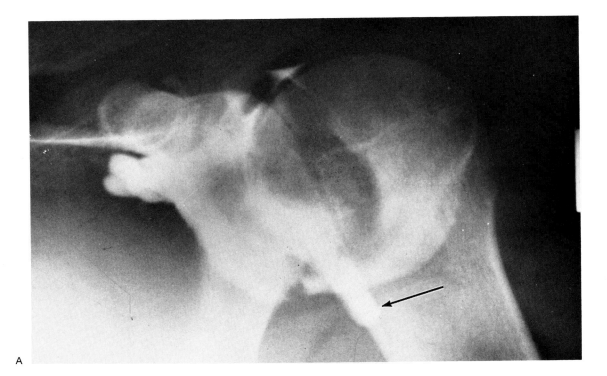

A

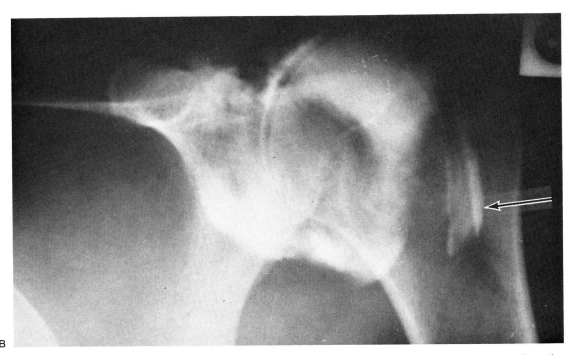

B

FIG. 15-9. Arthrograms of a normal joint in, A, internal rotation and, B, mild external rotation. Arrows show the outline of the biceps sheath.

cates with the shoulder joint between the superior and middle glenohumeral ligaments. A separate subcoracoid bursa does not communicate with the subscapular bursa. The subacromial bursa does not communicate with the shoulder joint (see Fig. 15-2A).

Normally, as the joint fills with dye a thin meniscus appears between the head of the humerus and glenoid cavity (Fig. 15-8).[21] The dye surrounds the head, fills the subscapular bursa beneath the coracoid, and usually collects in the most inferior recess of the articular capsule. As more dye is injected the synovial prolongation about the long biceps tendon is filled. If the humerus is externally rotated this projection may be confused with extravasated dye on the lateral side of the head below the greater tuberosity, when in reality it is the normal projection of dye along the biceps tendon (Fig. 15-9). The glenoid labrum may be seen as an area of lesser density extending vertically within the joint (Fig. 15-9B). There is no extension of the dye beyond the greater tuberosity in a normal patient. Also, there is a normal communication of the joint with the subscapularis bursa. Since the articular capsule is intimately related to the tendons of the rotator muscles, any disruption of the

cuff or of the synovial covering of the long head of the biceps will cause abnormal findings on arthrograms.[21,32,35] The normal volume of the average glenohumeral joint is 28 to 35 ml.[52,59] The normal adult joint will easily accept 16 to 20 ml. of fluid. Ordinarily 8 to 10 ml. of dye are used.

At the start of the examination, the patient should be asked to elevate his arm above his head, thereby depressing the humeral head and forcing dye from the inferior joint recess superiorly so that the entire joint cavity is well outlined. This should be done as soon as possible because the dye is water soluble and begins to be resorbed after 1 hour.

ABNORMAL ARTHROGRAPHIC FINDINGS. *Rotator Cuff Tear.* Dye will exude through a full-thickness tear in the rotator cuff, and appear beyond the normal cuff attachment (Fig. 15-10). The subacromial or subdeltoid bursa is normally separated from the glenohumeral joint. With a cuff tear, dye can appear above the cuff in the subacromial region, or around the attachment of the cuff at the greater tuberosity (Fig. 15-11).[21,29,32] Arthrograms indicative of rotator cuff tear do not indicate the degree of cuff tear.

Bicipital Pathology. The pencil-thin projection of dye within the synovial sheath

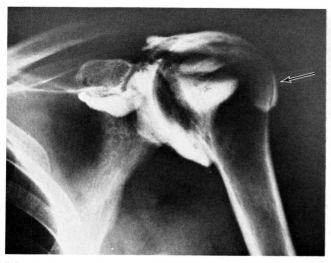 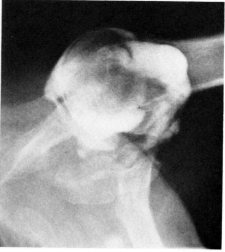

FIG. 15-10. A, A 56-year-old man complained of long-standing pain and stiffness in his left shoulder. A, An arthrogram shows the leakage of dye beyond the cuff attachment at the greater tuberosity (arrow). B, With his arm in abduction, note the disappearance of the dye from the inferior recess.

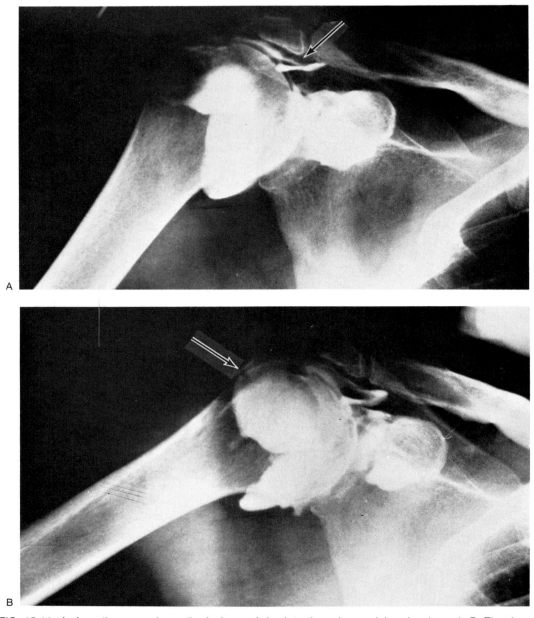

FIG. 15-11. A, An arthrogram shows the leakage of dye into the subacromial region (arrow). B, The dye also extended beyond the normal cuff attachment at the greater tuberosity (arrow).

along the long head of the biceps normally extends to a level just below the inferior border of the transverse bicipital ligament across the bicipital groove (see Fig. 15-1). Normally, dye will not be seen below this level. A tear of the transverse bicipital ligament, the long head of the biceps tendon, or its synovial reflection can be detected on arthrograms (Fig. 15-12). It may even be possible to detect subluxation of the long head of the biceps from its groove, usually medially.[50] Samilson and associates' report that as much as 8 percent of the patients with complete rupture of the long head of

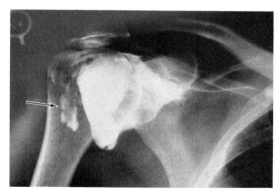

FIG. 15-12. An arthrogram shows an irregular dye pattern within the biceps sheath of a patient known to have bicipital tendinitis (arrow).

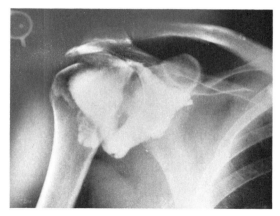

FIG. 15-13. A middle-age adult had recurrent anterior shoulder dislocations. An arthrogram demonstrates the larger-than-normal volume of dye, particularly in the subscapular bursa.

the biceps has associated tears of the rotator cuff appears to be correct.[62] When rotator cuff attrition occurs in the superior portion of the joint, the same degenerative changes often occur in the intra-articular portion of the long head of the biceps.

Dislocation of the Shoulder. Reeves stated that arthrography can demonstrate two types of dislocation.[59] In the first, there is a capsule rupture anteriorly or antero-inferiorly with an egress of dye into the axillary tissues. In the second type, the glenoid labrum or adjacent capsule becomes detached from the glenoid margin and the separation thereby allows dye to escape beneath the subscapularis in the region of its bursa.

Reeves showed by arthrography that in recurrent dislocation there was an enlargement of the subscapularis bursa.[59] Nelson and Razzano stated that 40 ml. of dye could be injected into recurrently dislocating shoulders[50] (Fig. 15-13). This statement is rational to any surgeon who has operated upon cases of anterior shoulder dislocation and has noted the pathologic alterations. Following successful Putti-Platt repair the anterior subscapular bursa is no longer present.

Adhesive Capsulitis (frozen shoulder). The joint volume shrinks in frozen shoulder to only 5 to 10 ml. (Fig. 15-14). Nelson and Razzano stated that a tear may be seen arthrographically in the inferior capsule following manipulation.[50]

Similarly, after repair of rotator cuff lesions the volume of the joint is diminished to 5 to 10 ml. Following the majority of cuff repairs, these operated-upon shoulders act like frozen ones, in my experience, and require considerable stretching exercises to achieve the maximum amount of motion postoperatively.

I do not believe that the arthrogram should be relied upon in deciding the degree of synovitis in a rheumatoid shoulder joint. This belief is in disagreement with the opinion of Weiss and co-workers.[67] For rheumatoid shoulders, clinical findings are best for diagnosis, especially if the surgeon contemplates surgical treatment.

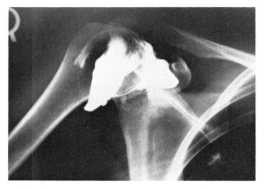

FIG. 15-14. A 38-year-old man had a long-standing history of frozen shoulder. An arthrogram shows the diminished volume of the joint. Note the decreased interval between the humeral head and acromion.

Nepomuceno and Miller showed that of 24 hemiplegic patients with pain, limitation of motion, or subluxation studied with arthrography, eight cases showed rotator cuff and transverse bicipital ligament tears.[51] Of the eight cases with abnormal findings on arthrograms, seven patients had left hemiplegia.

MANAGEMENT OF ROTATOR CUFF TEARS

Conservative Treatment

Most patients with shoulder pain, weakness of the arm on elevation, and even grating indicative of rotator cuff pathologic changes are treated by nonsurgical means. They can be treated with local anesthetic and steroid injection, often with good results, in that the inflammation is decreased and pain subsides. During the acute phase of pain the extremity is supported for 4 to 7 days in a sling. McLaughlin emphasized that the abduction position is unwarranted in the conservative care of a cuff tear because (1) incomplete ruptures are unaffected by posture; (2) retracted edges often are not approximated by abduction; (3) increased synovial fluid volume with anticoagulant activity that more easily escapes through a rent while the arm is in abduction lessens healing (an assumption not completely proven); and (4) the abduction position compresses the retracted tendon stump between the acromion and humerus, much to the detriment of the hypovascular tissues.[41] As the patient begins to feel comfortable, gentle pendulum exercises are started and increased later to passive and active motion exercises in forward flexion, abduction, external rotation, and internal rotation behind the back.

Occasionally, oral anti-inflammatory drugs produce symptomatic relief. Analgesics are prescribed for pain relief. I continue conservative treatment for 2 to 3 months or occasionally even longer, and inform the patient of the suspected diagnosis. When this form of treatment fails and the patient is desirous of relief, arthrography is recommended before attempting surgical repair.

Surgical Treatment

Early surgical repair is recommended for traumatic massive rotator cuff ruptures, especially those in which bone is avulsed from the region of the cuff attachment (see Fig. 15-5). In cuff tears showing attrition and fibrosis, surgical treatment is advocated when pain and other described symptoms become disabling and have failed to respond to adequate conservative treatment. Immediate operation in these cases shows no benefit over deferred repair in which the defect is obliterated. The ideal is to achieve repair and effective healing of the torn edges. There is enough evidence from published reports and from the personal experience of many to advise the reader that in any repair the degenerated hypovascular portion of the cuff should be excised if the patient is to benefit from operative treatment.[58, 60] I have seen numerous surgically repaired cases that have failed because "bad" tissue was repaired or the diseased tissue was excised and the defect was too great to close (Fig. 15-15). In the preoperative evaluation, the surgeon must decide whether or not repair can be reasonably expected to succeed, the goals of treatment being to relieve pain and restore active motion. A correct early assessment of such a case will lessen the need for multiple procedures, each of which further weakens shoulder girdle muscle power, and the lessened power thereby reducing the chance for success.

Following Codman's notable work in which he advised surgical repair of rotator cuff tears,[9, 10, 11, 13] Mayer described his method for repairing cuff tears in 1937.[39] He suggested not splitting the deltoid in order to obviate deltoid weakness after nerve injury. He used fascia to repair large rents in the capsule when the torn edges could not be approximated, and found that when the patient's arm was abducted excessively to prevent tension on the suture line an abduction contracture resulted. Although his

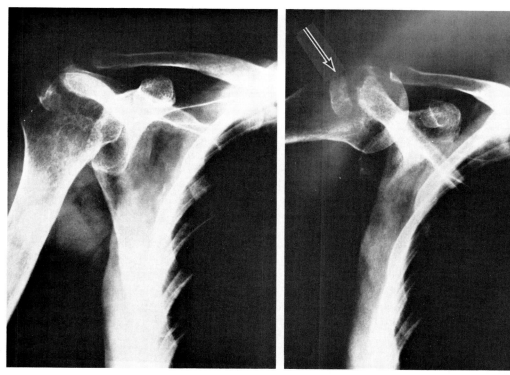

A

B

FIG. 15-15. A 68-year-old woman had a large rotator cuff tear for which she had had an unsuccessful repair. A, Note the superior subluxation of the humeral head and the nonunited acromial osteotomy site. The fragment is tilted downward, which is common and may cause symptoms. B, The arrow points to the nonunited acromial fragment with the arm abducted.

series of four cases is not large, his findings and suggestions are lucid and worthwhile.

In 1941, Bosworth reported on the operative findings in patients with tendon lesions about the rotator cuff in which 4 cases had complete avulsion of the short rotator cuff attachment and 17 cases related to laceration or avulsion of one or more short rotator tendon attachments.[4] He concluded that at times the attempted repair was far more radical and less satisfactory than shoulder fusion, a statement with which I agree. He believed that the tendinous structures first tore and then wore, and thus progressive degeneration and increasing symptoms could be expected.[4] In subsequent papers, Bosworth emphasized that at operation the superficial surface of the tendinous cuff may appear normal and still have a massive avulsion of the underlying tissue.[5,6] He stressed that exploration should not stop with the bursa but should include the deep

surface of the cuff. He recommended repair of supraspinatus and infraspinatus tears by transplantation into a raw wedge-shaped defect in the area of the greater tuberosity. He reiterated his recommendation that fusion of the shoulder is indicated for massive avulsion of the rotator cuff associated with massive fibrillation of the tendons and old crescentic tears.[5] Jones, in a discussion of Bosworth's paper, pointed out the importance of preserving the cuff mechanism by reinserting it into the diaphysis and obtaining good results even when the humeral head was discarded.[28] However, it should be emphasized that with present-day methods of total shoulder replacement, the latter method may give more worthwhile results than fusion.

In a series of excellent papers, McLaughlin provided the surgeon with insight as to the pathology and principles of the treatment of rotator cuff tears.[40-43] He stated that the requisites for successful repair do not necessitate anatomic reconstruction of a cuff tear for good function.[41] However, apposition of healthy tissues is necessary. The tissues must be cut back to strong and reasonably healthy tendon, and if needed, the cut edges of the healthy tendon must be inserted into a raw bone bed. The final repair should be free from tension while the arm is at the side. This is often difficult when the edges are retracted without abduction of the arm. If the arm must be abducted beyond 45 to 50 degrees, consideration should be given to another procedure, such as arthroplasty. In any event, after side-to-side repair any residual tendon defect should be as small as possible (see Fig. 15-18). McLaughlin correctly stated that continuity without tension should be achieved between the muscle bellies of the tendons and the humerus by reinsertion of the remaining edges of the defect into a V-shaped groove in the bone if necessary.[41] The superior surface of the repair should be smooth for movement beneath the acromion. If this cannot be attained, the anterior portion of the acromion should be excised. Neer restated the concept that with the arm in anatomic position the critical area is the part where degenerative tendinitis and rupture occur in the supraspinatus, and occasionally extends to involve the anterior part of the infraspinatus and long head of the biceps.[12,47,49] If painful impingement of the repaired cuff seems likely, resection of the anterior acromion, as suggested by Neer,[49] is recommended. I often follow this practice and obtain an excellent exposure of the cuff structures. It is not necessary in most cases to remove osteophytes on the undersurface of the acromioclavicular joint because they seldom cause impingement. Only in very select cases is complete acromionectomy warranted, as suggested by Armstrong[1] and by Hammond.[26] Occasionally, I find that the arm must be abducted to prevent tension on the new deltoid insertion into the raw acromial edge. Four weeks later the arm is slowly brought down to the side over a 2-week period (Fig. 15-16).

McLaughlin also advised that an enlarged and inflamed long head of the biceps tendon is not functionally needed and may cause symptoms if left behind.[41] In such an event, the intra-articular part should be removed and the distal end sutured to the roof of the bicipital groove. Lastly, it is best to attempt a watertight repair so that later motion will not force synovial fluid through an opening in the repair.

Eichler reported his experience of 24 cases on which he used the Bateman technique[2,3] for repairing a torn rotator cuff. He resected the anterior acromion with an osteotomy extending from a point just anterior to the posterior capsule of the acromioclavicular joint to the anterior and lateral corner of the acromion in order to achieve repair in difficult cases.[20] He removed the bone along with the coracoacromial ligament in order to expose the cuff and to decompress the cuff in the arc of motion of the repaired defect.[20] Bateman combined acromionectomy with resection of the outer fifth of the clavicle.[2] If needed, the coracoacromial ligament can be used to close a large gap.

Debeyre, Patte, and Elmelik reported their results of rotator cuff repair, using a posterosuperior approach, in which the whole supraspinatus muscle was advanced from its fossa laterally, if needed, to close a large gap.[16] Thus, a wide defect can be closed with little tension on the suture line (Fig. 15-17). The patient is placed in the prone position and the extremity is draped free. A transverse incision is made 1 cm. above the spine of the scapula, curved over the acromion, and extended 2.5 cm. beyond its lateral edge (see Fig. 15-20A). The trapezius is detached from the scapular insertion. An osteotomy of the acromion is performed transversely and obliquely outward and backward (Fig. 15-17B). The anterior segment is left connected to the clavicle by the acromioclavicular joint and the posterior part to the spine of the scapula.[16] The upper deltoid fibers are split, care being taken to avoid injury to the axillary nerve. The osteotomy site is kept open by a self-retaining retractor. The coracoacromial ligament is

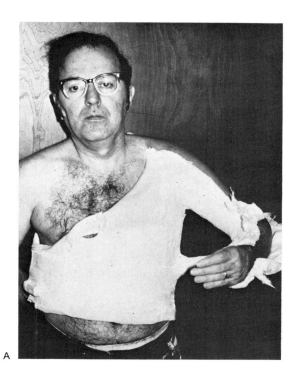

A

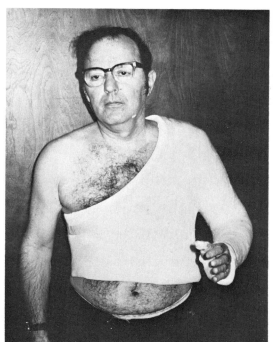

B

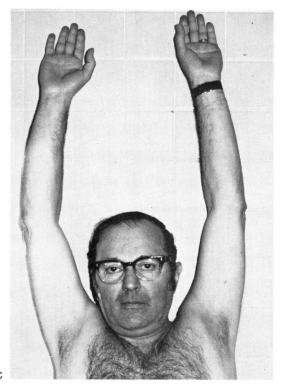

C

FIG. 15-16. A 50-year-old man underwent a repair of a torn rotator cuff. There was excessive tension on the suture line of the repair site. A, The day after surgery the extremity was placed in 45 degrees of abduction. B, At 4 weeks postoperatively, the arm was slowly brought down to the side over the next 2 weeks and motion exercises were started thereafter. C, Two years later, note the overhead motion. The result was excellent.

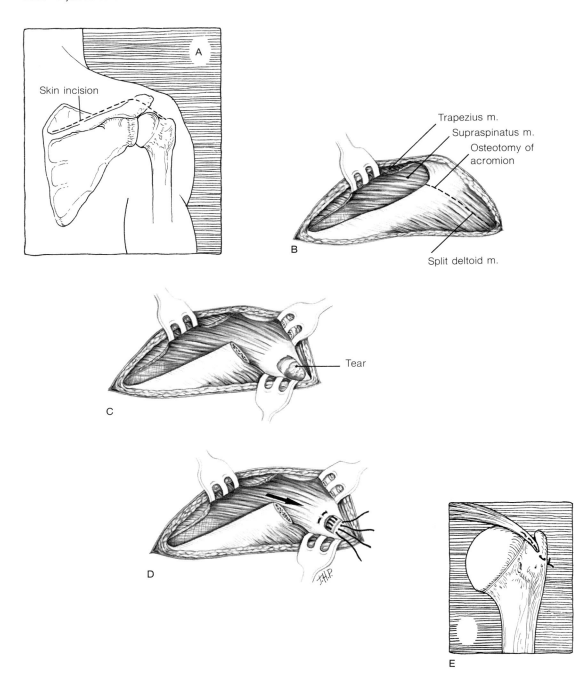

FIG. 15-17. Debeyre method for repair of the rotator cuff. (See text for discussion.)

divided and the subacromial bursa opened.

With small rents in the cuff, the supraspinatus tendon may be stretched to close the tear. For large ruptures, the supraspinatus muscle can be carefully elevated from its fossa, and its nerve and blood supply preserved so that the proximal end of the tendon can be reattached into bone (Fig. 15-17D and E). The trapezius is reattached, the deltoid edges are closed, and the osteotomy site is allowed to fall into place. Hemovac suction is recommended.

Aftercare requires a plaster of Paris spica cast with the arm abducted for 4 to 6 weeks, and then gradually increasing exercises are prescribed for 3 to 4 months. This method of treatment seems to have merit for large cuff tears.

Still other techniques have been devised to close rotator cuff defects. Neviaser described his method of closing a defect when the cuff edges cannot be approximated.[52] The patient is placed in a semireclining position and the arm is draped free. A saber-cut incision is made and an osteotomy of the outer portion of the acromion performed (see Fig. 15-20A and B). The deltoid is retracted after elevating it from the lateral portion of the clavicle (see Fig. 15-20C). Adhesions between the subdeltoid bursa and undersurface of the deltoid are freed by finger dissection or with a periosteal elevator to allow visibility of the cuff tear (Fig. 15-18). When the cuff edges cannot be approximated, Neviaser takes a free graft from the intra-articular portion of the long head of the biceps and sutures the distal end in its groove.[52] The free tendon graft is sectioned in a book-like fashion and stretched, and the smooth side is placed toward the joint and attached in place with Dexon, Vicryl, or nonabsorbable suture. Closure of the defect should be watertight. The deltoid is reattached to the acromion. A Velpeau dressing is applied. The patient is instructed in shoulder girdle elevation exercises the next day. The bandage is removed after 3 weeks, and gentle pendulum exercises are started with the arm in a sling for 1 week. Thereafter, motion exercises are increased. I have performed this operation and find that it is satisfactory in selected cases.

Wolfgang reported on a series of 65 surgical repairs in which the results tended to be worse when there were calcific deposits in the cuff, if the acromion was not reattached after osteotomy of the acromion, and if the repair required suturing of the proximal cuff into a trough in the humeral head.[71] He reported 14 cases in which the condition of the long head of the biceps did not appear to influence the results of cuff repair. The results of cuff repair in these 14 cases were slightly better than those in patients who underwent other types of repairs in the rest of the series.

Bush reported a transacromial surgical exposure. A V-shaped osteotomy of the acromion was performed and the acromion was subsequently repositioned using bone screws to hold it.[8] Bush repaired the cuff defect by performing a standard repair after the long head of the biceps tendon was reseated in a newly constructed, more laterally located trough in the humeral head (Fig. 15-19).

Postoperatively, the extremity is placed in Velpeau position or occasionally in a shoulder spica cast. The arm is slowly lowered to the side. Passive exercises are started after 3 weeks, and active exercises against gravity after 6 weeks. When large defects cannot be closed primarily, this procedure has merit in select cases.

Author's Management of Rotator Cuff Ruptures

I believe that when surgical treatment is needed to relieve pain and restore function in cases of rotator cuff tear, the sooner the repair is performed the better the result, because long delay often causes an increase in disuse atrophy of the rotator muscles. Furthermore, there is no single method that can be used to treat every case. Thus, every case should be individualized. Although strong shoulder girdle muscles are desirable, pain prevents exercising which builds muscle strength. For best postoperative results I also recommend exercises to attain as complete a passive range of motion preoperatively as is possible in those cases demonstrating frozen shoulder symptoms. However, when this is not possible, a successful operative result is not necessarily precluded (see Fig. 15-18). Moreover, whatever surgical method is selected, the principles enunciated by McLaughlin should be followed.[41] For example, Hauser described two cases of avulsed subscapularis tendon in which he effected repair of the defect by laterally advancing the muscle-tendon

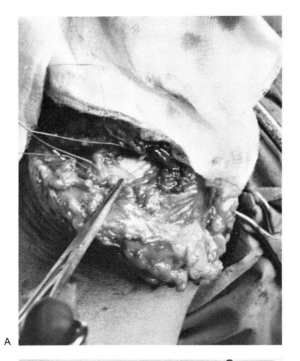

A

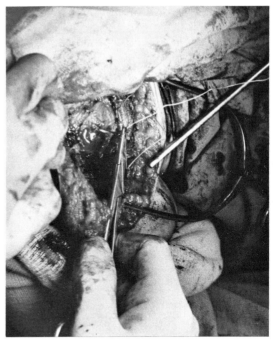

B

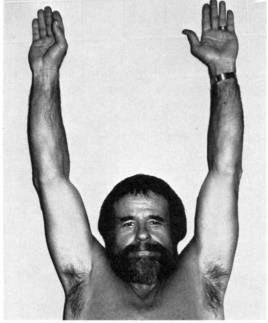

C

FIG. 15-18. A, A 44-year-old man had a frozen shoulder and torn rotator cuff. Note the defect. B, After resection of the avascular, degenerated tissue, the fresh cut edges were approximated. The enlarged defect, as well as the repair, is shown. C, His motion is demonstrated 4 years later. The result was excellent.

structure beneath the long head of the biceps and fixing it to the bone lateral to the bicipital groove.[27] The subscapularis may also be mobilized to cover anterosuperior defects. The methods of Bosworth,[4,6] McLaughlin,[41,42] Bateman,[2,3] Debeyre and associates,[16] and others[53,56,65,71] may be used to close a defect. Neviaser's method to bridge large gaps in the rotator cuff by using the long head of the biceps tendon works satisfactorily.[52]

When closing a large defect, the apex of

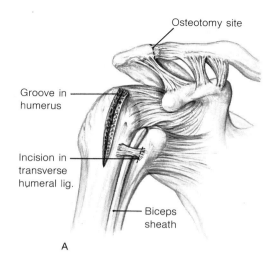

Osteotomy site

Groove in humerus

Incision in transverse humeral lig.

Biceps sheath

A

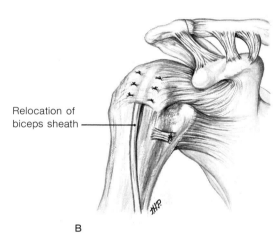

Relocation of biceps sheath

B

FIG. 15-19. Bush method for closing rotator cuff defects. A, An osteotomy of the acromion is performed in a V-shaped fashion and a trough made in the lateral proximal humeral cortex. B, The long head of the biceps is reseated into the trough and sutured in place, and the freshened torn cuff edges are sutured to the repositioned tendon.

the defect should be closed first. The edges of the gap are brought together as much as possible in the shape of a V, until a small gap results whose edges are then sutured into a raw bone trough in the humeral head. In my experience, when the arm must be abducted more than 45 to 50 degrees, it is better to consider a salvage procedure.

The patient is positioned in a semireclining position and the extremity draped free.[18] The shoulder is elevated on a sandbag placed behind the shoulder blade. I prefer a saber-cut incision starting at the posterosuperior edge of the acromion, and extend it over the top of the shoulder and downward just lateral to the acromioclavicular joint (Fig. 15-20A). It may be extended downward over the deltopectoral groove, if necessary. The skin flaps are freed medially and laterally to expose the deltoid origin. The acromial attachment of the deltoid with 1 to 2 mm. of bone is elevated from the lateral and anterior acromion, and outer inch of clavicle. The deltoid is retracted downward and any adherent deltoid muscle is freed from the underlying subacromial bursa. The arm is rotated inward and outward in order to observe a wide arc of the rotator cuff (Fig. 15-20C).

It may be difficult to locate the tear. In this case the wet, gloved finger may palpate the defect as the patient's arm is rotated. It may be necessary to open the floor of the subacromial bursa in order to define the gap. After the defect is located, the edges are cut back to healthy tissue (Fig. 15-20B). The edges are approximated with 2-0 suture (Dexon, Vicryl, or nonabsorbable), if possible (Fig. 15-20C). With large gaps in the torn rotator cuff, advancement of the supraspinatus after the method of Debeyre and coworkers is preferred.[16]

If it seems that a spur is present on the undersurface of the acromion, that later there might be an impingement between the humeral head and acromion, or that additional exposure is needed to fully repair the cuff defect, then partial acromionectomy is performed as described by Neer.[49]

In reattaching the deltoid muscle, small holes are drilled in the distal clavicle and acromion and heavy suture material is passed through the holes and the muscle is reattached. If any tension is present in the repaired defect or the reattached muscle-to-bone suture line, the arm can be abducted to 45 degrees following closure of the wound (see Fig. 15-16).

The patient's arm is kept abducted in a splint and a plaster of Paris spica cast applied the next day. After 3 to 4 weeks the arm is brought down slowly over the next 2 weeks. Gentle pendulum exercises with the

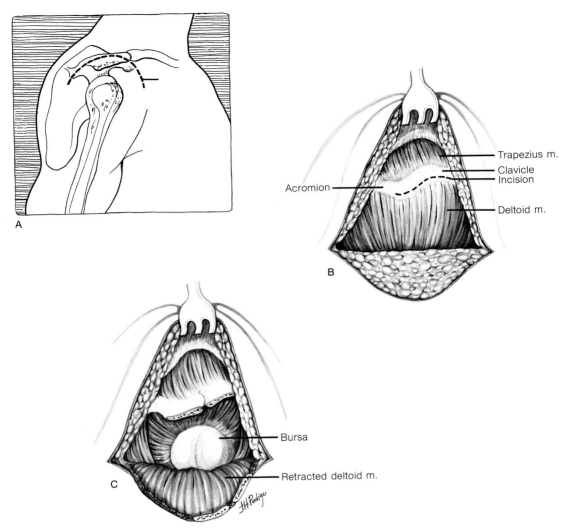

FIG. 15-20. Anterior surgical approach via a saber-cut incision. (See text for discussion.)

arm in a sling are started at 5 to 6 weeks, and passive motion exercises gradually increased. Later, active exercises are prescribed. The patient is weaned from the sling at 6 weeks postoperatively.

Complications of Surgical Repair

When excessive bone is removed from the lateral humeral head in an attempt to close the gap, the result is likely to be a disastrous one. Total acromionectomy should be avoided except in unusual cases because it is difficult to reattach the deltoid and the fulcrum for this muscle is then lost. Finally, it is important to have functioning rotator muscles that are necessary to stabilize the humeral head. Merely repairing large defects in the presence of weak or nonfunctioning rotator muscles will not allow a good result. In this event, a salvage procedure must be considered. These patients often complain of severe pain and unstable shoulder joints. They require a fixed fulcrum total shoulder replacement if arthroplasty is planned (see Chapter 10).

REFERENCES

1. Armstrong, J. R.: Excision of the acromion in treatment of the supraspinatus syndrome. J. Bone Joint Surg., 31-B:436–442, 1949.
2. Bateman, J. B.: The diagnosis and treatment of ruptures of the rotator cuff. Surg. Clin. North Am., 43:1523–1530, 1963.
3. Bateman, J. E.: The Shoulder and Neck. Philadelphia, W. B. Saunders Co., 1972.
4. Bosworth, D. M.: Analysis of 28 consecutive cases of incapacitating shoulder lesions radically explored and repaired. J. Bone Joint Surg., 22:369–392, 1940.
5. Bosworth, D. M.: The supraspinatus syndrome. Symptomatology, pathology and repair. J.A.M.A., 117:422–438, 1941.
6. Bosworth, D. M.: Muscular and Tendinous Defects of the Shoulder and Their Repair. American Academy of Orthopaedic Surgeons. Lectures on Reconstruction Surgery of the Extremities. Ann Arbor. J. W. Edwards, pp. 380–392, 1944.
7. Brown, J. T.: Early assessment of supraspinatus tears: Procaine infiltration as a guide. J. Bone Joint Surg., 31-B:423–425, 1949.
8. Bush, L. F.: The torn shoulder capsule. J. Bone Joint Surg., 57-A:256–259, 1975.
9. Codman, E. A.: Complete rupture of the supraspinatus tendon. Operative treatment with report of two successful cases. Boston Med. Surg. J., 164:708–710, 1911.
10. Codman, E. A.: Obscure lesions of the shoulder; Rupture of the supraspinatus tendon. Boston Med. Surg. J., 196:381–387, 1927.
11. Codman, E. A.: The Shoulder. Boston, Thomas Todd Co., 1934.
12. Codman, E. A.: Rupture of the supraspinatus, 1834 to 1934. J. Bone Joint Surg., 19:643–652, 1937.
13. Codman, E. A., and Akerson, I. B.: The pathology associated with rupture of the supraspinatus tendon. Ann. Surg., 93:348–359, 1931.
14. Cotton, R. E., and Rideout, D. F.: Tears of the humeral rotator cuff. A radiological and pathological necropsy survey. J. Bone Joint Surg., 46-B:314–328, 1964.
15. Dawbarn, R. H. M.: Subdeltoid bursitis: A pathognomonic sign for its recognition. Boston Med. Surg. J., CLIV:691, 1906.
16. Debeyre, J., Patte, D., and Elmelik, E.: Repair of rupture of the rotator cuff of the shoulder. With a note on advancement of the supraspinatus muscle. J. Bone Joint Surg., 47-B:36–42, 1965.
17. DePalma, A. F.: Surgery of the Shoulder. Philadelphia, J. B. Lippincott Co., pp. 125–136, 1950.
18. DePalma, A. F.: Surgical approaches to the region of the shoulder joint. Clin. Orthop., 20:163–184, 1961.
19. DePalma, A. F., Callery, G., and Bennett, C. A.: Variational Anatomy and Degenerative Lesions of the Shoulder Joint. American Academy of Ortho-paedic Surgeons. Instructional Course Lectures, 6:255–281, 1949.
20. Eichler, E. J.: Treatment of Ruptures of the Rotator Cuff (Bateman Technique). Proceedings of the Clinical Orthopaedic Society, Oct. 2–4, 1974.
21. Ellis, V. H.: The diagnosis of shoulder lesions due to injuries of rotator cuff. J. Bone Joint Surg., 35-B:72–74, 1953.
22. Golding, F. C.: The shoulder—the forgotten joint. Br. J. Radiol., 35:149–158, 1962.
23. Golding, C.: Radiology and orthopaedic surgery. J. Bone Joint Surg., 48-B:320–332, 1966.
24. Grant, J. C. B., and Smith, C. G.: Age incidence of rupture of the supraspinatus tendon. Anat. Rec., 100:666, 1948 (Abstr.).
25. Gray, H.: Anatomy of the Human Body, ed. by Goss, C. M., 29th ed. Lea & Febiger, Philadelphia, 1974.
26. Hammond, G.: Complete acromionectomy in the treatment of chronic tendinitis of the shoulder. A follow-up study of 90 operations on 97 patients. J. Bone Joint Surg., 53-A:173–200, 1971.
27. Hauser, E. D. W.: Avulsion of the Subscapularis Muscle. J. Bone Joint Surg., 36-A:139–141, 1954.
28. Jones, L.: The shoulder joint: Observations on the anatomy and physiology with an analysis of a reconstructive operation following extensive injury. Surg. Gynecol. Obstet., 75:433–444, 1942.
29. Kernwein, G. H., Roseberg, B., and Sneed, W. R.: Arthrographic studies of the shoulder joint. J. Bone Joint Surg., 39-A:1267–1274, 1957.
30. Keyes, E. L.: Anatomical observations on senile changes in the shoulder. J. Bone Joint., 17:953–960, 1935.
31. Killoran, P. J., Marcove, R., and Freiberger, R. H.: Shoulder arthrography. Am. J. of Roentgenol., 103:658–668, 1968.
32. Kotzen, L. M.: Roentgen diagnosis of rotator cuff tear—Report of 48 surgically proven cases. Am. J. Roentgenol., 112:507–511, 1971.
33. Laing, P. G.: The arterial supply of the adult humerus. J. Bone Joint Surg., 38:1105–1116, 1956.
34. Lewis, W. H.: The development of the arm in man. Am. J. Anat., 145:184, 1902.
35. Lindblom, K.: Arthrography and roentgenography in rupture of the tendons of the shoulder joint. Acta Radiol., 20:548–562, 1939.
36. Lindblom, K.: On pathogenesis of ruptures of the tendon aponeurosis of the shoulder joint. Acta Radiol., 20:563–577, 1939.
37. Lindblom, K., and Palmer, F.: Rupture of the tendon aponeurosis of the shoulder joint—The so-called supraspinatus rupture. Acta Chir. Scand., 82:133–142, 1939.
38. Linge, B., van, and Mulder, J. D.: Function of the supraspinatus muscle and its relation to the supraspinatus syndrome. J. Bone Joint Surg., 45-B:750, 1963.

39. Mayer, L.: Rupture of the supraspinatus tendon. J. Bone Joint Surg., 19:640–642, 1937.

40. McLaughlin, H. L.: Lesions of the musculotendinous cuff of the shoulder. I. The exposure and treatment of tears with retraction. J. Bone Joint Surg., 26:31–49, 1944.

41. McLaughlin, H. L.: Rupture of the rotator cuff. J. Bone Joint Surg., 44-A:979–983, 1962.

42. McLaughlin, H. L.: Repair of major cuff ruptures. Surg. Clin. North Am., 43:1535–1540, 1963.

43. McLaughlin, H. L., and Asherman, E. G.: Lesions of the musculotendinous cuff of the shoulder. IV. Some observations based upon the results of surgical repairs. J. Bone Joint Surg., 33-A:76–86, 1951.

44. Meyer, A. W.: Further evidence of attrition in the human body. Am. J. Anat., 34:241–267, 1924.

45. Meyer, A. W.: The minute anatomy of attrition lesions. J. Bone Joint Surg., 13:341, 1931.

46. Moseley, H. F.: Rupture of the Rotator Cuff. Springfield, Ill., Charles C Thomas, 1952.

47. Moseley, H. F.: Shoulder Lesions, ed. 3. Edinburgh, E. & S. Livingstone Ltd., pp. 75–81, 243–292, 1969.

48. Moseley, H. F., and Goldie, I.: The arterial patterns of the rotator cuff of the shoulder. J. Bone Joint Surg., 45-B:780–789, 1963.

49. Neer, C. S.: Anterior acromioplasty for the chronic impingement syndrome in the shoulder. A preliminary report. J. Bone Joint Surg., 54-A:41–50, 1972.

50. Nelson, C. L., and Razzano, C. D.: Arthrography of the shoulder. A review. J. Trauma, 13:136–141, 1973.

51. Nepomuceno, C. S., and Miller, J. M.: Shoulder arthrography in hemiplegic patients. Arch. Phys. Med. Rehabil., 55:49–51, 1974.

52. Neviaser, J. S.: Ruptures of the rotator cuff of the shoulder. New concepts in the diagnosis and operative treatment of chronic ruptures. Arch. Surg., 102:483–485, 1971.

53. Neviaser, J. S.: Arthrography of the Shoulder. The Diagnosis and Management of the Lesions Visualized. Springfield, Ill., Charles C Thomas, 1975.

54. Oberholzer, J.: Die Arthropneumoradiographie bei Habitueller Schulterluxation. Roentgenpraxis, 5:589–590, 1933.

55. Olsson, O.: Degenerative changes in the shoulder joint and their connection with shoulder pain. A morphological and clinical investigation with special attention to the cuff and biceps tendon. Acta Chir. Scand. (Suppl.), 181:1–130, 1953.

56. Packard, A. G.: Management of large tears of the rotator cuff of the shoulder. Clin. Orthop., 44:279–280, 1966.

57. Pettersson, G.: Ruptures of the tendon aponeurosis of the shoulder joint in anterior inferior dislocation. Acta Chir. Scand. (Suppl.), 77:1–184, 1942.

58. Rathbun, J. B., and Macnab, I.: The microvascular pattern of the rotator cuff. J. Bone Joint Surg., 52-B:540–553, 1970.

59. Reeves, B.: Arthrography of the shoulder. J. Bone Joint Surg., 48-B:424–435, 1966.

60. Rothman, R. H., and Parke, W. W.: The vascular anatomy of the rotator cuff. Clin. Orthop., 41:176–186, 1965.

61. Samilson, R. L., and Binder, W. F.: Symptomatic full thickness tear of the rotator cuff. An analysis of 292 shoulders in 276 patients. Orthop. Clin. North Am., 6:449–466, 1975.

62. Samilson, R., Raphael, R. L., Post, L., Noonan, C., Siris, E., and Raney, F.: Arthrography of shoulder joint. Clin. Orthop., 20:21–31, 1961.

63. Skinner, H. A.: Anatomical consideration relative to ruptures of the supraspinatus tendon. J. Bone Joint Surg., 19-A:137–151, 1937.

64. Smith, J. G.: Pathological appearances of seven cases of injury of the shoulder joint with remarks. London Med. Gazette, 14:280, 1834 (reported in Am. J. Med. Sci., 16:219–224, 1834).

65. Weiner, D. S., and Macnab, I.: Rupture of the rotator cuff: Follow-up evaluation of operative repairs. Can. J. Surg., 13:219–227, 1970.

66. Weiner, D. S., and Macnab, I.: Superior migration of the humeral head. A radiological aid in the diagnosis of tears of the rotator cuff. J. Bone Joint Surg., 52-B:524–527, 1970.

67. Weiss, J. J., Thompson, G. R., Doust, V., and Burgener, F. A.: Arthrography in the diagnosis of shoulder pain and immobility. Arch. Phys. Med. Rehabil., 55:205–209, 1974.

68. Wilson, C. L.: Lesions of the supraspinatus tendon: Degeneration, rupture, and calcification. Arch. Surg., 46:307–325, 1943.

69. Wilson, C. L., and Duff, G. L.: Pathological study of degeneration and rupture of the supraspinatus tendon. Arch. Surg., 47:121–135, 1943.

70. Wilson, P. D.: Complete ruptures of the supraspinatus tendon. J.A.M.A., 96:433–439, 1931.

71. Wolfgang, G. H.: Surgical repair of tears of the rotator cuff of the shoulder. J. Bone Joint Surg., 56-A:14–26, 1974.

16

Management of Open Wounds of the Shoulder

MELVIN POST

The shoulder joint and important neighboring structures are vulnerable to a variety of wounding agents. Most notable are those caused by sharp objects such as knives and those from missiles like bullets, shotgun pellets, and metal fragments. Serious open injuries are occasionally caused by industrial and vehicular accidents. It is essential to determine both the magnitude and mechanism of the injury. In the case of knife wounds, a discrete laceration can be recognized, whereas missile wounds usually cause latent tissue injury.

Carney and associates found an 8.9 percent incidence of gunshot wounds of the shoulder in comparison to the total number of joint wounds in one study of major joint injuries during World War II.[3] Moreover, these injuries resulted in a 66 percent infection rate. Such serious wounds not only are encountered during wartime, but are seen daily in civilian practice especially in the large cities. When the importance of the shoulder in relation to normal function of the whole upper extremity is considered, it is crucial that the most effective treatment be instituted from the very onset.

HIGH-VELOCITY BULLET WOUNDS

Rational treatment of open wounds caused by high-velocity bullets depends upon an understanding of the wounding capacity of various missiles.

Ballistic Considerations

The extent of a missile wound relates to a number of parameters, the more important of which include missile energy (ME) at impact and the type of missile employed.

Military bullet designs conform to Geneva Convention standards that differ from those of the expanding, hunting-type bullets used in civilian life. In any event, the wounding effects of any bullet may be explained by the now commonly accepted kinetic energy theory: the greater the energy of the missile at impact the greater is the degree of piercing, laceration, and contusion of the tissues penetrated. The amount of kinetic energy developed is equal to the mass of the missile (M) multiplied by the square of the velocity (V).[4,5] The energy force (E) may be expressed as $E = MV^2/2$. Accordingly, doubling the bullet weight doubles the energy, and doubling the velocity quadruples it. The energy imparted at impact causes tissue damage, so that different bullets with different energy levels permit varying degrees of injuries (Table 16-1).

Bullet velocity may be classified as low when the velocity is under 1000 ft./sec., medium between 1000 and 2000 ft./sec., and

329

Table 16-1. *Ballistics of Common Rifle Cartridges*

Caliber	Bullet Weight (gr.)	Velocity (ft./sec.)		Energy (ft-lb.)	
		Muzzle	100 Yards	Muzzle	100 Yards
Civilian Rifles					
.22 Hornet	46	2380	1710	578	289
.243 Winchester	100	3070	2790	2093	1729
.30-30 Winchester	170	2220	1890	1861	1349
.44 Magnum Remington	240	1850	1450	1820	1120
Military Rifles					
M-16 .223	55	3250	2869	1289	1004
M-14 .308	110	3340	2810	2730	1930
.303 British	180	2540	2340	2579	2189

Data from Barnes, F. C.: Cartridges of the World, 3rd ed. Ed. by J. T. Amber. Chicago, Follett Publishing Company, 1972; National Rifleman, March, 1968; DeMuth, W. E., and Smith, J. W.: High-velocity bullet wounds of muscle and bone: The basis of rational early treatment. J. Trauma, 6:744–755, 1966.

high above 2000 ft./sec. Most military ammunition delivers the bullet at a muzzle velocity between 2400 and 2900 ft./sec., and some bullets, such as the M-16 bullet, attain a muzzle velocity of about 3250 ft./sec. Hopkinson and Marshall have shown that when the bullet leaves the muzzle the velocity decreases, so that it is the velocity at impact that determines the amount of tissue damaged.[12]

Pistol bullet wounds are generally delivered by low-velocity bullets of varying weights (Table 16-2). The diminishing velocity of a rifle bullet may fall off so that at 100 yards or less a greater degree of wounding capacity is present than at ranges of 400 to 1000 yards. At the latter distances, the velocity (wounding capability) may be reduced to those seen with pistol bullets at shorter distances. When only the rifle caliber and bullet weight are known, accurate estimates of wounding capability cannot be made.

Bullet stabilization is greater when the missile spins. Therefore, a greater degree of spin increases the strike velocity, range, and consistency of the trajectory because of reduced air drag. Stability is achieved by spin imparted by rifling of the barrel. Residual velocity is that velocity which remains as the target is perforated, and energy expended within the organism is a function of the difference between impact and residual velocities. When a missile remains within the body all available energy has been absorbed. When the bullet is retained within the organism the severity of the wound is increased compared with that caused when the missile also has left the body. Other ballistic considerations, such as trajectory, yaw, bullet and barrel design, and the resulting spin and tumble of a bul-

Table 16-2. *Ballistics of Common Pistol Cartridges*

Cartridge Caliber	Bullet Weight (gr.)	Muzzle	
		Velocity (ft./sec.)	Energy (ft-lb.)
.38 Smith and Wesson	150	1065	382
.38 special	158	866	266
.45 Automatic (USA)	230	860	378
.22 Remington Jet	40	1710	261

Data from Barnes, F. C.: Cartridges of the World, 3rd ed. Ed. by J. T. Amber. Chicago, Follett Publishing Company, 1972: National Rifleman, March, 1968; DeMuth, W. E., and Smith, J. W.: High-velocity bullet wounds of muscle and bone: The basis of rational early treatment. J. Trauma, 6:744–755, 1966.

let help determine the final velocity at impact.

Pathology and Pathogenesis of Missile Wounds

High-velocity penetrating missiles cause laceration, crushing, shock waves, and temporary cavitation of deep tissues.[11] The penetrating missile causes tissue destruction or a permanent wound tract immediately after the missile passes. The track caused by a high-velocity missile is usually cylindrical or slightly conical, and the exit wound is often larger than the wound of entry. However, the surgeon must not rely on wound size to decide the point of exit or entry. The military bullet with a velocity over 1800 ft./sec. traverses a straight course. The low-velocity missile crushes and forces the tissue apart. The permanent cavity is filled with blood and macerated cells. As the high-velocity missile moves through the tissue, a large temporary cavity results. The cavity quickly subsides but may contain seriously damaged tissue. Increased pressure pulses lasting a few millionths of a second followed by a negative phase may rupture a gas-filled viscus such as the lung.[11] The negative force may suck clothing and dirt into the wounds. Low-velocity missiles do not produce cavitation and shock waves, and thus do not usually cause necrosis. Since the temporary cavity is determined by the energy, the behavior of the missile, and the elastic properties of the tissue, it is important to evaluate the kinds of tissues traumatized.

SHOTGUN INJURIES

Civilian fatality rates are higher with shotgun than with gunshot injuries even though the velocity of the missile is about one-third that of the army rifle. Shotgun wounds produce a wide variety of injuries which include massive tissue destruction. The degree of wounding depends upon barrel length, bore, choke, load, wadding, and range, among other factors. Sherman and Parrish divide such wounds into three types based on the fact that the close-range wound leads to greater tissue destruction.[18] Shotgun injuries from over 7 yards away lead to penetration of subcutaneous tissue or deep fascia (type I), wounds acquired from 3 to 7 yards (close-range) cause injury to blood vessels and nerves beneath the deep fascia (type II), and point-blank wounds, under 3 yards (type III), are characterized by massive tissue destruction. Type III wounds lead to massive primary hemorrhage and are the greatest cause of death.

Besides the clinical assessment of the wound, it is important to know such things as the gauge of the shell and its range if at all possible.

MUSCLE AND OTHER SOFT-TISSUE WOUNDS

Cavity volume is proportional to the energy delivered by the missile.[4] Muscle fibers may swell to an enormous degree, as much as five times normal. Interstitial extravasation of blood is common. Clotting of muscle cytoplasm may result in nonviable tissue. In addition, capillaries may rupture, whereas large arteries are resistant to such injuries. Connective tissue and skin resist the development of large permanent tracks because of the elasticity of these tissues, a property also shown by the lung. Fascial planes permit an explosive force to dissipate. However, muscle at a distance from the permanent track but adjacent to fascial planes may be severely injured.

Crushed muscle within an enclosed area serves as an excellent culture medium for the growth of many bacteria, particularly the gas-producing bacilli such as clostridia. Devitalized muscle often extends beyond what appears to be the obvious localized wound,[20] particularly in military injuries.

BONE INJURIES

Cortical bone has a higher specific gavity than muscle and is much more likely to be severely damaged. A long bone such as the humerus is composed of dense cortical

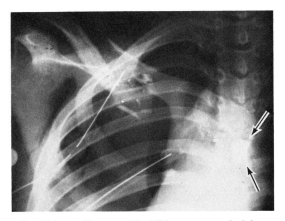

FIG. 16-1. A 13-year-old child was wounded by a .38 cal. bullet that struck the clavicle, driving the comminuted bone fragments into the lung and causing a pneumothorax secondary to a torn lung. Two chest tubes connected to a waterseal were needed to reexpand the lung. The bullet struck the thoracic spinal cord (arrows) causing a permanent paraplegia.

bone in its shaft and cancellous bone in its head. Flat bones such as the ribs and scapula contain considerable cancellous bone. The types of wounds produced in these structures will depend on where the impact force is struck. When cancellous bone is struck by high-velocity missiles, there is usually little comminution of the bone when compared to the same missile striking dense cortex (Figs. 16-1 and 16-2).

Fracture of a flat bone, like the scapula, produced by a high-velocity bullet does not generally cause great damage unless associated vital soft-tissue structures such as nerves and arteries are involved (Fig. 16-3). Similar injuries of the ribs are not significant unless the lung and major vessels are involved (Fig. 16-1).

NERVE AND ARTERY INVOLVEMENT

A wide range of nerve injuries about the shoulder can result from missile injury. For example, Carney and co-workers found axillary nerve paralysis in 1 out of 12 shoulder wounds.[3] In another study, associated nerve damage occurred in 95 percent of shoulder joint wounds caused by missiles.[1] The great disparity may be accounted for by the different types of missiles employed. Because of the closeness of major structures like the brachial plexus to the shoulder joint, a greater disability may be incurred than in a

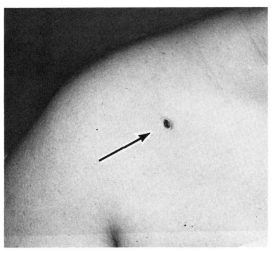

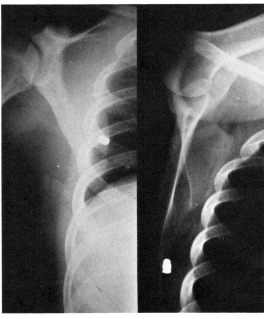

A B

FIG. 16-2. A, A woman was shot in the right infraclavicular region. B, A .22 cal. bullet struck the scapula outside the thorax and traveled to the inferior angle of the scapula. The patient was asymptomatic.

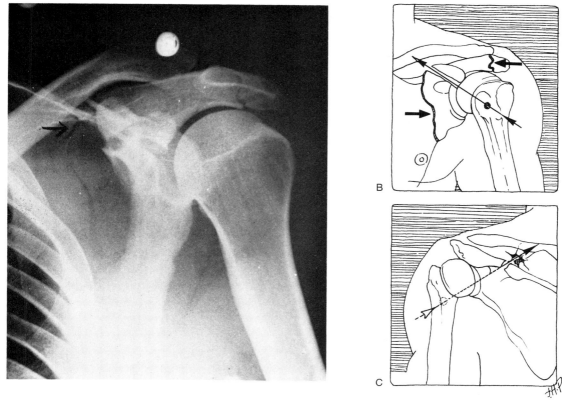

FIG. 16-3. A, An anteroposterior x-ray film of the left shoulder of a 23-year-old man shows fractures of the acromion, base of the coracoid, body of the scapula, and anterior glenoid sustained from a .38 cal. bullet. B, Diagram of anterior aspect of shoulder shows the path of the bullet. C, Diagram of posterior aspect of shoulder shows the exit site. The wounds of entry and exit were debrided and the extremity was immobilized in a sling for 2 weeks and then started on gentle passive motion exercises. The patient made an excellent recovery.

joint wound itself. The magnitude of nerve injury caused by a high-velocity missile ranges from neurapraxia to neurotmesis.[15] When the expected time interval for spontaneous recovery of the injured nerve has elapsed, surgical treatment should be considered without delay. With knife wounds assessment of the nerve involvement is certainly more easily made. The use of operating microscopes now makes it possible to attempt repair of proximal nerve injuries early in select cases of knife wounds. Because of the uncertain effects of shock waves up and down peripheral nerves from high-velocity missiles, similar early exploration should be deferred. Bateman states that a missile jarring force may sever nerve bundles without rupturing the sheaths, and although distal segment degeneration oc-

curs there is less tendency to intraneural fibrosis than with traction injury.[2]

Rich and associates found that in a series of 1000 cases of arterial trauma sustained in Viet Nam, major arterial injuries to the axillary and brachial arteries accounted for 34 percent of the injuries. Autogenous vein grafts were used for repair of major vessels most frequently (45.9 percent), and initial end-to-end anastomoses were employed in 37.7 percent of the cases. They also found a significantly low amputation rate of 5.7 percent for injuries to the brachial artery (16 amputations in 283 injuries) which compared favorably with an even lower amputation rate of 5.1 percent for injuries to the axillary artery (3 amputations in 59 injuries). Major complications after repair were most often caused by thrombosis followed by hemorrhage, the incidence decreasing with massive soft-tissue destruction, sepsis, and venous insufficiency. For patients with these complications, 42.5 percent had amputations of both the upper and lower extremities.

Associated injuries such as massive soft-tissue and osseous defects, complete denervation, and venous insufficiency often influence the final outcome of the vascular repair. Concomitant nerve injuries are particularly high in axillary artery injuries, in which more than 90 percent had associated nerve injuries.

PRINCIPLES OF WOUND MANAGEMENT

Treatment starts at the scene of injury. The patient's airway should be clear, and it should be ascertained that breathing and oxygenation are adequate. Major hemorrhage must be controlled, preferably with compression dressings. Wounds of the chest and abdomen should be covered. Fractures of the extremities must be adequately splinted after open wounds of the extremity are covered in order to prevent further contamination. The patient is quickly transported to a hospital where definitive treatment may be undertaken. Thereafter, rapid transfusion via multiple venous catheters is used to combat shock. Wounds acquired in military combat are exceptionally dirty in comparison to civilian wounds. Although the degree of debridement will vary accordingly, the principles of treatment remain the same, namely, to prevent sepsis and establish the conditions for optimum healing.

Hampton has shown that the factors that determine success in managing open injuries of the extremity are (1) optimum reduction of fractures, (2) minimum wound sepsis, (3) achievement of rapid wound healing, and (4) restoration of maximum functional recovery of the part.[8-10] Fortunately, the muscles about the humerus and scapula are excellently vascularized, which facilitates the covering and revascularization of bone denuded by wounding. The greater the degree of soft-tissue destruction about the shoulder region, the slower and less satisfactory will be the healing. Another important fact to remember is that maintenance of full arm length is not crucial for good function later. A soft-tissue injury takes precedence over bone fracture; therefore, the mechanical advantage of a lengthened humerus may be compromised in order to effect vascular continuity. Thus, humeral fractures that necessarily heal in a shortened position can still give a good result. Nevertheless, the arm acts as lever for the upper extremity which allows the hand to function, and everything should be done to restore function in the proximal arm about the shoulder without endangering vital structures.

General Evaluation

The whole patient must be examined for injuries in areas other than the upper extremity (see Figs. 16-1 and 16-2). Especially with high-velocity missile wounds about the shoulder extensive hemorrhages may occur, and secondary pulmonary effects of nonpenetrating injuries to the lung may result.[11] For this reason, adequate oxygenation of tissues must be ensured by treating any airway obstruction or lung tissue trauma. Arterial blood oxygen tensions must be evaluated to determine any perfusion defect.

In military injuries tetanus has not been a problem in recent conflicts. However, the same assurance cannot be given in civilian injuries because patients may not have received complete tetanus immunization. Therefore, tetanus toxoid boosters are routinely given to all combat patients, and civilian patients should receive simultaneous passive immunization with human immune globulin and initiation of active immunization with a clean syringe in another anatomic location.

After stabilization of the patient, an examination must include as complete a vascular and neurologic examination as is possible. When the physical examination has been completed, appropriate x-ray films of the injured parts are obtained. Multiple views are taken to document the true location of missiles (Fig. 16-4). All wounds of entry and exit should be counted, and an attempt made to correlate these with the wounding missile(s), including those that may have traversed the body, and those that may have taken a circuitous route. The surgeon must not rely on the size of the skin wound to determine the exit or entry. At times, it may be impossible to understand the actual missile course, and in this situation the surgeon must search near and far.

Local Wound Evaluation and Management

Evaluation of the extent of military wounds may be somewhat easier than that of civilian injuries because in the former usually more extensive debridement will demonstrate the state of the injured deep tissues. Often, when major vessel damage is not present about the shoulder in a civilian wound, "clean" wounds are merely treated by thorough cleansing and debridement of the wounds of entry and exit.

In cleaning the skin in the operating room for deep debridement, the wound is copiously irrigated with sterile saline solution. The skin is shaved after the open wound is covered with a sterile dressing. The rest of the extremity is washed with pHisoHex. The wound dressing is next removed and a second washing with pHisoHex performed. The skin is prepared with aqueous benzalkonium chloride (Zephiran).

When a wound requires deep debridement, customary incisions should be made in the longitudinal axis. If wounds approximate each other, incisions should be arranged to avoid a narrow base of skin between the wounds. In some cases, it may be necessary to connect the wounds by a curved incision. In any event, dirty wound edges should be excised and the wound left open. The aim of treatment is to achieve a clean granulating base that can be closed 4 to 7 days after injury by secondary closure of the skin edges or skin grafting. Seidenstein and co-workers believe that delayed primary wound closure is better on the fourth or fifth day.[17] In no case should skin grafts be placed over a necrotic or dirty base. In some cases, split-skin grafting may serve as a temporary cover in preparation for delayed flap grafting.

The underlying fascia should be opened longitudinally, deep debridement performed, and the wound should be left open to allow for drainage and to avoid compression of swollen injured muscle. In other situations, extensive fasciotomy may help keep the blood supply open to the distal part of the extremity. Fasciotomy may help restore venous blood return.

Whenever devitalized tissues are excised major nerves and blood vessels must be saved. Judgment must be individualized for each wound. Dziemian and associates have shown that low-velocity missiles produce permanent damage only in the area bordering the track, and despite great cavitation produced by a high-velocity missile, permanent damage occurs only in the tissues immediately surrounding the missile track provided the whole blood supply to the muscle or major blood supply is not destroyed.[6] Good results have been obtained in dirty military or similar severe wounds when they have been deeply debrided and left open for 4 to 7 days before secondary closure was performed.[17] Excellent results have been demonstrated at Cook County Hospital and Michael Reese Medical Center for the past 15 years when fresh civilian missile wounds are merely cleansed, irrigated superficially, perhaps a small rim of damaged skin tissue excised, and a sterile dressing applied if there is no major vascular damage. The entire extremity is immobilized in Velpeau position until the surface wound has healed. At that time, the joint or deep tissues are explored, if necessary. With extensive damage to the shoulder joint, plaster of Paris spica immobilization of the shoulder in a position consistent with shoulder joint fusion later is recommended if loss of joint function seems likely. In essence, civilian bullet wounds must be individually assessed, but the great majority do not require immediate extensive debridement.

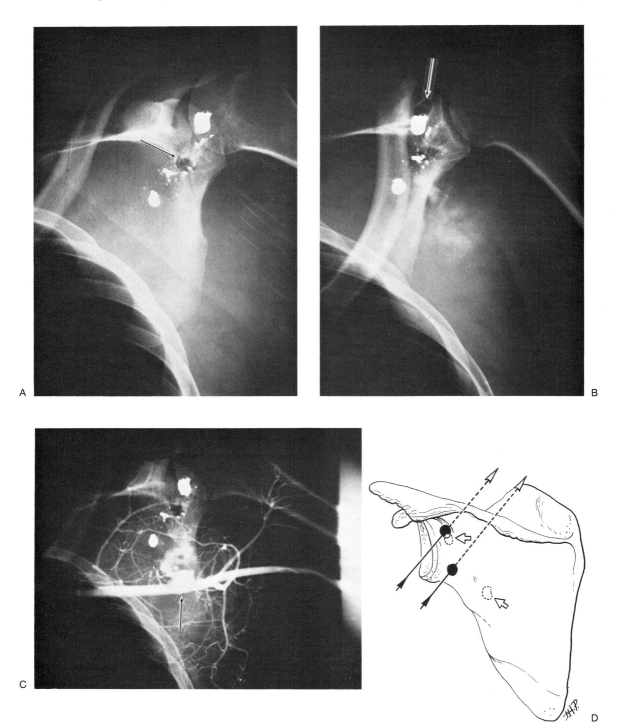

FIG. 16-4. A, Two .38 cal. bullets with parallel courses struck a young man from behind. One comminuted hole in the glenoid is visible (arrow). B, A slightly angled view shows a second bullet hole in the superior glenoid neck and the metal fragment away from the joint (arrow). C, There were no peripheral pulses. An arteriogram shows a bullet fragment almost completely occluding the axillary artery (arrow). The fragment was removed and the torn artery repaired. D, Diagram shows anteriorly directed bullet paths. Dotted circles show the final resting positions of the two main bullet fragments. Recovery was uneventful.

Unlike gunshot wounds, shotgun injuries are treated somewhat differently. Type III wounds with obvious massive tissue destruction, both superficial and deep, are widely debrided and left open to granulate (Fig. 16-5). At times, type II wounds may require debridement. If the chest is penetrated, blood is aspirated from the chest cavity, and rapid expansion of the lung accomplished by whatever means is needed. Again, as with any chest wound cardiorespiratory dysfunction must be immediately treated. Type I shotgun wounds are not operated upon. The surface wounds are cleansed and dressed. In no event should the surgeon explore the deep tissues with the idea of removing the metal pellets.

In older missile wounds with significant hematoma or containing dead tissue, drainage must be effected and debridement performed in order to lessen the chance of infection. If bone is obviously contaminated, it should be debrided with a sharp curette, and occasionally a rongeur. As much bone as possible should be saved, but devitalized and contaminated fragments should be removed.[13]

In some cities, bullets, metal pellets, and "wadding" surgically removed must be submitted to the police crime laboratory. If at all possible they should be removed with rubber-tipped forceps, and placed on a gauze square in the original condition. These objects should be placed in a sealed container bearing the names of the patient and institution, and the signature of the physician.

Management of Joint Injuries

In treating missile injuries about the shoulder joint, two points must be remembered: the shoulder joint is nonweight-bearing, and the articular surfaces of the glenohumeral joint do not have total contact as do articular surfaces of the hip. The cartilage surfaces actually touch over a small area at any given time in any position. Therefore, it is important to determine if an injury will interfere with painless function, and whether surgical treatment will improve the outcome. Missile injuries of the shoulder joint may be divided into nonpenetrating and penetrating wounds.

Nonpenetrating Wounds

Nonpenetrating wounds with no or negligible articular injury allow the best prognosis for recovery. The bullet does not seriously damage the joint surfaces. The head of the humerus and scapular neck contain cancellous bone which helps lessen the chance for comminution. Retained metal fragments in these regions will not impede function, and therefore need not be removed from civilian wounds. For military wounds, the joint injury should have more aggressive debridement. If there is a suggestion of debris within the joint or more extensive involvement, an arthrotomy should be performed.

Penetrating Wounds

Single articular surface injuries also carry a favorable prognosis if the joint surface is

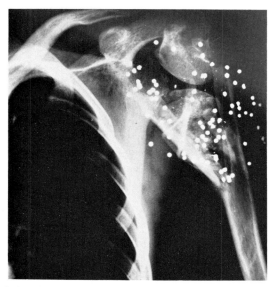

FIG. 16-5. A 13-year-old girl sustained a type III shotgun wound of the left shoulder. There was massive soft-tissue destruction involving the brachial plexus. The wound was widely debrided removing only destroyed tissue, left open, and allowed to granulate. A shoulder arthrodesis was planned because of the loss of deltoid and triceps function.

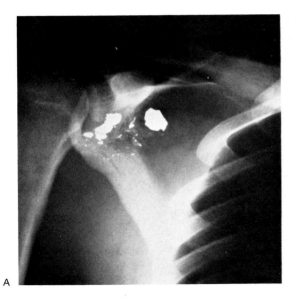
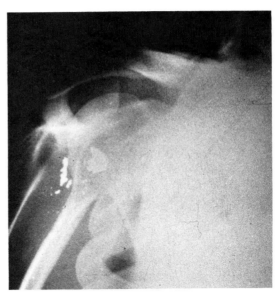

A   B

FIG. 16-6. A, A .38 cal. bullet struck a 20-year-old man from the front. The shattered metal fragments damaged the glenoid articular surface but left the humeral head and neurovascular structures uninjured. B, A tangential view of the scapula shows that the metal fragments are not in the joint. The patient made an uneventful recovery after debridement of the skin wound.

not extensively disrupted. Again, high-velocity missile wounds require extensive debridement, whereas low-velocity missile wounds may have deferred surgical treatment if deemed advisable (Fig. 16-6). If loose or projecting particles are present within the joint they should be removed. Like that for any joint injury, treatment should be directed toward preventing sepsis. Relatively large defects within the cancellous bone of the humeral head or scapular neck are not incompatible with good function in this nonweight-bearing joint. If the humeral head is irreparably damaged later consideration may have to be given to a reconstructive procedure in the most severe injuries.

When *both articular surfaces* of the shoulder joint are damaged, the prognosis depends upon the location of the articular injury (Fig. 16-7). If the bullet completely traverses the joint at the periphery and little or no debris or metal remains in the joint, arthrotomy need not be performed for civilian injuries (Fig. 16-8). Considerable judgment must be exercised in deciding which wound needs arthrotomy, and

whether it should be done from the anterior or posterior approach.

Acromioclavicular and Sternoclavicular Joint Injuries

When the articular surfaces of the acromioclavicular and sternoclavicular joints are damaged and later produce pain, the lateral or medial end of the clavicle may be resected. With the increasing numbers of bullet wounds now observed in children it should be recalled that the clavicular epiphysis lies medially and should be preserved if at all possible.

Management of Nerve Damage

Brachial plexus injury commonly occurs concomitantly with injuries to other systems.[14] When such nerve trauma accompanies chest wounds, for example, the chest wounds that endanger life may overshadow the nerve injury that leads to serious loss of function. In fact, a nerve wound may not be discovered for a few days.

Regardless of the mechanism of trauma

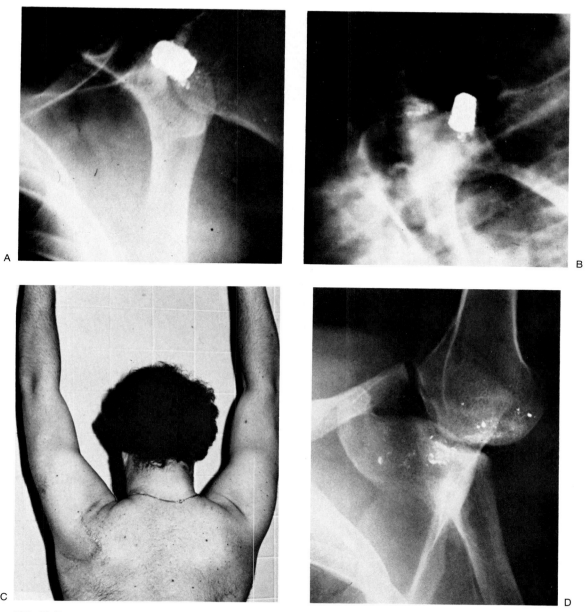

FIG. 16-7. A police officer sustained a gunshot wound from the front. A, Anteroposterior and, B, lateral views of the shoulder show the .38 cal. bullet lodged in the posterior joint space. The entry wound was debrided. Nine days later the bullet was removed through a posterior surgical approach. Both joint surfaces were damaged. C, Six years later the patient had a full range of painless motion. D, Note the remaining metal fragments and irregularity of the joint surfaces.

to the nerves, the level and degree of injury must be precisely documented. Missile wounds causing nerve deficit should not be immediately explored,[14] as was stated previously. Incomplete lesions or partial laceration may lead to a good result without exploration.[15] Precise, periodic clinical evaluation and electromyographic testing may help the surgeon decide whether to explore the nerve(s) 4 to 6 months after injury if there is no evidence of recovery. Too early exploration may cause additional

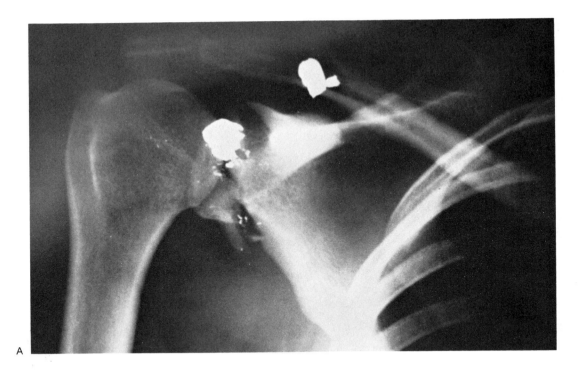

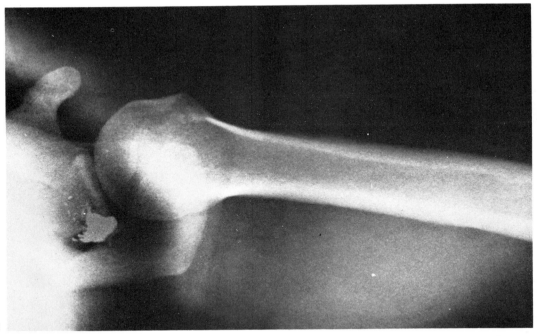

FIG. 16-8. A, Roentgenogram shows a comminuted fracture of the glenoid following a bullet injury. One metal fragment traveled to the clavicular region where it was allowed to remain. B, An axillary view shows the metal fragment posteriorly. Through a posterior surgical approach, the metal fragment and many small loose osteocartilaginous fragments were removed. A small screw was used to hold a large, inferior glenoid fragment. The extremity was immobilized in Velpeau position for 3 weeks. Recovery was uneventful.

nerve injury. During this waiting period shoulder motion exercises and strengthening of functional muscle groups should be instituted.

For definite nerve laceration, as with a knife, early or even initial repair may be undertaken by a competent surgeon skilled in nerve repair. Newer techniques of nerve repair increase the chance for success.

When brachial plexus injuries associated with fracture are caused by missile trauma, such things as shortening of the humerus or resection of a neuroma may be required to effect nerve continuity in some instances. In any event, a major injury should take precedence over a fracture.

With an existing bone defect in the arm and nerve injury, the nerve should be repaired before the bone is reconstructed. Such a defect may facilitate nerve mobilization. Despite nerve recovery joint stiffness may persist. Therefore, great detail should be directed toward preventing contractures of all upper extremity joints.

CHEMOTHERAPY OF SHOULDER WOUNDS

A chief goal of management of all joint wounds is to prevent sepsis. From the moment of missile wounding the deep tissues must be considered contaminated irrespective of whether debridement is superficial or deep. Prophylactic intravenous antibiotic therapy should be started from the onset and certainly preoperatively.[7] The antibiotic of choice depends upon the environment at the time of wounding. Soil-borne bacteria, including clostridia, pseudomonas, and proteus, as well as skin-borne organisms like staphylococcus are found in the deep tissues. The most effective antibiotics are described in Chapter 6, Antimicrobial Therapy.

When the joint is already exposed to the surface or an arthrotomy is performed, the liberal use of saline solution alone or preferably lavage with saline-polymixin-B/bacitracin/neosporin solution is recommended.

As stated previously, exceptionally dirty wounds are not closed but allowed to drain. Rigid tube suction treatment may be employed in established deep wound and joint sepsis. Continuous antibiotic irrigation-suction is not more effective than open treatment methods nor more effective than the other nonantibiotic solutions if closed irrigation-suction treatment is used.

CLOSTRIDIAL INFECTION

The surgeon must constantly be alert to the danger of true gas gangrene. Six species of clostridia can cause gas gangrene in man.[19] Gas gangrene has occurred in urban areas after trauma and following elective surgery. Because other organisms such as bacteroides, coliforms, and anaerobic streptococci can produce gas in tissues, the surgeon should not rely on this finding alone to make a diagnosis of gas gangrene.

A distinction should be made between the less severe anaerobic cellulitis caused by clostridia, with an incubation period of 3 to 4 days, and the serious clostridial infection causing anaerobic myonecrosis (gas gangrene). In the latter infection the incubation periods may range from hours to 6 weeks.[19]

The surgeon must be familiar with the fulminating and lesser effects of gas gangrene. Death may be rapid because of renal shutdown due to acute tubular necrosis or intoxication.

In managing such cases fluid and electrolyte balance must be carefully monitored at all times and vasoconstricting drugs to combat shock avoided since these interfere with the perfusion of tissues. Only surgery and the use of hyperbaric oxygen (100 percent oxygen at a pressure of 3 atmospheres) have proved of value in saving life. The adjunctive use of large doses of penicillin is recommended (see Chapter 6, Antimicrobial Therapy). The effectiveness of antitoxin is unproved in the presence of infection.

POSTOPERATIVE MANAGEMENT

If wounds of the shoulder joint remain "clean" postoperatively, the joint may be mobilized when there is soft-tissue healing to the degree that movement will not adversely affect the outcome. With irreparable glenohumeral joint damage the extremity should be placed in a plaster of Paris spica cast in a position used for arthrodesis. If later reconstruction is required it should be undertaken when enough time has elapsed so that there is little chance for exacerbation of sepsis. Excessive delay for planned surgery about the shoulder should be avoided because atrophy of muscles often precludes a good result no matter how well the procedure is executed.

REFERENCES

1. Bailey, H., Editor: Surgery of Modern Warfare, Vol. II, 2nd ed. Edinburgh, E. and S. Livingstone, 1942.
2. Bateman, J. E.: Trauma to Nerves in Limbs. Philadelphia, W. B. Saunders Co., 1962.
3. Carney, P. W., Fitts, W. T., Jr., and Kirby, C. K.: Gunshot wounds of major joints. J. Bone Joint Surg., 28-A:607–615, 1946.
4. DeMuth, W. E., Jr.: Bullet velocity as applied to military rifle wounding capacity. J. Trauma, 9:27–38, 1969.
5. DeMuth, W. E., Jr., and Smith, J. W.: High-velocity bullet wounds of muscle and bone: The basis of rational early treatment. J. Trauma, 6:744–755, 1966.
6. Dziemian, A. M., Mendelson, J., and Lindsey, D.: Comparison of the wounding characteristics of some commonly encountered bullets. J. Trauma, 1:341–353, 1961.
7. Fogelberg, E. V., Zitzmann, E. K., and Stinchfield, F. E.: Prophylactic penicillin in orthopaedic surgery. J. Bone Joint Surg., 52-A:95–98, 1970.
8. Hampton, O. P., Jr.: Wounds of the Extremities in Military Surgery. St. Louis, C. V. Mosby Co., 1951.
9. Hampton, O. P., Jr.: The indications for debridement of gun shot (bullet) wounds of the extremities in civilian practice. J. Trauma, 1:368–372, 1961.
10. Hampton, O. P., Jr.: Management of open fractures and open wounds of joints. J. Trauma, 8:475–478, 1968.
11. Harvey, E. N., Kerr, I. M., Oster, G., and McMillen, J. H.: Secondary damage in wounding due to pressure changes accompanying the passage of high velocity missiles. Surgery, 21:218–239, 1947.
12. Hopkinson, D. A. W., and Marshall, T. K.: Firearm injuries. Br. J. Surg., 54:344–353, 1967.
13. Keggi, K. J., and Southwick, W. O.: Early Care of Severe Extremity Wounds: A Review of the Viet Nam Experience and its Civilian Application. Instructional Course Lectures, Vol. 19, Chap. 12. St. Louis, C. V. Mosby Co., 1970.
14. Nelson, K. G., Jolly, P. C., and Thomas, P. A.: Brachial plexus injuries associated with missile wounds of the chest: A report of 9 cases from Viet Nam. J. Trauma, 8:268–275, 1968.
15. Omer, G. E., Jr.: Injuries to nerves of the upper extremity. J. Bone Joint Surg., 56-A:1615–1624, 1974.
16. Rich, N. M., Baugh, J. H., and Hughes, C. W.: Acute arterial injuries in Viet Nam. J. Trauma, 10:359–369, 1970.
17. Seidenstein, M., Newman, A., and Tanski, E. V.: Some clinical factors involved in the healing of war wounds. Arch. Surg., 96:176–178, 1968.
18. Sherman, R. T., and Parrish, R. A.: Management of shotgun injuries: A review of 152 cases. J. Trauma, 3:76–86, 1963.
19. Weinstein, L., and Barza, M. A.: Gas gangrene. N. Engl. J. Med., 289:1129–1131, 1973.
20. Ziperman, H. H.: The management of soft tissue missile wounds in war and peace. J. Trauma, 1:361–367, 1961.

17

Injuries to the Shoulder Girdle

MELVIN POST

There are few locations in the human body where a loss of function causes more disability than in the shoulder. Similarly, any loss in shoulder function impairs hand function. As a general rule, the longer the shoulder is in disuse the greater is the resultant disability. After trauma a chief goal of fracture treatment is to attain the earliest optimum return of painless motion that injured tissue will permit. The surgeon should consider the effect of injury on other soft tissues and treat the whole patient.

PRINCIPLES OF FRACTURE CARE

An expeditious union of fractured bone requires an adequate blood supply, anatomic reduction, and effective immobilization at the fracture site.[16] The common causes for delayed union and nonunion are:

1. Loss of blood supply
2. Distraction of fragments
3. Inadequate immobilization
4. Interposition of soft tissue
5. Infection

Anything that interferes with revascularization of bone ends impedes normal healing. Loss of blood supply not only hinders the normal exchange of oxygen, nutriments, and toxic products but retards normal histologic repair and remineralization of fractured bone. If the bone fragments on both sides of a fracture are viable, Charnley has shown that absolute immobilization is not essential for union and rigid immobilization is futile if both fragments are ischemic.[4]

Regardless of the kind of treatment given, nothing should be done that will further damage the available blood supply at the fracture site. Care must be taken to do everything that will encourage early healing. Consequently, gaps should be avoided between bone fragments whether it be by excessive traction, through the injudicious use of internal fixation devices, or by actual loss of bone substance. Particularly in the humerus, some shortening does not compromise good function of the upper extremity. When a gap results between the fracture fragments, a longer period of time is needed for bone cells and blood vessels to close the defect than when the fragments are in continuity. Moreover, more time is required for bone tissue to become mineralized with hydroxyapatite crystals.

Inadequate immobilization increases the incidence of delayed union and nonunion. Effective immobilization should be continued until there is clinical evidence of sound union to the degree that mobilization of the shoulder will not result in reinjury or deformity at the fracture site. This does not mean that absolute rigid fixation is needed in every situation, as evidenced by the high rate of union of clavicular and humeral fractures treated conservatively, for example. Although a delay of weeks to months before final healing occurs does not preclude union, protracted healing is detrimental to a normal return of function. Should this occur a greater degree of muscle atrophy about the shoulder and joint stiffness secondary to soft-tissue contracture ensues, which makes recovery difficult. As soon as it is determined that a plateau of delayed union or nonunion is reached, appropriate surgical treatment must be taken to remedy this complication in order to obviate further atrophy and contracture of the surrounding tissues. It is important to select a definitive operation early and avoid multiple procedures that postpone early use of the shoulder. However, it should be stressed that most fractures about the shoulder can be managed by nonoperative methods.

If the bone ends are precluded from touching one another because of interposed soft tissue, this diagnosis must be established early, as bone cells are not capable of traversing a solid wall of tissue. In this event, operative intervention becomes necessary to permit bone ends to contact one another.

Infection at the site of fracture or about the shoulder joint itself must be avoided, since infectious material compromises the blood supply and increases the formation of fibrous tissue which thus prevents the normal repair and mineralization of fractured bone. Scar tissue in and about a joint ultimately leads to permanent loss of normal motion. For this reason open injuries must be meticulously cared for in a clean area such as an operating room. If doubt exists as to the cleanliness of a wound, the surgeon should avoid the introduction of foreign objects such as screws, plates, and rods during the acute phase of treatment, except under the most strict precautions. As a general rule, the use of bone grafts should be deferred in the presence of obvious infection. In this instance, a period of 1 year should elapse from the time of infection without recurrence before proceeding with bone grafting operations. Even then, careful consideration of this procedure should be given in the light of residual upper extremity function.

INJURIES OF THE THORAX

Because the upper extremity is suspended from the chest wall, its normal activity depends upon the integrity of the chest cage. The thorax houses the vital cardiopulmonary organs. What may appear to be a slight trauma to the rib cage may produce extreme physiologic changes that require immediate treatment. In the face of a horrendous injury to the shoulder, it is easy for the surgeon to defer treatment of a "trivial" chest injury. The surgeon who undertakes the management of chest cage injuries must be cognizant of the danger inherent with such trauma, understand the consequences of dire cardiopulmonary abnormalities, and know effective management methods. Serious damage to the great vessels, heart, and lungs requires appropriate consultative services.

Anatomy

The chest cage consists of 12 thoracic vertebrae to which articulate 12 slender, elastic curvilinear ribs which enclose the thoracic space. The upper 7 ribs attach to the sternum indirectly through costal cartilages interposed between the ribs and sternum. The eighth, ninth, and tenth ribs are attached to the cartilage of the seventh rib by fibrous tissue. The anterior ends of the eleventh and twelfth ribs are not fixed anteriorly.

The head of each rib has two articular facets for the body of its corresponding thoracic vertebra, and each rib tubercle has an articular facet for the transverse process of its vertebra. The neck of the rib is a flattened portion between the head and tubercle. The long, curved diaphysis is smooth on its undersurface and roughened on the outer surface. The ribs are designed for great flexibility.

Centered in the anterior midline is the broad, flat sternum composed of an upper manubrium, a middle body, and an inferior, thin xiphoid tip. In youth the xiphoid is cartilaginous but may ossify in the adult. The lateral border of the upper manubrium contains a depression for the first costal cartilage. The manubrium is thickened and contains facets for articulation with the clavicle superiorly. On either side of the body are articulations for the second through seventh costal cartilages. The manubrium and body of the sternum are united by a synchondrosis which may ossify late in adult years.

Rib Fractures

Rib fractures occur often, and it is common for more than one rib to break at one time. Laustela found that traffic accidents were the most common cause of thorax injury,[10] and Nordlund reported that falls were the cause of many thorax injuries incurred by elderly persons.[11] In recent years the incidence of stabbings and gunshot wounds involving the thorax has increased. Rib fractures are rarely seen before puberty, because of the great elasticity of the rib cage.

MECHANISM OF INJURY. The manner in which a rib fractures is important in deciding treatment. A penetrating chest wound is managed differently from a closed blunt injury. The fracture may be direct or indirect. In general ribs tend to fracture at the point of applied force as from a direct blow. However, a crushing force may cause the rib(s) to break at its angle when the force is transmitted backward along the rib shaft, the extent and number of ribs broken depending on the actual force. Multiple rib fractures are often caused by a compressive force which tends to produce more than one fracture in each rib. They may lead to chest wall instability, a condition known as "flail chest," in which the unstable chest wall moves paradoxically, and is sucked in with inspiration and is expanded with expiration (Fig. 17-1A and B). Expired air from the lung on the unaffected side is displaced into the lung on the fractured side, which increases the volume of dead space and decreases the efficiency of ventilation.

In injuries of direct violence, displaced fractures of even a single rib may cause a tear of the parietal pleura. The lung may be

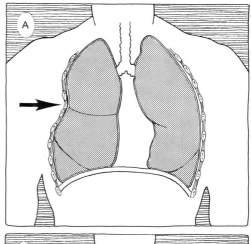

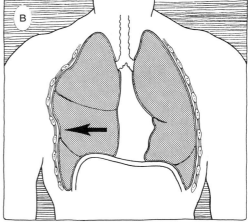

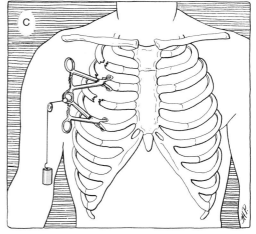

FIG. 17-1. Paradoxical movement of flail chest wall during, A, inspiration and, B, expiration. C, Towel clip method for stabilizing a flail chest segment.

damaged at the site of impact of the fractured end.

The last two ribs are rarely broken by a delivered force because of their great mobility.

It is rare for the first two ribs to be broken because they are protected by the shoulder and clavicle.[12] Joshi and associates reviewed the literature on first rib fractures and suggested that indirect trauma accounted for most of the injuries causing severe muscular action on the first rib[9] (Figs. 17-2 and 17-3). Violent traumas causing such fractures are associated in a high percentage of cases with tear of the tracheobronchial tree.[1]

Finally, once considered uncommon open rib fractures in civilian life are now seen with increasing frequency because of gunshot wounds.

DIAGNOSIS. While a precise history is being obtained and a clinical examination is being performed, the patient should be fully undressed. Some of the important areas with which the examiner should be concerned are whether the patient fell against a sharp object, received a hard blow, or sustained a crushing chest injury as with the force of a steering wheel violently pressed against the chest wall. If there is an open chest wound, can the examiner hear air being sucked into the chest cavity? Is the heart contused? Serial electrocardiograms may help determine any adverse effects.

With one or two closed rib fractures the patient is usually able to localize the pain. Pain is more severe with flail chest injuries. Breathing is shallow and any attempt to inspire deeply, cough, or sneeze exacerbates the chest pain. With first and second rib fractures, the patient may complain of shoulder pain causing him to support his extremity (Fig. 17-2). Sudden arm movement such as abduction produces increased pain that may radiate to the inner arm. As with other rib fractures, coughing or sneezing may cause localized pleuritic pain at the root of the neck or in the axilla. Unless the surgeon considers this injury as a possibility it can easily be overlooked.

The patient should be observed for paradoxical breathing and cyanosis. The examiner should not attempt to localize the patient's pain by compressing the chest wall. However, light palpation may detect the crunching sensation of air in the subcutaneous space, the crepitus of the movement of fractured bone ends, or the site of localized tenderness. Abnormalities in tactile fremitus may be found. By auscultation the surgeon should recognize any evidence of diminished breath sounds, after a thorough evaluation of all systems. Clear roentgenograms are taken in the anteroposterior, lateral, and oblique planes whenever possible. Often, reliance on excellent films is necessary for a correct diagnosis. However, an undisplaced rib fracture may be difficult to detect on the roentgenograms. Even a single rib fracture may cause serious intrathoracic injury such as pneumothorax and hemothorax.

TREATMENT. The chief goals in treating rib fractures are to relieve pain, stabilize an unstable chest wall if present, and allow adequate air ventilation so that blood can remain oxygenated. Anything that impedes normal pulmonary function, including muscular and postural interference, and respiratory excursions ultimately has an adverse effect on pulmonary function. Overmedication, tight bandaging, and adhesive strapping of the chest wall to control pain interfere with air exchange, limit lung expansion, and are not recommended. Recumbent positions, especially in the elderly, hinder postural changes needed for gravitational drainage of the bronchopulmonary system. Fixed positions cause accumulations of bronchial secretions, lead to edema in the most dependent segments of the lung, and further diminish air exchange. For example, abdominal distention or peritoneal inflammation may compromise normal ventilation.

Young and middle-age patients with uncomplicated rib fractures need not be admitted to the hospital if they are otherwise healthy. Outpatient treatment with analgesics alone can be undertaken if the physician knows that other complicating factors such as pneumothorax are not present. The

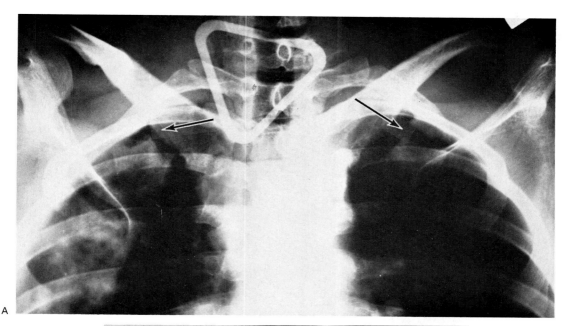

A

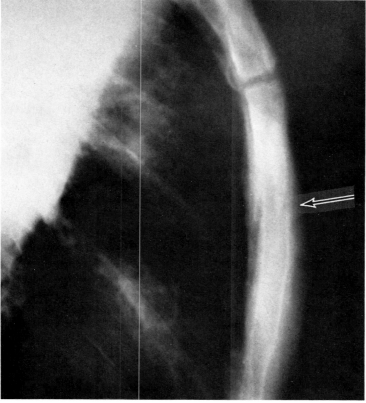

B

FIG. 17-2. A, A 21-year-old man was involved in an automobile accident and sustained a right clavicular fracture and bilateral first rib fractures (arrows). B, A sternal fracture was visible on the lateral sternal film but was almost missed because the chief complaint was shoulder pain. The patient had severe dyspnea and changes on electrocardiograms that subsequently cleared. A figure-eight harness was ineffective in relieving pain. Recovery was complete.

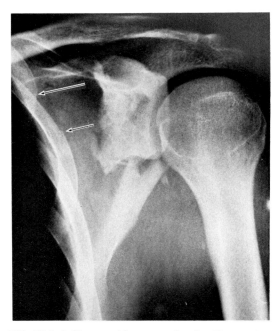

FIG. 17-3. A 38-year-old man was involved in a motorcycle accident and sustained fractures of the first and second ribs (arrows) and a severe compression fracture of the scapular neck. The patient had severe difficulty in breathing. After 4 weeks in a sling gentle motion exercises were started. Recovery was uneventful. The functional result was good.

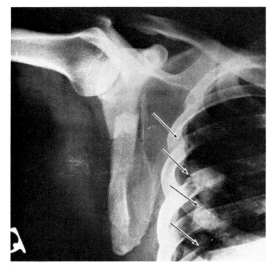

FIG. 17-4. A young adult sustained multiple rib fractures (arrows) in an automobile accident. The patient had difficulty in breathing and was admitted to the hospital. A tangential roentgenogram shows a displaced, comminuted fracture of the scapula that was not visible on the anteroposterior film.

physician should watch for late complications by performing another clinical and roentgenographic examination of the patient within 48 hours. Instructions should be given the patient regarding coughing and deep breathing exercises if it is possible. Patients with more serious fractures should be admitted to the hospital for treatment (Fig. 17-4).

When the costal cartilages are contused or fractured, treatment is the same as that for rib fracture.

Local anesthetic injection of the intercostal nerves is not usually worthwhile, except for unusual cases with discrete rib fractures and uncontrolled pain, because pain relief may not last for more than a few hours, if at all. The judicious use of analgesics and an elastic external rib support in stable fractures for short periods to minimize pain are preferred.

Rib Cage Instability (Flail Chest)

If several or more ribs are broken and the rib cage is unstable enough to produce decreased pulmonary function and subsequent hypoventilation that cannot be controlled, fixation methods should be employed to stabilize the chest wall. Once the chest wall is stabilized, continuous positive pressure ventilation can be instituted especially if the patient is comatose or there is associated trauma.[2] The positive pressure helps maintain reduction of the broken ribs and keeps the chest cage expanded. Barrett stressed the importance of treating respiratory problems immediately.[3] For rib fractures causing a flail upper rib cage that does not require prolonged immobilization, or when the surgeon wishes immediate and temporary chest wall stabilization, a $\frac{3}{32}$-in.-diameter smooth wire can be inserted beneath the pectoralis major muscle mass under local anesthesia, and light upward traction used to prevent the chest wall from collapsing. When rib cage fractures are extensive, and especially when they are bilateral and likely to require several weeks of continued traction, the traction methods of

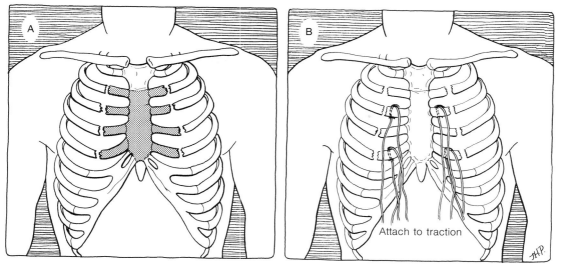

FIG. 17-5. A, Bilateral flail chest. B, Gibson and associates' method for stabilizing a flail chest using wire or heavy suture. Heavy trocar needles are used to place the suture material about the rib.

Richardson and Jones[14] on the sternum or the costal traction technique of Gibson and co-workers[7] may be employed (Figs. 17-1C and 17-5B). Other techniques including towel clip traction may be satisfactorily applied.[13] However, recent experiences with the newer methods of accomplishing adequate air ventilation and keeping the airway clear have lessened the need for these fixation methods. Flail chest must be managed immediately by whatever methods are necessary to establish an effective air exchange.[17,18]

Endotracheal Intubation

If nasotracheal suction does not suffice to clear secretions, a controlled airway may be established by endotracheal intubation through which oxygen can be administered directly and secretions aspirated when necessary. The tube may be left in place for 48 to 72 hours with safety and may be attached to a mechanical ventilator. In this event, trained personnel who understand pulmonary physiology and the capacity of the equipment must continually observe the patient.

If prolonged intratracheal ventilation is necessary tracheostomy should be per-

formed.[6] In the unconscious patient, a patient-triggered artificial respirator should be used, but only under the most stringent criteria. Most cases can be treated by endotracheal intubation. It should be recalled that intubation or tracheostomy methods (1) allow the entry of airborne microorganisms and dust into the tracheopulmonary tree, (2) cause severe drying of the surface mucous membrane, with resulting inspissated mucus, (3) increase the insensible water loss from the lung, and (4) eventually may damage the lung tissue. Therefore, these methods should be used only when inadequate air ventilation is life threatening, as in tracheal obstruction, massive aspiration, pulmonary hemorrhage, respiratory burns, or wounds of the head, neck, and face. The surgeon should not rely on clinical assessment alone to determine the need for such measures. Whenever there is a suspicion of disturbed respiratory function, the levels of blood gases should be determined, day or night, because the information they can provide is so valuable.

Patients who have sustained trauma, have had repeated blood transfusions, who are in shock, or who have chronic cardiac or chronic pulmonary problems are good candidates for arterial blood gas analysis.

Baseline values of Po_2, Pco_2, and pH levels can be crucial for effective management of the patient with chest trauma, especially when comparisons of later laboratory data are needed.[5] In addition to blood gas values, the inspired oxygen concentration and the patient's position in bed must be known for accurate assessment. Other essential information should include the fractional concentration of inspired oxygen, the time of sampling, and the patient's age and temperature. All these factors affect the values and their interpretation. The Po_2 ordinarily decreases with age and is higher when the patient sits than when he is recumbent. The surgeon must know if the report is corrected for body temperature. Moreover, the fractional concentration of inspired oxygen must be known because an arterial oxygen of 80 mm. of mercury may be normal for a given patient, but not if the patient is breathing 50 percent oxygen.

Patients who receive oxygen therapy, especially those with chronic lung damage (chronic emphysema), may go into respiratory acidosis and respiratory failure even in the presence of normal oxygen tensions. If post-traumatic pulmonary insufficiency is suspected, the arterial Pco_2 should be measured periodically and interpreted in the light of the pH and Po_2. An isolated "normal" Pco_2 value of 40 mm. Hg has no meaning. In otherwise healthy patients, the arterial oxygen should be kept in the range of 80 to 100 mm. Hg. In individuals who have demonstrated hypoxia secondary to chronic pulmonary disease, levels of oxygen as low as 60 mm. of mercury can be tolerated, if the circulation and hematocrit are adequate.

Complications

Like other fractures, rib fractures are less important than concomitant complications from trauma to the surrounding soft tissues. Injuries to the chest wall that cause complications may often be life threatening. Complications include pneumothorax, interstitial emphysema, hemothorax, lung injury, heart contusion, anoxemia secondary to traumatic tracheal obstruction, paralytic ileus, and empyema.

PNEUMOTHORAX. Traumatic pneumothorax may result from penetrating or nonpenetrating wounds. In either type, there is some degree of hemothorax. In the first instance, air enters the pleural cavity from the outside, whereas in the closed-type injury air fills the pleural space after a lung injury. As air enters the pleural space the lung on that side collapses, the degree of collapse determining the loss in pulmonary function. Simple pneumothorax in an otherwise healthy patient may be tolerated. However, if there is an open wound of the chest wall acting as a one-way valve, air may be sucked into the pleural space during inspiration and cause the air to accumulate under pressure (tension pneumothorax).

If the roentgen examination shows a simple pneumothorax of less than 20 percent, the blood gases are normal, and ventilation apparently is normal, the patient can be observed. A pneumothorax of greater degree requires a chest tube that should be inserted in the second intercostal space anteriorly and connected to a water-seal system. Most simple cases show cessation of bubbling before 7 days. Beyond that time surgical intervention by a thoracic surgeon may be needed.

In tension pneumothorax it is crucial to immediately close the leak in the chest wall, first by applying a sterile petrolatum dressing or any other external seal, and later by surgery. From the onset, the pressure between the atmosphere and pleural cavity should be equalized by the insertion of a percutaneous needle into the pleural space. It may be necessary to insert a chest tube as described previously.

INTERSTITIAL EMPHYSEMA. When pneumothorax is associated with rib fractures, air may be forced through a tear in the parietal pleura into the tissues of the chest wall. In palpating the chest wall a characteristic soft-tissue crepitus may be felt. If the amount of air is large it may spread and cause pain. In most patients soft-tissue emphysema resolves spontaneously.

If a bronchus is injured, air may escape

into the tissue of the lung and mediastinum, a serious complication requiring immediate endotracheal intubation and repair of the bronchus by a thoracic surgeon.

HEMOTHORAX. Blood in the pleural cavity is not usually associated with uncomplicated fractures of the ribs. It may be caused by gunshot wounds that lacerate the lung and the intercostal vessels (see Fig. 16-1). If blood loss into the pleural cavity is large, the cause of the hemorrhage should be sought and corrected and a chest tube with an appropriate water-seal inserted.

LUNG INJURY. The lung may be lacerated by a fractured rib or by violent compression of the chest wall. In addition to chest pain, cardiopulmonary signs may become ominous. The patient may become dyspneic, and signs of shock may increase.

CONTUSION OF THE HEART. If the heart is contused when it forcibly strikes the sternum, as in a steering wheel injury, serious problems may arise. Serial electrocardiograms should be obtained to check the patient's status. Bed rest is ordinarily all that is needed for complete recovery. More serious sequelae such as cardiac tamponade, valve damage, or tears of the coronary arteries require the immediate services of a cardiac surgeon.

ANOXEMIA SECONDARY TO TRAUMATIC TRACHEAL OBSTRUCTION. Sudden, severe compression of the abdominal and thoracic cavities may cause complete cessation of respiration. Characteristically, the skin of the face, upper chest, and arms is purplish, and there are numerous petechiae. The conjunctivae are reddened. This complication is caused by a sudden backward pressure of blood in the areas affected. The patient should have immediate endotracheal intubation and positive pressure control of breathing.

PARALYTIC ILEUS. On occasion, paralytic ileus may result from severe injury to the chest wall. In this event a gastrointestinal tube should be inserted and nothing given by mouth. Appropriate intravenous therapy is instituted.

EMPYEMA. Pus in the pleural cavity may rarely result from an open rib fracture or a laceration of the lung. This complication is not commonly seen because the pleura has a high resistance to infection.

Prolonged drainage with a chest tube is required along with adequate antibiotics. In some cases the lung surface may need to be decorticated 6 weeks later when the fibrous inelastic layer is thick enough to peel.

Fractures of the Sternum

Fractures of the sternum are uncommon, occurring in 17 patients out of 304 cases of major chest trauma reported by Laustela.[10] They usually result from direct violence as in a direct force applied to the chest wall.[8] The mortality rate is high, ranging from 25 percent or more from serious associated injuries.

Most of the fractures are transverse and occur in the body of the sternum. Gibson and associates reported that in 80 patients with sternal fracture 25 fractures were displaced or overriding, with anterior displacement of the distal fragment occurring most often.[7] Other common associated injuries encountered are rib fractures, distant fractures, head injury, and intrathoracic injury (see Fig. 17-2A and B).

DIAGNOSIS. A complete examination should include a detailed evaluation of the chest wall and its cavity to rule out injuries other than to the sternum. In isolated fractures of the sternum there is localized pain and tenderness. In very lean patients displaced fractures may occasionally be palpated. As soon as possible oblique and lateral films of the sternum should be obtained to assess the fracture accurately. The lateral view best shows displacement of the fracture fragments (Fig. 17-6). In any event, an undisplaced sternal fracture should not be interpreted as an insignificant injury since there may be associated serious intrathoracic trauma.

TREATMENT. Undisplaced or displaced fractures of the sternum showing no associated injuries may be treated with bed rest until there is subsidence of pain and the patient can sit comfortably in a chair. Most patients do not require adhesive strapping

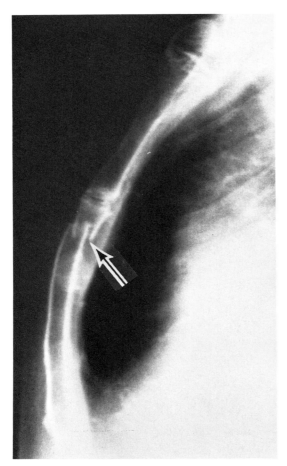

FIG. 17-6. A 60-year-old woman fractured the body of the sternum (arrow) when her chest struck the steering wheel in an accident. The patient was treated with bed rest as an inpatient until transient changes on electrocardiograms disappeared.

wire suture or plate to secure the fragments may be accomplished under general anesthesia.[15] The fracture may be exposed through a vertical midline incision (Fig. 17-7).

If traction methods are used to fix flail segments, 3 to 5 pounds of weight or rarely more are needed to stabilize the chest wall in the adult. Usually 3 weeks of traction treatment is enough to effect stabilization of the chest wall. A small number of patients may develop persistent post-traumatic pain.

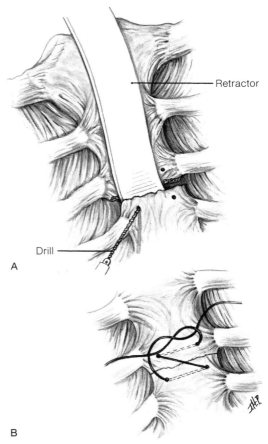

FIG. 17-7. Method for stabilizing a sternal fracture with heavy suture. A, A malleable retractor is used to protect the anterior mediastinal contents from the drill tip. B, I prefer to suture diagonally across the fracture rather than vertically, as this lessens the possibility of the sutures' pulling from the bone, especially when the bone is osteoporotic. (Redrawn from Gibson, D. L., Carter, R., and Hinshaw, D. B.: Surgical significance of sternal fracture. Surg. Gynecol. Obstet., 114:443–448, 1962.)

of the chest wall, figure-eight harness immobilization of the shoulders, or sandbag immobilization for comfort.

Complete evaluation and care are essential for satisfactory recovery of these fractures, the physician making certain there is no airway obstruction or other physiologic disturbance. Local anesthetic injection of the fracture site may give temporary relief of pain. If there is marked overriding of the fragments, closed reduction may be attempted. If there is failure, open reduction may be tried if deemed necessary to effect stabilization of the anterior chest wall. To fix a flail segment, open reduction using heavy

INJURIES OF THE SHOULDER REGION

Fractures of the Scapula

The scapula is a large, irregular flat bone the main function of which is to provide the shallow glenoid for articulation with the humeral head and to give leverage for the attachment of muscles such as the deltoid which move the arm and shoulder. Its only connection with the trunk is by muscles except for its indirect articulation with the skeleton by the clavicle. Furthermore, its posterior linear spinous crest and anterior thick, headlike bony process, the coracoid, arising from the anterior part of the neck of the scapula, serve for the attachment of important muscles and ligaments which allow stability of the shoulder girdle. The scapula is well covered by a relatively large number of muscles which cushion the bone and serve to protect it from injury. Injuries of the scapula may go unnoticed when there are associated injuries (see Fig. 17-3). The surgeon should not dismiss fractures of the scapula as unimportant with the mistaken idea that they all heal without disability (Fig. 17-8).

MECHANISM OF INJURY. Fractures of the scapula are uncommon, comprising 1 percent of all fractures. Fractures of the upper part are especially rare.[21,32] Most patients sustain fractures of the scapula by severe force, either direct or indirect.[35] Automobile and motorcycle accidents account for a large percentage of the total number seen. Oftentimes the patient does not recall the precise direction of a blow to the shoulder. However, localized findings may suggest a direct blow either anteriorly or posteriorly to the shoulder. Commonly, there are other associated injuries which take precedence over the fractured scapula. In one study at a naval hospital the age range for fractures of the scapula was 17 to 56 years, with a mean age of almost 28 years.[24] However, another report stated fractures of the scapula in the population occurred most often between 40 to 60 years.

DIAGNOSIS. If the patient is not in coma and carefully examined, there is little difficulty in discovering a scapular fracture. The

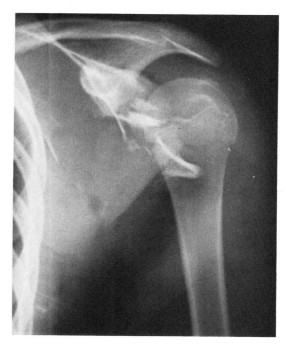

FIG. 17-8. An 11-year-old child had received a direct blow to the shoulder during an automobile accident. Note the severe shattering of the glenoid and scapular neck as well as comminution of the scapular body. There was a permanent brachial plexus injury. The result was poor because of the neurologic deficit.

patient tends to splint the arm at the side or keep the extremity slightly abducted, avoiding all movements especially when there is extensive comminution of the body and spine of the scapula. The patient usually lies tilted away from the injured side with fractures of the body and spine. Tenderness, ecchymosis, hematoma, and even abrasions are often found at the site of fracture. Occasionally, with extensive comminution of the body of the scapula, the patient may complain of increased pain during deep inspiration. During the acute phase of injury it is often impossible to test muscle power about the shoulder because of muscle spasm and local hemorrhage. In fact, muscle paralysis should be ruled out[32] (Fig. 17-8).

Whenever fractures of the scapula are suspected roentgenograms should be taken in the anteroposterior neutral, tangential, and axillary positions with the arm gently

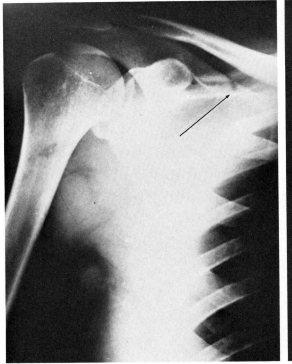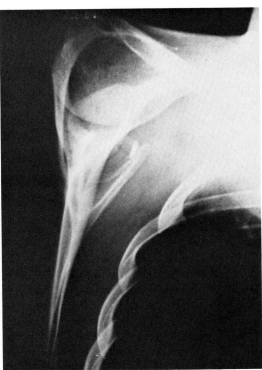

A

B

FIG. 17-9. A, A 36-year-old man fractured the spine of the scapula (arrow). B, A comminuted, displaced fracture of the body was not suspected until a lateral view of the scapula was obtained. The patient was treated in a sling for 18 days before he started gentle motion exercises. Recovery was uneventful.

abducted, if possible (Figs. 17-9 and 17-10). I find the axillary view much more valuable than the lateral transthoracic view. In the former superimposition of the ribs and other bones is avoided. The axillary film demonstrates the glenoid very well. Anteroposterior roentgenograms demonstrate the axillary border and inferior angle of the scapula.

Fractures of Spine and Body of Scapula

Fractures of the spine and body of the scapula require only symptomatic treatment. The surgeon should examine the patient for other injuries to the rib cage, lungs, local neurovascular system, and vertebral column. Rib fractures almost always all heal without disability, even when markedly displaced (Figs. 17-9 to 17-11). The surgeon should not strive for anatomic reduction since the means do not justify the result.

Reliance should be placed on effective immobilization of the extremity and shoulder blade. This can usually be accomplished with a sling or Velpeau immobilization. After 10 to 14 days, or longer, gentle motion exercises may be started and increased until normal shoulder function is attained. Generally, only time and reassurance are needed to ensure a satisfactory result.

Complications have not been encountered at our Center although they have been reported by other authors. Should pain about the scapula persist after healing occurs and there are no abnormal findings, rarely, the supraspinatus nerve may be compressed as it traverses the suprascapular notch. Electromyographic testing may be of help in evaluating the problem.

Intrathoracic Dislocation of Scapula

First described by Key and Conwell,[25] this injury was postulated to result from force-

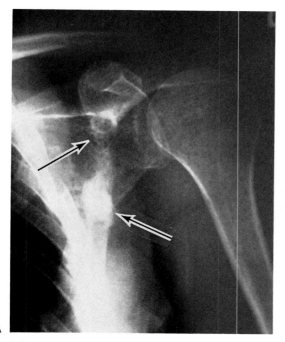

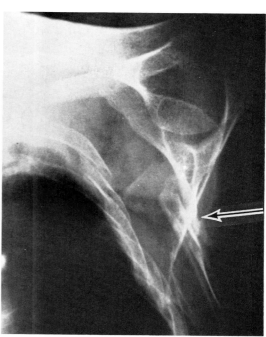

A

B

FIG. 17-10. A, An anteroposterior film shows a fracture of the scapular body and neck (arrows) of a 40-year-old woman. B, A tangential view demonstrates the extent of displacement (arrow). The patient was treated in a sling for 3 weeks. The result was excellent.

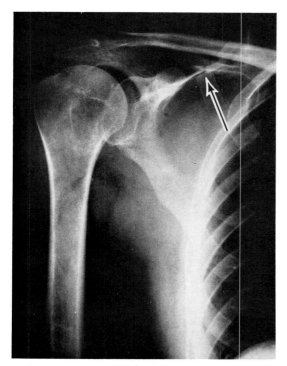

FIG. 17-11. A fracture of the scapular spine (arrow) was seen on the anteroposterior film only after prevention of the superimposition of the ribs and clavicle.

ful outward traction on the arm or from direct force applied to the back surface of the scapula. The dislocation is exceptionally rare. Nettrour and co-workers reported a case of intrathoracic scapular dislocation associated with ipsilateral sternoclavicular separation and rib fracture in which the inferior angle of the scapula locked between the fourth and fifth ribs.[31] The diagnosis was established 6 weeks after injury. During open reduction, the serratus anterior and subscapularis muscles were released from the inferior angle of the scapula and reattached more superiorly under less tension. After 6 weeks of immobilization with the arm held in anatomic position at the side and 6 additional weeks of exercises recovery was complete.

Fractures of the Acromion

Fractures of the acromion usually occur from a severe downward blow on the process.

Ordinarily, fractures of the acromion require only rest and sling immobilization until pain subsides (Fig. 17-12). This is true of undisplaced or slightly displaced acromial fractures. Rarely, the fractured acromion may rotate downward and narrow the space between the superior portion of the humeral head and undersurface of the acromion (Fig. 17-13). In this event abduction motion may decrease. When a nonunited acromial epiphysis is suspected contralateral shoulder roentgenograms should be taken for comparison to rule out a fracture, since a nonunited acromial epiphysis or os acromiale occurs bilaterally in 62 percent of the cases.[29] Liberson believed bilateral views taken in the superoinferior position were best to observe this anomaly[29] (see Fig. 18-32C).

Closed reduction methods which include forceful upward displacement or wide abduction of the humerus usually fail to reduce displaced acromial fractures or to hold them in a reduced position (see Fig. 17-17C). The patient should be forewarned that open reduction is indicated in such

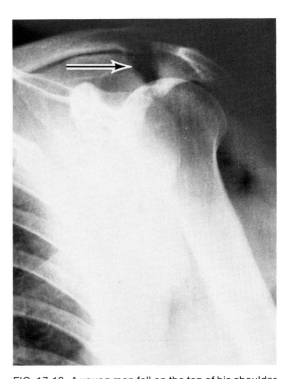

FIG. 17-13. A young man fell on the top of his shoulder and fractured the acromion (arrow). Note the downward displacement of the acromion. The space between the acromion and head of the humerus was decreased. The patient refused an open reduction. The result was poor in that pain persisted and significant overhead shoulder motion was lost.

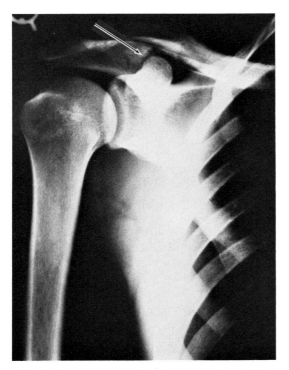

FIG. 17-12. A young adult fell from a height onto the top of his shoulder. Note the slightly displaced fracture of the base of the acromion (arrow). He was treated in a sling for 4 weeks. Recovery was complete.

injuries when closed reduction methods fail. These fractures may be held in the reduced position by screw fixation or two smooth Steinmann pins crossing the fracture site and bent at the outer end to prevent migration. If the acromial fragment is small, especially if there is malunion, it is probably better to remove the fragment.

McLaughlin stated that bony union will occur if the fragments are in apposition.[30] Fibrous union may result if there is interposed soft tissue. Nonunions have not been observed even in those uncooperative young adults who removed their slings early and used their extremities if the fracture fragments were in continuity. However, this statement is not true in older persons who have undergone osteotomy of the acromial edge during shoulder operations, and who have developed asymptomatic fibrous union of the osteotomy site.

Conservative and postoperative treatment are the same. The extremity should be held in a sling or Velpeau position for 3 to 4 weeks. Thereafter, gentle motion exercises are started.

Fractures of Glenoid Fossa and Neck of Scapula

Sir Astley Cooper described the clinical picture of fracture of the scapular neck which included prominence of the acromion, flattening of the shoulder contour, and easy reduction of inferior displacement of the shoulder by support of the elbow.[23]

However, two of three cases he described were in reality humeral neck fractures.

The injury usually results from a blow directed from the front, back, or directly over the point of the shoulder. The patient may hold the arm in slight abduction. Any attempted movement of the extremity is painful, including compression of the humeral head against the glenoid. Loss of shoulder contour may be observed if local swelling is not great.

Fractures of the glenoid and neck of the scapula may be undisplaced, displaced, or burst injuries (Figs. 17-8, 17-14, and 17-15). When the glenoid rim is avulsed in trau-

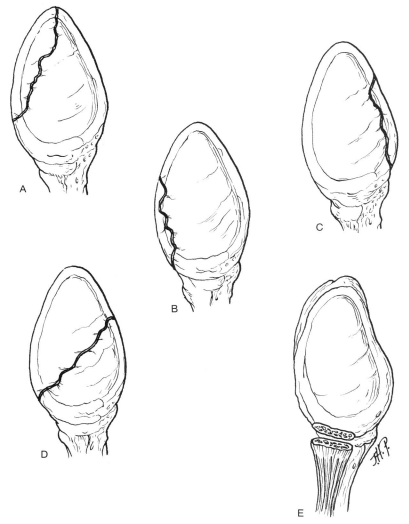

FIG. 17-14. Various types of fractures of the glenoid. A, Anterosuperior glenoid rim fracture. B, Anterior glenoid rim fracture. C, Posterior glenoid rim fracture. D, Glenoid face fracture. E, Inferior glenoid rim fracture.

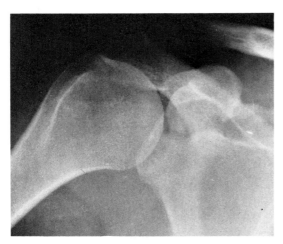

FIG. 17-15. An adult man sustained a displaced fracture of the glenoid. He was treated in a Velpeau sling for 4 weeks, followed by increasing gentle motion exercises for 6 weeks. The functional result was excellent, and the patient was free of pain. (Reprinted from Post, M., and Haskell, S.: Fractures and Dislocations of the Shoulder Girdle, Ribs, and Sternum, Chapter 8. In Practice of Surgery, Volume 2, Orthopedics, 1973 revision with permission of the Medical Department, Harper & Row, Publishers, Inc., Hagerstown, Md.)

matic shoulder dislocations the small fragment may be observed on the axillary view if not clearly seen on the anteroposterior roentgenogram. With posterior or anterior dislocations the posterior and anterior rims, respectively, may be avulsed. Avulsion of the inferior lip may be caused by violent contraction of the triceps muscle. These avulsion injuries may account for recurring shoulder dislocations.

Velpeau immobilization is recommended for a 4-week period as in an acute shoulder dislocation, particularly when the mechanism of injury of any part of the rim is known to have been caused by traumatic dislocation (Fig. 17-16). However, large glenoid fractures associated with anterior dislocation should not be treated as are small chip or rim fractures.[19] They may lead to chronic dislocation.[27] Moreover, when small glenoid rim fractures are associated with other fractures, such as those of the acromion, they should be anatomically reduced and internally fixed. Otherwise, there is

danger that a chronic dislocation will result (Fig. 17-17).

Fractures of the neck of the scapula involving the glenoid fossa may be difficult to diagnose if excellent roentgenograms are not studied (see Fig. 17-3). As a general rule, these injuries may be treated closed except when a large segment of the glenoid is displaced in a steplike fashion. Depression or separation of 2 or 3 mm. will not cause disability (Fig. 17-15). The surgeon should remember that the glenohumeral joint is not a weight-bearing or total contact joint.

Impacted comminuted neck fractures are caused by a direct blow from one of several directions on the point of the shoulder (see Fig. 17-3). The patient holds the extremity in a neutral or slightly abducted position. Considerable swelling may exaggerate the shoulder contour unless there is a dislocation. Ecchymosis may ensue. There may be severe tenderness about the shoulder.

Scapular neck fractures do not require open treatment for a satisfactory result even with glenoid involvement. Sling or Velpeau immobilization for 3 to 4 weeks is all that is needed for undisplaced fractures, followed by a gradual increase of gentle motion exercises until normal shoulder function is restored.

For highly comminuted or displaced fractures of the neck of the scapula involving the articular surface, it is safer and more comfortable for the patient to be placed in a plaster shoulder spica for 6 to 8 weeks. Traction treatment does not appear to help reduce the fragments or affect the outcome. Remember that the vast majority of cases do well with nonoperative treatment. Therefore, it is only in the very exceptional situation of marked displacement of a large segment of the glenoid articular surface leading to instability that an open reduction may be necessary.

Fractures of the Coracoid

Fractures of the coracoid are uncommon. They may result from a severe blow to the shoulder, the bone being avulsed by sudden

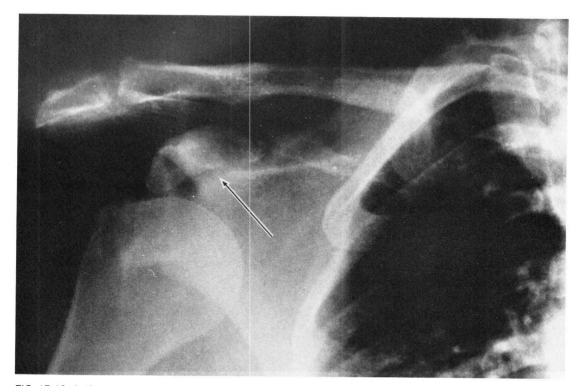

FIG. 17-16. A 43-year-old man sustained an anterior shoulder dislocation. There was an associated fracture of the base of the coracoid process (arrow). After closed reduction, an anteroposterior film showed a fracture of the rim of the inferior glenoid. The patient was treated in Velpeau immobilization for 5 weeks. The functional result was excellent and the patient was free of pain.

forceful traction of the muscles that attach to it or by the impact of a dislocated humeral head[20,28,34] (Fig. 17-16). Boyer described a case of stress fracture of the coracoid process caused by the repeated use of a shotgun.[22]

During the acute phase of the injury, there is localized tenderness. Any forced pull, including forced adduction, of the muscles that attach to the coracoid process increases the patient's pain. Pain may also increase on deep inspiration. The force of the fracture may contuse the cords of the brachial plexus positioned on the medial side of the base of the coracoid. Unless they are suspected, minimal neurologic changes may be missed.

Anteroposterior roentgenograms often will show a fractured coracoid. Angled axillary views show the length of the coracoid process and are more likely to demonstrate the fracture. Accessory ossification centers may occur at the proximal and distal parts of the process and should not be interpreted as a fracture[26] (Fig. 17-18).

Treatment should be conservative in most cases, immobilizing the extremity for 2 to 3 weeks until there is significant pain relief. All markedly displaced symptomatic fractures may be treated open by excising the fragment and reattaching the conjoined tendon. Open treatment also is indicated for the acute case in which neurologic deficit results from brachial plexus injury. If the acromioclavicular joint is dislocated the dislocation and the coracoid fracture may be treated by open reduction and internal fixation. It is especially important to recognize a coracoid fracture when the surgeon plans to hold a dislocated lateral clavicle to the coracoid either by Dacron tape or by a Bosworth screw.[33]

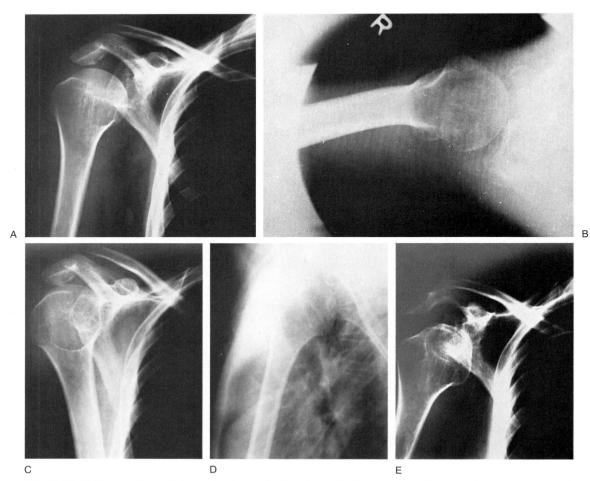

FIG. 17-17. A 25-year-old man fell onto the top of his shoulder while his arm was abducted. A, Anteroposterior and, B, axillary roentgenograms show an acromial fracture with downward tilt and anteroinferior dislocation. A small anterior rim fracture was present. C, Anteroposterior and, D, lateral transthoracic roentgenograms show the apparent reduction of the dislocation but not the acromial displacement. Note the slight disruption in the parabolic curve. The patient refused surgical treatment. E, Two years after injury, note that there is a chronic anteroinferior shoulder dislocation. The acromion healed in malalignment. There was severe pain and stiffness of the joint.

Fractures of the Clavicle

The clavicle is a strut that serves as a support connecting the upper extremity to the rest of the skeleton. It adds to the stability of the shoulder. The clavicle is a long, curved bone placed almost horizontally at the upper anterior portion of the thorax immediately above the first rib. It supports the shoulder and keeps it away from the chest wall. The clavicle is the first bone to ossify in utero. In the child it has one epiphyseal plate at the medial end which articulates with the manubrium. The outer end

of the clavicle articulates with the acromion. The clavicle lies subcutaneously in its entire length thereby accounting for its easy injury. The middle portion of the clavicle is composed of tubular cortical bone, whereas the outer clavicle is flattened. The sternocleidomastoid and anterior portion of the trapezius attach to the clavicle, and their actions are countered by the clavicular origins of the pectoralis major and anterior part of the deltoid muscles below. The clavicle is fixed at the outer end to the coracoid and acromion, and at its long axis during shoulder motion. Moreover, its close ana-

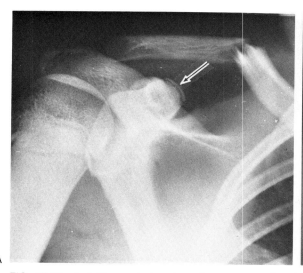

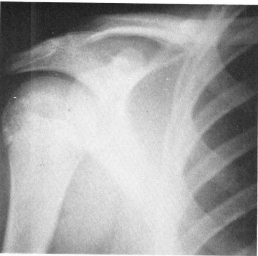

A   B

FIG. 17-18. A, Anteroposterior view shows an angulated fracture of the clavicle of a teenage boy. Note the coracoid ossification center (arrow). B, Following reduction the fracture was immobilized for 8 weeks in a plaster of Paris spica cast, after the fracture had slipped twice during the first week. The result was excellent. (Reprinted from Post, M., and Haskell, S.: Fractures and Dislocations of the Shoulder Girdle, Ribs, and Sternum, Chapter 8. In Practice of Surgery, Volume 2, Orthopedics, 1973 revision with permission of the Medical Department, Harper & Row, Publishers, Inc., Hagerstown, Md.)

tomic relationship to the first rib and major neurovascular structures may occasionally cause serious problems during injury.

MECHANISM OF INJURY. The clavicle is one of the most frequently broken bones. This is especially true in childhood when fracture of this bone may be incomplete or unrecognized (Fig. 17-19). Considerable force directed against the clavicle at its outer end tends to push the shoulder inward toward the chest and causes a sheering fracture in its midportion. The bone may be fractured by a fall from a height or on the outstretched hand, elbow, or shoulder in which the shoulder is forcefully pushed inward toward the chest wall.[42] Fracture often results from direct violence, as during contact sport activity in which force on the point of the shoulder may cause fracture at the outer end.

Allman has classified fractures into three groups.[36] Group I represents fractures of the middle third, the most frequent site, where the clavicle is unsupported by ligaments (Figs. 17-18, and 17-20). The region of greatest frequency of fracture is just medial

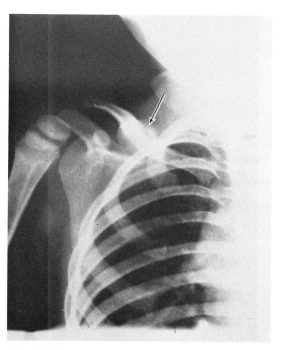

FIG. 17-19. A 22-month-old child developed a tender "lump" over the right midclavicle (arrow). This anteroposterior roentgenogram shows an exuberant mass of callus about an undisplaced fracture. The mother was reassured.

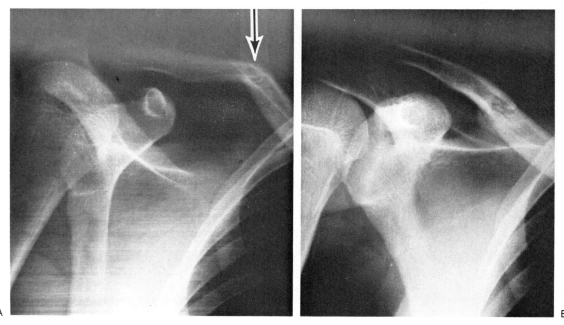

A
B

FIG. 17-20. A, Anteroposterior view shows angulated fracture of the clavicle of a 15-year-old boy who fell on the point of the shoulder. Arrow indicates direction of force used to reduce the fracture under 1 percent lidocaine (Xylocaine) local injection. B, Note the callus formation about the fracture after he was treated in a figure-eight harness for 4 weeks. The result was excellent.

to the attachment of the coracoclavicular ligament. In elderly patients the bone tends to be comminuted when broken (Fig. 17-21). The inner fragment is often elevated by the sternocleidomastoid muscle (Fig. 17-22). The bone may angulate markedly, so that the apex of the fracture is positioned superiorly and causes a marked prominence beneath the skin (Fig. 17-20).

Comprising 10 percent of clavicle fractures, group II fractures involve the clavicle lateral to coracoclavicular ligament and are caused by direct violence. They occur less often than fractures of the middle third because the outer fragment is fixed to the acromion and the inner fragment is held to the coracoid process by the coracoclavicular ligament. Fractures of the clavicle distal to the coracoclavicular ligament often do not unite. Neer has divided these injuries into two types.[46] Type I injuries include fractures in which the coracoclavicular ligament remains intact with little tendency toward displacement. Type II fractures are associated with rupture of the coracocla-

vicular ligament and a marked tendency toward displacement of the clavicle (Fig. 17-23). The forces that cause displacement include (1) the trapezius muscle pulling the medial fragment posteriorly; (2) the weight of the arm pulling on the lateral fragment with its attachment to the trapezoid ligament and acromion; (3) the trunk muscles which displace the lateral fragment medially toward the apex of the thorax; and (4) the scapular ligaments which may rotate the lateral fragments as much as 40 degrees with arm movement.

Group III fractures involve the medial end of the clavicle but are rarely caused by direct violence. If the costoclavicular ligament remains intact there is little or no displacement.

DIAGNOSIS. The patient with a fractured clavicle splints the involved extremity at his side, holding it close to his body. Any movement of the extremity elicits pain. The area over the fracture site is swollen and tender. With severe displacement associated with tearing of soft tissues ecchymosis may be

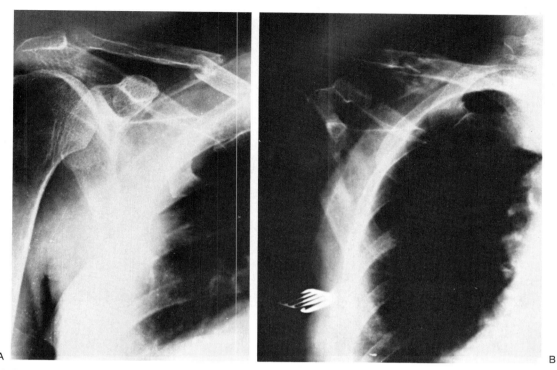

FIG. 17-21. A, Comminuted fracture of the midportion of the clavicle in an 80-year-old woman. B, The patient was treated for 5 weeks in a figure-eight harness and sling. Note the exuberant callus about the fracture site. The functional result was excellent. (Reprinted from Post, M., and Haskell, S.: Fractures and Dislocations of the Shoulder Girdle, Ribs, and Sternum, Chapter 8. In Practice of Surgery, Volume 2, Orthopedics, 1973 revision with permission of the Medical Department, Harper & Row, Publishers, Inc., Hagerstown, Md.)

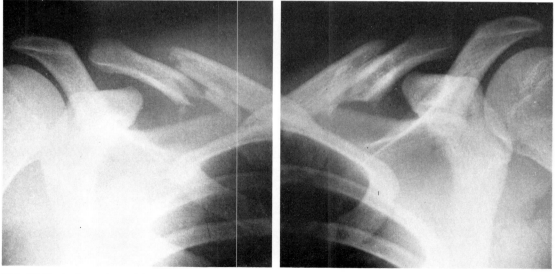

FIG. 17-22. A, Comminuted fracture of the midportion of the clavicle of a teenage girl. Following reduction and immobilization the patient inappropriately removed the harness 3 weeks after reduction. B, At 8 weeks the fracture was clinically solid but the clavicle was shortened. The patient regretted the raised area over her healed fracture. The functional result was excellent. (Reprinted from Post, M., and Haskell, S.: Fractures and Dislocations of the Shoulder Girdle, Ribs, and Sternum, Chapter 8. In Practice of Surgery, Volume 2, Orthopedics, 1973 revision with permission of the Medical Department, Harper & Row, Publishers, Inc., Hagerstown, Md.)

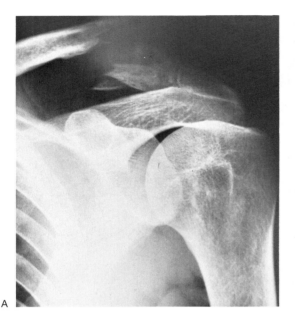

A

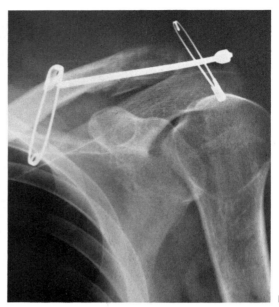

B

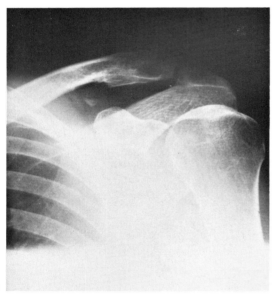

C

FIG. 17-23. A, Anteroposterior view shows a comminuted, displaced lateral clavicle fracture (group II, type II) in an adult man. B, A $\frac{3}{32}$-in. smooth wire was used to hold the open reduction. The extremity was kept in a figure-eight splint and sling for 6 weeks and the wire then was removed. C, One year postoperatively, observe the healed fracture. The result was excellent.

observed. Crepitus may be palpated when there is displacement. The greater the injury the more evident are the complaints and findings.

On occasion, when the diagnosis is in doubt, additional roentgenograms should be taken 7 to 10 days after injury. In any event, at least two films of the clavicle should be taken in order to establish a correct diagnosis. These should include an an-

teroposterior film and an oblique anteroposterior roentgenogram.

TREATMENT. The principal goal in treating fractures of the clavicle is to restore a healed strut in an anatomic position as normal as possible. Once this position is attained, it provides stability to the shoulder girdle. The choice of treatment for achieving optimum healing depends on the age of the patient.

A fractured clavicle in the newborn sustained during birth merely requires gentle care and quiet in order to avoid pain, and heals easily within 2 weeks without additional treatment. Healing of a clavicle deformed by overriding, displacement, or angulation will in time remodel it to a normal shape.

In a child the clavicle should be immobilized in a figure-eight splint made from cotton stockinet into which have been placed several layers of sheet wadding or in a figure-eight harness. The patient should be seen at least weekly and the stretched, cotton splint tightened each time. A new one should not be applied with each visit because it becomes impossible to maintain the desired retraction of the shoulder blades. For incomplete clavicular fracture in older cooperative children, a sling can be used in lieu of a figure-eight splint.

Roentgenograms should be taken on the seventh and fourteenth days following manipulation in order to be certain that the positions of the fracture fragments are satisfactory. The younger the child, the less time is required for immobilization. For example, in a 3-year-old child healing will have occurred within 3 to 4 weeks, whereas in a 10-year-old child 6 to 8 weeks of immobilization will be necessary. Although the splint may be removed at the end of these periods energetic competitive play should be avoided until in the judgment of the surgeon bone healing is truly solid. Parents should be forewarned that at least in younger children who still have significant growth potential the raised area formed at the fracture site during the healing phase usually molds with growth (Fig. 17-24).

In teenagers the problem is to maintain reduction. Although it is often difficult to keep the bone fragments in satisfactory position under the best circumstances, the impatience of youth may complicate matters. The patient should be instructed to

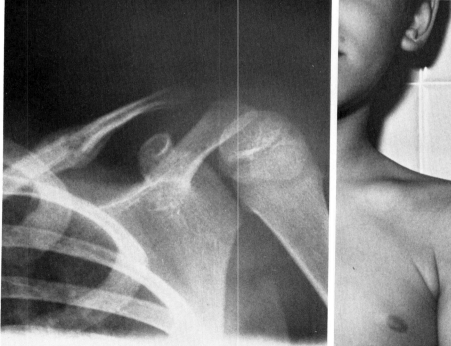
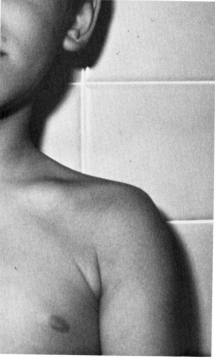

A

B

FIG. 17-24. A, Anteroposterior view shows a healing midclavicular fracture in a 6-year-old boy. B, At 8 weeks after injury, note the raised area overlying the healing fracture of the left clavicle. Two years later the lump had disappeared.

curtail all activities, and to rest for several weeks if there is marked displacement since clavicular fractures that are easily reduced may displace. These patients may be treated with a figure-eight harness which forces the shoulders back and keeps the bone aligned Reinjury to the same bone does not preclude this method of treatment or satisfactory healing (Fig. 17-25). In active or uncooperative individuals a plaster of Paris shoulder spica cast may be applied. A shoulder spica cast is comfortable because it affords a safer degree of immobilization. The plaster yoke or figure-eight harness used in young patients may not provide effective immobilization.

Fractures sustained by adults are more difficult to treat than those of children. The bones tend to displace more easily and take longer to heal. Fractures may be treated with a plaster of Paris shoulder spica cast.[50] To apply a cast, have the patient lie supine on a long, smooth, narrow plate that is suspended between two tables. Gravity will draw the shoulders backward. After the cast has been applied, the metal plate is withdrawn. In adults, immobilization of the fracture fragments should be maintained

for at least 6 to 8 weeks or longer. In teenagers and adults, local injection of 1 percent lidocaine (Xylocaine) into the fracture hematoma permits relatively painless manipulation of the bone fragments.

Patients treated with a figure-eight stockinet splint or harness may develop an irritation of the axilla or compression of the great vessels and nerves in the axilla. The patient may complain not only of irritated skin but also of tingling and numbness in the fingertips. The surgeon should instruct the patient to place his hands on his hips or head, or to lie down and externally rotate his arms in an abducted position. These positions cause the shoulders to retract, help maintain length at the fracture site, and allow the arm to be brought away from the splint in the axillary region, thus lessening any pressure effects on the neurovascular bundle.

Open reduction is seldom justified because surgical treatment, especially in women, can cause an objectionable scar and even become a factor in nonunion (Fig. 17-26). In one exceptional case in a child who had sustained a midclavicular fracture after severe trauma, an open procedure was

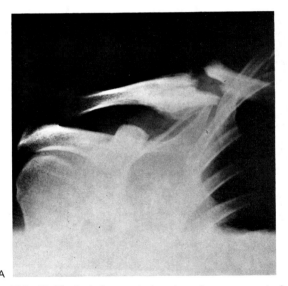
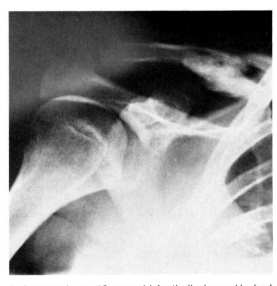

A

B

FIG. 17-25. A, Anteroposterior view shows an acute fourth fracture in an 18-year-old football player. He had sustained the first fracture at 14 years of age. The patient was treated in a figure-eight harness for 6 weeks. B, Anteroposterior view of healing after 6 weeks in the harness. After 16 weeks he returned to competitive sports. The result was excellent.

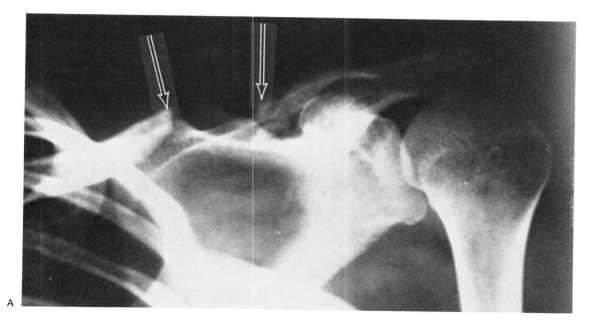

A

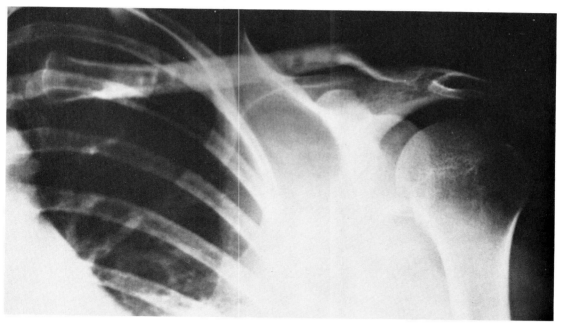

B

FIG. 17-26. A 26-year-old woman with nonunion was inappropriately treated with an open reduction and ineffective intramedullary pins which were removed 12 weeks postoperatively. A, Three years later, note the large gap between the bone ends (arrows). A plate and screws were used to fix the bone ends and an iliac bone graft was employed to fill the large defect because the patient had much pain and an unsightly tenting of the skin when she moved her arm. B, Note the healed clavicle 18 months after bone grafting and plate removal. The result was excellent. Initial conservative treatment would have obviated any surgical procedure.

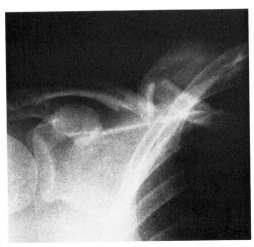

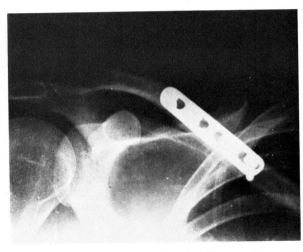

A

B

FIG. 17-27. A, Anteroposterior view shows a midclavicular fracture with severe overriding in a 37-year-old woman. B, An open reduction and internal fixation were performed 14 days after a closed reduction failed and signs and symptoms of brachial plexus compression increased. The result was excellent.

needed to reduce the lateral end of the medial fragment that had buttonholed through the platysma and had tented the subclavian vein. Even repeated fractures of the same bone can be treated nonoperatively with good results (Fig. 17-25). In certain cases in which there is marked displacement and angulation of the fracture fragments or clinical evidence of increasing neurovascular compression, open reduction with intramedullary pinning or plating may become necessary in the adult (Fig. 17-27). The patient should be placed in a semireclining position with the shoulder slightly elevated on the injured side. A 7.5-cm. linear incision is made parallel to and centered just above the clavicular fracture. Care must be taken in exposing the fragments in order to avoid injuring the subclavian vessels or nerves of the brachial plexus. Only as much of the periosteum should be stripped as necessary. To pin an acute fracture, a $3/32$-in. smooth pin is drilled through the medullary canal of the outer fracture fragments until it pierces the skin behind the acromion.[38] The pin is drilled outward until its medial end is at the fracture site. The bone fragments are reduced, and the pin is then driven across the fracture site for a distance of 2 to 3 cm. until it strikes the cortex of the middle third of the clavicle. Although the blunt end of the pin is not likely to penetrate the cortex, it should be bent laterally to preclude migration. External support such as a plaster of Paris cast is needed for 4 weeks or longer and provides greater certainty of healing (Fig. 17-28). The lateral end of the bent pin is cut beneath the skin so that it may be removed at 6 to 8 weeks, or longer if deemed necessary.

Roentgenograms should be taken periodically to check the position of the pin and the degree of healing. Blind pinning, as suggested by some authors,[43] is dangerous and is not justified.

Treatment of Types I and II Fractures. Type I fractures of the distal clavicle may be treated with a figure-eight bandage. Type II acute fractures should be treated open in most adults, because external immobilization such as adhesive strapping is often ineffective in maintaining the position of the fragments (Fig. 17-29). Open treatment methods include insertion of one or two $3/32$-in. pins across the acromion and fragment of lateral clavicle into the reduced fragment of the medial clavicle, in a manner similar to that described if external support is to be utilized for 8 weeks postoperatively.[45] The lateral cut ends of the pins should be bent beneath the skin in order to prevent migration. At the end of 8 to 10

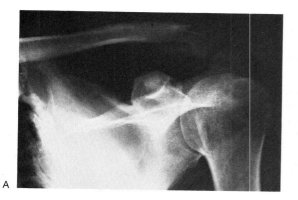

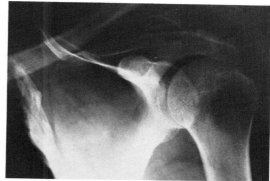

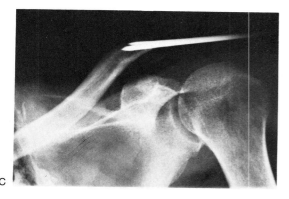

FIG. 17-28. A, Anteroposterior view shows a comminuted, undisplaced fracture (type II) of the lateral clavicle of a 38-year-old man. B, Anteroposterior view shows ineffectiveness of a figure-eight harness when the clavicle is displaced. C, Roentgenogram 10 days later shows the reduction held by 2 smooth pins bent laterally. The pins were removed 6 weeks postoperatively. The result was excellent.

weeks the pins can be removed and gentle motions of the extremity started. In acute or old cases of unreduced displaced fracture of the lateral clavicle, internal fixation of the medial fragment to the coracoid with Dacron tape and autogenous bone grafting is

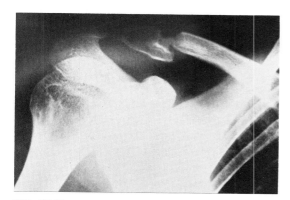

FIG. 17-29. Anteroposterior view of type II fracture of the lateral clavicle 5 months after injury. The fracture was treated with adhesive strapping. A painful nonunion developed. Movement of fragments could be palpated.

worthwhile, as performed for grade III acromioclavicular dislocation. In the uncommon event that the surgeon is confronted with a previously excised short fragment of lateral clavicle and a superiorly dislocated medial clavicle fragment resulting from rupture of the coracoclavicular ligament, control of this section of the clavicle can be achieved by transferring the coracoid with its active short biceps and coracobrachialis to the clavicle, as is performed in the treatment for a chronic acromioclavicular dislocation (see Acromioclavicular Dislocation).

COMPLICATIONS. *Nonunion.* Nonunion is an unusual complication of fractures of the clavicle treated nonoperatively.[44] Should nonunion of the clavicle result, autogenous iliac bone grafts should be placed about the raw area of the fracture site after internal fixation with a plate is accomplished[40] (see Fig. 17-26). Sakellarides recommended the use of an onlay iliac bone graft fixed with screws and packed with cancellous iliac bone between the ends.[48] He advised the use of a spica cast postoperatively. Mild compression of transverse fractures of the midclavicle with internal fixation plates has given good results. Care must be exercised in this area so as not to penetrate the periosteum with the drill points or screw ends. In the elderly or poor-risk patient, a state of nonunion is compatible with good function and comfort. In these cases acceptance of the nonunion is wise.

Malunion. Marked deformity of the midclavicle may be unacceptable in a young woman (Fig. 17-30). If the patient insists on correction, osteotomy and realignment of the clavicle should be performed. Internal fixation with a plate and the addition of iliac bone about the raw site is recommended. However, it should be explained to the patient that nonunion may result and that obviously there will be a scar that can be more disfiguring than the original malunion. In any event, malunions are compatible with a good functional result.

Neurovascular Disturbances. Although uncommon, neurovascular disturbance has been reported when there is encroachment of the space between the clavicle and the first rib. When compression of the subclavian vessels or brachial plexus is present and causing symptoms whether it results

from injury, exuberant callus, or malunion, the pressure phenomenon should be relieved.[41] It may be necessary to resect the first rib or clavicle, or in the case of nonunion internally fix the clavicle and add a bone graft.[37,47] It must be remembered that although resection of the clavicle will not result in great disability, removal of the clavicle is not harmless because this bone does help to stabilize the shoulder.[39]

In the rare event that there is tearing of large vessels, immediate surgical exploration is mandatory. In order to gain adequate exposure as much of the clavicle as needed should be excised in order to isolate and repair the injured major vessels. For example, if repair of the subclavian artery is impossible and it is ligated, it is not necessary to ligate the subclavian vein. However, ligation of the subclavian artery in elderly patients is dangerous since circulation to the upper extremity on the injured side may be imperiled. In this case every effort by a skillful vascular surgeon must be made to repair the vessel.

Associated Upper Rib Fractures

Occasionally, the upper ribs may be fractured along with the clavicle[49] (see Fig. 17-2). There may be associated head and neck injuries. The scalene anticus muscle attaches on a tubercle of the first rib. On either side of this tubercle lies a groove for the subclavian vein anteriorly and the subclavian artery posteriorly. Posterior to the groove for the subclavian artery lies a roughened area for the attachment of the scalene medius muscle. These two muscles elevate the first rib during inspiration. The serratus anterior, arising from the outer surfaces of the upper eight ribs, tends to fix the rib posteriorly during inspiration. These structures may be important in the production of combined injuries of the clavicle and first rib. Fracture of the upper ribs during clavicular fracture may occur through a number of mechanisms: (1) an indirect force transmitted via the manubrium, (2) avulsion fracture at the weakest portion of the rib produced by the scalene anticus,

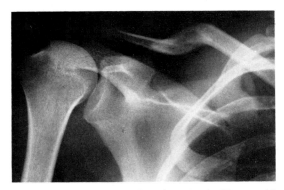

FIG. 17-30. Anteroposterior view in an 18-year-old woman shows a malunion of a fractured clavicle that occurred because she removed her figure-eight harness 3 days after injury. She was displeased with the poor cosmetic result, but decided against surgical correction when advised about possible postoperative complications.

and (3) injuries to the lateral clavicle that cause an acromioclavicular separation when the subclavius muscle transmits an indirect force to the costal cartilage and anterior aspect of the first rib and fractures the posterior portion of the first rib. Therefore, it seems reasonable that the surgeon should look for fractures of the upper ribs when there are severe acromioclavicular injuries and type II fractures of the lateral clavicle. This is best done by observing anteroposterior roentgenograms of the cervical spine and a lateral film of the dorsal spine which best demonstrates the upper ribs.

REFERENCES

Fractures of the Rib Cage

1. Anderson, I., Halkier, E., Poulsen, T., and Westengård, E.: Traumatic lesions of the thorax: A clinical study of the relative frequency of various injuries and their therapy. Acta Chir. Scand. (Suppl.), 332:7–179, 1965.
2. Avery, E. E., Mörch, E. T., and Benson, D. W.: Critically crushed chests; A new method of treatment and continuous mechanical hyperventilation to produce alkalotic apnea and internal pneumatic stabilization. J. Thorac. Surg., 32:291–311, 1956.
3. Barrett, N. R.: Early treatment of stove-in chest. Lancet, 1:293–295, 1960.
4. Charnley, J.: The Closed Treatment of Common Fractures, ed. 3. Edinburgh, E. & S. Livingston, Ltd., 1966.
5. Comroe, J. H.: Physiology of Respiration, Chicago, Year Book Medical Publishers, Inc., 1970.
6. D'Abreu, A. L.: Thoracic injuries, J. Bone Joint Surg., 46-B:581–597, 1964.
7. Gibson, D. L., Carter, R., and Hinshaw, D. B.: Surgical significance of sternal fracture. Surg. Gynecol. Obstet., 114:443–448, 1962.
8. Helal, B.: Fracture of the manubrium sterni. J. Bone Joint Surg., 46-B:602–607, 1964.
9. Joshi, S. G., Panday, S. R., Parulkar, G. B., and Sen, P. K.: Bilateral fracture of the first rib. J. Bone Joint Surg., 47-B:283–285, 1965.
10. Laustela, E.: Thorax traumatology. Acta Chir. Scand. (Suppl.), 332:17–22, 1964.
11. Nordlund, S.: Chest injuries. Acta Chir. Scand. (Suppl.), 332:23–29, 1964.
12. Powell, F. I.: Fractures of the first rib; Its occurrence and clinical diagnosis. Br. Med. J., 1:282–285, 1950.
13. Proctor, H., and London, P. S.: The stove-in chest with paradoxical respiration. Br. J. Surg., 42:622–633, 1955.
14. Richardson, E. P., and Jones, T. B.: Traction on the sternum in the treatment of multiple fractured ribs. Surg. Gynecol. Obstet., 42:283–286, 1926.
15. Sillar, W.: The crushed chest. J. Bone Joint Surg., 43-B:738–745, 1961.
16. Watson-Jones, R.: Fractures and Joint Injuries, ed. 4. Baltimore, Williams & Wilkins Co., Vol. 1, 1957.
17. Williams, G.: The management of stove-in chest. J. Bone Joint Surg., 46-B:598–601, 1964.
18. Williams, M. H.: Severe crushing injury to the chest. Ann. Surg., 128:1006–1011, 1948.

Fractures of the Scapula

19. Aston, J. W., and Gregory, C. F.: Dislocation of the shoulder with significant fracture of the glenoid. J. Bone Joint Surg., 55-A:1531–1533, 1973.
20. Benton, J., and Nelson, C.: Avulsion of the coracoid process in an athlete. J. Bone Joint Surg., 53-A:356–358, 1971.
21. Bonnin, J. G.: A Complete Outline of Fractures. New York, Grune & Stratton, 1946.
22. Boyer, D. W.: Trapshooter's shoulder: Stress fracture of the coracoid process. J. Bone Joint Surg., 57-A:862, 1975.
23. Cooper, A.: Lectures on Principles and Practice of Surgery, ed. 3. Boston, Lilly & Walt, 1831.
24. Imatani, R. J.: Fractures of the scapula: A review of 53 fractures. J. Trauma, 15:473–478, 1975.
25. Key, J. A., and Conwell, H. E.: Fracture, Dislocations and Sprains, ed. 5. St. Louis, C. V. Mosby Co., 1951.
26. Köhler, A., and Zimmer, E. A.: Borderlines of the Normal and Early Pathologic in Skeletal Roentgenology, Amer. ed. 3. New York, Grune & Stratton, 1968.
27. Kummel, B. M.: Fractures of the glenoid causing chronic dislocation of the shoulder. Clin. Orthop., 69:189–191, 1970.
28. Landoff, B. A.: Hitherto undescribed injury of the coracoid process. Acta Clin. Scand., 89:401–406, 1943.
29. Liberson, F.: Os acromiale—Contested anomaly. J. Bone Joint Surg., 19:683–689, 1937.
30. McLaughlin, H. L.: Trauma. Philadelphia, W. B. Saunders Co., 1959.
31. Nettrour, L. F., Krufky, E. L., Mueller, R. E., and Raycroft, J. F.: Locked scapula: Intrathoracic dislocation of the inferior angle. A case report. J. Bone Joint Surg., 54-A:413–416, 1972.
32. Nunley, R. C., and Bedini, S. J.: Paralysis of the shoulder subsequent to a comminuted fracture of

the scapula: Rationale and treatment methods. Phys. Ther. Rev., 40:442–447, 1960.

33. Protass, J. J., Stampfli, F. V., and Osmer, J. C.: Coracoid process fracture diagnosis in acromioclavicular separation. Radiology, 116:61–64, 1975.

34. Rounds, R. C.: Isolated fracture of the coracoid process. J. Bone Joint Surg., 31–A:662–663, 1949.

35. Rowe, C. R.: Fractures of the scapula. Surg. Clin. North Am., 43:1565–1571, 1963.

Fractures of the Clavicle

36. Allman, F. L.: Fractures and ligamentous injuries of the clavicle and its articulation. J. Bone Joint Surg., 49-A:774–784, 1967.

37. Howard, F. M., and Shafer, S. J.: Injuries to the clavicle with neurovascular complications. J. Bone Joint Surg., 47-A:1335–1346, 1965.

38. Lee, H. G.: Treatment of fracture of the clavicle by internal nail fixation. N. Engl. J. Med., 234:222–224, 1946.

39. Lusskin, R., Weiss, C. A., and Winer, J.: The role of the subclavius muscle in the subclavian vein syndrome (costoclavicular syndrome) following fracture of the clavicle: A case report with a review of the pathophysiology of the costoclavicular space. Clin. Orthop., 54:75–83, 1967.

40. Mayer, J. H.: Non-union of fractured clavicle. Proc. R. Soc. Med., 58:182–184, 1965.

41. Miller, D. S., and Boswick, J. A.: Lesions of the brachial plexus associated with fractures of the clavicle. Clin. Orthop., 64:144–149, 1969.

42. Mosely, H. F.: Athletic injuries to the shoulder region. Am. J. Surg., 98:401–422, 1959.

43. Murray, G.: A method of fixation for fracture of the clavicle. J. Bone Joint Surg., 22:616–620, 1940.

44. Neer, C. S.: Nonunion of the clavicle. J.A.M.A., 172:1006–1011, 1960.

45. Neer, C. S.: Fracture of the distal clavicle with detachment of the coracoclavicular ligaments in adults. J. Trauma, 3:99–110, 1963.

46. Neer, C. S.: Fractures of the distal third of the clavicle. Clin. Orthop., 58:43–50, 1968.

47. Penn, I.: The vascular complications of fractures of the clavicle. J. Trauma, 4:819–831, 1964.

48. Sakellarides, H.: Pseudarthrosis of the clavicle. J. Bone Joint Surg., 43-A:130–138, 1961.

49. Weiner, D. S., and O'Dell, H. W.: Fractures of the first rib associated with injuries to the clavicle. J. Trauma, 9:412–422, 1969.

50. Young, C. S.: The mechanisms of ambulatory treatment of fractures of the clavicle. J. Bone Joint Surg., 13:299–310, 1931.

18

Fractures of the Proximal Humerus

MELVIN POST

The proximal humerus is one of the pivotal points for the normal function of the upper extremity. Correct treatment of fractures of this region not only depends upon an accurate diagnosis of the injury but also requires an appreciation of the local functional anatomy and the dynamics of the injury.

The humerus is the largest bone in the upper limb. Its hemispherical head articulates with the shallow glenoid cavity of the scapula. The slightly constricted circumference of the articular surface is termed the anatomic neck in contradistinction to the surgical neck located at the tapered area below the tubercles.

OSSIFICATION

The entire humerus ossifies from eight centers. The center for the body appears near the middle of the bone in the eighth week of fetal life. Thereafter, it extends toward each end of the bone so that at birth it is almost fully ossified. There are three centers of ossification for the proximal end of the humerus. The major, or central, center appears between 4 and 6 months of age. The ossification center for the greater tuberosity can be seen on roentgenograms during the third year and the center for the lesser tuberosity makes its appearance dur-

ing the fifth year. By the sixth year and in most cases by the seventh year, all three ossification centers coalesce into one ossification center.[17,22] No injuries separating these centers have been reported.

The abundant cancellous trabecular network in the proximal humerus often serves to cushion the head from serious injury in the young. As osteoporosis in the elderly advances, the proximal humerus is less able to withstand even minimal force, thus accounting for the higher incidence of fracture in this region in older persons.

CLASSIFICATION

Although most fractures of the proximal humerus can be treated conservatively some displaced fractures or fracture-dislocations require specialized treatment. In 1934, Codman showed that the fracture lines about the humeral head follow the old epiphyseal lines delineating the tuberosities and anatomic head from the diaphysis.[6] He suggested that the head of the humerus be divided into four main segments or combinations of the four parts, namely, the humeral head, the lesser tuberosity, the greater tuberosity, and the shaft. Other classifications based on the anatomy and mechanism of injury attempted unsuccessfully to simplify the treatment of proximal humeral fractures.[17,18] Neer has elegantly refined the classification of proximal humeral fractures.[14] His classification is based on the displacement of one or more of the described four major segments (Figs. 18-1 and 18-2). The systematization of the different kinds of displaced fractures, forecasting the status of the vascular supply and determining the effects of the muscle attachments and the continuity of the articular surfaces of the proximal humerus, now permits a greater degree of sound treatment to be instituted.

MINIMUM DISPLACEMENT. This group stands alone and includes all fractures, regardless of the level or number of fracture lines, in which no segment is displaced more than 1 cm. or angulated more than 45 degrees (Fig. 18-1A). These fractures account for a majority of those of the proximal humerus, about 85 percent. They are considered 1-part fractures. The bone fragments are usually held together by soft tissues or are impacted and permit early motion exercises (Fig. 18-3).

ARTICULAR SEGMENT DISPLACEMENT. Displacement fractures at the anatomic neck without separation of the tuberosities are rare (Fig. 18-1B). It is easy to overlook this 2-part injury (Fig. 18-4). Good quality roentgenograms should be obtained in both the anteroposterior and lateral transthoracic or true axillary planes in order to identify the injury. It may be of help to compare roentgenograms of the injured shoulder with those of the opposite shoulder if doubt exists. Disability may result from malunion or from avascular necrosis, the latter occurring often.

SHAFT DISPLACEMENT. The fracture occurs just beneath the tuberosities at the level of the surgical neck (Fig. 18-1C). The fragments are displaced more than 1 cm. or angulated more than 45 degrees in this lesion (Figs. 18-5 and 18-6). Although fracture lines may be seen proximally in this injury, the rotator cuff attachments are intact. For this reason in most cases the humeral head is maintained in neutral position (Figs. 18-7 and 18-8). In exceptional cases malunion may result (Fig. 18-9). If open reduction is

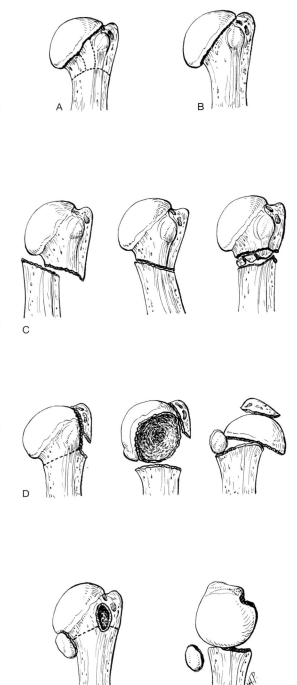

FIG. 18-1. Neer classification of fractures of the proximal humerus. A, Minimal displacement. B, Anatomic neck. C, Surgical neck. D, Greater tuberosity. E, Lesser tuberosity. (Redrawn from Neer, C. S., II: Displaced proximal humeral fractures. Part I. Classification and evaluation. J. Bone Joint Surg., 52-A:1077–1089, 1970.)

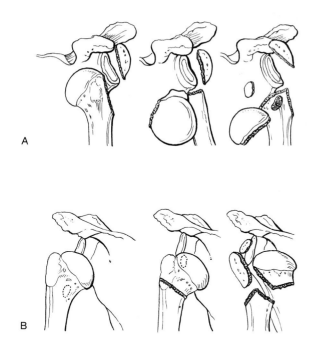

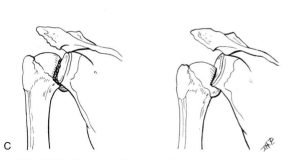

FIG. 18-2. Neer classification of fractures of the proximal humerus (continued). A, Anterior fracture-dislocation. B, Posterior fracture-dislocation. C, Articular surface. (Redrawn from Neer, C. S., II: Displaced proximal humeral fractures. Part I. Classification and evaluation. J. Bone Joint Surg., 52-A:1077–1089, 1970.)

attempted, occasionally avascular necrosis of the head of the humerus may result (see Fig. 10-17). After closed reduction, the fracture may be stable with an intact periosteum or it may be unstable and result in nonunion secondary to instability and the interposition of soft tissues (Fig. 18-10).

GREATER TUBEROSITY DISPLACEMENT. The greater tuberosity contains the three facets for the tendon attachment of the rotator cuff. Any one of the facets or the entire tuberosity may be retracted more than 1 cm. from the lesser tuberosity (Fig. 18-11). If the bone fragment with its attached tendinous tissue is retracted superiorly, it is usually difficult to maintain the reduced fragment by closed methods (Fig. 18-11A). In this case there is ordinarily a longitudinal tear in the rotator cuff in this 2-part injury.

If a fracture occurs through the surgical neck of the humerus, then a 3-part injury results (Fig. 18-1D). If not significantly displaced, the articular segment remains in a normal relationship to the shaft. With significant displacement at the surgical neck, along with retraction of the tuberosity, the articular segment rotates internally because of the action of the subscapularis muscle (Fig. 18-12).[15] The rotator cuff defect allows rotation of the articular segment in a posterior direction. In this situation the blood supply to the head of the humerus is preserved because of soft-tissue attachment.

LESSER TUBEROSITY DISPLACEMENT. A 2-part lesion results when there is an isolated avulsion fracture of the lesser tuberosity (Figs. 18-1E, 18-13, and 18-14). It is equivalent to the isolated avulsion of the lesser tuberosity seen with epiphyseal injuries (see Fig. 18-31). The injuries are uncommon.[23] Three-part lesions occur when there is an associated fracture of the surgical neck. In 3-part lesions, displacement at the surgical neck allows the articular segment to be externally rotated and abducted by the external rotators of the shoulder, thereby interfering with closed reduction (Fig. 18-1E). In this event the articular surface faces anteriorly. The head segment retains an adequate blood supply through the posterior soft-tissue attachments. In 4-part fractures both tuberosities may be retracted. In this instance, the blood supply to the head is lost.

FRACTURE-DISLOCATION. This injury is a true dislocation in which the head loses all continuity with the glenoid. It occurs after the capsule and ligamentous structures are torn. Baker and Leach reported three unusual cases of fracture-dislocations with

(Text continues on page 383)

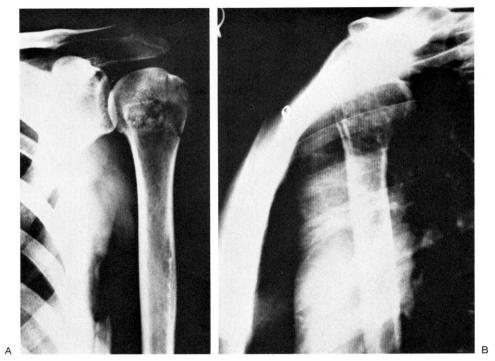

FIG. 18-3. A, Anteroposterior and, B, lateral transthoracic films of a comminuted fractured humeral head and neck with minimal displacement in a 30-year-old woman. The patient was treated with Velpeau sling immobilization for 3 weeks. Thereafter, gentle motion exercises were gradually increased. At 2 months the shoulder was free of pain and overhead motion was excellent. (Reprinted from Post, M., and Haskell, S.: Fractures and Dislocations of the Upper Extremity, Chapter 7. In Practice of Surgery, Volume 2, Orthopedics, 1973 revision, with permission of the Medical Department, Harper & Row, Publishers, Inc., Hagerstown, Md.)

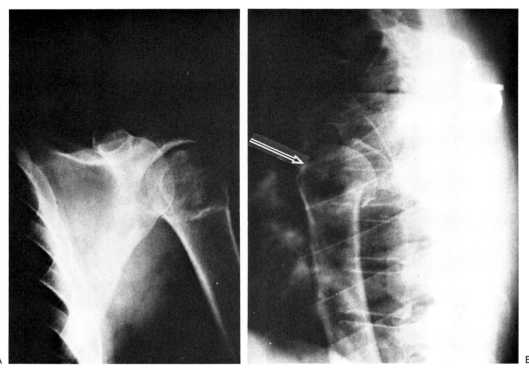

FIG. 18-4. A, Anteroposterior and, B, lateral transthoracic views of a 39-year-old man show a fracture of the anatomic neck. The head is rotated slightly posteriorly. Fracture level is shown on lateral film (arrow). The fracture was immobilized 4 weeks in a sling. The result was excellent.

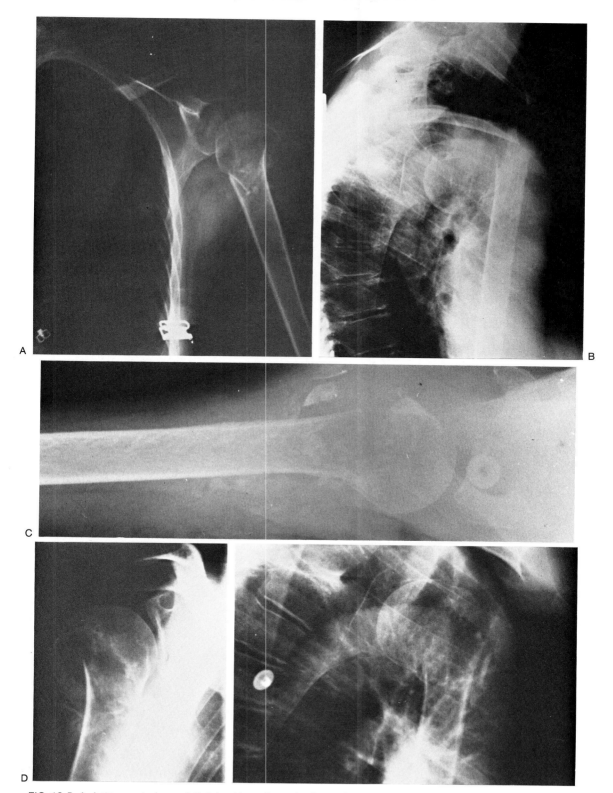

FIG. 18-5. A, Anteroposterior and, B, lateral transthoracic views of the shoulder show a comminuted fracture of the surgical neck of the humerus of a 54-year-old woman. Note the marked posterior angulation of the humeral head on the lateral film. C, After 5 weeks in skeletal traction the humeral head and shaft are well aligned. After 6 weeks, gentle motion exercises were begun with the extremity in a sling. D, Roentgenograms show some rotation of the head. Serious medical problems precluded a Nicola stabilization procedure. The result was satisfactory. (Reprinted from Post, M., and Haskell, S.: Fractures and Dislocations of the Upper Extremity, Chapter 7. In Practice of Surgery, Volume 2, Orthopedics, 1973 revision, with permission of the Medical Department, Harper & Row, Publishers, Inc., Hagerstown, Md.)

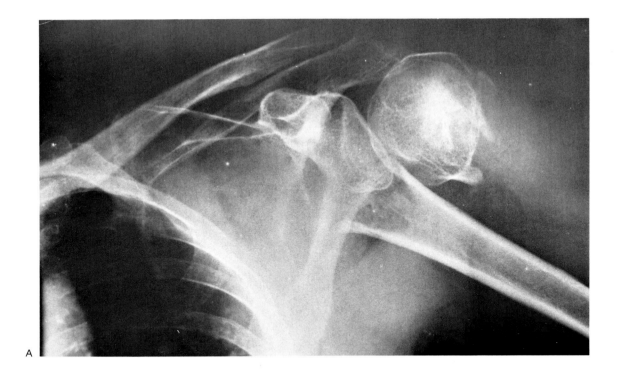

A

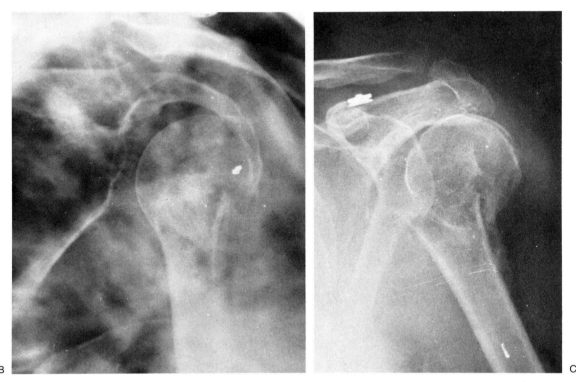

B

C

FIG. 18-6. A, Anteroposterior view shows a highly displaced surgical neck fracture. B, Lateral transthoracic and, C, anteroposterior views show the reduction achieved by manipulation under image intensifier. The patient was kept in traction 25 days and then in Velpeau immobilization another 3 weeks. The functional result was excellent.

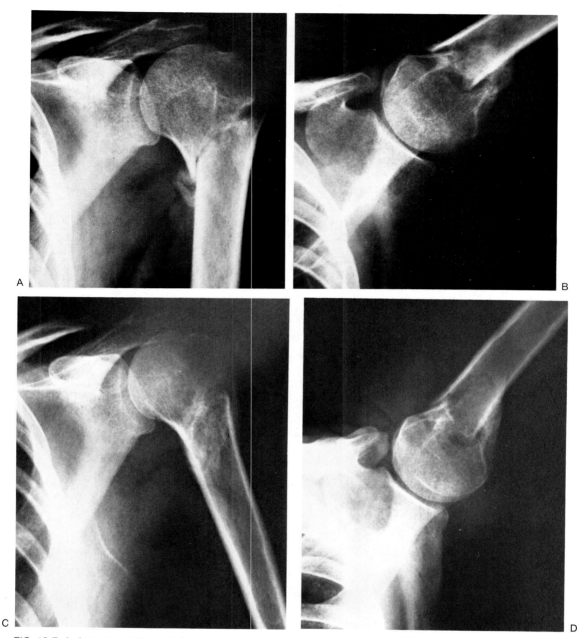

FIG. 18-7. A, Anteroposterior and, B, overhead lateral views show a surgical neck fracture in a 33-year-old woman who also had a femoral shaft fracture. The extremity was treated in Velpeau immobilization for 5 weeks. C, Anteroposterior and, D, lateral views of the humerus show progressive healing at 8 weeks. The result was excellent.

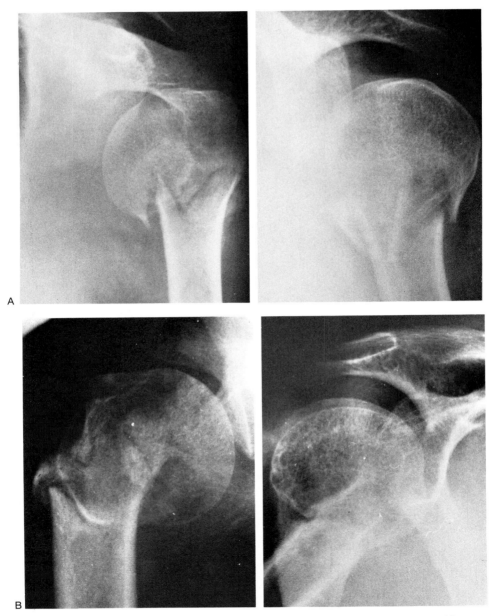

FIG. 18-8. A, Anteroposterior roentgenograms taken at two different angles show a comminuted fracture through the surgical neck of the humerus. The extremity was correctly treated in a Velpeau sling but incorrectly mobilized too early (at 3 weeks) because the fracture was unstable. B, Roentgenograms show healed valgus malunion at 10 weeks. There was marked limitation of abduction and elevation of the extremity. (Reprinted from Post, M., and Haskell, S.: Fractures and Dislocations of the Upper Extremity, Chapter 7. In Practice of Surgery, Volume 2, Orthopedics, 1973 revision, with permission of the Medical Department, Harper & Row, Publishers, Inc., Hagerstown, Md.)

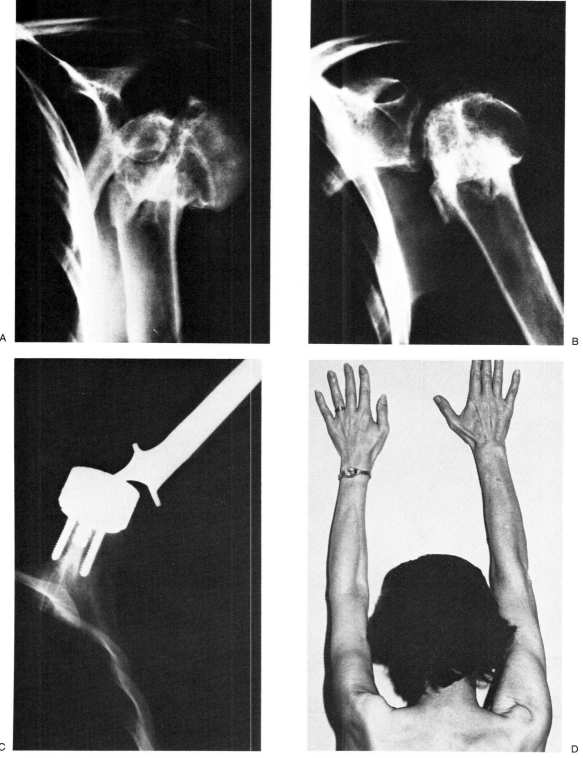

FIG. 18-9. Anteroposterior views in, A, neutral and, B, internal rotation show a severe malunion of a surgical neck fracture in a 50-year-old woman who had had an open reduction 2 years previously. There was a nonfunctioning rotator cuff, and severe humeral head degeneration was discovered at operation. C, A total shoulder replacement was performed with good results. Note the artificial joint in the overhead position. D, Two years after joint replacement, observe the extent of passive motion. Deltoid function was ineffective at the time of the second operation. There is also severe atrophy of the left supraspinatus and infraspinatus muscles.

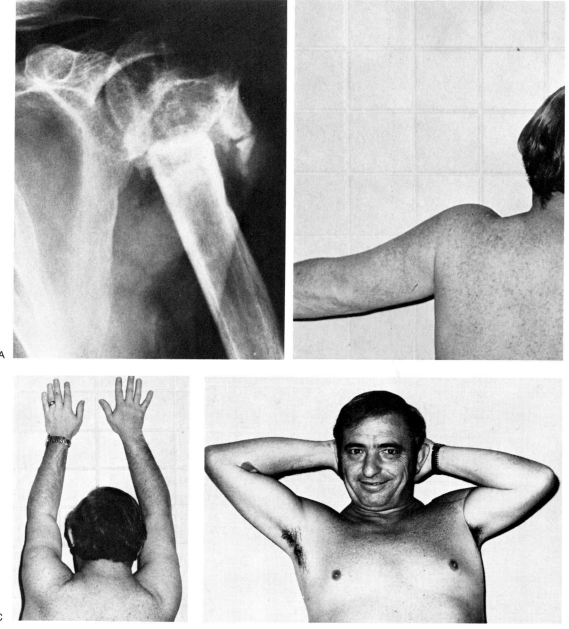

FIG. 18-10. A, Anteroposterior roentgenogram shows a nonunion and failed bone graft in a 40-year-old man. The nonunion occurred after conservative treatment. B, Note the patient's inability to actively abduct his left extremity. There was deltoid atrophy. A total shoulder replacement was performed because of intractable pain. There was a nonfunctioning rotator cuff. C and D, The extent of active motion is shown 18 months later. Thus far, the result is excellent.

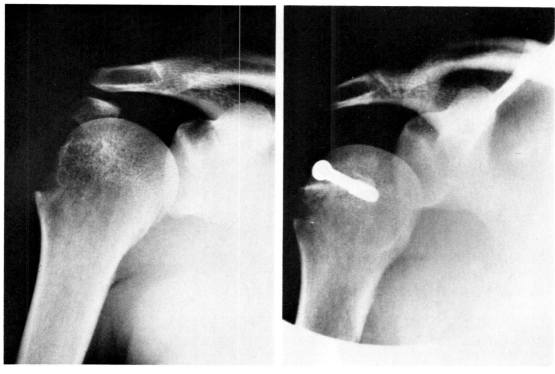

A   B

FIG. 18-11. A, Anteroposterior roentgenogram shows a 2-part avulsion fracture of a portion of the greater tuberosity with severe upward displacement of the fragment. B, Anteroposterior roentgenogram shows the reduction after operation and the transient subluxation. The result was excellent.

rotator cuff avulsions.[2] The head may be displaced anteriorly (Fig. 18-2A) or posteriorly (Fig. 18-2B). In 2-part and 3-part fracture-dislocations, the blood supply to the humeral head is usually adequate because one of the tuberosities and soft-tissue attachments remain in continuity with the articular segment (Figs. 18-2A and 18-15). The lesser tuberosity almost always remains attached to the humeral head in 3-part anterior fracture-dislocations. In exceptional cases the head of the humerus may be devoid of any soft-tissue attachment (Fig. 18-16).

In posterior fracture-dislocation of the humeral head it is the lesser tuberosity that is usually displaced. In a rare 2-part posterior fracture-dislocation where the fracture occurs high on the neck, the blood supply to the head may be adequate (Fig. 18-17). In 3-part posterior fracture-dislocation the greater tuberosity provides circulation to the head. In 4-part anterior or posterior fracture-dislocation both tuberosities are detached and the head has no blood supply. It is here that complications in the vascular supply to the humeral head are common.

When the articular cartilage is crushed by the force of the head striking against the glenoid, some of the fragments of the cartilage may be extruded from the glenoid fossa (Fig. 18-18). Commonly, an impression fracture is seen with a posterior dislocation (Fig. 18-19, see also Fig. 10-15A). This defect rarely occurs to any significant degree with an anterior dislocation.

DIAGNOSIS

An accurate history will help determine the mechanism of injury. Most fractures of the proximal humerus occur because of a force transmitted along the arm.[9]

Local pain is the sine qua non for the

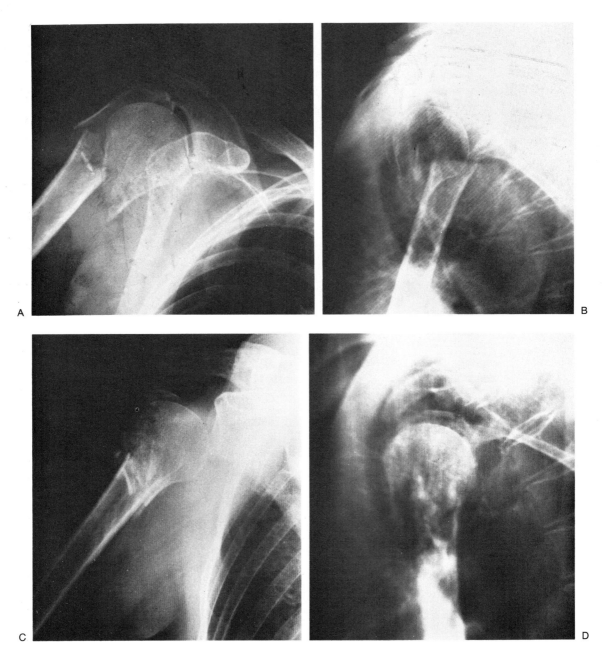

FIG. 18-12. A, Anteroposterior and, B, lateral transthoracic views of a 24-year-old man show a displaced 3-part fracture of the greater tuberosity. C, Anteroposterior and, D, lateral transthoracic post-reduction views show improved alignment of the fracture fragments. A portion of the greater tuberosity is still retracted. The patient was treated in a Velpeau cast after he refused operation. The result was fair because of recurring shoulder pain.

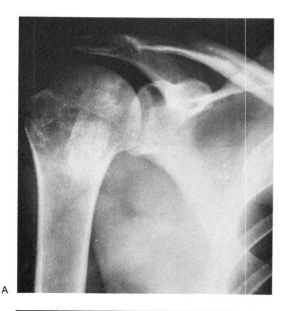

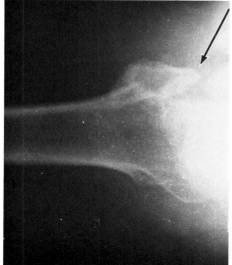

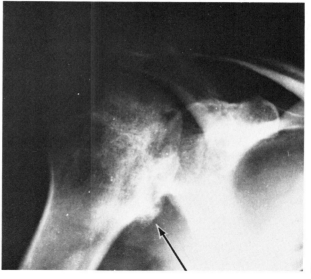

FIG. 18-13. A, Anteroposterior roentgenogram of a 47-year-old man shows a sclerotic area at the surgical neck with the arm in neutral position. B, Axillary and, C, anteroposterior views with the arm in 60 degrees of internal rotation show a healed undisplaced avulsion fracture of the lesser tuberosity (arrows). The patient was treated in a sling for 4 weeks. The result was excellent.

confirmation of significant shoulder trauma. Especially in a well-developed or obese individual, it may be impossible to detect abnormalities in the regional anatomy by physical means alone. The surgeon must then rely on excellent quality roentgenograms for a correct diagnosis. Only later will such findings as ecchymosis become apparent. When the shoulder is dislocated anteriorly or posteriorly, the surgeon should familiarize himself with the disappearance of normal landmarks. A thorough vascular and neurologic examination should be conducted, since fractures in the proximal shaft can be associated with neurovascular complications.

TREATMENT

Closed Methods

The surgeon should individualize the treatment for each case, selecting the method that best serves the needs of the

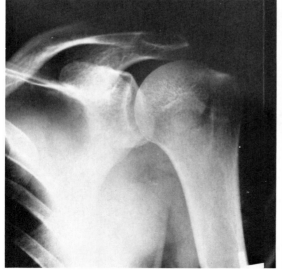

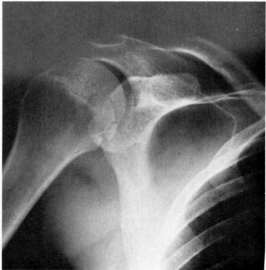

A

B

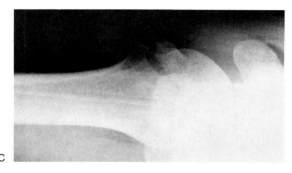

C

FIG. 18-14. Anteroposterior views in, A, neutral and, B, internal rotation demonstrate a slightly displaced lesser tuberosity fracture in a 28-year-old man. C, Lateral view better illustrates the 2-part fracture fragments. The result was excellent following 3 weeks immobilization in a sling.

patient. Hanging cast treatment is not recommended for most proximal humeral fractures. Its use may cause inferior subluxation of the humeral head especially when atony of the shoulder muscles exists (Fig. 18-20). Furthermore, in unimpacted fractures it can be difficult to maintain alignment of the long distal shaft with the head (Fig. 18-21). The method has been used occasionally in young adults, who are better able than elderly patients to tolerate such treatment, to permit the reduction of an angulated, impacted surgical neck fracture. Gravity without excessive weight added to the cast is important in the successful use of such treatment if distraction is to be avoided.[7]

The best results have been obtained with manipulation, Velpeau immobilization, shoulder spica casts, and occasionally traction methods (see Figs. 18-5 and 18-6). In the last-named method, prolonged excessive traction may lead to stiffness of the elbow and shoulder. Whenever traction is used the elbow should be flexed and skeletal traction used if feasible, as in the patient with multiple injuries. Only enough traction weight to maintain reduction of the fracture is added. Continuous traction with the limb in adduction, or occasionally abduction, may be required to maintain satisfactory position of the fracture fragments (see Fig. 18-5).

When manipulation is used to reduce displaced or angulated fractures, the surgeon should consider the deforming forces of muscles on the fracture segments. Gentle manipulation should be performed while the patient is under anesthesia. For example, when the humeral shaft is significantly displaced from its head, the long distal shaft

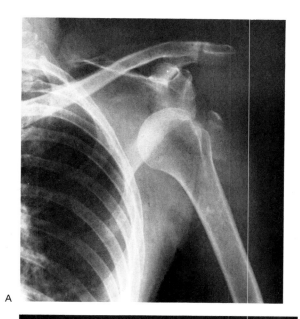

A

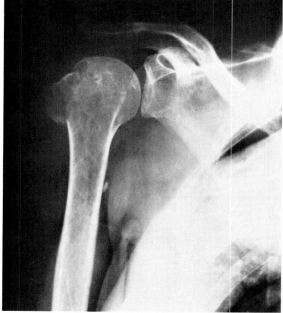

B

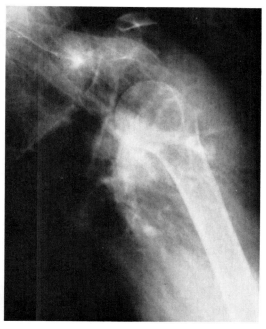

C

FIG. 18-15. A, Anteroposterior view shows a 2-part anterior fracture-dislocation of the proximal humerus. B, Anteroposterior and, C, lateral transthoracic views of the closed reduction. The extremity was placed in a Velpeau cast for 5 weeks in 20 degrees of abduction and internal rotation. The result was excellent.

is moved into alignment with its head because motion in the proximal head segment cannot be controlled. Even some fracture-dislocations that seem to require open reduction may be treated closed with good results[4] (Fig. 18-22).

Regardless of the method of treatment, enough bone healing must have occurred before early motion is initiated or else an-gulation at the fracture site will occur (see Fig. 18-8). If the surgeon is uncertain as to the degree of healing it may be helpful to obtain laminograms.

The surgeon's decision as to when to achieve a better reduction and when to leave a fracture alone requires solid judgment based on knowledge. In an elderly, ill patient it is usually better to accept some

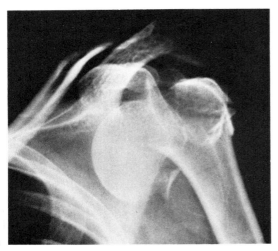

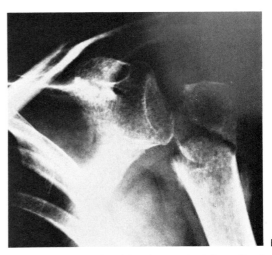

A   B

FIG. 18-16. A, Anteroposterior view shows a 3-part anterior fracture-dislocation involving the greater tuberosity of a 48-year-old woman. B, At operation, the surgeon removed the free-lying humeral head and reattached the rotator cuff to the fractured proximal humerus. The result was poor. A hemiarthroplasty was indicated.

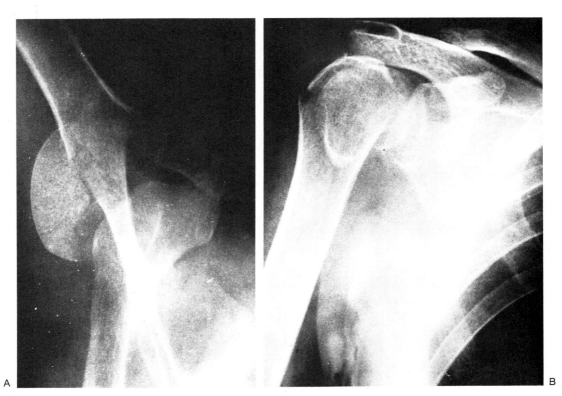

A   B

FIG. 18-17. A, Anteroposterior and, B, modified axillary views show a 2-part posterior fracture-dislocation of the shoulder sustained during electroshock treatment. The patient was treated by open reduction and a Nicola procedure.

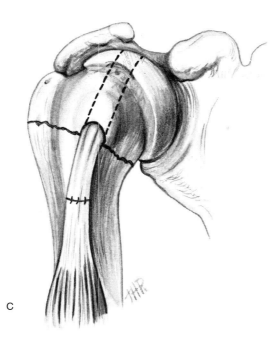

C

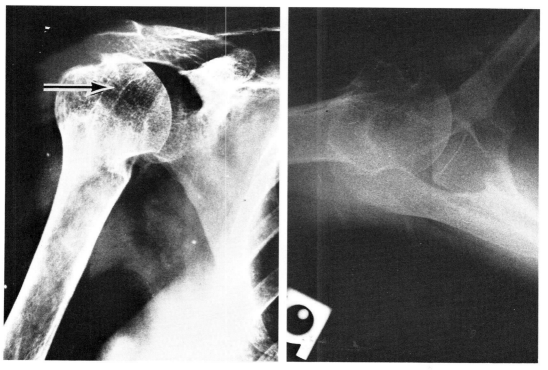

D

FIG. 18-17 continued. C, Nicola's method for holding humeral head to the shaft by threading the long biceps tendon through the humeral head and reattaching it distally. D, One year later, notice the bony tract through which the long biceps tendon traverses (arrow). The result was excellent. (A, B, and D reprinted from Post, M., and Haskell, S.: Fractures and Dislocations of the Upper Extremity, Chapter 7. In Practice of Surgery, Volume 2, Orthopedics, 1973 revision, with permission of the Medical Department, Harper & Row, Publishers, Inc., Hagerstown, Md.)

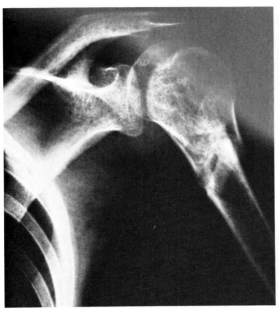
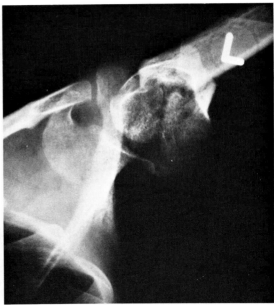

A   B

FIG. 18-18. **A,** Anteroposterior and, **B,** modified axillary roentgenograms of a middle-age adult show the reduction of a 3-part posterior fracture-dislocation with a split humeral head. The patient had severe pain and stiffness in the shoulder. A hemiarthroplasty would have given a better result.

functional loss rather than to subject such a patient to open treatment.

Open Methods

If open reduction is necessary either because of an interposed biceps tendon[7] or an inability to maintain reduction by closed means, it can be readily achieved by a variety of methods, including (1) internal fixation methods; (2) head resection and reposition of the rotator cuff to the shaft[13] (see Fig. 18-16); and (3) prosthetic replacement of the humeral head when the head is irrevocably damaged and there is a functioning rotator cuff (Fig. 18-23). In recent years, head resection has lost popularity because of the loss of good active overhead motion and the frequent persistence of discomfort and weakness about the shoulder. The use of prosthetic replacement of the severely damaged head has been more successful during the acute phase than during the chronic phase of fracture,[10] because a few months after injury a torn rotator cuff may scar and cause a less successful result in late prosthetic replacement of the head.

For most fractures of the proximal humerus requiring open treatment, the anterior surgical approach to the shoulder allows the best exposure. The deltoid may be removed from its clavicular origin if needed. The incision can be extended upward and downward as far as necessary. Commonly, some form of internal fixation is necessary. The methods of internal fixation include (1) a Rush nail driven through the proximal segment into the shaft to stabilize the humeral head, a method that may be used for acute injuries or for nonunions; (2) a lag screw to provide stability and allow early motion exercises; (3) multiple screws; (4) an AO shoulder plate; and (5) a Nicola procedure[3] (see Fig. 18-17). An anterior surgical approach is used in the Nicola procedure (Fig. 18-17C). The long head of the biceps tendon is transected in its groove and allowed to remain attached at the superior aspect of the glenoid fossa. The proximal end is threaded through a hole made in the humeral head that opens near the proximal end of the bicipital groove. The hole should be just large enough to receive the tendon. The threaded end is then secured to the

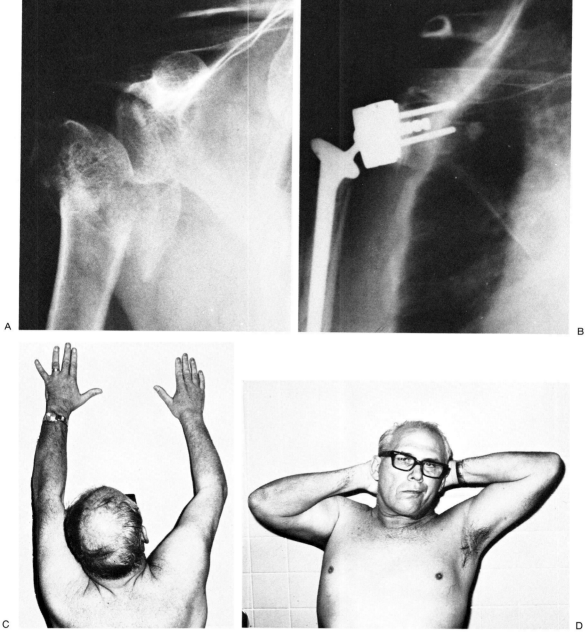

A

B

C

D

FIG. 18-19. A, Anteroposterior view shows a highly comminuted 3-part anterior fracture-dislocation of the shoulder of a 58-year-old man. At operation there was extensive tearing of the rotator cuff. B, A total shoulder replacement (series I) was performed. C and D, The extent of active shoulder motion is shown 10 weeks postoperatively. At 18 months postoperatively, motion had improved but was not complete. The patient returned to his regular job as a flute player. The result was very satisfactory.

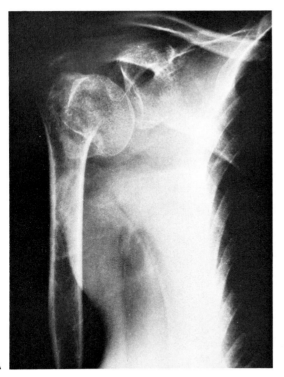

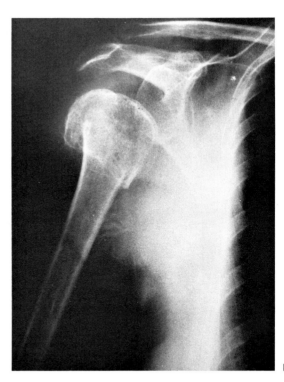

A

B

FIG. 18-20. A, Anteroposterior view shows a 3-part surgical neck fracture in a 58-year-old man 1 week after hanging cast treatment. Note the inferior subluxation. B, Anteroposterior view 4 weeks later after the hanging cast was removed and the patient placed in Velpeau immobilization.

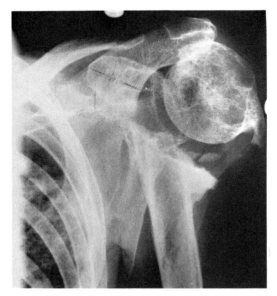

FIG. 18-21. Anteroposterior roentgenogram shows the poor end result of an unstable surgical neck fracture in a 76-year-old woman whose arm was allowed to hang.

shaft distally. This method should not be used when the head is markedly osteoporotic or has multiple small fractures because the tendon will not maintain reduction. The first three methods usually require external support for varying periods of time until enough tissue healing has occurred to maintain the fracture fragments.

The Rush rod technique may be used occasionally to maintain reduction of a badly displaced surgical neck fracture. The proximal deltoid muscle fibers are split near their anterolateral acromial origin. The rod is inserted through the proximal head fragment at the constricted anatomic neck, but the articular surface of the head is avoided by moving the head into valgus using a special hand reamer with a diameter equal to that of the rod and placed in a retrograde manner. The Rush rod will then follow the reamer tip and should be inserted until the beveled end is seen at the fracture site. The

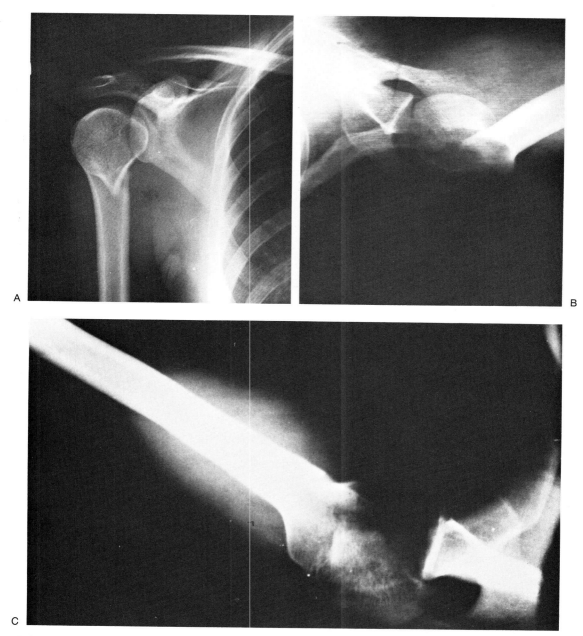

FIG. 18-22. A, Anteroposterior and, B, modified axillary views show a 2-part posterior fracture-dislocation in a 24-year-old man. C, A true axillary view shows the actual posterior dislocation.

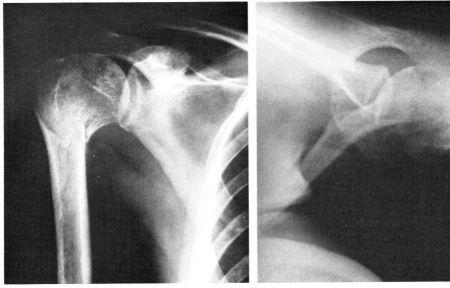

D   E

FIG. 18-22 continued. D, Anteroposterior and, E, modified axillary views after manipulation. With the patient under local anesthesia and in a sitting position, Bell's method[4] of reduction was achieved by adducting the extremity, using traction in the long axis, and applying pressure over the humeral head at the infraspinatus region. The patient was kept in a Velpeau cast for 4 weeks and sling for 2 additional weeks. The result was excellent.

shaft is adducted and rotated into a reduced position with its head, and the rod
then driven downward. The beveled end
should at first face the cortex and near the
end of insertion be rotated to face the canal.

When the intramedullary canal is obliterated it is first necessary to create a new
canal using needle-tip curettes and power
reamer in order to avoid forcing the rod tip
through the cortex.

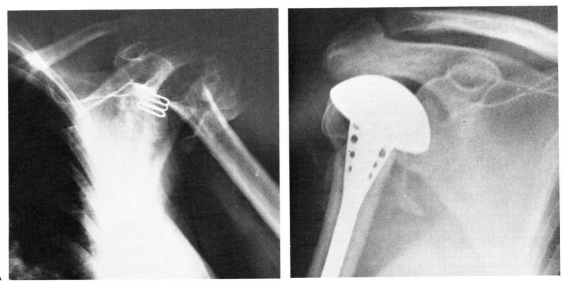

A   B

FIG. 18-23. A, A 65-year-old man sustained a highly comminuted fracture of the humeral head and surgical neck fracture. B, A Neer prosthesis was inserted with good results. The tuberosity fragments with their cuff attachments were fixed to the shaft.

In elderly patients I have drilled a ¼-in. hole through the midportion of the acromion. Keeping the bone fragments aligned I drive the rod from above downward across the reduced fracture site. Intraoperative roentgenograms in two planes should be obtained to determine the rod's position.

Specific Treatment
Minimal Displacement

Fractures of the proximal part of the humerus with minimal displacement, irrespective of the level or number of fractures, can be treated conservatively with a sling and early functional exercises (see Fig. 18-3). Minimally displaced impacted fractures of the surgical neck and head are usually stable and are usually well healed after 6 weeks, at which time early gentle pendulum exercises can be started. When the pain threshold permits, motion exercises are increased. Overhead motion is more easily achieved if, while reclining on his back, the patient grasps a 1-in.-diameter piece of dowel with both hands and reaches overhead. For young patients a ¼- to ½-pound weight may be taped to the center of the dowel after they regain some overhead motion. Rotation exercises and pulley exercises at home can be done early. The patient who is uncooperative in performing exercises may not attain maximum motion for 6 months or more.

Anatomic Neck Fracture

Fractures of the articular segment are rare but the incidence of avascular necrosis is high in this 2-part injury. When there is severe displacement the fracture should be reduced and internally fixed, preferably by two screws. If the displacement is minimal the fracture should be treated closed by merely immobilizing the extremity for 4 or 5 weeks or until it appears that there is sufficient healing to permit motion exercises. Prosthetic replacement is not recommended immediately because occasionally a good result is obtained when the humeral head is saved (see Fig. 18-4).

Surgical Neck Fracture
(Shaft Displacement)

Most of these fractures can be treated closed. Impacted fractures are usually stable and, if the fracture is not badly displaced, the patient can be treated with Velpeau immobilization. At 3 weeks, gentle motion exercises are started with the arm in a sling and then gradually increased. With severely displaced and angulated impacted fractures, the fracture is manipulated while the patient is under anesthesia, and traction is placed on the arm in order to reduce impaction and correct any angulation. The extremity is immobilized in Velpeau position for 3 or 4 weeks or longer, until enough healing has occurred to start gentle motion exercises.

When a surgical neck fracture is severely displaced, indicating extensive tearing of the periosteal cuff and surrounding soft tissues, it can often be treated by closed methods (see Fig. 18-6). Under an image intensifier the shaft can be manipulated into a reduced position and the arm internally rotated across the chest and then immobilized in Velpeau position (see Fig. 18-5). A flat soft axillary pad should be used. However, care should be taken to avoid bunching the pad because in a few cases neurapraxia of the major nerves in the axilla has been observed.

Inadequate immobilization of unstable fractures will lead to severe displacement and failure of treatment (see Fig. 18-21). The great majority of 2-part displacements, with the exception of inadequately reduced greater tuberosity fractures and unstable or poorly aligned surgical neck fractures, can be treated by closed methods.

If the fracture cannot be reduced, especially if there are multiple injuries, traction treatment employing an olecranon pin with the elbow flexed is often effective (see Fig. 18-5).

For 3-part surgical neck fractures it is often best to perform an open reduction to suture the fragments together accurately and to repair the cuff. Postoperative immobilization is the same as that for other displaced 2-part surgical neck fractures.

When the surgical neck is comminuted and reduction cannot be maintained by closed methods, or when there is an interposed biceps tendon, then open reduction may become necessary.[7]

Greater Tuberosity Displacement

Occasionally, a superiorly displaced greater tuberosity segment can be maintained in a reduced position by closed means. However, most cases require open reduction and internal fixation in order to prevent the mechanical blocking of abduction and to repair a rotator cuff defect associated with this injury (see Fig. 18-11). This can be done through either a saber-cut or an anterior surgical approach. In the former approach, the repair can be effected by detaching only a portion of the deltoid from its acromion and lateral clavicle (see Fig. 15-20).

When the lesser tuberosity is also fractured no special additional treatment is needed. However, when the surgical neck is fractured and displaced and the lesser tuberosity remains attached, the head internally rotates and it is difficult, if not impossible, to achieve reduction by closed means. In this event the fracture should be opened through an anterior surgical approach, and as recommended by Neer, the tuberosities stitched with 20-gauge wire loops or heavy nonabsorbable suture, in anatomic position.[15] The soft-tissue tear is then repaired. The use of a plate and screws is not recommended in elderly persons, because the screws can easily pull out from the osteoporotic bone even with the arm immobilized. When enough healing has occurred gentle motion exercises are started.

When 4-part fractures exist the articular part has no blood supply. Dewar and Yabsley reported good results by scooping the cancellous bone from the head and replacing the articular shell (osteochondral implant) on a reshaped proximal shaft.[8] I have not had experience with this technique. Initial replacement is preferred, reattaching the tuberosities by wire loop, thus effecting a cuff repair (see Fig. 18-23). This method

does allow early motion exercises. At first only passive exercises are allowed. When enough healing has occurred in the soft tissues active exercises are started, usually after 3 weeks.

Fracture-Dislocation

The chief goal of treatment with this injury is to reduce the dislocated humeral head as soon as possible. It is essential to determine whether the injury is anterior or posterior and the number of segments involved by obtaining excellent roentgenograms. Gentle reduction should be performed while the patient is under anesthesia in order to preserve any residual blood supply to the head. The neurovascular status of the extremity should be determined before and after manipulation.

ANTERIOR FRACTURE-DISLOCATION. In anterior fracture-dislocation with greater tuberosity displacement, closed gentle reduction can usually be accomplished while the patient is under anesthesia by placing traction on the arm and gradually abducting the extremity (see Fig. 18-15). Occasionally, it is difficult to achieve reduction and in this event I have found that gently rotating the humerus externally while maintaining traction allows reduction. Attempting to lift the humeral head into the glenoid fossa alone during traction will not permit reduction. Most of the time the greater tuberosity falls into place. The extremity is then placed in a Velpeau plaster of Paris spica cast for 4 weeks. After 1 to 2 additional weeks, exercises are started in a sling and gradually increased.

If the greater tuberosity remains displaced following reduction of the dislocated humeral head, it is wise to perform an open reduction of the tuberosity and repair the torn rotator cuff.

Three-part anterior fracture-dislocations are best treated by open reduction, suture of the reduced fragments, and repair of the torn rotator cuff. Aftercare in a Velpeau spica cast is the same as that for similar 3-part injuries without dislocation.

When 4-part anterior fracture-dislocations occur it is probably best to initially replace the head with a prosthesis and start early motion exercises.

POSTERIOR FRACTURE-DISLOCATION. This rare lesion may result from direct trauma or other violence caused by convulsive disorders.[16,19] Posterior fracture-dislocation with avulsion of the lesser tuberosity may be treated closed like any other similar injury. With the patient relaxed under anesthesia traction is placed on the extremity while the arm is gradually forward flexed, adducted,[10] and in some cases gently internally rotated. Some pressure may be placed on the humeral head from behind. This causes the humeral neck to be levered outward, thereby unlocking the head from behind the glenoid rim. The arm is immobilized at the side in slight external rotation for 4 weeks. If this method fails the method of Bell may be successful[4,5] (see Fig. 18-22).

In 3-part posterior fracture-dislocations closed reduction may be attempted, but with failure an open reduction should be performed and the bone fragments sutured back into place.

Four-part posterior fracture-dislocations are rare and best treated in the acute stage by prosthetic replacement of the humeral head because of the high incidence of osteonecrosis of the head.

In the elderly, poor-risk patient it may be better to treat the patient symptomatically with a sling and early motion.

Impression Defect

An impression defect located in the posterolateral head surface caused by anterior dislocation seldom creates the serious problem seen with defects caused by posterior fracture-dislocation. If less than 20 percent of the articular surface is impressed in a posterior fracture-dislocation, it may be reduced and immobilized as described previously, with satisfactory results. If 20 to 40 percent of the head has an impression defect, redislocation occurs in most cases unless the main articular fragment is stabilized, usually by transplanting the subscapularis tendon into the anteromedial

defect of the head.[11,12] When more than 50 percent of the cartilage surface is involved, the joint is unstable and will dislocate no matter what surgical reconstruction is performed. In this instance a prosthesis may be used to replace the head if the rotator cuff structures are functioning. However, recent experience has shown that in long-standing chronic dislocations it is better to perform a fixed fulcrum total shoulder replacement in symptomatic cases, except when the patient is subject to recurrent convulsive seizures.

Fragmented Head

When the humeral head is highly fragmented it can be replaced with a prosthesis (see Fig. 18-23).[1] The results of such treatment vary with the status of the shoulder muscles, particularly the deltoid and external rotators, and the time of implantation following trauma. In one extraordinary case, a total joint replacement was performed initially with good results (see Fig. 18-19). In these cases early pendulum exercises are avoided. Rather, early passive motion exercises in forward flexion, abduction, and internal rotation behind the back are encouraged (see Chapter 10, Part B).

When the humeral head has been split it should be treated like a fragmented head, replacing it with a prosthetic device and starting early motion.

COMPLICATIONS

Malunion

When malunion causes significant disability, reconstruction should be performed. A retracted greater tuberosity reduces elevation and external rotation and needs to be removed and the cuff defect repaired. Considerable scar and adhesions that may involve the articular surface may preclude a satisfactory result. If the fragment can be repositioned anatomically the rotator cuff defect must still be repaired. The arm should not be immobilized in more than 45 degrees of abduction in a plaster spica. At 4 weeks the arm should be slowly brought to

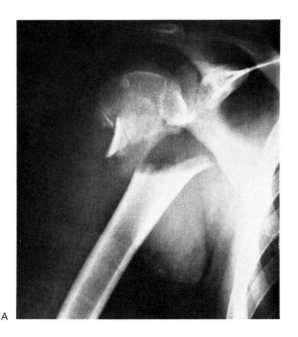
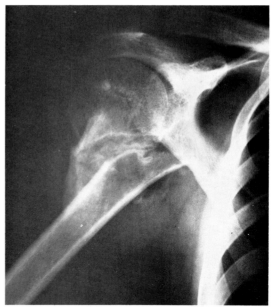

A

B

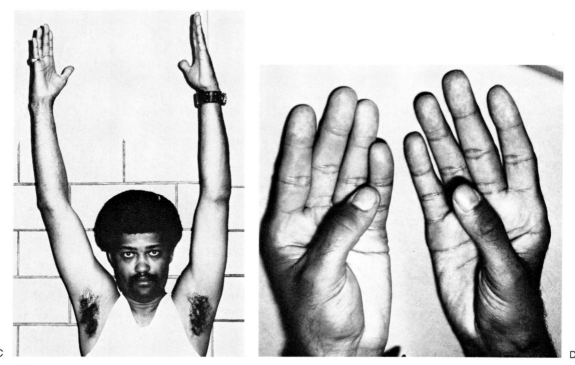

C

D

FIG. 18-24. A, Anteroposterior roentgenogram shows a displaced, highly comminuted surgical neck fracture that could not be reduced by closed methods because the biceps tendon was interposed. The patient refused surgical treatment. B, Seven months later, anteroposterior view in abduction shows the malunited fracture. C, Although the patient had excellent active motion, he was bothered by tingling, numbness, and weakness in the right hand. D, The patient was unable to fully oppose the right thumb and had atrophy of the thenar muscles and first dorsal interossei.

the side over a 10-day period. Gentle exercises are then started.

Some malunions may cause little difficulty (Fig. 18-24).

In old malunions of the surgical neck, the procedure of osteotomy and bone grafting is seldom successful. In such cases more extensive reconstruction such as prosthetic head replacement or total shoulder replacement may be needed if the rotator cuff is nonfunctioning (see Chapter 10, Part B). As a last resort, arthrodesis can be considered depending upon the needs of the patient.

Nonunion

If the fragments of a surgical neck fracture are not in continuity nonunion usually results (Fig. 18-25). It may result from distraction of the fragments caused by a hanging cast or traction. Another cause is interposition of the long head of the biceps. If there is interposed soft tissue, it must be released and the bone ends aligned (Fig. 18-25). If overriding of the fragments exists, rather than perform excessive stripping and cutting it is better to shorten the distal fragment as much as 2.5 cm. in order to align the fragments. Cases with angulation and nonunion can be treated similarly. In each case, a Rush rod with iliac bone graft is recommended. The extremity should be immobilized in a Velpeau spica postoperatively. Exercises are started when enough healing has occurred, at 8 to 10 weeks or longer.

Joint Stiffness

Adhesions about the injured bone and surrounding soft tissues are the most common cause of joint stiffness.[7] They are best managed by a persistent program of vigorous motion exercises. On rare occasions, manipulation while the patient is under

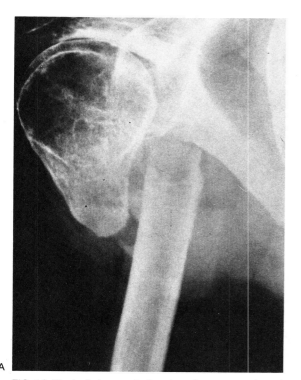
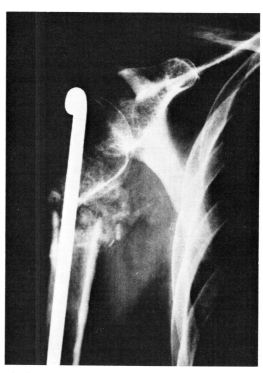

A

B

FIG. 18-25. A, Anteroposterior view shows nonunion of a surgical neck fracture with overriding bone fragments. B, Anteroposterior view shows result of open reduction, Rush rod procedure, and iliac bone grafting. A Velpeau cast was applied for 8 weeks. Despite the technical errors that resulted in tilting of the proximal fragment and a gap between the bone ends, there was uneventful healing.

general anesthesia, followed by an exercise program, may be beneficial. I have never seen an open lysis of adhesions produce a satisfactory result. If the surgeon does choose manipulation as a method to increase shoulder motion, especially in the elderly, it is easy to cause iatrogenic fracture of the humerus with too forceful manipulation. The procedure should be performed while supporting the whole length of humerus, and excessive rotational force must be avoided.

Atony

During the treatment period the humeral head may inferiorly subluxate (see Fig. 18-20). This results from the laxity of the capsule and ligaments and the atony of the inactive deltoid and rotator cuff muscles. With increasing exercises the condition soon clears.

Neurovascular Deficit

Occasionally, unreduced surgical neck fractures or fracture-dislocations may cause significant neurologic deficit (see Fig. 18-24). These same fractures may cause an injury such as an aneurysm to the surrounding vessels. The patient should have a thorough neurovascular examination at the time of injury and after treatment. Each patient should be managed according to nature of the lesion.

Osteonecrosis

Four-part fractures and displaced anatomic neck fractures commonly result in osteonecrosis of the head segment. Occasionally, surgical neck fractures that have been operated upon may develop osteonecrosis of the humeral head. If this condition ensues and produces symptoms, the head should be resected and replaced with a prosthetic device if the rotator cuff is functioning or with a fixed fulcrum total shoulder joint if the rotator cuff is nonfunctioning.

Myositis Ossificans

I have seen this complication occur usually with dislocation and only seldom with seemingly uncomplicated proximal humeral fractures. Usually, the excess bone matures. Rarely, and especially in drug addicts or alcoholics, the bone mass may increase and cause major disability (Fig. 18-26). If a resection of excess bone is considered it should not be performed before the bone is mature. This may take at least 1 year. However, I have never seen a successful result after such an excision.

METHYL METHACRYLATE IN FRACTURES

When conservative treatment fails as in the case of an interposed biceps tendon,

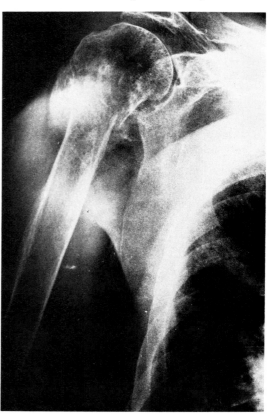

FIG. 18-26. Anteroposterior view shows a healed surgical neck fracture with exuberant bone in the surrounding tissues in an elderly woman. There was severe limitation of motion following sling immobilization.

when there is a pathologic fracture in an elderly, debilitated patient, or when there is an imminent or pathologic fracture, newer methods of treatment may be tried in highly selected cases (Fig. 18-27). Methyl methacrylate and the insertion of an intramedullary rod is a definitive procedure that permits immediate use of the extremity. This technique should not be used in the young adult with normal bone, but should be reserved for the elderly or the individual with a pathologic fracture whose life expectancy is shortened.

FRACTURE OF PROXIMAL HUMERAL EPIPHYSIS

Fractures of the proximal humeral epiphysis are relatively uncommon injuries, and seldom occur during infancy.[24,27] Because the growth plate is involved and the events that follow such injuries are so different

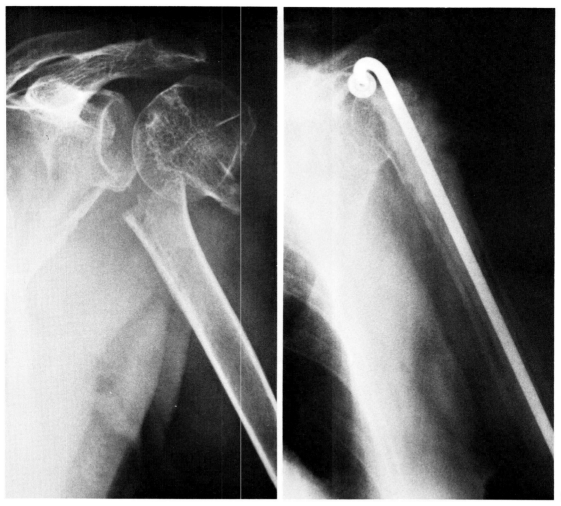

A   B

FIG. 18-27. A, Anteroposterior roentgenogram shows a 6-month-old fracture of the surgical neck of an 84-year-old woman. B, Open reduction with Rush rod fixation and the use of cement was performed when her pain became intolerable. At operation, the rod was placed into the proximal fragment and a trial reduction attempted before methyl methacrylate was injected into both fragments with a wide-bore plastic syringe. The procedure permitted use of the extremity the following day. The result was excellent.

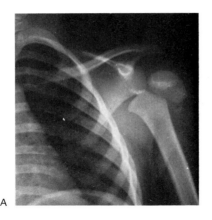

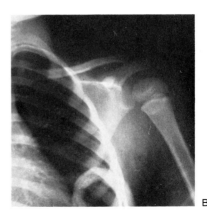

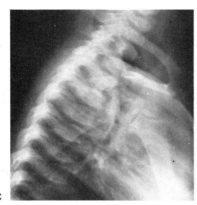

A

B

C

FIG. 18-28. A, Anteroposterior view of the shoulder of a 3-year-old child who had fallen from a table shows a Salter-Harris type I markedly displaced fracture of the humeral head. B, Anteroposterior and, C, lateral transthoracic films show excellent replacement of the fracture by manipulation. The patient was treated with a sling and swath for 3 weeks. The result was excellent. (Reprinted from Post, M., and Haskell, S.: Fractures and Dislocations of the Upper Extremity, Chapter 7. In Practice of Surgery, Volume 2, Orthopedics, 1973 revision, with permission of the Medical Department, Harper & Row, Publishers, Inc., Hagerstown, Md.)

from those that follow the corresponding adult injury, an understanding of the mechanism of injury and of the appropriate management at various ages is required.

MECHANISM OF INJURY. Dameron and Reibel showed that, like other epiphyseal injuries, the proximal humeral epiphyseal plate fractures through the zone of hypertrophy in an infant when the shaft is extended and adducted.[22] The deforming pull of the muscles attached to the proximal fragment causes it to flex, abduct, and slightly rotate externally. These investigators discovered that it was easy to reduce the fragments by manipulation, and that at least in the infant the biceps tendon would not interpose at the fracture site without force. In similar fractures of older children, Brashear found that a triangular piece of bone remained with the epiphysis (Salter-Harris, type II[26]) in contradistinction to the more common type I injuries seen in in-

fants[21] (Figs. 18-28 and 18-29). The other types (III, IV, and V) have not been seen in a relatively large number of children with proximal humeral fractures treated at Michael Reese Medical Center over the past 20 years. Moreover, traumatic separation of the centers of ossification has not been reported.[22]

DIAGNOSIS. Diagnosis is based on the history, physical examination, and age of the patient. When swelling occurs at the shoulder it may be impossible to palpate abnormal prominences or displacement. In this event the surgeon must rely on roentgenograms taken in at least two planes and compared with those of the opposite joint. If the proximal epiphysis is completely separated, the arm is shortened and the axis of the humerus is altered. Roentgenograms of the distal humerus should also be studied if findings suggest possible trauma (Fig. 18-30). False motion may be demonstrated.

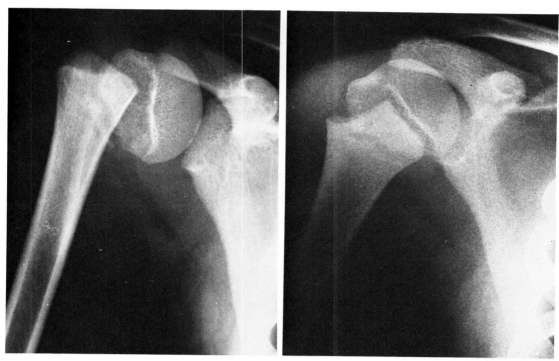

A

B

FIG. 18-29. A, An anteroposterior view of the shoulder of a 12-year-old boy who was tackled in football shows a Salter-Harris type I markedly displaced fracture of the humeral head. B, Following manipulation, roentgenogram shows an excellent reduction. The patient was treated in a Velpeau cast for 25 days. The result was excellent.

In the infant, the diagnosis is especially difficult since the epiphysis may not be seen on the roentgenograms. Thus, the diagnosis is made more easily after the appearance of the epiphysis.

TREATMENT. In older children a triangular fragment of the metaphysis usually remains attached to the posteromedial portion of the epiphysis (Fig. 18-31). In children up to 5 years of age, anatomic reduction of the fracture is not needed. These fractures may be treated by manipulation or traction in abduction. Following manipulation the arm may be immobilized at the side with the forearm across the chest. Hanging cast treatment is not recommended (see section on Hanging Cast Treatment). Roentgenograms should be made in two planes to be certain of the reduction.

After 5 years of age and increasing with age, there is less potential for remodeling. If there are more than 20 degrees of angulation at 11 years of age, for example, the fracture should be manipulated so that a more accurate reduction produces a satisfactory end result. Following closed reduction, immobilization in a plaster of Paris shoulder spica cast is preferred to other methods whenever possible. The extremity should be maintained in the position of abduction and rotation that allows the greatest stability of the fracture.

Closed manipulative reduction in young age groups has been found to be consistently successful without the need for open methods of treatment. In the older adolescent, open reduction and internal fixation are rarely necessary because precise fracture alignment is almost never needed for good results. When the mobile humeral head cannot be controlled, stability may be accomplished by overhead traction for 3 or 4 weeks and plaster cast treatment for 2 additional weeks, during which time the arm is gradually brought to the side. Thereafter, gentle motion exercises are started. It

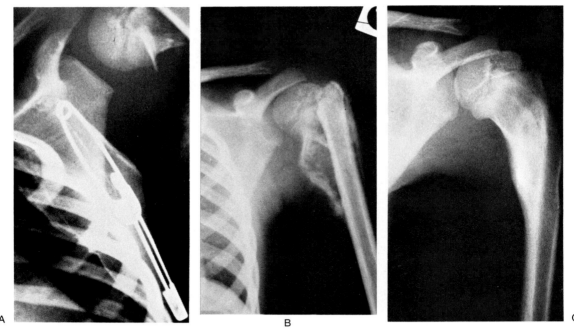

A   B   C

FIG. 18-30. A, A 6-year-old child sustained extensive third-degree burns and a highly displaced proximal humeral fracture visible on this anteroposterior view. There were also a supracondylar and wrist fracture on the same side. B, Serious burns of the extremity and rest of the body precluded effective orthopaedic treatment. At 5 weeks after injury, note the exuberant callus formation. C, Twenty months later, molding at the healed fracture site is shown. Shoulder function was normal.

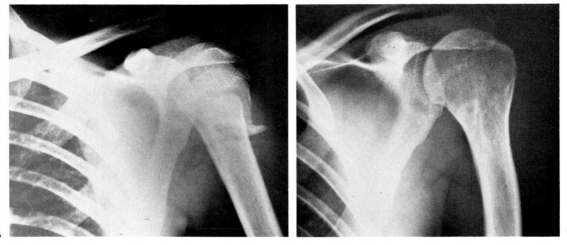

A   B

FIG. 18-31. A, Anteroposterior view of a proximal humeral fracture (Salter-Harris type II) in a 15-year-old boy. Nine days after injury, a Rush rod was inserted because of malalignment and an interposed long head of the biceps. The rod was removed 5 weeks later. B, Anteroposterior view taken 5 years later shows the healed fracture. The result was excellent.

is the exceptional case that requires open reduction (Fig. 18-31).

ISOLATED AVULSION FRACTURE OF THE LESSER TUBEROSITY

Although isolated avulsion fracture of the lesser tuberosity is exceptionally rare,[23] it may pose a problem in establishing a correct diagnosis. These injuries may be confused with calcific tendinitis of the rotator cuff.

The teenager or young adult in whom it is usually seen should be carefully questioned. The patient does not ordinarily recall any specific trauma. However, the patient usu-ally recalls using the extremity violently as in gymnastics or pitching hardballs.

The patient complains of progressive pain and discomfort in the shoulder made worse with activity. Point tenderness in the rotator cuff is usually present. Results of motion testing may be normal but pain is increased during testing abduction against resistance.

Roentgenograms should be taken in several planes of rotation in order to avoid missing the lesion,[20] which shows a calcareous density at the proximal humeral epiphysis which may confuse the surgeon (Fig. 18-32).

TREATMENT. When the lesion is suspected and merely observed, the fracture will heal

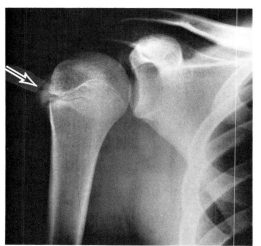

A

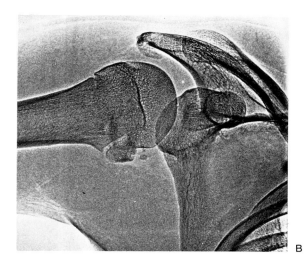

B

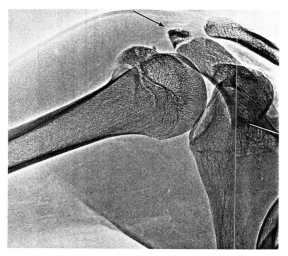

C

FIG. 18-32. A, Anteroposterior view of the humerus in external rotation shows a healing avulsion injury of the lesser tuberosity in a 16-year-old boy (arrow) taken 4 weeks after strenuous hardball pitching. B, Lateral xeroradiogram of the fracture. Note the fine detail of the healing fracture. C, Twelve weeks after injury, a xeroradiogram of the humerus shows the healed fracture site. Arrow shows acromial epiphysis.

with rest, if all violent activities are avoided. In time, new bone crosses the epiphyseal plate (Fig. 18-32C). The lesion may be classified as a type VI epiphyseal injury wherein the periosteum or perichondral ring has been damaged.[25] This lesion has not been observed in young children. However, with the increasing emphasis on competitive sports in our society such a lesion in a youth can occur and results in growth arrest and progressive angular deformity in the young child.

REFERENCES

Fractures of the Adult Proximal Humerus

1. Aufranc, O. E., Jones, W. N., and Turner, R. H.: Bilateral shoulder fracture-dislocation. J.A.M.A., 195:1140–1143, 1966.
2. Baker, D. M., and Leach, R. E.: Fracture-dislocation of the shoulder. Report of three unusual cases with rotator cuff avulsion. J. Trauma, 5:659–664, 1965.
3. Baker, L. D.: The Nicola operation: A simplified technique. J. Bone Joint Surg., 22:118–119, 1940.
4. Bell, H. M.: Posterior fracture-dislocation of the shoulder—A method of closed reduction. J. Bone Joint Surg., 47-A:1521–1524, 1965.
5. Chattopadhyaya, T.: Posterior fracture-dislocation of the shoulder. J. Bone Joint Surg., 52-B:521–523, 1970.
6. Codman, E. A.: The Shoulder. Boston, Thomas Todd, 1934.
7. DePalma, A. F., and Cantilli, R. A.: Fractures of the upper end of the humerus. Clin. Orthop., 20:73–93, 1961.
8. Dewar, F. P., and Yabsley, R. H.: Fracture-dislocation of the shoulder: Report of a case. J. Bone Joint Surg., 49-B:540–543, 1967.
9. Hoyt, W. A.: Etiology of shoulder injuries in athletes. J. Bone Joint Surg., 49-A:755–766, 1967.
10. Knight, R. A., and Mayne, J. A.: Comminuted fractures and fracture-dislocation involving the articular surfaces of the humeral head. J. Bone Joint Surg., 39-A:1343–1355, 1957.
11. McLaughlin, H.: Trauma. Philadelphia, W. B. Saunders Co., 1959.
12. McLaughlin, H. L.: Posterior dislocation of the shoulder. J. Bone Joint Surg., 34-A:584–590, 1952.
13. Michaelis, L. S.: Comminuted fracture-dislocation of the shoulder. J. Bone Joint Surg., 26:363–365, 1944.
14. Neer, C. S., II: Displaced proximal humeral fractures. Part I. Classification and evaluation. J. Bone Joint Surg., 52-A:1077–1089, 1970.
15. Neer, C. S., II: Displaced proximal humeral fractures. Part II. Treatment of three-part and four-part displacement. J. Bone Joint Surg., 52-A:1090–1103, 1970.
16. Prillaman, H. A., and Thompson, R. C.: Bilateral posterior fracture dislocation of the shoulder. J. Bone Joint Surg., 51-A:1627–1630, 1969.
17. Roberts, S. M.: Fractures of the upper end of the humerus. An end result study which shows the advantage of early active motion. J.A.M.A., 98:367–373, 1932.
18. Sever, J. W.: Fracture of the head of the humerus. Treatment and results. N. Engl. J. Med., 216:1100–1107, 1937.
19. Shaw, J. L.: Bilateral posterior fracture-dislocation of the shoulder and other trauma caused by convulsive seizures. J. Bone Joint Surg., 53-A:1327–1440, 1971.

Fractures of the Proximal Humeral Epiphysis

20. Bowerman, J. W., and McDonnell, E. J.: Radiology of athletic injuries: Baseball. Radiology, 116:611–615, 1975.
21. Brashear, H. R., Jr.: Epiphyseal fractures. A microscopic study of the healing process in rats. J. Bone Joint Surg., 41-A:1055–1064, 1959.
22. Dameron, T. B., and Reibel, D. B.: Fractures involving the proximal humeral epiphyseal plate. J. Bone Joint Surg., 51-A:289–297, 1969.
23. LaBriola, H. J., and Mohaghegh, H. A.: Isolated avulsion fracture of the lesser tuberosity of the humerus. J. Bone Joint Surg., 57-A:1011, 1975.
24. Nilson, S., and Svartholm, F.: Fractures of upper end of the humerus in children. Acta Chir. Scand., 130:433–439, 1965.
25. Rang, M. (Ed.): The Growth Plate and Its Disorders. Edinburgh: E. & S. Livingstone, Ltd., 1969.
26. Salter, R. B., and Harris, W. R.: Injuries involving the epiphyseal plate. J. Bone Joint Surg., 45-A:587–622, 1963.
27. Smith, F. M.: Fracture-separation of the proximal humeral epiphysis. A study of cases seen at the Presbyterian Hospital from 1929–1953. Am. J. Surg., 91:627–635, 1956.

19

Fractures of Shaft of the Humerus

MELVIN POST

The humerus acts as a lever that permits the hand to be placed in myriad positions. Although some shortening of this bone can be tolerated without great disability, its integrity is vital for the normal function of the hand. This chapter details those methods of treatment that have been found most effective in management of fracture of the humeral shaft.

ANATOMY

In cross section, the shaft of the humerus may be compared to a cylinder in its upper half, being almost straight in its long axis. Its distal portion is flattened and broad. On the anterior surface are the deltoid, the biceps brachii, and brachialis anticus muscles. Posteriorly are the deltoid and triceps brachii. The single deltoid tendon inserts on the deltoid tuberosity lateral to the midshaft of the humerus.

Intermuscular septa dip between the anterior and posterior muscle groups to attach to the bone medially and laterally and divide the arm into anterior and posterior compartments.[7] The anterior compartment contains the biceps brachii, coracobrachialis, brachialis anticus, and the neurovascular bundle, the latter coursing along the medial border of the biceps. The posterior compartment contains the triceps brachii

and the radial nerve. The nerve lies along the course of a shallow groove on the posterior and lateral surfaces of the medial and upper thirds of the shaft of the humerus, separated from the bone by 1 to 5 cm. of muscle averaging 3.4 cm.[9,30] Only at the lateral supracondylar ridge is the nerve in direct contact with the humerus where it pierces the lateral intermuscular septum before passing onto the surface of the brachialis muscle.

When the supracondylar process is present, the median nerve and the brachial artery are positioned behind the process and then pass forward through a fibrous band connecting the process and epicondyle.[29]

Finally, the main nutrient artery enters the humerus at the junction of the middle and lower thirds of the shaft.[15] Fracture at this site will disturb the blood supply to the bone.

MECHANISM OF INJURY

Fractures of the humeral shaft are not uncommon but not as common as those in the upper end of the bone. In the vast majority of cases the mechanism of injury is direct violence, such as a fall with the arm at the side. A direct blow, crushing injury, or gunshot wound may result in an open fracture (Fig. 19-1). Less often, the hu-

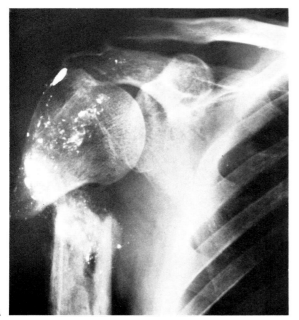

A

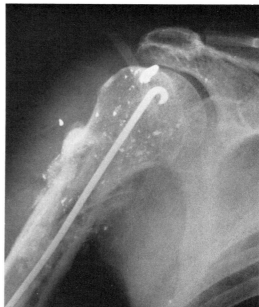

B

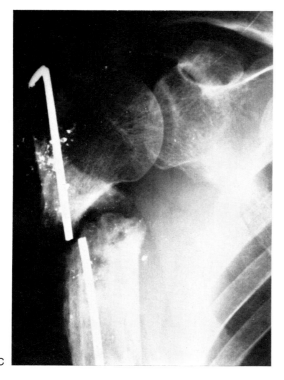

C

FIG. 19-1. A, Anteroposterior roentgenogram shows a 6-month-old comminuted fracture caused by a gunshot wound. The patient failed to return for treatment until his pain increased. B, A small-size Rush rod was incorrectly used, along with an iliac bone graft and plaster spica cast for 10 weeks. C, Anteroposterior view shows eventual breakage of the inadequate intramedullary nail from metal fatigue. The intramedullary canal should have been enlarged with flexible reamers and a stout nail used, if this was the surgeon's desire. The bone does not know the "average" time for complete healing and this average period should not be relied upon.

merus may be fractured by indirect violence, such as a fall on the hand or the elbow (Fig. 19-2). The shaft also may be broken by violent muscular action.[6]

Fractures caused by direct violence tend to be transverse (Fig. 19-3) or comminuted, whereas fractures related to indirect violence or muscular action are usually oblique or spiral. The fragments may separate and angulate with little or no displace-

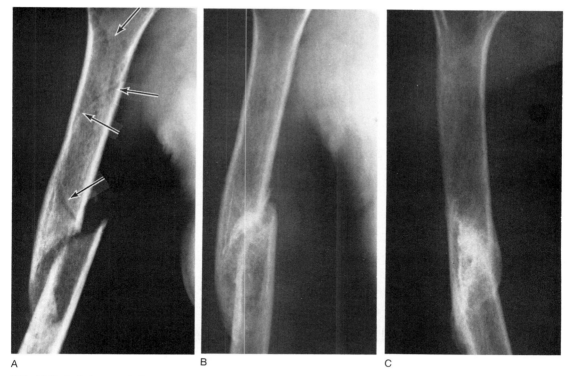

A   B   C

FIG. 19-2. A, Anteroposterior roentgenogram shows a displaced spiral fracture of the shaft of a 37-year-old man who fell on his outstretched hand. Arrows show the fracture line of a longer undisplaced segment. A radial nerve neurapraxia was present. The fracture was treated in a hanging cast that was maintained for 11 weeks. The nerve recovered in 7 weeks. B, Anteroposterior and, C, lateral views of the healed fracture. The result was excellent.

ment (Fig. 19-4), or they may be displaced and slide past one another (Fig. 19-5). The lower fragment may be drawn upward by contraction of the arm muscles. Shortening is ordinarily less than 2.5 to 5 cm. Whether the lower fragment is displaced inward or outward depends upon the site of fracture. When the shaft is broken above the deltoid insertion, the muscle, being attached to the lower fragment, causes this fragment to be drawn outward (Fig. 19-6A). The pectoralis major inserts on the lateral lip of the bicipital groove with the latissimus dorsi and the teres major all pulling the proximal fragment inward (Fig. 19-6A).

If the fracture is below the deltoid insertion the deltoid muscle and coracobrachialis tend to draw the upper fragment outward and forward, whereas the lower fragment is drawn upward by the arm muscles (Fig. 19-6B). Usually, the proximal frag-

ment remains in midposition because of gravity and the fact that the arm and forearm tend to lie across the chest. Depending upon the activity of muscle contraction, various other combinations of positions may be seen.

DIAGNOSIS

Fracture of the humeral shaft occurs most often in persons over 50 years of age.[19,24,25] The diagnosis is obvious when there is displacement of the humeral shaft. When documentation of the degree of shortening is desired, comparison lengths can be obtained by measuring the distances from the tips of both the acromial processes downward to the external condyles. The neurovascular status of the extremity should be determined at the initial examination. Specifically, the surgeon should de-

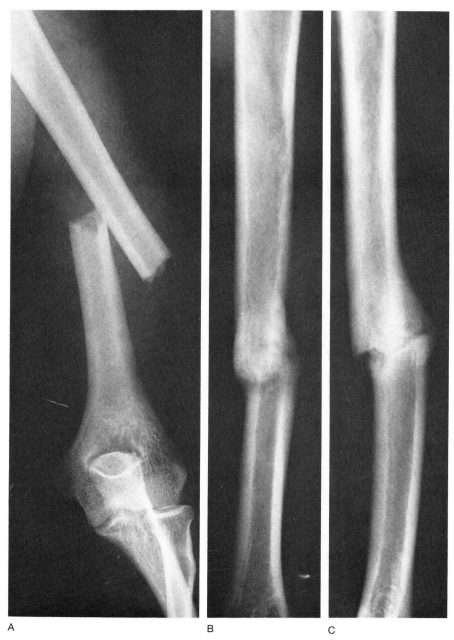

A   B   C

FIG. 19-3. A, Displaced fracture of the humeral shaft of a 28-year-old man. Excellent alignment and healing are shown in the, B, anteroposterior and, C, lateral views after 10 weeks of hanging cast treatment. The patient was started on gentle pendulum exercises with the arm in a sling. An excellent result was achieved. (Reprinted from Post, M., and Haskell, S.: Fractures and Dislocations of the Upper Extremity, Chapter 7. In Practice of Surgery, Volume 2, Orthopedics, 1973 revision, with permission of the Medical Department, Harper & Row, Publishers, Inc., Hagerstown, Md.)

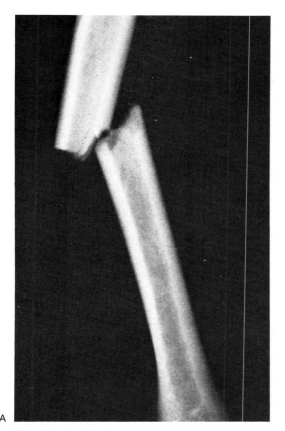
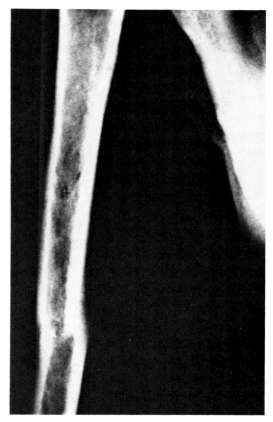

A   B

FIG. 19-4. A, A displaced transverse midshaft fracture is shown in a 48-year-old woman. The fracture was treated in a hanging cast, which was removed after 10 weeks. B, The healed fracture. Gentle pendulum exercises were started after 3 weeks while the arm was in the hanging cast. The result was excellent.

termine if there is a radial nerve injury, since this is the most common peripheral nerve lesion complicating these fractures. Swelling and tenderness help to establish the diagnosis. Gentle manipulation performed only once easily demonstrates whether there is crepitus. When there is interposed soft tissue, there will be no crepitus (Fig. 19-7).

In children, especially those with incomplete fracture, the diagnosis is more difficult, and greater reliance should be placed on roentgenograms for diagnosis. In general, roentgenograms must include the entire humeral shaft and at least one joint above and below, depending on the physical findings, in order to avoid missing associated injuries[1] (Fig. 19-8).

TREATMENT

Conservative Methods

I prefer to treat humeral shaft fractures by closed methods and in a hanging cast whenever possible, since operative treatment of the shaft is not often required and can be a cause of delayed union or nonunion.[13] The results of the hanging cast method are excellent if the surgeon follows the principles enunciated by Caldwell[3] and others.[4,10,23,28] Results of one study showed that when the hanging cast was used for humeral shaft fractures 96 percent of the patients achieved union in an average healing time of 10 weeks.[25] Even when there is some deformity after healing, more than 20 degrees of anterior bowing or varus of 30

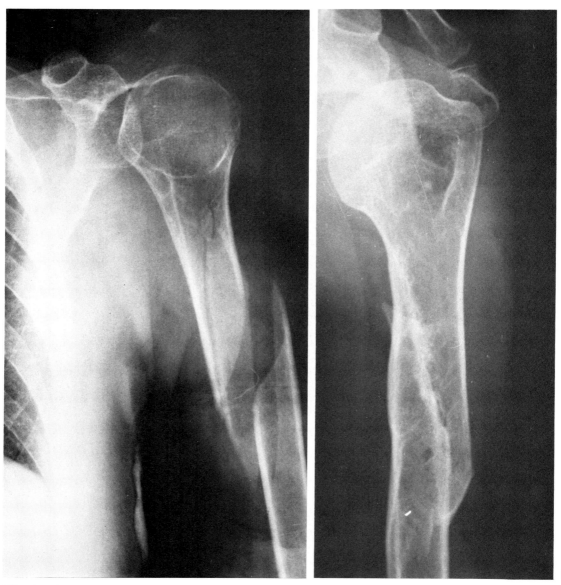

FIG. 19-5. A, An anteroposterior roentgenogram shows a comminuted spiral fracture of the shaft of the humerus below the deltoid insertion in a 71-year-old woman. The patient was treated with the extremity in a hanging cast for 6 weeks. Gentle motion exercises were subsequently started with the arm in a sling. B, After 1 year, an anteroposterior film shows excellent union, with overriding of the fracture fragments. There was no obvious deformity and the result was excellent.

degrees must usually be present before it is clinically apparent.[13] This deformity does not interfere with function (Fig. 19-9).

Hanging Cast Method[3,31]

With the patient's elbow flexed to 90 degrees, a well-padded circular plaster of Paris cast is applied from just below the axillary fold to the wrist. The hand down to the metacarpophalangeal joints should be included in the cast (Fig. 19-10). The forearm is held in neutral but may be held in various degrees of rotation as desired. If the hanging cast is used for fractures of the distal third of the shaft, the forearm should

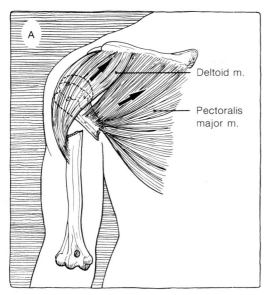 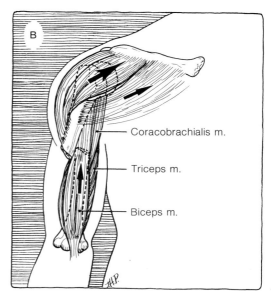

FIG. 19-6. A, Dynamics of muscle pull when the fracture is above the deltoid insertion. B, Dynamics of muscle pull when the fracture is below the deltoid insertion.

be immobilized in pronation in order to help overcome the pull of the supinators which can tilt the distal fragment outward. A plaster loop is incorporated into the cast at the wrist to which a padded sling is attached for suspension from the neck. Abduction pads can be placed on the inner side of the cast to help control angulation but should be used cautiously to avoid compression of the neurovascular structures. Furthermore, anterior or posterior angulation is easily controlled by shortening or lengthening the sling. The cast should be light not heavy, since it is gravity that helps maintain the fracture fragments in a reduced position.[31]

Although the hanging cast is indicated in fractures of the middle and lower thirds of the humeral shaft, the surgeon must exercise good judgment for best results. It has been used occasionally for fractures of the proximal third of the humerus. For example, in this method the patient cannot take a recumbent position. Therefore, other associated injuries that require the patient to be recumbent preclude this method. Hanging cast treatment is not effective in the very young or uncooperative child, because this method demands that the patient must co-

operate and remain in an upright or semi-reclining position to carry out prescribed exercises. For the same reasons, this method is not applicable for the patient who is senile, psychotic, or unconscious. The elbow should not be supported.

A hanging cast will not ordinarily correct a severely displaced fracture. In this case the fracture should be manipulated prior to the application of the cast. If the fracture does not align then treatment is doomed to failure. In summary, the hanging cast method may be used (1) for humeral shaft fractures in which the fragments are in good position with little tendency toward displacement; (2) for humeral shaft fractures without marked displacement but with some angulation of the lower fragment; (3) for fractures with displacement after adequate reduction has been attained; and (4) for certain open fractures in which wound treatment has been successful.

The patient should be advised that during the first 10 days of hanging cast treatment there will be significant pain and crepitation of the fracture fragments. The patient should be instructed not to disturb the length of the sling support. When a padded stockinet sling is used, it should be pre-

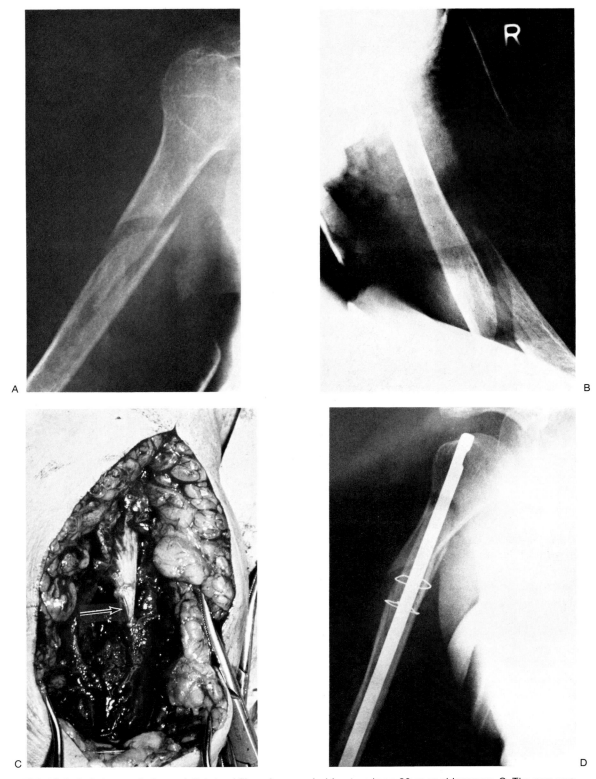

FIG. 19-7. A, Anteroposterior and, B, lateral films show a spiral fracture in an 80-year-old woman. C, The arm was explored through a Henry surgical approach when there was no crepitus and the fracture failed to align in a hanging cast. Arrow shows the proximal spike of humerus that had telescoped through the belly of the biceps muscle. D, The alignment of the fracture is shown postoperatively. In addition to the Küntscher intramedullary nail, an encircling wire was needed to control a comminuted segment. The extremity was kept in a sling for 6 weeks. There was uneventful healing.

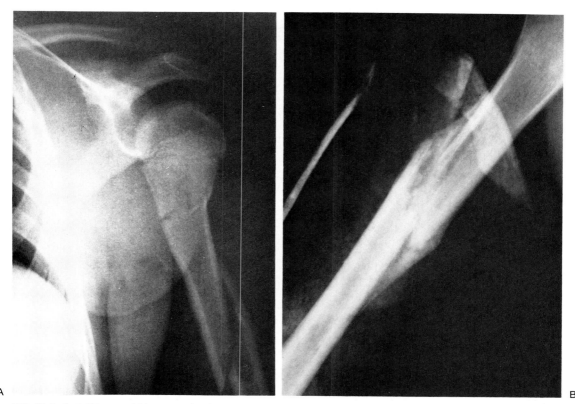

FIG. 19-8. A, A 15-year-old boy sustained a segmental fracture of the humerus. The proximal fracture was missed initially on films that included only the elbow. Tenderness was present at the upper lateral arm. B, The healing fracture is shown after 6 weeks in a hanging cast. The cast was removed after 8 weeks and exercises were started. The result was excellent.

stretched to minimize any change in the length of the suspension system. In addition, the patient should be as ambulatory as possible, and should perform circumduction exercises as soon as feasible in order to prevent atony of the extremity muscles and shoulder stiffness. Even when the hand is included in the cast, omission of the plaster bridge between the thumb and index finger will allow performance of some wrist exercises.

The extremity of the child who is incapable of cooperating should be placed in a plaster spica cast rather than in a hanging cast. Holm suggested an open Velpeau cast for children and older adults who cannot cooperate with hanging cast treatment.[8] The hanging cast method should not be used for obese individuals or women with large, pendulous breasts, as the extremity cannot hang in a straight position near the body.

Sugar Tong Method

The sugar tong technique has been used successfully for fractures of the middle and lower thirds of the shaft in children in whom the periosteal cuff is intact, and in adults when the hanging cast caused distraction of the bone fragments. A slab of plaster is applied over the lightly padded arm in a U-shaped fashion from the axilla around the elbow to the upper arm laterally, and held with a gauze roller bandage. The elbow should be padded to protect the bony prominences and the ulnar nerve in its groove. The forearm is suspended by a col-

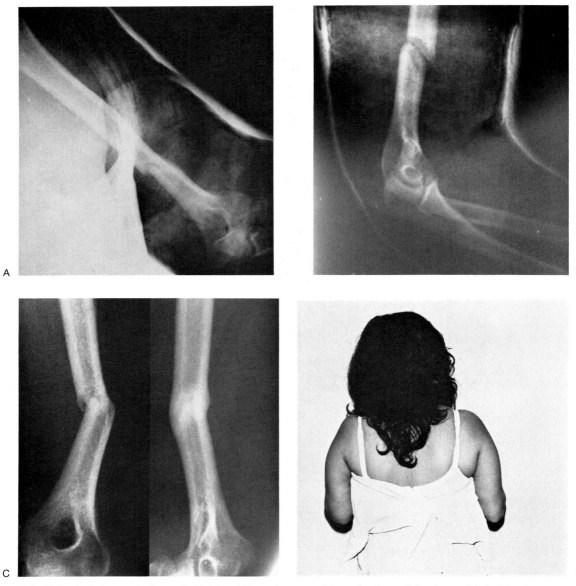

FIG. 19-9. A, Anteroposterior and, B, lateral films show an oblique fracture of the lower third of the humerus aligned in a plaster spica cast. The patient demanded removal of the spica cast at 6 weeks and treated herself in a sling for another 6 weeks. C, X-ray films in two planes show malunion of the fracture. D, Function was excellent, but there was slight visible varus deformity of the left arm.

lar and cuff. This method is not recommended for adults with highly unstable fractures.

Shoulder Spica Cast Method

If the methods already described do not permit adequate fracture alignment or can-

not be tolerated, a plaster spica cast may be used in adults or children. In those patients with delayed union, this method is preferred for a greater degree of immobilization. It is especially useful in proximal humeral shaft fractures in which the upper fragment is displaced outward and the lower fragment must be moved and aligned in the

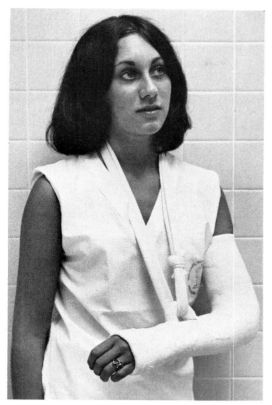

FIG. 19-10. A hanging cast. The cast should be light and extend to the level of the metacarpophalangeal joints. Fracture alignment can be controlled by shortening or lengthening the stockinet sling (see text for discussion).

same position as that of the upper fragment. It should not be used routinely in the elderly, the obese, or in warm weather when skin hygiene may interfere with treatment.

Sling Treatment

Occasionally, a sling may be all that is needed to maintain the aligned fragments, such as in proximal shaft fractures when the inward pull of the pectoralis major is not great. An elderly patient may be kept comfortable if a swath is included for a greater degree of immobilization. Caution should be exercised not to cause a decrease in respiratory excursion of the chest cage.

Traction Method

For the recumbent patient, skeletal traction by a wood screw or Steinmann pin may be used to maintain fracture reduction, especially when there is comminution or an open wound. The elbow is kept at 90 degrees, usually with the arm abducted. If the area about the elbow cannot be employed for pin traction because of fracture, for example, the distal humerus may be used, care being taken to avoid injury to the ulnar nerve.

Lam showed that delayed internal fixation of tibial and femoral shaft fractures was worthwhile and did not delay union in femoral shaft fractures, and gave a lesser incidence of nonunion in the tibia.[16] Similar conclusions can also be drawn for humeral shaft fractures in which delayed internal fixation is necessary for a variety of reasons (see Figs. 19-15 and 19-18).

Operative Treatment

Open reduction of humeral shaft fractures is seldom indicated. Only when closed methods fail to maintain adequate bony contact, length, and alignment are open reduction and internal fixation methods contemplated[21] (Fig. 19-11). Open reduction is considered on rare occasions when interposition of soft tissues, like the radial nerve, interferes with reduction, especially in the long oblique and spiral fracture of the lower half of the humerus (see Fig. 19-7). Internal fixation is not needed to provide rigidity, since rigidity is not necessary in the usual shaft fracture, provided adequate external fixation is accomplished by a hanging cast or shoulder spica cast.

The use of internal fixation devices in all open fractures, such as the insertion of an intramedullary rod, retards the rate of healing and increases the incidence of nonunion. When needed, I prefer rigid internal plate fixation in preference to intramedullary rod methods whenever possible. When applicable, a compression technique is preferred. However, when the plate and screws are later removed, the extremity should be

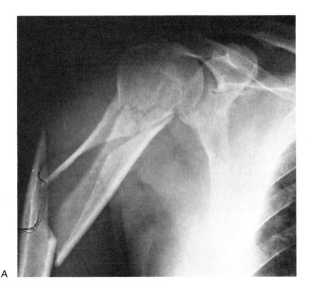

A

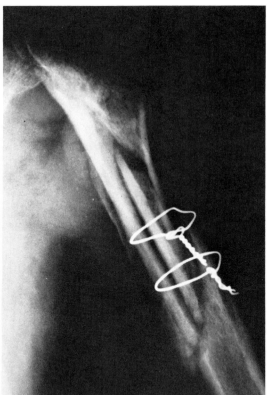

B

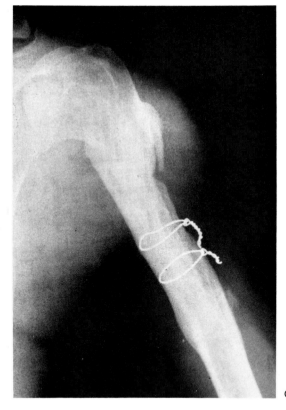

C

FIG. 19-11. A, Highly splintered upper humeral shaft fracture involving the surgical neck of a 56-year-old man. A hanging cast did not improve the position of the fragments. B, Postoperative alignment is shown after an open reduction was performed, and wire used to hold the numerous fragments. The two large spikes of bone completely pierced the deltoid. The patient was treated in a plaster of Paris spica cast for 12 weeks. Pendulum exercises were continued with the arm in a sling for 4 weeks. C, The healed fracture 2 years postoperatively. Except for slight loss of overhead shoulder motion the result was excellent. (Reprinted from Post, M., and Haskell, S.: Fractures and Dislocations of the Upper Extremity, Chapter 7. In Practice of Surgery, Volume 2, Orthopedics, 1973 revision, with permission of the Medical Department, Harper & Row, Publishers, Inc., Hagerstown, Md.)

exercised carefully for a period of time to avoid fracture through the holes in the bone created by the screws.

The use of Küntscher intramedullary rod may be advantageous when the surgeon wishes to achieve anatomic alignment and have the patient start early motion when closed methods fail (see Fig. 19-18). However, blind insertion of the rod is not recommended for the novice. A rod of appropriate diameter should be selected so as to prevent rotation at the fracture site.[14]

Other worthwhile methods include the use of multiple screws for a long spiral fracture with plaster cast, whereas a well-applied plate and screws or a compression plate is best for a transverse fracture[20] (Fig. 19-12). The use of other types of intramedullary nails, such as a Rush rod,[24] or the rare use of encircling wires (Fig. 19-11) to maintain a highly comminuted fracture has merit, provided external support is employed postoperatively (Fig. 19-13). Occasionally, there is excessive motion at the fracture site and additional internal fixation is needed in addition to a rod (Fig. 19-14).

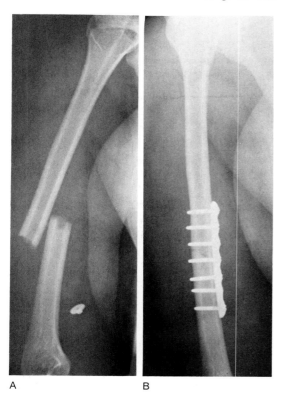

A   B

FIG. 19-12. A, Highly displaced shaft fracture of the humerus of a 30-year-old man. B, The fracture was treated with a compression plate because the patient could not tolerate a hanging cast. The fracture line was completely obliterated after 4 months. The result was excellent. (Reprinted from Post, M., and Haskell, S.: Fractures and Dislocations of the Upper Extremity, Chapter 7. In Practice of Surgery, Volume 2, Orthopedics, 1973 revision, with permission of the Medical Department, Harper & Row, Publishers, Inc., Hagerstown, Md.)

When osteoporotic bone is unable to accept a plate and screws, it is wise to allow some shortening and telescoping of the fragments and utilize an intramedullary nail. The use of plate and screws is recommended for a displaced comminuted fracture with butterfly fragment.

When external immobilization is required, it should be maintained until there is solid healing, as determined both clinically and by roentgenographic evidence. Following cast removal, the arm is supported in a sling and gentle motion exercises at the wrist, elbow, and shoulder are initiated, scrupulous attention being paid to rebuilding muscle strength. After 2 weeks the sling may be removed and the patient gradually allowed to resume active exercises of all upper extremity joints.

When open reduction is performed the utility incision of Henry is recommended when the radial nerve is not involved (see Fig. 10-4). If there is radial nerve paralysis, the incision should follow the course of the nerve. The preoperative and postoperative neurovascular status should be determined. If a major vessel is repaired, the fracture must first be stabilized by rigid internal fixation even allowing an inch or slightly more of bone shortening in order to effect vessel repair. If a large amount of soft tissue has been lost, the wound must be closed with pedicle flaps or free skin grafts in order to prevent subsequent infection. Contaminated or high-velocity missile wounds should be left open and several days later be closed secondarily. When a great loss of soft tissue has occurred, especially muscle, supplemental external support with the hanging cast may cause an overpull at the fracture site and should be avoided. In this event the shoulder spica cast is preferred.

COMPLICATIONS

Neurologic Injury

The most common nerve injury in humeral shaft fracture is radial nerve injury, occurring in 5 to 10 percent of humeral shaft fractures. It is recognized by the loss

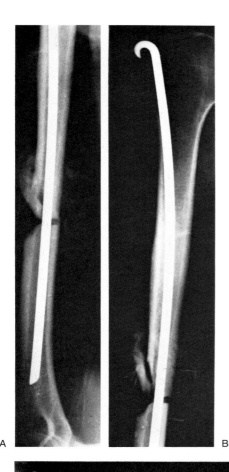

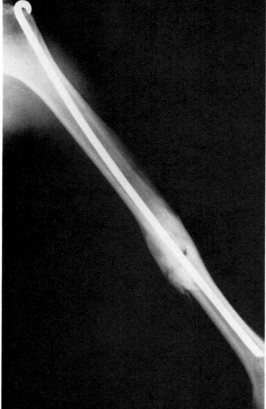

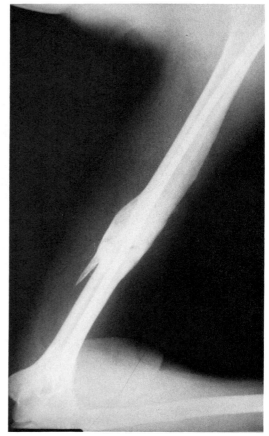

FIG. 19-13. A, Anteroposterior and, B, lateral views show a fractured humeral shaft of a 40-year-old woman who could not tolerate a hanging cast. A Rush rod was used to immobilize the fracture fragments. Iliac bone was added about the fracture site, and the extremity was placed in Velpeau sling immobilization. Note the gap at the fracture site. C, Anteroposterior and, D, lateral views at 12 months demonstrate the degree of healing at the fracture site. Gentle motion exercises were started at 12 weeks. The rod was subsequently removed. The result was excellent. (Reprinted from Post, M., and Haskell, S.: Fractures and Dislocations of the Upper Extremity, Chapter 7. In Practice of Surgery, Volume 2, Orthopedics, 1973 revision, with permission of the Medical Department, Harper & Row, Publishers, Inc., Hagerstown, Md.)

A

B

C

D

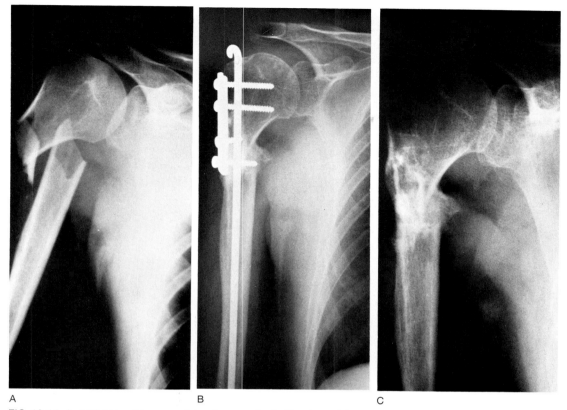

A   B   C

FIG. 19-14. A, A 56-year-old man sustained a comminuted fracture of the proximal shaft. B, An open reduction was performed 12 days later because of poor fracture alignment. An interposed long biceps tendon was found. A rod was inserted and a short plate added to control rotational movement of the bone fragments. C, The rod, plate, and screws were removed after 12 months and the degree of healing is shown. The result was excellent.

of active wrist extension. With incomplete paralysis active wrist extension power is diminished. More rarely, the median and ulnar nerves may be injured. Newman reported median nerve symptoms, resulting from fracture of the supracondylar process.[22]

Most radial nerve injuries are the result of stretching or contusion, and the nerves tend to recover function within days to several months.[12] Uncommonly, the nerve may be severely compressed within the fracture site or, in one personal experience, completely pierced by a thin bone spike pointing upward in the lowest third of the shaft. However, when a reasonable period has elapsed so that there is no return of function, based on the recovery rate of 1 mm. a day after wallerian degeneration occurs (6 weeks), then exploration is justified.[26]

If the radial nerve is believed to be interposed between the bone fragments or to be severed, an open reduction should be performed. When the nerve is crushed the neuroma should be resected, the ends then approximated in correct rotation, and neurorrhaphy performed. If the surgeon is experienced he should undertake the primary repair of a severed nerve. However, repair delayed several months gives excellent results, often superior to those of primary repair.

If the surgeon elects to observe the patient after radial nerve paralysis, it is useful to obtain results of nerve conduction velocity and electromyographic studies starting 3 weeks after injury. If there is no evidence at all of nerve recovery after 8 to 10 weeks, exploration is indicated. This delay obviates unnecessary operations in most patients in whom spontaneous recovery will occur. In unusual cases palsy may develop several weeks after fracture. In this case it may be suspected that the nerve is entrapped in callus formation. If there is no relief from or there is progression of the palsy, a decompression should be performed. In this event, exploration of the nerve is indicated. In all cases of radial nerve palsy the wrist and fingers should be treated with a dynamic splint to prevent joint contracture.

Vascular Injury

Vascular injury complicating humeral shaft fracture demands immediate treatment. Major vessel laceration should be repaired. In rare instances, the brachial artery or vein is injured and thrombosis results, with loss of the radial pulse. Subsequently, gangrene develops if the problem is not quickly treated. Aneurysm may follow vessel injury and can produce an enormous localized swelling due to extravasation of blood into the soft tissues (see Figs. 2-5 and 2-6). An aneurysm of a major vessel requires repair, whereas a smaller vein or artery may be ligated. A surgeon untrained in such procedures would be wise to consult a vascular surgeon.

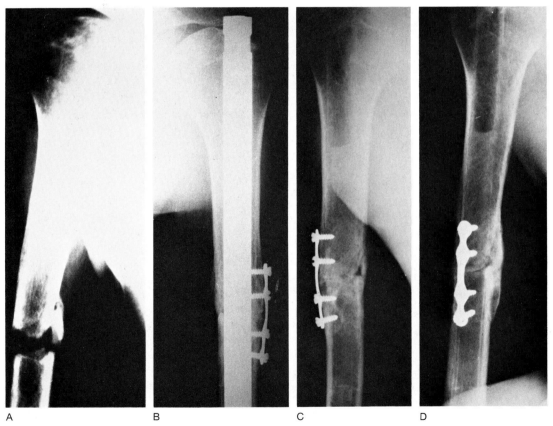

A   B   C   D

FIG. 19-15. A, Failure of hanging cast treatment in a fractured humeral shaft. B, Four months following injury, the distracted fragments were treated with a Küntscher rod and small bone plate, prior to the advent of compression devices, to prevent rotation of the fracture fragments. An iliac bone graft was added. The extremity was kept in Velpeau sling immobilization for 10 weeks. C, Anteroposterior and, D, lateral views 11 months postoperatively after rod was removed when fracture had healed. The result was excellent. (Reprinted from Post, M., and Haskell, S.: Fractures and Dislocations of the Upper Extremity, Chapter 7. In Practice of Surgery, Volume 2, Orthopedics, 1973 revision, with permission of the Medical Department, Harper & Row, Publishers, Inc., Hagerstown, Md.)

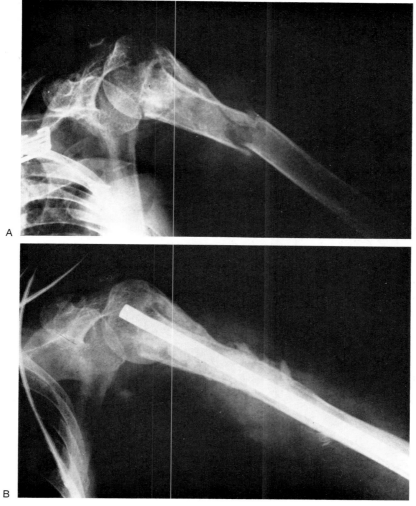

FIG. 19-16. A, A 54-year-old woman sustained a pathologic fracture of the midhumerus. Note the previous, healed surgical neck fracture. B, A Küntscher rod and methyl methacrylate were used to stabilize the fracture and other impending fractures in the same bone. The patient lived in comfort for another 14 months.

Delayed Union and Nonunion[2]

Delayed union and nonunion are frequent complications of fracture of the humeral shaft, occurring most often in transverse fractures of the midportion of the diaphysis. Although factors such as interposition of soft tissue, distraction of the fracture ends, and stripping of the periosteum following open reduction predispose to this complication, it may occur even when treatment is excellent[5] (Fig. 19-15). Conservative treatment should be continued 4 to 5 months before the surgeon decides that a plateau of delayed union or nonunion has been reached.

To achieve rapid healing there must be contact of the bone ends, rigid internal fixation, and the application of an autogenous cancellous bone graft. For transverse fractures, I prefer a compression plate, remembering that slight shortening of the shaft of the humerus is compatible with good function. However, it is not necessary to disturb the nonunion site itself as long as the bone ends are in continuity and the bone graft is applied to the raw bone surfaces. The outer bone cortex should be gouged to raw bleed-

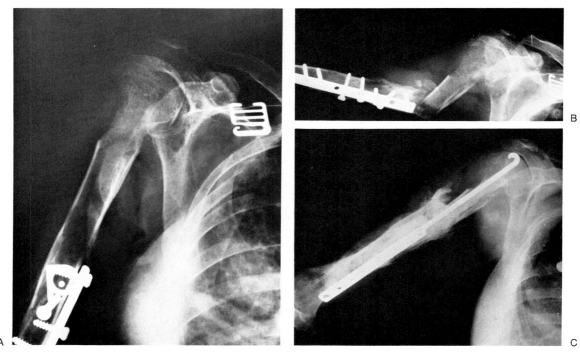

FIG. 19-17. A, A 50-year-old woman had plate fixation of a lower humeral fracture 6 months before another lytic lesion was discovered more proximally in the shaft. B, The bone fractured just above the plate before operation could be performed. C, The screws were removed, but the plate that was surrounded by some bone was left to act as additional support. A rod and methyl methacrylate were used to stabilize the whole shaft. The result was excellent.

ing bone, and the cancellous bone graft applied to this site. In some cases it may be better to use an intramedullary rod of appropriate size and cancellous bone graft rather than a plate (see Fig. 19-1). Here, the intramedullary canal should be opened by reaming above and below the nonunion site. When nonunion is present in the proximal shaft where the canal is wide, it may be necessary to use a small bone plate in conjunction with an intramedullary rod and bone graft in order to decrease rotational movement (Fig. 19-15). Whatever method is decided upon to attain healing, additional external support in the form of a plaster shoulder spica cast or Velpeau should be considered, especially when absolute rigid fixation is not possible.

To avoid shoulder and elbow stiffness following inactivity, passive and active motion exercises should be initiated as soon as sufficient healing has occurred at the non-union site. If a compression plate and screws are later removed, guarded activities for 10 to 12 weeks must be enforced to preclude a possible fracture through one of the screw holes.

Pathologic Fracture

When the humeral shaft is affected with tumor, pathologic fracture may occur. If the patient is not expected to live for an extended time and a fracture is imminent or has already resulted, it may be treated with plaster of Paris technique methods. If the patient is disabled and has intractable local pain, internal fixation methods as described herein should be performed (Fig. 19-16).[11,18,27] Occasionally, the ability to ambulate may depend upon stabilization of the humerus. An intramedullary nail is preferred to a plate because a second fracture may occur above or below the plate and

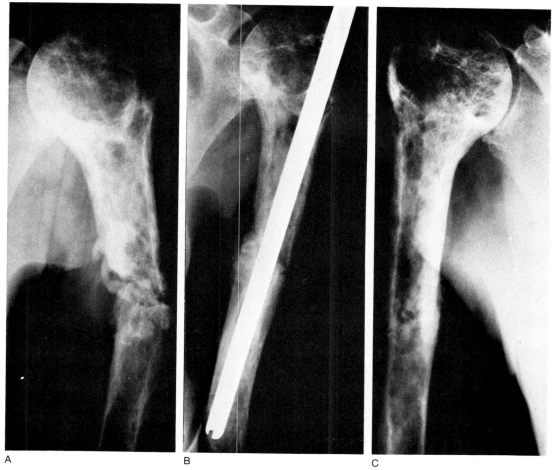

A   B   C

FIG. 19-18. A, Nonunion of a fractured humeral shaft 3 months after injury in an 80-year-old man with Paget's disease. B, The fracture fragments were immobilized with a Küntscher nail, and an iliac bone graft was placed about the nonunion site. The extremity was kept in Velpeau sling immobilization for 10 weeks. C, After 14 months the rod was removed and union was complete. The result was excellent. The patient was still well 10 years later. (Reprinted from Post, M., and Haskell, S.: Fractures and Dislocations of the Upper Extremity, Chapter 7. In Practice of Surgery, Volume 2, Orthopedics, 1973 revision, with permission of the Medical Department, Harper & Row, Publishers, Inc., Hagerstown, Md.)

necessitate a second operation (Fig. 19-17). Once they are stabilized, pathologic fractures may go on to bone union following treatment with chemotherapy and/or radiation.

In some patients even when not expected to live for a prolonged time and immediate rigid fixation of a pathologic fracture is needed, excellent results with relief of pain and restoration of function have been accomplished with the use of an intramedullary rod and methyl methacrylate cement (Figs. 19-16 and 19-17). When radiation

therapy is planned the use of cement and metal rods will not interfere with treatment.[11,32] Internal fixation should be used even in special circumstances such as a pathologic fracture due to Paget's disease and delayed union or nonunion (Fig. 19-18). It is also wise to fix impending fractures internally (Fig. 19-19).

Iatrogenic Fracture

When a humeral fracture is healing, too vigorous physical therapy to restore joint

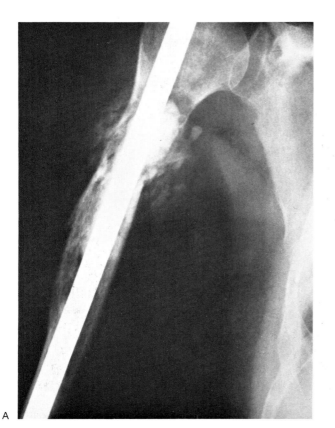

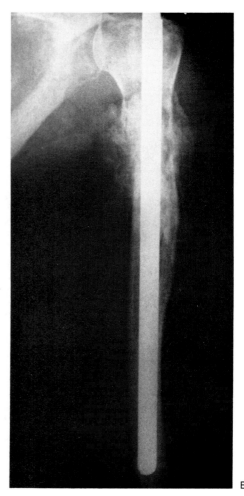

A

B

FIG. 19-19. Six months after an impending pathologic fracture of the upper third of the humeral shaft of a 48-year-old woman was treated with methyl methacrylate and a Küntscher rod. The result was excellent.

motion should be avoided to obviate another injury (Fig. 19-20). The surgeon should instruct the physical therapist and patient how to support the humerus and elbow while the exercises are being performed, especially during early exercise therapy when the musculature is atrophic.

REFERENCES

1. Baker, D. M.: Fractures of the humeral shaft associated with ipsilateral fracture dislocation of the shoulder: Report of a case. J. Trauma, 11:532–534, 1971.
2. Bennett, G. E.: Fractures of the humerus with particular reference to nonunion and its treatment. Ann. Surg., 103:994–1006, 1936.
3. Caldwell, J. A.: Treatment of fractures in the Cincinnati General Hospital. Ann. Surg., 97:161–176, 1933.
4. Christensen, S.: Humeral shaft fractures, operative and conservative treatment. Acta Chir. Scand., 133:455–460, 1967.
5. Fenyö, G.: On fractures of the shaft of the humerus. Acta. Chir. Scand., 137:221–226, 1971.
6. Gregersen, H. N.: Fractures of the humerus from muscular violence. Acta Orthop. Scand., 42:506–512, 1971.
7. Hollinshead, W. H.: Anatomy for Surgeons, vol. 3, 2nd ed. (The Back and Limbs). New York, Hoeber-Harper, 1958.
8. Holm, C. L.: Management of humeral shaft frac-

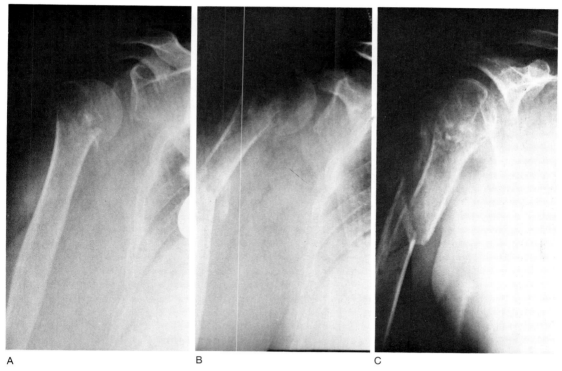

A   B   C

FIG. 19-20. A 35-year-old man was treated for a surgical neck fracture with Velpeau immobilization. A, An anteroposterior roentgenogram shows the fracture at 7 weeks. B, While performing vigorous shoulder motion exercises he fractured the shaft. C, The new fracture was treated in a hanging cast for 9 weeks. There was uneventful healing. However, shoulder stiffness persisted for several months.

tures. Fundamentals of nonoperative techniques. Clin. Orthop., 71:132–139, 1970.

9. Holstein, A., and Lewis, G. B.: Fractures of the humerus with radial nerve paralysis. J. Bone Joint Surg., 45-A:1382–1388, 1963.

10. Hudson, R. T.: The use of the hanging cast in treatment of fractures of the humerus. South. Surgeon, 10:132–134, 1941.

11. Jensen, T. M., Dillon, W. L., and Reckling, F. W.: Changing concepts in the management of pathological and impending pathological fractures. J. Trauma, 16:496–502, 1976.

12. Kettelkemp, D. B., and Alexander, H.: Clinical review of radial nerve injury. J. Trauma, 7:424–432, 1967.

13. Klenerman, L.: Fractures of the shaft of the humerus. J. Bone Joint Surg., 48-B:105–111, 1966.

14. Küntscher, G.: The Küntscher method of intramedullary fixation. J. Bone Joint Surg., 40-A:17–26, 1958.

15. Laing, P. G.: The arterial supply of the adult humerus. J. Bone Joint Surg., 38-A:1105–1116, 1956.

16. Lam, S. J. S.: The place of delayed internal fixation of the treatment of fractures of the long bones. J. Bone Joint Surg., 46-B:393–397, 1964.

17. Laustela, E.: Thorax traumatology. Acta Chir. Scand. (Suppl.), 332:17–22, 1964.

18. MacAusland, W. R., Jr.: Management of metastatic pathological fractures. Clin. Orthop., 73:39–51, 1970.

19. Mann, R., and Neal, E. G.: Fractures of the shaft of the humerus in adults. South. Med. J., 58:264–268, 1956.

20. Müller, M. E.: Treatment of nonunions by compression. Clin. Orthop., 43:83–92, 1965.

21. Naiman, P. T., Schein, A. J., and Siffert, R. S.: Use of ASIF compression plates in selected shaft fractures of the upper extremity. A preliminary report. Clin. Orthop., 71:208–216, 1970.

22. Newman, A.: The supracondylar process and its fractures. Am. J. Roentgenol. Radium Ther. Nucl. Med., 105:844–849, 1969.

23. Raney, R. B.: The treatment of fractures of the humerus with the hanging cast. North Carolina Med. J., 6:88–92, 1945.

24. Rush, L. V., and Rush, H. L.: Intramedullary fixation of fractures of the humerus by the longitudinal pin. Surgery, 27:268–275, 1950.

25. Scientific Research Committee, Pennsylvania Orthopaedic Society. Fresh midshaft fractures of the humerus in adults. Penn. Med. J., 62:848–850, 1959.

26. Seddon, H. J.: Nerve lesions complicating certain closed bone injuries. J.A.M.A., 135:691–694, 1947.

27. Sim, F. H., Daugherty, T. W., and Ivins, J. C.: The

adjunctive use of methylmethacrylate in fixation of pathological fractures. J. Bone Joint Surg., 56-A:40–48, 1974.

28. Stewart, M. J., and Hundley, J. M.: Fractures of the humerus. A comparative study in methods and treatment. J. Bone Joint Surg., 37-A:681–692, 1955.

29. Terry, R. J.: A study of the supracondyloid process in the living. Am. J. Phys. Anthropol., 4:129–139, 1921.

30. Whitson, R. O.: Relation of the radial nerve to the humerus. J. Bone Joint Surg., 36-A:85–88, 1954.

31. Winfield, J. M., Miller, H., and LaFerte, A. D.: Evaluation of the "hanging cast" as as method of treating fractures of humerus. Am. J. Surg., 55:228–249, 1942.

32. Yablon, I. G.: The effect of methylmethacrylate on fractures. Clin. Orthop., 114:358–363, 1976.

20

Dislocations of the Shoulder

MELVIN POST

From the beginning of recorded history throughout the time of the Pharaohs and the centuries that followed, choice management of shoulder dislocations has eluded physicians.[22,53,86,91,110] Although methods for reducing acute dislocations have not changed appreciably from ancient times, a better understanding of the functional and pathologic anatomy and of the mechanism of injury has allowed orthopaedic surgeons to achieve better results with their present knowledge and techniques.

The three joints of the shoulder girdle, glenohumeral, acromioclavicular, and sternoclavicular, may dislocate most commonly after trauma and also from other causes that will be considered in this chapter.

GLENOHUMERAL JOINT

Traumatic dislocation of the shoulder joint is seen more frequently than fracture of the neck of the humerus in the 17- to 30-year age group. The great majority of cases occur in young males. Even though an increasing number of athletic injuries in females are now seen, experience shows that dislocation of the shoulder in females is still not as common as that in males.

Rowe stated the importance of classifying patients with recurrent dislocations of the shoulder into a traumatic group, accounting for 85 percent, and an atraumatic group, constituting 15 percent of the cases.[93-96] The latter group includes the rare voluntary type. As you will note later, results of treatment depend upon the cause of the dislocation.

Dislocations of the glenohumeral joint may be divided into four groups: anterior, posterior, inferior, and superior. Depending upon the degree and mechanism of injury, gradations of trauma from sprain and subluxation to complete joint dislocation may ensue.

Anterior Glenohumeral Dislocation

Anterior dislocation of the shoulder constitutes approximately 95 percent of all shoulder dislocations. The final resting position of the humeral head following dislocation depends primarily upon the mechanism of injury and the delivered force. The most common variety is subcoracoid anterior dislocation in which the head of the humerus rests anterior to the coracoid process (Fig. 20-1). Subglenoid anterior dislocation is the next most common type, although it occurs infrequently. Here the head of the humerus is anterior and beneath the inferior glenoid fossa. Other rare forms of anterior shoulder joint dislocation are the subclavicular and intrathoracic types. In the former type, the humeral head is medial to the coracoid and below the midclavicle. In the latter, an exceptionally rare dislocation, a medially directed force drives the humeral head between the ribs into the thoracic cavity.

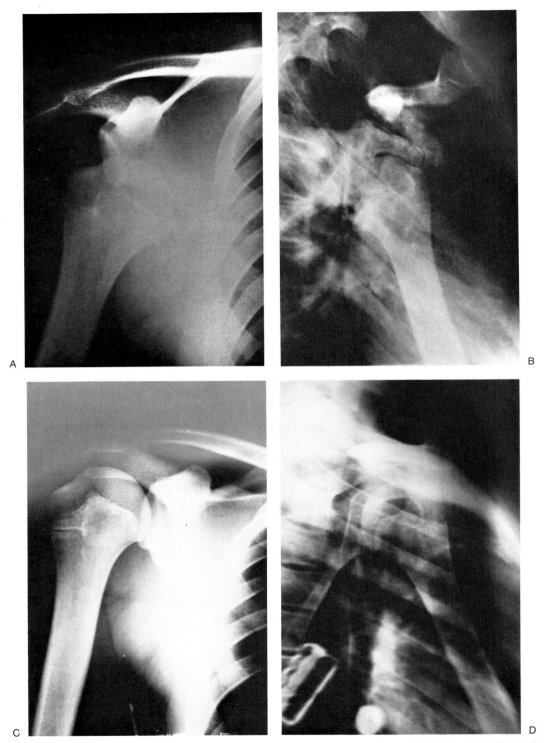

FIG. 20-1. A, Anteroposterior and, B, lateral transthoracic views show a subcoracoid anterior shoulder dislocation in a 16-year-old boy. Note the break in the smooth parabola on the lateral film. C, Anteroposterior and, D, lateral transthoracic roentgenograms after reduction. Note the continuity of the parabolic line on the lateral film. Any break in this line is abnormal.

INCIDENCE. The incidence of dislocation has been reported as five times greater in males than in females. Experience at Michael Reese Medical Center indicates that the frequency of acute anterior dislocation is four to five times greater in males than in females, at least in the young age groups. Without defining the age group, others have stated that in their practice the ratio is not so great. However, this may simply reflect demographic variation among medical centers. At Michael Reese Medical Center acute anterior dislocation is most common in patients between 20 and 30 years of age. However, the frequency has been reported to be highest between 51 and 70 years of age.[56] Rowe studied 500 dislocations of the glenohumeral joint and found that 96 percent was caused by trauma and 4 percent was atraumatic.[92] He discovered that the incidence was the same in patients older than 45 years as in those in the younger age groups.

Kazár and Relovszky reported a 27 percent recurrence rate of dislocation.[56] Rowe and Sakellarides believed that dislocations recurred in 94 percent of patients younger than 20 years of age and in 74 percent of those between 20 and 40 years.[98] They found that after the age of 40 years the recurrence rate dropped to 14 percent and that there was an overall recurrence rate of 42 percent.

Because of the wide variation of reports and lack of correlation of statistics, inferences should not be drawn.

MECHANISM OF INJURY. In most cases of anterior dislocation there is a history of a fall or blow upon the abducted arm. Thus, the humeral head is forced against a weakened anterior or anteroinferior aspect of the capsule when the force is transmitted on the outstretched hand with the elbow in an extended position. As the elbow buckles during the fall, the head of the humerus tilts downward and forward while the extremity is in an abducted and externally rotated position. The greater the degree of hyperabduction, the more the head is forced downward upon the inferior part of the capsule. This may be accomplished indirectly by leverage of the arm or by a direct force applied to the back of the shoulder. As the fall is completed the arm may momentarily be extended, and at this point the posterolateral portion of the humeral head comes in contact with the glenoid rim (Fig. 20-2). Less forceful similar trauma is required to cause recurrence. Eventually, merely turning in bed or elevating and hyperabducting the arm can cause a dislocation. Often, the patient will voluntarily hold the arm at the side in order to protect against such a happening.

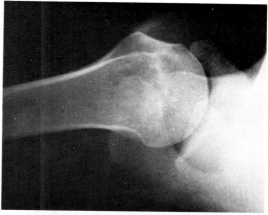
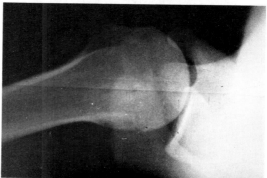

FIG. 20-2. Modified axillary views taken from a cine film of a 25-year-old man who complained of his shoulder dislocating during elevation of his arm. Note the increasing degree of subluxation of the humeral head as it passes over the anterior rim of the glenoid. This condition was treated by the Bankart procedure, with excellent results. (Reprinted from Post, M., and Haskell, S.: Fractures and Dislocations of the Shoulder Girdle, Ribs, and Sternum, Chapter 8. In Practice of Surgery, Volume 2, Orthopedics, 1973 revision, with permission of the Medical Department, Harper & Row, Publishers, Inc., Hagerstown, Md.)

The exact resting position of the head of the humerus depends upon the amount of force, its direction, and the movement of the arm during the dislocation, as described. In some cases, the humeral head may dislocate while the shoulder is in abduction.[26] Moseley stated that there is a greater incidence of greater tuberosity fracture of the humerus and a higher incidence of rotator cuff avulsion with subglenoid dislocation than with other types[69] (Fig. 20-3). Baker and Leach reported three cases of rotator cuff avulsion associated with fracture-dislocation.[7] In such cases, when the dislocation is reduced and the extremity properly immobilized there is less likelihood of recurrent dislocation.

PATHOLOGY AND PATHOGENESIS. It is probable that there is no single cause for recurrent dislocation.[101,102] Rather, there is an alteration in the normal anatomic structures that maintain the humeral head in the shallow glenoid fossa. Perthes[82] and Bankart[8,10] believed that the anterior capsule with or without the glenoid labrum became detached from the margin of the glenoid fossa following dislocation. Bankart believed that although a tear in the fibrous capsule heals rapidly, a detached capsule fails to unite spontaneously with the fibrocartilage, thereby creating a permanent defect that permits the head of the humerus to move to and fro over the anterior rim of the glenoid with the slightest force.[8-10] Thus, he believed that the detached labrum or torn capsule from the anterior rim of the glenoid fossa was the "essential lesion," and it has been termed the "Bankart lesion." Cotton and Morrison showed that the anterior capsule of the shoulder joint was deficient.[25] Gallie and LeMesurier believed the commonest lesion in anterior dislocation of the shoulder was separation of the anterior ligaments from the bone with insufficient healing to prevent recurrence.[40] Reich[89] and others[33,87-89,105] thought that an insufficient subscapularis was a contributing factor in dislocation. DePalma stated that there were significant laxity of the musculotendinous cuff in all cases and varying de-

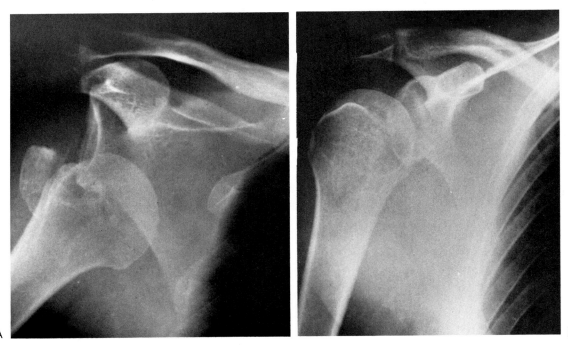

A　　　　　　　　　　　　　　　　　　　　　　　　　　　　　　　　B

FIG. 20-3. A, Anteroposterior view of an anterior subglenoid dislocation with a fracture of the greater tuberosity of a 53-year-old man. B, Anteroposterior film shows anatomic closed reduction of the bone fragment. After 4 weeks of Velpeau immobilization followed by exercises, the result was excellent.

grees of erosion and eburnation of the anterior margin of the glenoid fossa in those in which labral detachment was found,[31,32] agreeing with the findings of Bost and Inman.[17]

In an illuminating paper, Saha restated his belief that there are three types of glenoid joints: namely, types A and B, in which the humeral head has contact with a good portion of the glenoid articular surface in all positions of movement, and type C, in which the humeral head rides on the glenoid rim and labrum.[101] The first two types help to retain the head. Saha also believed that in some normal shoulders and in all with recurrent anterior dislocations that he studied the normal retrotilt of 2 to 12 degrees of the glenoid fossa was reversed, the anterior tilt thereby increasing the chance for anterior subluxation. He also stated that an increased retrotorsion of the proximal humerus may be a factor in causing recurrent anterior dislocation. Finally, the power of the subscapularis, infraspinatus, and teres minor may be inadequate to check subluxation of the humeral head.

Hermodsson showed that a defect in the humeral head occurred in many cases at the time of the first dislocation and did not change significantly with subsequent dislocations.[49] In a classic paper, Hill and Sachs reported that a navicular or wedge-shaped defect that did not change with later dislocations could be found in the posterolateral portion of the humeral head.[50] They thought the defect was caused by compression of the cancellous bone of the head as it passed forcibly over the anterior glenoid rim and could be correlated with the size of the head and the "line of condensation," represented by a sharp, vertical, dense medial border of the groove defect. Earlier, Caird was able to produce these defects in experiments on cadavers.[23]

In 1966, Reeves showed arthrographically and by tensile strength measurements of the subscapularis tendon in cadavers that capsule and subscapular tendon rupture occurred in the elderly because these were the weakest portions that resulted with increasing age, whereas intracapsular dislocation resulted in younger patients because the weakest point in this age group was at the glenoid labral attachment.[87,88] Thus, he emphasized the strength of the tissues rather than the mechanism of injury as being the essential factor in anterior dislocation.

Moseley and Overgaard[70] and Symeonides[105] further clarified the importance of the subscapularis mechanism. Symeonides, from experiments on cadavers, stressed that the subscapularis muscle and the posterior border of the greater tuberosity form a musculotendinous system that helps prevent dislocation. Moreover, stretching of the subscapularis in recurrent dislocation decreases its power, and results in lengthening and laxity which predispose to dislocation. He believed that the capsule is detached from the anterior glenoid fossa in 80 percent of cases of recurrent dislocation. Although this occurs in the first dislocation, it is not the sole cause of recurrent dislocation.

In summarizing the sequence of events that are important in recurring dislocation, it appears that an abnormal force causes the head of the humerus to be driven out of the shallow glenoid socket. Often, the capsule is stripped from the anterior scapular neck and the labrum may become detached.[77] The posterolateral humeral head may be compressed by the anterior bony glenoid rim, producing an indentation or a notch.[38] Finally, during dislocation the subscapularis tendon may be overstretched and remain lax. There is no absolute evidence that any one of the factors causes dislocation.[38] It is probable that the laxity of the subscapularis and torn capsule adds greatly toward diminishing the normal restraints that help confine the humeral head in its socket. Poppen and Walker have demonstrated a delicate relationship of the humeral head to the glenoid fossa, in that normally there is less than 1.5 mm. of excursion in the superoinferior plane between each 30-degree arc of motion.[85] Significant previous injury may alter the normal mechanism of the glenohumeral joint and the excursion values. Studies like this point to the great importance of the musculotendinous structures and their dynamic relationship to one another in maintaining the integrity and normal function of the shoulder joint.

DIAGNOSIS. The surgeon should take a careful history, asking the patient if he has had previous incomplete dislocations. After the first acute dislocation the patient may complain of subluxation or dislocation when simply abducting the arm.[14] In order to prevent recurrences the patient may limit external rotation movements. Also, dislocation frequently accompanies a convulsive seizure (Fig. 20-4).

Anterior dislocation of the humeral head may be surmised clinically when the normal rounded contour of the shoulder disappears and is replaced by a flat, sharp outline over the lateral part of the shoulder joint[61] (Fig. 20-5). The acromion is prominent. Palpation reveals a depression or concavity beneath the acromion. Usually, the patient has considerable pain. But in a chronically dislocated shoulder there may be little discomfort. The extremity is slightly abducted and the patient may tilt toward the affected side in order to keep the arm in a vertical position. All attempts to bring the arm to the side are resisted by the patient. In a thin patient before severe muscle spasm has occurred, the humeral head may be palpated anteriorly in its final resting position. At the first examination the surgeon should record any abnormal neurovascular findings.

Interpretation of Roentgenograms. Roentgenograms should be obtained in two planes (Figs. 20-1 and 20-5). In addition to the anteroposterior film, either an axillary or a lateral transthoracic roentgenogram must be obtained in order to be certain not only that the suspected diagnosis is correct but also that there are no associated fractures at the glenohumeral joint (Fig. 20-3). Although the axillary view gives specific and accurate information about the direction of dislocation, the surgeon should also learn to interpret the transthoracic view because it may be more difficult and painful for the patient to cooperate in obtaining the axillary film. Remember that the normal parabolic curve formed by the outline of the neck of the humerus and the axillary border of the scapula is disrupted with dislocation (Fig. 20-1). In anterior dislocation the humeral head is displaced anteriorly or downward, depending on the kind of anterior dislocation. Mere inferior displacement should cause suspicion that no ordinary dislocation has occurred (Fig. 20-6).

The surgeon should look for the notch or crease defect present in 80 to 90 percent of the cases of anterior shoulder dislocation.[1,81] It is found in the posterolateral surface of the humeral head when the arm is internally rotated between 50 and 80 degrees[1,2,30] (Fig. 20-4). It is best for the surgeon to supervise the taking of the films.

Roentgenograms may also reveal an erosion and fragmentation of the glenoid rim[42] (Fig. 20-4), false joint formation on the anterior aspect of the scapula,[24] and loose bodies (Fig. 20-7). Loose bodies occur in about 8 percent of the cases.[20]

MANAGEMENT. *Sprains of Glenohumeral*

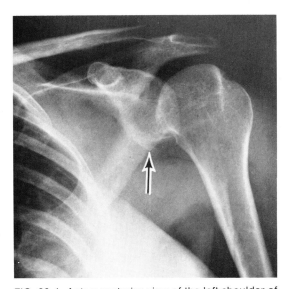

FIG. 20-4. Anteroposterior view of the left shoulder of a 45-year-old epileptic woman shows a Hill-Sachs lesion and a healed avulsion fracture of the inferior glenoid rim (arrow) following a convulsive seizure. A modified Putti-Platt procedure, in which the tendon of the subscapularis was transferred laterally, gave an excellent result.

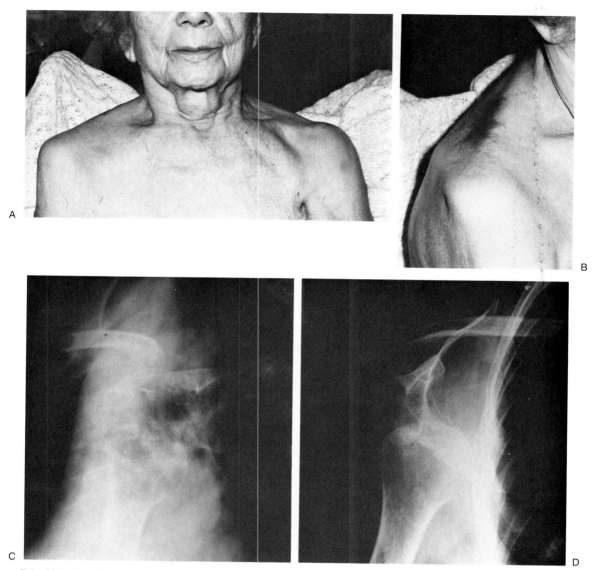

FIG. 20-5. A and B, Different views of an anteriorly dislocated shoulder in a 78-year-old woman. The normal rounded shoulder contour is replaced with lateral flattening and the prominence of the acromion. C, Lateral transthoracic and, D, anteroposterior views show an anterior subglenoid dislocation.

Joint. Like sprains of other joints, these injuries may be classified as mild, moderate, or severe.[3] In the mild type a small number of fibers of the ligament are torn, in the moderate type more fibers are disrupted but usually no instability results, whereas complete tearing and instability are observed in the severe type. The findings in the mild form indicate localized tenderness that increases in the moderate form and

becomes more generalized and harsh with severe sprain. With a severe sprain there is increased swelling. A severe sprain implies a more serious prognosis and requires additional treatment.

For mild sprain ice packs should be applied to the joint for 6 to 12 hours. A sling support should be used for 4 to 7 days to permit the pain to subside. Thereafter, gentle motion exercises can be initiated. It may

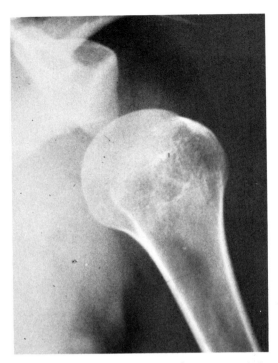

FIG. 20-6. Anteroposterior view shows marked inferior subluxation of the humeral head of a 20-year-old man. Lateral views showed neither anterior nor posterior displacement. Evaluation proved the patient was a factor VIII deficient mild hemophiliac. He was treated with a sling and factor replacement therapy with complete resolution of the subluxation. Manipulation or attempted aspiration is contraindicated.

take as long as 3 weeks for a satisfactory recovery.

With moderate sprain a sling support or immobilizer should be worn for 3 weeks to allow adequate healing of the torn ligament fibers. When the pain is severe but there is no instability, the surgeon may decide to apply a Velpeau shoulder cast for 2 or 3 weeks and then start the patient on gentle motion exercises.

When there is complete tearing of the anterior ligaments and capsule, the injury should be treated like an anterior shoulder dislocation in order to avoid instability later (Fig. 20-8).

Acute Anterior Dislocation. Before treating any dislocation the surgeon should accurately assess the injury and have information regarding the following factors:

(1) the precise position of the humeral head, determined both clinically and roentgenographically; (2) the condition of the humeral head and glenoid fossa and whether there are any associated fractures; (3) whether the dislocation is primary or recurrent and also whether any rare congenital conditions that might influence treatment are present (Fig. 20-6); (4) the length of time the shoulder had been dislocated before it was seen by the surgeon;

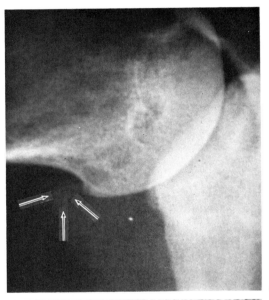

A

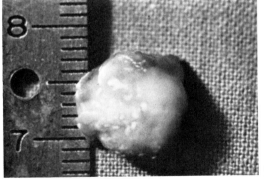

B

FIG. 20-7. A, Anteroposterior view of the shoulder, with the arm abducted, of a 26-year-old man who complained of recurring "locking" of his shoulder following an old dislocation. Arrows show a radiopaque loose body. B, An arthrotomy was performed and a detached labrum and loose body were found. A Bankart procedure was performed with excellent results.

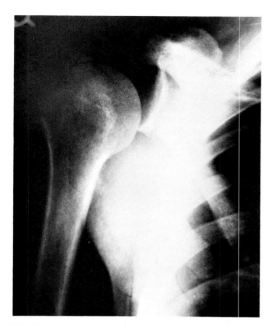

FIG. 20-8. Anteroposterior view shows inferior sub-luxation with light traction on the extremity of a 55-year-old man who continued to complain of pain and instability in his shoulder after an injury that was not immobilized. This represents an old grade III sprain injury.

and (5) whether there is vessel or nerve injury.

As a general principle a dislocated shoulder should be reduced as soon as possible. Delay causes pain and makes reduction more difficult because of increased muscle spasm. It is often possible to gently reduce a dislocation early without resorting to general anesthesia. However, force must never be used to accomplish a reduction.[106,109] Undue force may cause joint, vessel, or nerve injury or iatrogenic fracture.

Following reduction of the dislocation the patient must be examined, particularly as to any change in neurovascular status. Post-manipulation films in two planes must be obtained to prove the reduction.

In any event when relaxation of the shoulder muscles is desired in order to achieve a reduction of the dislocation, this may be accomplished with relative ease using intravenous meperidine (Demerol) and hydroxyzine (Vistaril), or thiopental sodium (Pentothal Sodium), administered

slowly over 2 minutes. In a young healthy adult, 100 mg. of meperidine and 25 mg. of hydroxyzine are mixed and slowly injected intravenously. In the elderly the doses are much reduced. In more difficult cases, general anesthesia is occasionally required in order to effect reduction.

I have successfully used the following methods with and without general anesthesia in achieving reduction of shoulder dislocation. If the cooperation of the patient is obtained, general anesthesia is seldom needed.

Kocher's method has been used less often in recent years but is still an excellent method for reducing an anterior dislocation[53,72,86] (Fig. 20-9). In this maneuver, intended only for acute dislocation, the patient's elbow is flexed and the arm is pressed close to the side of the body and externally rotated until a resistance is met[72,86] (Fig. 20-9A). The externally rotated arm is flexed forward and slowly rotated inward (Fig. 20-9B and C). Excessive force should be avoided. The greater tuberosity of the humerus contacts the glenoid rim to act as a fulcrum. Flexion of the externally rotated arm relaxes the upper part of the capsule. Nash rejected this method because clinical, roentgenographic, and autopsy evidence did not support Kocher's beliefs with respect to the role played by the muscle, capsule, and greater tuberosity.[72] Regardless of the merit of Nash's argument, Kocher's maneuver or modifications of it do work (Fig. 20-10). In fact, it appears that simple traction to fatigue the muscles and gentle external rotation are all that are needed in most cases to permit easy reduction. The following methods have also been found to be useful for reducing an anterior dislocation.

1. While the patient is sitting with the arm at the side in slight abduction and the elbow flexed to 90 degrees, the surgeon places his hand in the cubital fossa and presses downward, gradually increasing the pressure. The force is maintained for a few moments, and then the surgeon slowly rotates the patient's arm outward by moving the wrist with his other hand. Following

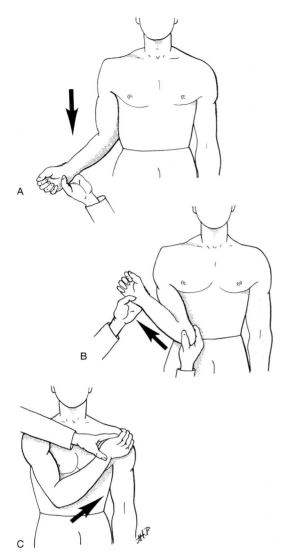

FIG. 20-9. Kocher's method of closed reduction of an anterior shoulder dislocation (see text for discussion).

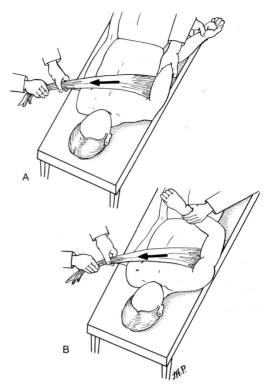

FIG. 20-10. Following reduction by straight traction, or by a modified Kocher maneuver shown here, the arm is placed in internal rotation and immobilized. A, During countertraction, force is placed on the externally rotated arm. B, Following reduction the arm is internally rotated.

reduction the arm is internally rotated and immobilized.

2. With the patient supine, a sheet is placed high in the involved axilla and about the chest wall. The two ends of the sheet are grasped by an assistant, and countertraction is applied slowly and firmly (Fig. 20-11A). Simultaneously, the surgeon applies steady traction in moderate abduction to the involved arm with the elbow straight or flexed to 90 degrees. The surgeon may place his hand in the axilla and guide the head of the humerus into position (Fig. 20-11A). It is helpful to increase external rotation gently during manipulation in order to achieve reduction. Following reduction the arm is internally rotated and immobilized in Velpeau position.

3. Still another method involves turning the patient into a prone position while the involved extremity is allowed to hang over the side of a table (Fig. 20-11B). Five to ten pounds of weight are applied to the dislocated extremity, and the extremity is allowed to hang for 5 to 10 minutes. This often accomplishes reduction when the spasm of the shoulder muscles is overcome.

Regardless of the method used to effect reduction of an acute dislocation, the extremity should be supported with a Velpeau plaster cast or Velpeau sling and swath. For

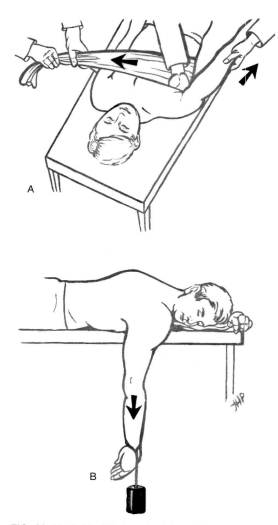

FIG. 20-11. A, Modified method for reducing an anterior shoulder dislocation. B, Stimson's method for reduction of an anterior shoulder dislocation. (Reprinted from Post, M., and Haskell, S.: Fractures and Dislocations of the Shoulder Girdle, Ribs and Sternum, Chapter 8. In Practice of Surgery, Volume 2, Orthopedics, 1973 revision, with permission of the Medical Department, Harper & Row, Publishers, Inc., Hagerstown, Md.)

patients younger than 50 years of age the shoulder should be immobilized for 4 weeks in order to allow sufficient healing of the soft tissues. McLaughlin and MacLellan reported that prolonged immobilization did not change the incidence of recurrence according to age.[63] However, I believe too early motion may result in a higher incidence of recurrent dislocation. After 4 weeks gentle pendulum exercises are instituted, and the extremity is protected in a sling for 2 additional weeks during periods of rest and sleep. Thereafter, motion exercises are increased. Rehabilitation should be aimed not only toward restoring motion but toward building the strength of the atrophied muscles about the shoulder girdle. In some cases a "frozen shoulder" results following treatment. In this event it may require a longer period of time than usual to regain full motion. Early violent extremes of motion and manipulation should be avoided. Patience and frequent encouragement of progressive exercises are the key to good results.

After the age of 50 years the incidence of recurrence is lessened, and the shoulder may be immobilized for 2 or 3 weeks in elderly patients. Pendulum exercises and increased motion exercises are started at the end of this time. It should be remembered that the incidence of recurrence is highest in the second and third decades of life.

Irreducible Acute Anterior Dislocation. Rarely, an acute anterior dislocation of the shoulder may not be reduced by manipulation while the patient is under anesthesia. Although I have not seen such a case, Lam reported one case of irreducible anterior shoulder dislocation that required division of the subscapularis because this stretched, taut muscle locked the humeral head within a notched defect over the anterior glenoid rim.[57]

Atraumatic Voluntary Dislocation. With atraumatic or spontaneous shoulder dislocation the patient is able to dislocate his shoulder either anteriorly or posteriorly at will. Most persons give no history of trauma. These cases start early in life and may be bilateral (Figs. 20-12 and 20-13). Rarely, the patient is able to dislocate the shoulder voluntarily both anteriorly and posteriorly (Fig. 20-14). In most situations there is little or no discomfort, and the patient can spontaneously reduce the dislocated shoulder at will. Occasionally there is discomfort and the patient may require help during the reduction. Many of the pa-

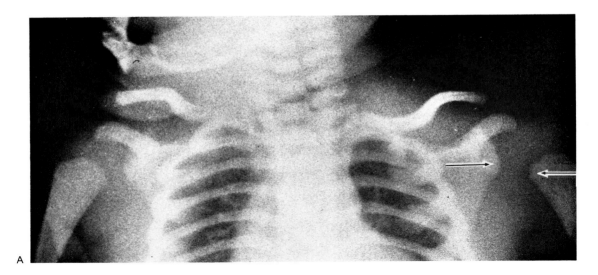

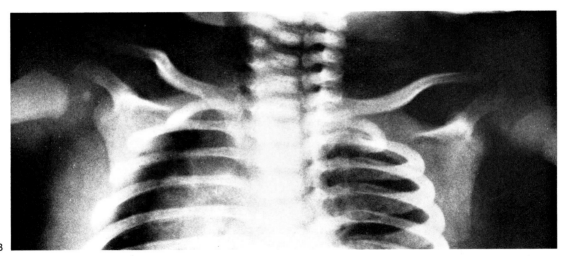

FIG. 20-12. A, Anteroposterior view of both shoulders of an infant whose mother claimed the left shoulder "dislocated" often without apparent pain. Arrows show increase in joint space during one such episode. B, Normal-appearing joints of same infant. Voluntary dislocation has subsequently continued.

tients have emotional disorders and may demonstrate a tic. Some patients show congenital joint laxity such as in Ehlers-Danlos syndrome and will not benefit from surgical correction.

Surgery is ordinarily unsuccessful in this group of patients, especially in those with emotional problems. They should receive psychiatric help.[97,99] Patients with spontaneous dislocation who are not afflicted with emotional problems should be started on a program of rehabilitation to strengthen the shoulder abductors and rotators. If the patient is physically troubled with voluntary shoulder dislocation that has not responded to conservative treatment, and there is no psychiatric problem, surgical repair can be successfully performed, preferably after the teenage period.

In one small series of cases with familial joint laxity, Carter and Sweetman found that generalized joint laxity is not common.[127] They did report that sporadic cases of recurrent dislocation of the shoulder are

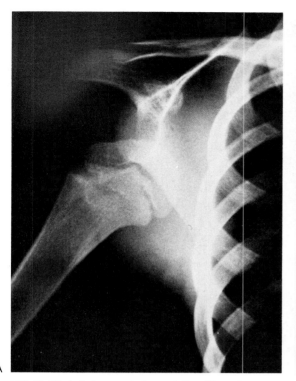 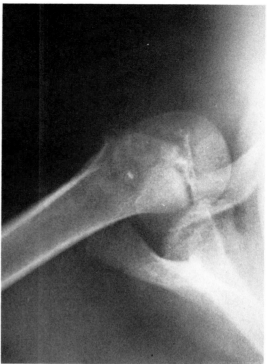

A   B

FIG. 20-13. A, Anteroposterior and, B, axillary views show voluntary anterior subglenoid dislocation in a 5-year-old boy. The condition was bilateral and painless.

rarely caused by familial joint laxity, except when a familial history of recurrent shoulder dislocation is present.

Congenital Dislocation. Congenital dislocation of the shoulder is quite uncommon. Grieg[43] and Cozen[27] have reviewed the literature. Many causes exist for this condition, notably birth trauma, muscle contractures, and true congenital dislocation. Manipulative treatment does not succeed in these cases. In the event that contractures or birth injury is the cause, procedures to correct this problem are described in the section dealing with obstetric trauma (Chapter 9). For true congenital dislocation, "masterful neglect" is recommended until the epiphyses are closed, at which time surgical treatment should be undertaken for serious disability only.

Chronic or Unrecognized Dislocation. Chronic or unrecognized anterior dislocation of the shoulder is not rare. Posterior dislocation is more easily missed than is the anterior type unless the diagnosis is suspected. There may be associated fractures and neurologic deficit. Closed manipulation may be attempted as long as 6 weeks after injury, with a chance that function may be restored.[13,45] The earlier the reduction after injury, the better is the result. However, the surgeon should not assure the patient of a good result even if reduction is accomplished within the 6-week period. On the other hand, others have reported a rare satisfactory result with closed manipulation of an older chronic anterior shoulder dislocation. In any event force must never be used, and repeated manipulations should be avoided.

After 6 weeks, if closed manipulation fails, open reduction in the young patient can be performed as long as 6 months after dislocation. Only the most experienced surgeon should attempt this procedure, for an extensive dissection of the surrounding scarred structures is required.[73,74] The gle-

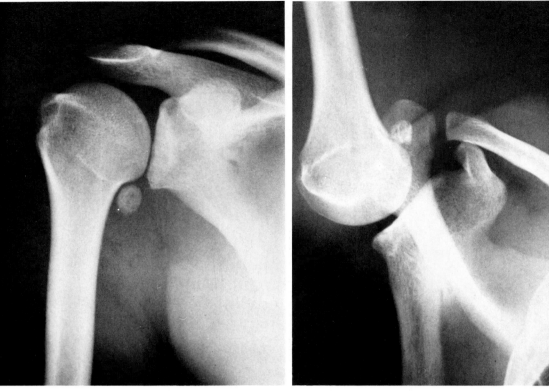

FIG. 20-14. A, Anteroposterior and, B, modified axillary views show overhead motion and loose body in an adult who since childhood could voluntarily dislocate the joint forward and backward.

noid fossa must be cleared before the humeral head can be replaced into it. Although this may be accomplished, a good result may not be achieved.

If open reduction fails and there is severe disability, other procedures have been employed, including humeral head resection and the new techniques of total shoulder replacement. In the elderly patient it is better to avoid surgical treatment unless there is disabling, intractable pain.

Anterior Dislocation and Fracture of Acromion. In some unusual cases of anterior dislocation of the shoulder associated with fracture of the acromion it is important to reduce the dislocation and any inferior angulation displacement of the acromion (see Fig. 17-17). Failure to reduce the acromial fracture will block glenohumeral reduction and overhead motion. Anatomic reduction of the acromion should be ac-

complished even if an open reduction and internal fixation must be performed. Occasionally, the humeral head may be superiorly displaced. Although the humeral head and fractured acromion may be reduced, the tendon cuff may be sufficiently torn so that operative repair and internal fixation are needed.[62]

Anterior Dislocation and Fracture of Greater Tuberosity. When an anterior dislocation of the shoulder is associated with a fracture of the greater tuberosity that is displaced upward and the fragment does not reduce, open reduction and internal fixation should be performed. Otherwise, the closed reduction should be accepted (Fig. 20-15).

Anterior Dislocation and Glenoid Rim Fracture. Anterior glenoid rim fractures are frequently associated with recurrent shoulder dislocation. Small rim fragments

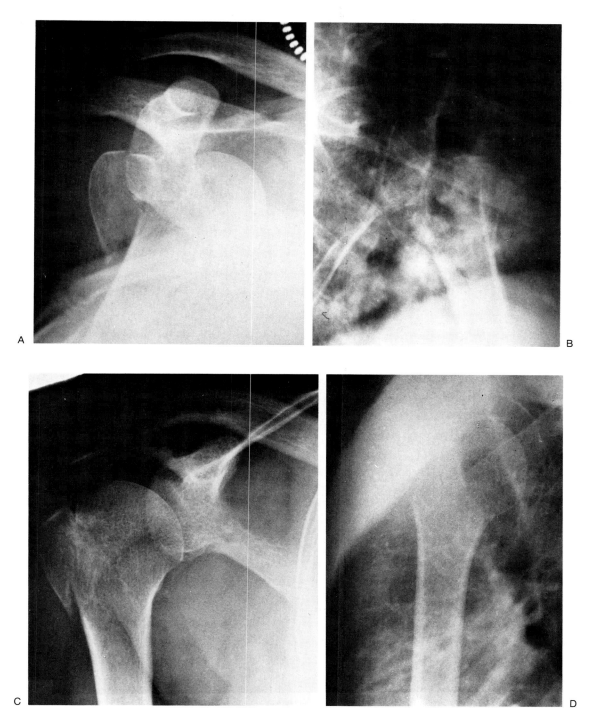

FIG. 20-15. A, Anteroposterior and, B, transthoracic lateral views show anterior shoulder dislocation with displaced fracture of the greater tuberosity. C, Anteroposterior and, D, lateral transthoracic roentgenograms taken after closed reduction show the healed fracture. The fragment was displaced downward slightly. If it had been displaced upward instead, an open reduction would have been indicated. The result was excellent. (Reprinted from Post, M., and Haskell, S.: Fractures and Dislocations of the Upper Extremity, Chapter 7. In Practice of Surgery, Volume 2, Orthopedics, 1973 revision, with permission of the Medical Department, Harper & Row, Publishers, Inc., Hagerstown, Md.)

should be treated closed. Larger rim fragments, those more than 5 or 6 mm. in thickness, should be treated surgically.

Recurrent Anterior Dislocation. The initial damage sustained and the type of treatment given determine future dislocations for the traumatic group. Operative treatment is indicated when the patient has had three or more dislocations in a reasonably short period of time. However, if there is a history of dislocation following trauma that occurred some years previously but not another dislocation following a severe trauma until years later, the surgeon would be prudent to observe whether dislocation recurs. If it does, surgical repair may be undertaken. When the patient complains of recurrent subluxation or dislocation that has not been observed, the surgeon should attempt to document this complaint to be certain that it is true shoulder dislocation, and if it is, whether it is anterior or posterior. This can be accomplished by asking the patient to attempt to dislocate his shoulder, which he may do with ease.[90] At this time a cine film frequently aids in documenting the patient's complaint (see Fig. 20-2). Also, roentgenograms should be studied for the notch defect in the posterolateral part of the humeral head seen with anterior dislocation, or a similar defect in the anteromedial head observed with posterior dislocation. This is presumptive evidence that dislocation has occurred in the past.

The aim of surgical treatment is to obtain a stable shoulder with a functional range of motion.[95] Some operations once popular, such as the Nicola,[52,75,76,78] Henderson,[47,48] and others,[28,83,84] have been discarded because of the significantly higher recurrence rate of dislocation following these procedures than that following other procedures described herein. Combined procedures have been successfully employed in order to reduce the recurrence rate.[5] New methods have been devised in the hope of further improving the overall results of surgical correction.[44] For example, Saha transferred the latissimus dorsi posteriorly into the infraspinatus insertion by routing the detached tendon of the latissimus dorsi

between the long head of the triceps and the deltoid.[100,101] Although he employed this procedure for the paralytic flail shoulder, he reported no recurrence in 45 cases of spontaneous and post-traumatic anterior recurrent dislocation. Du Toit and Roux used a stapling procedure,[36] and Boyd and Hunt employed a similar method that nailed the capsule to the bone which permitted early motion exercises.[18] If performed correctly these newer operations give less than a 4 percent recurrence rate.[1,15,36,39,46,65,66,79,91,92]

In many instances the recurrence rate is below 2 percent. However, Morrey and Janes disclosed a recurrence rate of 11 percent for long-term follow-up after the Bankart and Putti-Platt procedures.[67] In these failures, occurring more than 2 years after operation, they believed important factors in redislocation were youth, athletic activity, inadequate immobilization, a history of contralateral dislocation, and a family history of shoulder dislocation. They suggested that the Bankart and Putti-Platt procedures may not always be adequate when there is erosion of the glenoid rim or a Bankart lesion is present. The pathologic condition of each case should be studied and a number of parameters considered, such as age and needs of the patient, before an operation is selected.

Whatever method is chosen to correct the problem of recurrent dislocation, certain principles must be adhered to in order to achieve a good result. Accordingly, anterior capsule defects must be closed or buttressed by scar tissue or glenoid bone blocks. Moseley employed a metal glenoid rim to accomplish this goal.[68] Extremes of external rotation must be controlled, as by capsular reefing, and effective postoperative immobilization must be assured even if it means using a plaster Velpeau cast. Table 20-1 summarizes the methods that have been found to be worthwhile in preventing recurring anterior dislocation of the shoulder. I personally attempt to study the pathologic change at operation and use a procedure or its modification that is best for the patient. For example, if there is marked

Table 20-1. *Surgical Repairs for Recurrent Anterior Shoulder Dislocation*

Method	Author(s)	Operation
Repair of anterior capsule mechanism (Bankart)	Perthes (1906) Bankart (1923, 1928)	Reattachment of anterior capsule to anterior glenoid
Shortening of subscapularis (Putti-Platt)	Osmond-Clarke (1948)	Transection of lateral part subscapularis and attachment of lateral inch of tendon to anterior rim
Transfer of subscapularis (Magnuson-Stack)	Magnuson-Stack (1940)	Transfer of subscapularis tendon distally and laterally across bicipital groove
Anterior glenoid bone block (Eden-Hybbinette)	Eden (1918) Hybbinette (1932) Palmer-Widén (1948)	Iliac grafts to buttress the anterior glenoid
Coracoid transfer (Bristow-Helfet)	Helfet (1958)	Transfer of coracoid and conjoined tendon to anterior glenoid
Fascial repair	Gallie and LeMesurier (1927, 1948)	Use of autogenous fascia lata to reconstruct new ligaments between anterior-inferior capsule and neck of humerus

eburnation and rounding of the anteroinferior glenoid rim, it is worthwhile to consider a bone block procedure.

All surgical repairs for recurring anterior dislocations of the shoulder are performed with the patient in a semireclining position of 30 degrees. A roll or sandbag is placed behind the involved shoulder, the whole extremity including the shoulder and extremity, axilla, adjacent chest wall, and neck is surgically prepared, and the extremity is draped free. A tilted half screen has been found useful in permitting an assistant to stand at the head of the table.

Following the classic work of Bankart,[8-10] numerous modifications of the original operation have appeared in the literature.[35,71] Dickson and Devas reviewed 50 cases operated upon by Bankart and concluded that this procedure was successful.[34] I teach this method to residents in training as a basic and reliable method in preventing recurrent anterior dislocation for the traumatic group.

In the *Bankart repair* an incision is directed from the anterolateral aspect of the acromion to the lateral clavicle and then downward across the coracoid process distally along the surface overlying the deltopectoral groove[8-10,107] (Fig. 20-16). I prefer

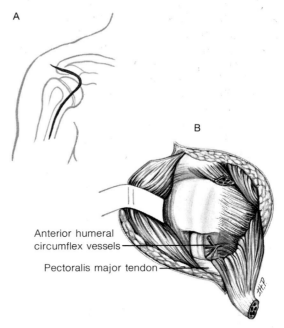

Anterior humeral circumflex vessels

Pectoralis major tendon

FIG. 20-16. A, Line of incision used in anterior approach to the shoulder joint. B, View of the subscapularis muscle following osteotomy of the coracoid process and retraction of the deltoid muscle. (Reprinted from Post, M., and Haskell, S.: Fractures and Dislocations of the Shoulder Girdle, Ribs, and Sternum, Chapter 8. In Practice of Surgery, Volume 2, Orthopedics, 1973 revision, with permission of the Medical Department, Harper & Row, Publishers, Hagerstown, Md.)

this surgical approach rather than the anterior axillary surgical approach for this operation. The cephalic vein is either ligated above and below or preserved and retracted medially with the pectoralis major. Several smaller veins in the depths of the wound should be ligated or coagulated. In a thin patient or in an individual who does not possess large muscles it is not necessary to elevate the deltoid from its clavicular origin to gain adequate exposure to the glenohumeral joint. At no time should the deltoid muscle fibers be split, for this may result in damage to the axillary nerve. Similarly, it is usually not necessary to perform an osteotomy of the coracoid process with its attached coracobrachialis and short head of the biceps in order to provide exposure of the deeper structures. However, exposure is facilitated by carrying out the following steps, if needed.

If coracoid osteotomy is needed, a $\frac{7}{64}$-in. hole is first drilled in the long axis of the coracoid process to facilitate later anatomic reattachment. The hole of the lateral fragment is enlarged to $\frac{9}{64}$ in. The process is cut just distal to the insertion of the pectoralis minor. The conjoined tendon is retracted downward to the penetration of the musculocutaneous nerve into the coracobrachialis, usually 6 cm. below the coracoid. In some cases the nerve may enter quite high, and careful dissection and gentle retraction will help one to avoid injury to the nerve. All dissection should be performed on the lateral side of the conjoined tendon because there is danger of injuring the neurovascular bundle if dissection is carried out on the medial aspect.

The extremity is externally rotated by an assistant, and the subscapularis muscle identified (Fig. 20-17A). At its lower border the transversely placed anterior humeral circumflex vessels are seen, and just beneath these vessels the thin portion of the pectoralis major tendon is noted. Neither of these structures needs to be touched. However, as much as a $\frac{3}{8}$-in. segment of the pectoralis major tendon may be cut to provide additional exposure.

A blunt dissector is passed beneath the

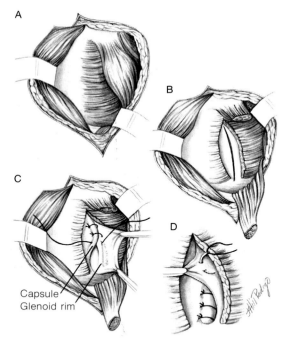

FIG. 20-17. Bankart's repair. A, View of subscapularis muscle following retraction of short biceps muscle medially and deltoid muscle laterally. B, Longitudinal transection of subscapularis and separation from its capsule. A separate incision is made in the capsule. C, The capsule and the detached labrum are sutured to the bony anterior glenoid rim via drill holes in the rim. D, The medial capsular flap is then imbricated. (Reprinted from Post, M., and Haskell, S.: Fractures and Dislocations of the Shoulder Girdle, Ribs, and Sternum, Chapter 8. In Practice of Surgery, Volume 2, Orthopedics, 1973 revision, with permission of the Medical Department, Harper & Row, Publishers, Inc., Hagerstown, Md.)

subscapularis tendon. The tendon is then divided near its insertion on the lesser tuberosity (Fig. 20-17B). If it is adherent, the tendon is dissected from the underlying capsule. The subscapularis is retracted medially. If the capsule is intact it is incised over the glenoid rim. The joint is inspected for loose bodies. Exposure of the joint and anterior rim is made easier by use of special retractors now manufactured by a number of companies. The anterior glenoid rim and front of the neck of the scapula are made raw, preferably by using small curved gouges. With an angular dental drill three or four holes are made in the anterior rim at least ¼-in. apart. Heavy nonabsorbable suture is passed through the holes, and the lateral margin of the cut capsule and the detached labrum are sutured to the glenoid rim (Fig. 20-17C). The medial capsule flap is plicated over the attached lateral flap (Fig. 20-17D). Thus, the defect is closed and a barrier is formed at the anterior and inferior glenoid rim. The subscapularis muscle is reattached to its original site. At this point I prefer to modify the procedure by advancing the subscapularis muscle laterally and slightly inferiorly, as in the modified Magnuson-Stack procedure. Here, the shaft periosteum is incised longitudinally lateral to the bicipital groove. The bone is gouged raw, and heavy suture is placed through the periosteum and surrounding tissues, or the tendon may be fixed into a bone slot (see Fig. 20-20B and C).

The coracoid is reattached to its original site with a screw or heavy suture if the coracoid has been inadvertently fractured. If it has been previously detached, the deltoid aponeurosis is reattached to the clavicle by passing sutures through small holes drilled through the clavicle. The subcutaneous layers and skin are closed. A 4-0 Dexon or Vicryl subcuticular suture, which is left in place, is preferred because it appears to minimize unsightly spreading of the scar.

The extremity is kept in Velpeau position with a sling and swath for 4 weeks. Thereafter, gentle motion exercises are started. Within 8 weeks gentle activities may be carried out. In general, it may take as long as 6 months to regain excellent motion, particularly if the modification method of lateral subscapularis advancement is used. In this event the patient should be forewarned that there will be limitation of external rotation.

Neither Putti nor Platt reported the excellent *Putti-Platt method.*[67,79] It was Osmond-Clarke who described it in 1948 but gave credit to these renowned surgeons for having independently conceived the idea.[79] Brav reviewed his extensive experience with this procedure.[19-21] He reported a 7.5 percent recurrence rate in contrast to the lower incidence of recurrence found by Osmond-Clarke.[79] My personal experience is in accord with that of the latter author.

The surgical approach is the same as that used for the Bankart repair, except that the subscapularis muscle and its underlying adherent capsule are cut longitudinally 2.5 cm. from its insertion into the lesser tuberosity (Figs. 20-16 and 20-18A). No attempt is made to separate the muscle and capsule if they are adherent. The subscapularis is retracted medially and the joint is inspected for loose bodies (Fig. 20-18B).

The bone surface over the anterior glenoid rim and scapular neck is gouged raw. Three or four sutures on a small, heavy trocar needle are placed through the intact glenoid labrum when present, or into the surrounding periosteal tissue. Occasionally, holes must be made through the glenoid

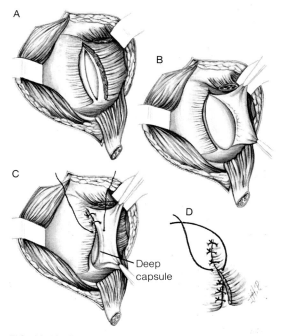

FIG. 20-18. Putti-Platt repair. A, One incision is made through subscapularis muscle and its capsule 2.5 cm. from its insertion. B, Retraction of medial flap. C, Suture of lateral flap of subscapularis tendon and capsule into glenoid labrum. D, Imbrication of medial flap of subscapularis muscle. (Reprinted from Post, M., and Haskell, S.: Fractures and Dislocations of the Shoulder Girdle, Ribs, and Sternum, Chapter 8. In Practice of Surgery, Volume 2, Orthopedics, 1973 revision, with permission of the Medical Department, Harper & Row, Publishers, Inc., Hagerstown, Md.)

rim along the scapular neck (Fig. 20-18C). The suture ends are then placed through the lateral subscapularis tendinous mass and capsule, the extremity is internally rotated, and the sutures are tied tightly (Fig. 20-18C). The medial portion of the subscapularis is imbricated over the attached lateral tendon capsule mass to the anterior glenoid region (Fig. 20-18D). Following the repair it should be possible to rotate the arm externally to a neutral position. The shorter the lateral subscapularis stump, the less is the amount of external rotation at the close of operation.

Aftercare is the same as that for the Bankart repair. After the classic Putti-Platt repair, external rotation is more limited than that after the Bankart procedure, but is not a problem if the patient is advised of this fact in advance.

In a *modification of the Putti-Platt procedure,* I prefer to transect the subscapularis tendon mass longitudinally to within 2 cm. of the medial lip of the bicipital groove, and then to undercut the short lateral tendinous mass carefully from a portion of its insertion to avoid injury to the long biceps tendon. This allows extra length to be gained in the lateral subscapularis tendon, and still permits the surgeon to transfer the medial cut end of the subscapularis laterally across the bicipital groove, as in a Magnuson-Stack repair. Although external rotation is slightly more limited, and a longer period of motion exercises is needed to regain overhead motion, the results are gratifying (Fig. 20-19).

Magnuson and Stack believed that the normal subscapularis formed a broad heavy ligamentous support around the head of the humerus.[4,18,41,64,65,93] When pulled taut it was adequate to hold the humeral head against the pull of the pectoral and adductor muscles. When the subscapularis muscle is weakened and thinned, and the arm is abducted and extended, the subscapularis muscle has a tendency to slip upward between the humeral head and glenoid fossa, or between the humeral head and coracoid. The purpose of the operation is to place a heavy anteroinferior portion of the subscapularis at the point where the humeral

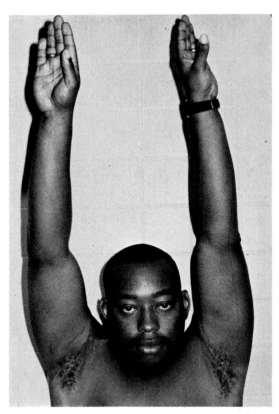

FIG. 20-19. Extent of overhead motion in a 26-year-old football player 4 months after he had had a modified Putti-Platt procedure, wherein the subscapularis tendon was also transferred laterally and slightly inferiorly across the bicipital groove. The patient lacked 15 degrees of external rotation of the operated-upon right shoulder in comparison to the normal left side. The result was excellent.

head commonly dislocates. The procedure also corrects any laxity in the subscapularis muscle-tendon structure. The authors stated that a disturbance in the normal synchronization of the relaxed subscapularis and the external rotators was a factor in causing recurrent dislocation. They correctly reasoned that transferring the subscapularis laterally to the tuberosity would correct the problem. Later, the tendon mass was also transferred slightly inferiorly in order to prevent any possibility of upward slippage during abduction and extension of the arm. Modifications in the method of fixation of the cut subscapularis tendon to the bone were subsequently made by Giannestras,[41] who employed a bone slot, and by Augustine,[4] who used a boat nail. Still others used staples.[29] I prefer the bone slot method when the Magnuson-Stack procedure alone is performed.

The surgical approach is the same as that in the other repairs described (Fig. 20-16). An osteotomy of the coracoid is not essential in this procedure.

The subscapularis tendon is isolated. Following longitudinal transection at its insertion, the borders of the tendon-muscle mass are dissected superiorly and inferiorly medialward in order to permit a flap to be lifted (Fig. 20-20A). The original operation required that 1 or 2 mm. of bone be elevated from the lesser tuberosity. However, this is unnecessary especially if the bone slot method is used. The tendon is usually firmly adherent to the underlying capsule, and no attempt is made to separate these structures.

The arm is internally rotated, the tendon-muscle mass is pulled laterally and slightly inferiorly, and then an area is selected below the greater tuberosity where a slot is made in the bone cortex using a power saw (Fig. 20-20B). Several holes are drilled in the lateral lip of the trough (Fig. 20-20B). Three or four heavy nonabsorbable sutures are used to secure the cut tendon edge into the bone slot (Fig. 20-20C). Care should be taken not to overstretch the transferred muscle. When the arm is in neutral position the subscapularis muscle should be taut following reconstruction.

Aftercare is the same as that in the other described procedures except that external rotation exercises are avoided for 8 weeks postoperatively. The patient should be forewarned that external rotation will be limited but that overhead motion is usually complete if the patient cooperates and performs the exercises as instructed.

I prefer this method of repair in the elderly patient, particularly when there is obvious thinning and stretching of the subscapularis.

Hybbinette[54] *and Eden*[37] independently described similar methods for preventing recurrent dislocation of the shoulder, in which a bone graft was placed into a periosteal pocket at the anterior glenoid rim.[37,51,54,78,81] In 1943, Ilfeld and Holder performed a similar operation but com-

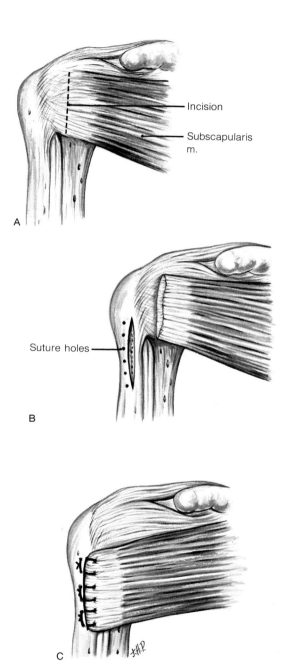

FIG. 20-20. Magnuson-Stack repair. A, Dotted line indicates the transection of the subscapularis tendon. B, Position of bone slot. C, Subscapularis tendon is sutured into bone slot.

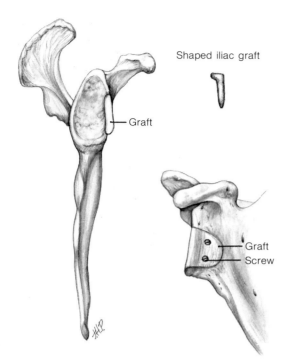

Shaped iliac graft

Graft

Graft
Screw

FIG. 20-21. Eden-Hybbinette repair. Sagittal and anterior views of the bone graft procedure. Note that the iliac graft is shaped in the form of an inverted J.

bined it with a transplantation of the biceps tendon.[55] Palmer and Widén described their modification of this method in 1948[81] (Fig. 20-21). It is especially indicated when recurrent anterior dislocation is associated with a false joint cavity into which the humeral head dislocates, when there is marked erosion and eburnation of the anterior rim, or when a humeral head notch defect tends to slip over the anterior rim.

Hindmarsh and Lindberg reported an increased risk of arthrosis in the glenohumeral joint a long time after the operation, but believed that this did not constitute a disadvantage considering the good clinical results.[51] Øster, in a long-term study, found a recurrent rate of 18 percent but stated that other methods did not give better results.[80] He believed the operation was not indicated in young patients since many of the redislocations occurred before 20 years of age. Moreover, the iliac graft tends to decrease in size and be resorbed to some extent after 1 or 2 years, indicating that the

chief benefit of this operation may be in the degree of scarification that results.

The surgical approach is the same as that described previously for other procedures (Fig. 20-16). The conjoined tendon is retracted medially, and the arm is externally rotated to expose the subscapularis tendon. The subscapularis tendon and underlying capsule are transected longitudinally $\frac{1}{4}$-in. from its insertion. With a special glenohumeral retractor the humeral head is drawn back from the anterior glenoid rim. The joint is inspected for loose bodies. A subperiosteal pocket is created with a sharp curette. If any labrum is present the pocket is placed between the rim and labrum (Fig. 20-21). An area on the anterior scapular neck is gouged raw for the reception of the bone graft.

An autogenous iliac graft, measuring 2.5 by 1.3 cm., is taken from the outer iliac crest, and after shaping, it is pressed into the subperiosteal pocket (Fig. 20-22). I agree with Rockwood, who reported that he prefers to fix the graft in place with small screws.[91] The subscapularis tendon is reattached, or in a modification it may be advanced laterally and slightly inferiorly. The wound is then closed.

Four weeks of immobilization in a Velpeau position are recommended, although Palmer and Widén prefer sling immobilization for only 2 weeks before gentle motion exercises that do not include external rotation are started.[81] If the subscapularis is advanced laterally, then the aftercare is as that described for the Magnuson-Stack procedure.

In 1958, Helfet described his method of preventing recurrent anterior dislocation by *transplantation of the coracoid process* and its attached conjoined tendon through an opening in the subscapularis to the anteroinferior aspect of the glenoid rim.[46] He gave credit for the procedure to Bristow. Bonnin, fearing resorption of the graft in the Eden-Hybbinette procedure, thought that coracoid transfer was a better method for preventing redislocation postoperatively.[15,16] In his original description Helfet merely sutured the raw surface of the coracoid to an

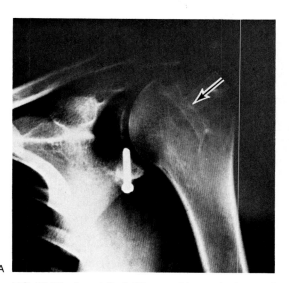

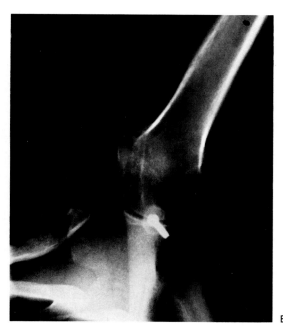

A

B

FIG. 20-22. A and B, A 50-year-old man had recurring anterior shoulder dislocation following a failed Nicola procedure that had been performed many years before. Arrow shows old tract for transplanted biceps tendon. Note the bone block effect of the coracoid 15 months after a Bristow-Helfet procedure was performed. The result was excellent.

abraded area in front of the neck of the scapula. Later, screw fixation came into vogue and produced good results.[60,66] In either case, after 6 weeks a bone block "effect" results when the coracoid attaches by firm fibrous or solid bone union (Fig. 20-22).

The surgical approach is the same as that for other procedures (Fig. 20-16), may be performed in the manner to be described, or may be performed in the manner described by Leslie and Ryan[58] and by Levy[59] who use an anterior axillary incision (Fig. 20-23A and B). An osteotomy of the coracoid process and its conjoined tendon is performed in the manner described for the Bankart repair. Dividing the clavicular origin of the deltoid facilitates exposure but need not be performed in thin patients. The conjoined tendon is cautiously retracted downward, care being taken to avoid injury to the musculocutaneous nerve which may enter the coracobrachialis quite high.

A longitudinal incision is made in the middle two thirds of the musculotendinous junction of the subscapularis and capsule (Fig. 20-23C). The capsule is usually adherent to the undersurface of the subscapularis. The joint is inspected for loose bodies. The adjacent surfaces of capsule and tendon are dissected apart. The glenoid rim is exposed, and any labrum attached where an abraded area, $\frac{3}{4}$-in. in diameter, is to be made over the anteroinferior region of the scapular neck close to the rim is cut and elevated. The capsule defect is closed. The coracoid process is placed through the opening of the subscapularis, and a bone screw is passed through the previously made $\frac{9}{64}$-in. hole in the coracoid and $\frac{7}{64}$-in. hole in the anterior glenoid fossa to a depth of 2 cm. into the scapula (Fig. 20-23D). If the coracoid fractures it may be sutured in place to the surrounding tissues as originally reported. Sutures are placed through the slit edges of the subscapularis and the conjoined tendon. The wound is closed.

Aftercare requires 6 weeks immobilization in Velpeau position. Thereafter, gentle motion exercises are started. Early vigorous motion exercises can result in the coracoid

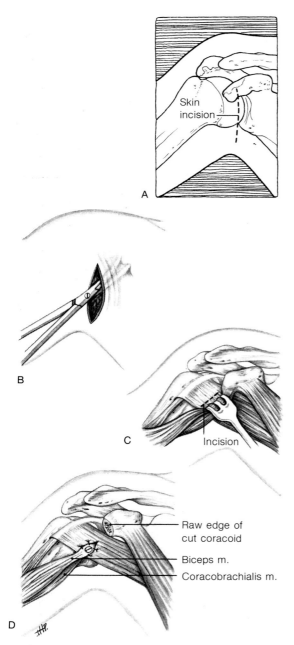

FIG. 20-23. Helfet-Bristow procedure. A, Axillary skin incision. B, Method of subcutaneous dissection. C, Retraction of the short head of biceps and incision in subscapularis muscle (dotted line). D, Transfer of coracoid into anterior glenoid.

or the screw pulling away from the glenoid fossa (see Fig. 20-27). In this case immobilization in a plaster of Paris Velpeau spica should be continued for 6 weeks from the time of this complication. In several instances of this kind in drug addicts and alcoholics, an excellent outcome still resulted following plaster cast immobilization.

I prefer May's[66] modification of the coracoid transplantation, which also was described by others[60],[104] (Fig. 20-24). May uses a saber incision. The subscapularis is sectioned 1.3 cm. from its insertion and the muscle split transversely between its middle and lower one third. The capsule is separated and opened transversely to expose the glenohumeral joint. The subscapularis split is carried medially for 5 cm. (Fig. 20-24A). An area over the anterior scapular neck is gouged raw. A 1.9-cm. bone screw is placed through a 3.2-mm. hole in the coracoid and a 2.8-mm. hole in the anterior scapular neck for rigid fixation of the conjoined tendon. While the arm is internally rotated the transected ends of the subscapularis are plicated using heavy suture (Fig. 20-24B). The wound is closed.

The shoulder is immobilized in Velpeau position for 4 weeks. Thereafter, shoulder exercises including gentle circumduction exercises are initiated and gradually increased.

Fascial repair (Gallie and LeMesurier) for recurring anterior dislocation of the shoulder is predicated on the idea that this method corrects a defect in the ligaments of the glenohumeral joint that permits dislocation.[11],[12],[39],[40] Numerous methods of fascial repair to prevent recurring dislocation have been tried,[47],[48] and have been discarded because of the high recurrence. Gallie and LeMesurier reported excellent results with their method.[39],[40] Bateman confirmed that this procedure was worthwhile and performs this operation with his own modifications, reporting a recurrence rate of 2.1 percent.[11],[12] I have had no experience with this method and believe it is not popular in the United States because of the poor results with the Nicola method and the generally good results with other methods.

The shoulder is elevated by placing a large roll or sandbag behind the scapula. The shoulder joint is reached through an anterior surgical approach (Fig. 20-16). The

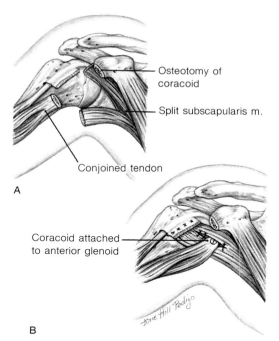

Osteotomy of coracoid

Split subscapularis m.

Conjoined tendon

A

Coracoid attached to anterior glenoid

B

FIG. 20-24. May's modification of the Helfet-Bristow procedure. A, The sectioned subscapularis is split at its lower and middle thirds. B, The coracoid and its conjoined tendon are fixed to the raw scapular neck through the split in the subscapularis. Thereafter, the transected ends of the subscapularis are plicated while the patient's arm is internally rotated.

deltoid and pectoral-biceps-coracobrachialis muscles are separated. The lower border of the subscapularis is retracted upward to expose the anterior glenoid rim. At a point 1.3 cm. above the inferior glenoid border, a $^3/_{16}$-in. drill is pushed through the detached anterior ligaments and a hole directed posteriorly, upward, and slightly outward made in the scapular neck (Fig. 20-25A). A 1.3 cm. skin incision over the posterior shoulder permits exposure of the drill point. A fascia lata strip 2.5 cm. wide and 25 cm. long is knotted at one end and oversewn to prevent loosening of the knot. A heavy suture is placed through the free end of the fascial strip, and the suture is passed through the eye in the drill point. The strip is pulled through the hole. The knot should lie next to the posterior scapular neck (Fig. 20-25B).

A tunnel is created through the head of the humerus and in the tip of the coracoid.

The fascial strip is pulled taut through these holes while the patient's arm is held in internal rotation (Fig. 20-25C). The end of the new ligament is split, and one tail is pulled through the biceps tendon and tied to the other tail. External rotation is limited to about 25 degrees. The wounds are closed.

The extremity is immobilized in Velpeau position for 4 weeks. Thereafter, motion exercises are gradually increased. The patient is not permitted to ambulate for 10 days in order to permit healing of the fascia lata in the thigh.

COMPLICATIONS. *Rotator Cuff Injury.* Rotator cuff tear is not uncommon with anterior shoulder dislocation. When the humeral head is severely displaced the rotator cuff is most certainly torn.[63,88] If full function is not restored, pain persists following treatment, or a massive rotator cuff tear is suspected, early confirmation may be obtained by arthrograms.

Pettersson showed, in a series of patients with first-time traumatic dislocations who had undergone arthrography, that 43.5 percent had no rotator cuff rupture, whereas 31.3 percent exhibited rupture without bone injury.[83] The average age of the latter group was 63 years compared with an average age of 45 years in the former group. In fact, Pettersson believed that it is the condition of the rotator cuff that determines the type of joint injury associated with traumatic dislocation.

Vascular Injury. Injury to the axillary artery occurs almost exclusively in elderly patients who show arteriosclerotic changes.[115] It may also occur in the young from excessive manipulation and traction of the extremity. The most common sites of injury are in the second and third parts of the axillary artery where the vessel is fixed by the pectoralis minor.[114] An aneurysm may form, there may be an avulsion of the axillary artery,[119] or there may be a complete rupture. Similar trauma may affect the axillary vein.

Diagnosis should be suspected when there are persistent pain and severe swelling in the shoulder (see Figs. 2-4 and 2-5). A bruit may be heard over the site of an aneu-

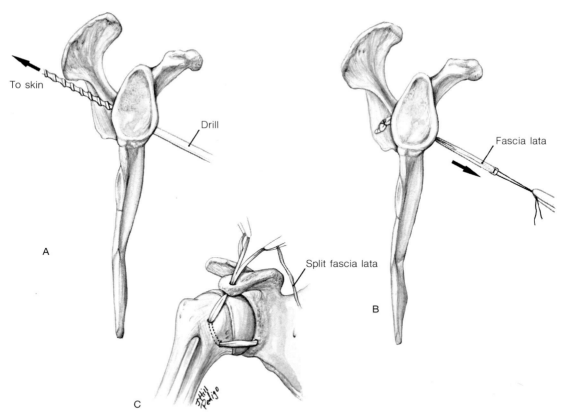

To skin

Drill

Fascia lata

Split fascia lata

A

B

C

FIG. 20-25. Gallie-LeMesurier repair. A, A tunnel is created in the scapular neck. B, Fascia lata strip, knotted posteriorly and oversewn, is pulled through the tunnel. C, The fascial strip is pulled taut through a tunnel in the head of the humerus, then through a hole in the coracoid (see text for discussion).

rysm. The extremity may become hypesthetic and even paralyzed. The radial pulse will disappear with complete rupture. Diminished circulation to the hand may cause cyanosis and the extremity to become cold.

An arteriogram should be obtained in order to confirm the diagnosis, locate the exact site of vessel injury, and determine the extent of trauma to the vessel. However, the surgeon must not base his decision of what he should do solely on the arteriogram.

Whenever possible every effort should be made to repair the torn vessel in order to restore circulation to the distal parts.[117,118] This may be impossible at times, necessitating ligation of the torn ends of the axillary artery. In this event enough collateral circulation may be present to ensure a successful result. However, in the elderly pa-

tient the risk is great and ligation may not allow adequate blood flow distally.[120]

Nerve Injury. Injuries to nerves are not uncommon.[116] The incidence of nerve injuries has been reported as being 10.5 percent for acute dislocations and 2 percent for recurrent dislocations.[63] Rowe reported a 5.4 percent nerve injury rate and spontaneous recovery in 23 of 27 cases.[92] If every patient who is seen for shoulder dislocation was carefully examined for nerve injury, the incidence of such complications would rise. This would entail follow-up assessment with electromyographic examination. As an example, Blom and Dahlback showed that merely examining for the sensory distribution of the axillary nerve when injury is suspected is unreliable.[112]

When an isolated nerve injury occurs the damage is usually transitory, the nerve recovering within weeks to months. The axillary nerve is most often injured. Milton reported that downward traction may injure the axillary, radial, and musculocutaneous nerves, and that the pull on the nerves is increased by internal or external rotation.[121]

The axillary nerve is vulnerable when it is stretched over the humeral head while the arm is hyperabducted during dislocation. Other injured nerves may be the ulnar, radial, musculocutaneous, median, combinations of these, or the whole of the brachial

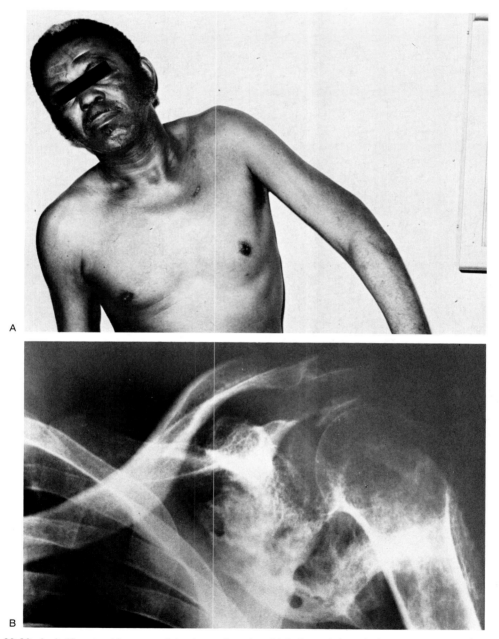

A

B

FIG. 20-26. A, A 45-year-old man sustained a serious brachial plexus injury during an acute anterior shoulder dislocation. He had no motion in the glenohumeral joint 15 months later. There was atrophy of the deltoid. B, Anteroposterior film shows myositis ossificans.

plexus.[111,113] Multiple nerve injuries tend to be more severe and permanent (Fig. 20-26).

Stiff Shoulder. Loss of motion and painful disability may follow treatment of a shoulder dislocation. For example, adhesive capsulitis following reduction is not uncommon in patients over 40 years of age. However mild, there may be some loss of overhead motion. This has not been observed in young adults and teenagers with first dislocations. Another cause is myositis ossificans (Fig. 20-26B).

Postoperative Complications. In an uncooperative patient the soft-tissue repair may be disrupted or the coracoid and its conjoined tendon may be pulled from the transplantation site. (Fig. 20-27). If the shoulder is immobilized for an extended period the situation may still be saved.

Postoperative infections may be disastrous and cause much functional loss (Fig. 20-28).

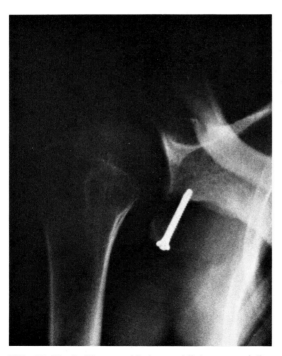

FIG. 20-27. A 20-year-old drug addict removed the Velpeau dressing 18 days after a Bristow-Helfet repair had been performed. The screw and coracoid pulled away from the glenoid rim. The patient was placed in a Velpeau cast for 6 weeks under supervision. The result was excellent.

Other complications include osteonecrosis and cartilage necrosis of the humeral head.

Posterior Dislocation

Posterior dislocation of the shoulder is the most often missed diagnosis of all the major joints in the body and may go unrecognized for months or years.[128] Because the sequelae of misdiagnosis can be so disabling, this condition requires special study so that the surgeon who is acquainted with it is less likely to make an error.

INCIDENCE. Posterior dislocation of the shoulder is rare. Rowe reported a 2 percent incidence in 500 cases,[92] and McLaughlin reported a 3.8 percent incidence in his series of 581 shoulder dislocations.[136] It is difficult to determine the true incidence in view of the fact that in a significant number of cases the diagnosis may be missed and remain unreported. In one recent year alone, five cases were referred to Michael Reese Medical Center more than 3 to 12 months after the initial trauma during which time the condition was not suspected. The chief cause of error in diagnosing the condition is the surgeon's acceptance of inadequate roentgenograms following a cursory physical examination.[103]

The reasons that posterior dislocation is seen less frequently than anterior dislocation relate to the protection of the archlike effect of the acromion, the spine of the scapula, the forward position of the scapula upon the thoracic cage, and the shape and tilt of the glenoid fossa itself.[142]

Like other joints, the posterior shoulder joint may sustain a mild, moderate, or severe sprain. All three types of sprain can be treated conservatively. The question of how much instability results from the trauma depends upon the amount of ligament tearing and the extent of healing. If there is poor healing of the soft tissues the patient will experience recurrent posterior dislocations merely by adducting and internally rotating the extremity in certain positions.[151]

CLASSIFICATION. Types of posterior dislo-

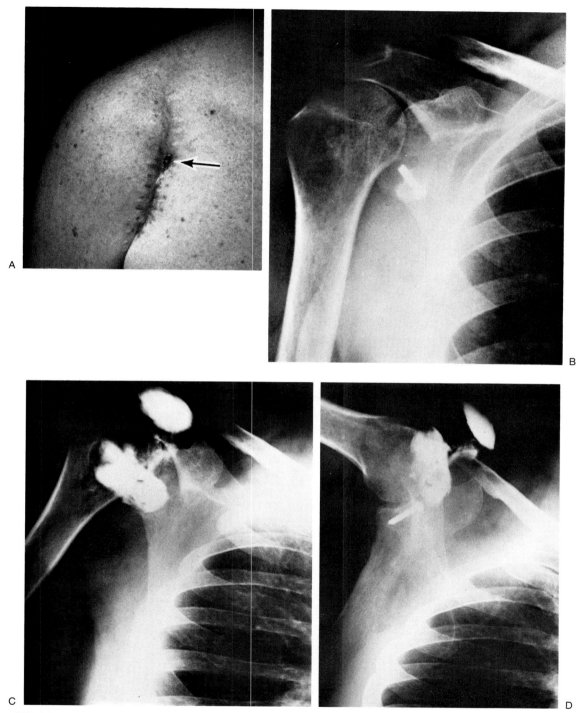

FIG. 20-28. A, A 33-year-old man had a failed Bankart procedure and a Bristow-Helfet operation 1 year later. Coagulase-positive Staphylococcus aureus pus drained postoperatively (arrow). B, Anteroposterior view shows superior subluxation of the humeral head and a diminution in the normal glenohumeral joint space. C, During a dye study, roentgenograms of the shoulder in C, neutral and, D, abducted positions show the distribution of the agent. At operation an extensive sinus tract was removed. The screw was removed, and a synovectomy was performed. This cured the infection but his shoulder stiffness was permanent.

cation of the shoulder based on the position in which the head of the humerus comes to rest were classified by Nobel as (1) subacromial, (2) subglenoid, and (3) subspinous.[142] I have not seen the third type of posterior dislocation in which the head comes to rest below the spine of the scapula. In the subacromial type, accounting for the vast majority of posterior dislocations of the shoulder, the humeral head comes to rest behind the glenoid and below the acromion.

Nobel reported a case of subglenoid posterior dislocation of the shoulder. In this rare type the humeral head comes to rest posterior and inferior to the glenoid fossa.[142] This is most unusual, considering the blocking origin of the long head of the triceps at the infraglenoid tuberosity of the scapula. Nobel believed that once the head is forced into the subglenoid position it may then pass through the subacromial stage into a subspinous position.

As that of anterior dislocations, it is important to recognize the cause of posterior dislocations of the shoulder so that appropriate treatment may be instituted. A classification of posterior dislocation based on etiology is:

    I. Traumatic dislocations
        A. Acute
        B. Recurrent
        C. Chronic
        D. Unreduced
    II. Atraumatic dislocations
        A. Acute
        B. Recurrent
        C. Voluntary
        D. Miscellaneous (cerebral palsy)[133]
    III. Congenital dislocations
        A. Glenoid defects
        B. Soft-tissue defects

In voluntary dislocations, one or both shoulders may dislocate. In the congenital type, defects may exist in the glenoid fossa or the capsule (Ehler-Danlos syndrome), or an excessive retrotilt of the glenoid fossa may exist. Kretzler and Blue have described the treatment for posterior dislocation of the shoulder in children with cerebral palsy in which they prefer osteotomy of the scapular neck.[133]

MECHANISM OF INJURY. The amount and direction of a force and the integrity of the posterior anatomy determine whether or not a posterior dislocation occurs. In most instances, the patient relates a history of an indirect force in which there is a fall on the outstretched hand causing sudden internal rotation, adduction, and flexion of the arm.[146] I have seen cases of posterior dislocation associated with epilepsy and electroshock therapy. Pear reported two patients with bilateral posterior fracture-dislocation of the shoulder who had convulsive seizures.[144] Not all cases of posterior fracture-dislocation need be operated upon to obtain correction. Bell reported a method of closed reduction for such cases that produced good results[123] (see Fig. 18-22).

A second rare mechanism of injury is direct trauma, in which a force applied directly to the front of the shoulder displaces the humeral head posteriorly.

PATHOLOGY AND PATHOGENESIS. As stated previously, there is no single cause of posterior dislocation. A sequence of pathologic changes occur that may or may not be associated with congenital abnormalities. Pathologic features observed with posterior dislocation include (1) detachment and laxity of the posterior part of the capsule; (2) detachment or erosion of the posterior labrum (a posterior or reverse Bankart lesion); (3) a grooved defect in the anteromedial part of the humeral head; (4) fracture of the posterior glenoid fossa; (5) congenital defects of the glenoid fossa (excessive retrotilt) or excessive retroversion of the head of the humerus.[142] With traumatic posterior dislocation the lesser tuberosity may be avulsed.

The humeral head may dislocate into a sac or recess following detachment or relaxation of the posterior capsule as a result of trauma. The subscapularis is stretched across the anterior glenoid rim during dislocation. The grooved defect in the anterior humeral head results from impaction of the hard posterior glenoid rim against the spongy head of the humerus.

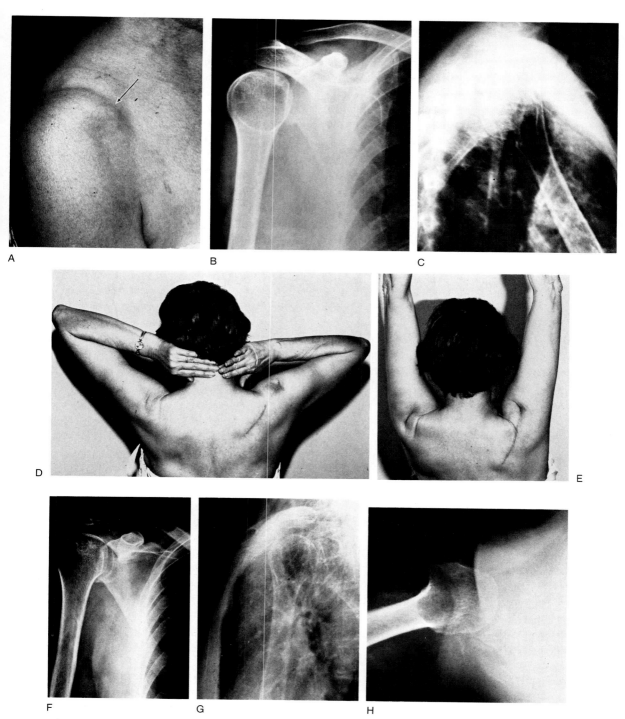

FIG. 20-29. A, A 65-year-old woman was severely disabled by recurring posterior shoulder dislocations. Note the flattening of the anterior aspect of the shoulder and the prominence of the coracoid (arrow). B, Anteroposterior and, C, lateral transthoracic views show a posterior dislocation. Note the increased space between the anterior glenoid rim and medial part of the humeral head, the disappearance of the normal "half-moon" overlap, and the break in the smooth parabolic curve in the lateral transthoracic film. A posterior glenoid osteotomy (Scott) was performed with excellent results. D and E, Note the excellent motion of the right shoulder 5 months postoperatively. F, Anteroposterior, G, lateral transthoracic and, H, axillary views show the shoulder 5 months after operation. The glenoid face is now tilted anteriorly. Note the spur formation at the inferior aspect of the healed glenoid osteotomy site.

459

Damage to the neurovascular structures has not been observed because the humeral head is displaced away from the anterior vessels and nerves. Therefore, except for the possibility of an injury caused by a force directed from the front to the back, the anterior neurovascular structures are not stretched or contused.

DIAGNOSIS. The surgeon must suspect the condition if he is to make the correct diagnosis of posterior dislocation of the shoulder.[130,148] Even if not considered, a thorough examination may point out the true lesion. First, both shoulders should be compared while the patient sits in a chair. The examiner should view both shoulders from the front, above, and behind. Whereas there is flattening of the lateral shoulder contour in anterior dislocation, the contour may appear normal if not actually compared to that of the contralateral shoulder. In posterior dislocation the anterior aspect of the shoulder is flattened (Fig. 20-29), whereas the posterior part may be more prominent when viewed from the back. The coracoid may be more pronounced than it usually is and is easily palpated[144] (Fig. 20-30), except in the individual who is obese or who has heavy musculature. These findings are not difficult to detect. In the classic case, the extremity is held in a neutral or a fixed internally rotated position with the arm adducted.[138,140] The arm cannot be abducted. In the subglenoid and subspinous types the extremity is internally rotated and held rigidly in slight abduction. However, further abduction and external rotation are not possible. Next, any attempt to move the extremity during the acute phase will cause an exacerbation of pain in an already painful joint. In recurrent dislocation there may be relatively little pain in some cases. One should not rely on measuring the distances between the tips of the acromion and the olecranon in hope that a discrepancy in the length of the arms will be found. Remember, the surgeon who truly examines the patient, and reexamines when in doubt, is not likely to miss the diagnosis.

Interpretation of Roentgenograms. Often, correct analysis of multiple roentgenograms wholly determines the diagnosis. For this reason, it is essential first to understand the normal roentgenographic anatomy before the abnormal becomes apparent.[149] Under no circumstances should one depend upon an anteroposterior film alone even though a careful inspection of this single roentgenogram may provide valuable information.

With the arm in anatomic position the humeral head and short anatomic neck are in 25 degrees of retroversion (see Diagnosis, Chapter 2). Accordingly, the usual *anteroposterior film* does not reveal the maximum length of the anatomic neck. As the arm is externally rotated, a greater length of the anatomic neck is seen along with an increased profile of the greater tuberosity. It is apparent that if one sees little of the anatomic neck on the anteroposterior film then the humeral head is in neutral or internal rotation. In posterior dislocation the humeral head is internally rotated and the anatomic neck is not visible (Figs. 20-31 and 20-32).

A second important finding has been named the positive "rim" sign. The scapula is positioned on the thoracic cage at approximately a 45-degree angle in the frontal plane. Thus, the face of the glenoid fossa faces anteriorly. When the humeral head is internally rotated in posterior dislocation, an increased space may be visible between the anterior glenoid rim and medial portion of the humeral head[145] (Fig. 20-32). Arndt and Sears believe that a measurement of more than 6 mm. between the medial aspect of the humeral head and the anterior glenoid rim is present only in posterior dislocation and therefore is significant.[122] If the posterior glenoid rim is fractured and displaced, the increased space may not be visible even though a posterior dislocation exists. It is worthwhile for the surgeon to supervise the taking of the films, because posterior rotation of the body will cause the glenoid fossa to be perpendicular to the film rather than in the angled position. This will hide the finding of a widened joint space.

A third important finding of posterior dislocation in the anteroposterior film is the

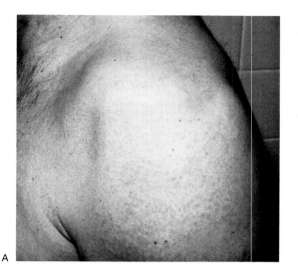

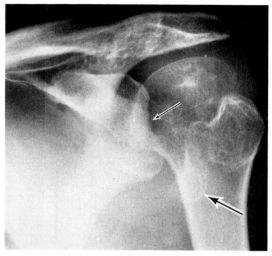

A

B

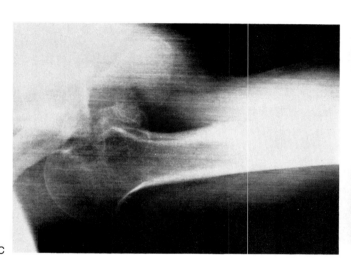

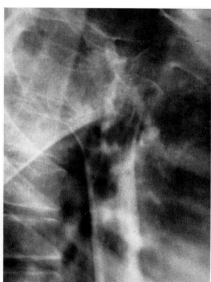

C

D

FIG. 20-30. A, A 53-year-old truckdriver sustained a posterior shoulder dislocation that was untreated for 14 months. Note the flattening of the anterior aspect of the shoulder, the prominence of the coracoid, and the bulge in the posterior shoulder caused by the dislocated humeral head. B, Anteroposterior, C, axillary and, D, lateral transthoracic views show the increased space between the anterior glenoid margin and medial part of the humeral head, the disappearance of the normal half-moon overlap, the fracture of the posterior rim and its loose bone fragment (arrows), the severe impression defect in the anteromedial head resting on the posterior glenoid rim, and the break in the parabolic curve. Preoperatively, the patient had excellent internal rotation behind the back but severe limitation of overhead, external rotation, and abduction motion. What is demonstrated is scapular motion. Pain was severe. A fixed fulcrum total shoulder replacement was performed with excellent results. The patient returned to his former job as a truckdriver.

disappearance of the normal half-moon overlap (Figs. 20-31 and 20-32). However, an angled projection of the normal shoulder may also cause its disappearance.

In posterior dislocation the anteropos-terior view may show the humeral head to be lower or higher than that of the normal shoulder (Fig. 20-33).

The medial portion of the humeral head may appear flattened. However, this may be

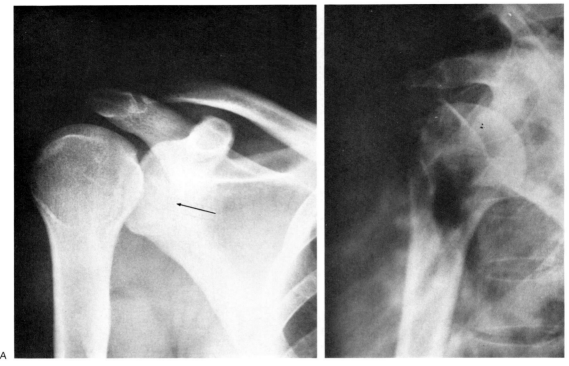

FIG. 20-31. A, Anteroposterior and, B, lateral transthoracic views show the relative absence of anatomic neck in a patient with posterior shoulder dislocation. Observe the increased space between the medial portion of the humeral head and the anterior glenoid rim (arrow). Note the disappearance of the normal half-moon overlap and the break in the smooth parabolic curve.

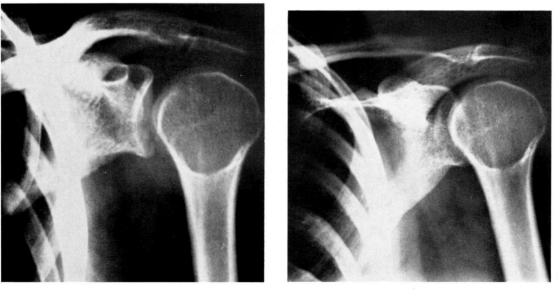

FIG. 20-32. A 44-year-old woman sustained an acute posterior shoulder dislocation. A, Anteroposterior view shows the widening of the space between the medial portion of the humeral head and the anterior glenoid rim and the disappearance of the normal half-moon overlap. B, Following reduction, note the normal relationships between the humeral head and the glenoid when compared to the dislocated state.

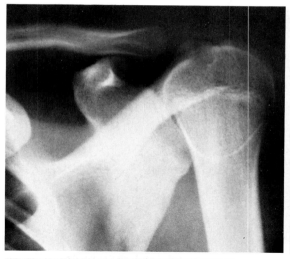
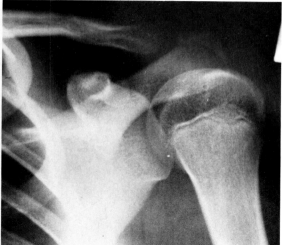

A

B

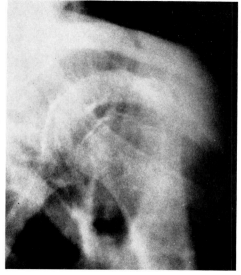

C

FIG. 20-33. A 14-year-old boy sustained a posterior shoulder dislocation and an ipsilateral posterolateral elbow dislocation when he fell from a third floor window. A, Observe the severe upward displacement of the humeral head, the widened space between the medial portion of the humeral head and the anterior glenoid rim, and the disappearance of the normal half-moon overlap. Following closed reduction, B, anteroposterior and, C, lateral transthoracic views show the restored normal joint relationships.

related to a fracture of the head, which can vary in size and shape (Fig. 20-34).

The *lateral transthoracic roentgenogram* may not disclose an abnormality. When the shoulder is abnormal the normal parabolic curve is lost (Figs. 20-30 and 20-31). Especially in obese patients the view is difficult to interpret and should not be relied upon.[225]

The true *axillary view* and to a lesser extent modifications of this view are the most reliable films that permit a correct diagnosis of posterior dislocation (Figs. 20-30C, 20-34C, and 20-35). Because it is not always possible for the patient to abduct his shoulder dur-

ing the acute phase of injury which is necessary to direct the tube and its ray into the axilla with the film over the top of the shoulder, or to place a curved cassette in the axilla and direct the ray downward, Bloom and Obata have suggested an angle-up view with the cassette placed parallel to the long axis of the thorax and posterior to the shoulder joint[124] (Fig. 20-35B and D). The pateint may be supine, seated, or standing. These modified films definitely provide diagnostic information.

The Velpeau axillary view is more difficult to obtain. A film is placed on a waist-high table. With his back to the table and looking

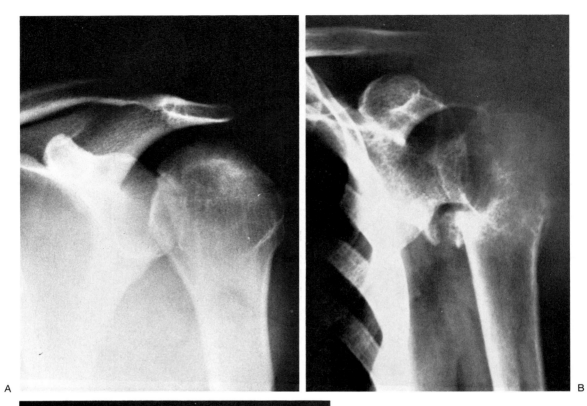

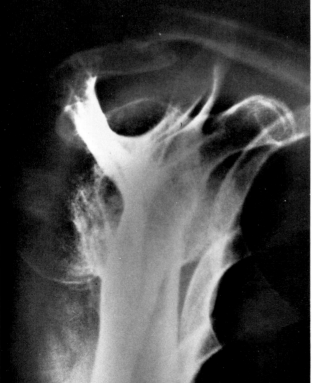

A

B

C

FIG. 20-34. A, Anteroposterior view shows an impression defect in the anteromedial aspect of the humeral head of a 38-year-old woman who sustained a posterior shoulder dislocation. Note the flattening of the humeral head and the widening of the joint space. B, Anteroposterior view shows a posterior shoulder dislocation with an enormous impression defect in the anteromedial head of the humerus in a 65-year-old woman. Undoubtedly, demineralized bone was related to the larger impression defect in the head. This injury was 8 months old and remained untreated since the patient had little discomfort. C, A Y view shows the humeral head beneath the acromial limb.

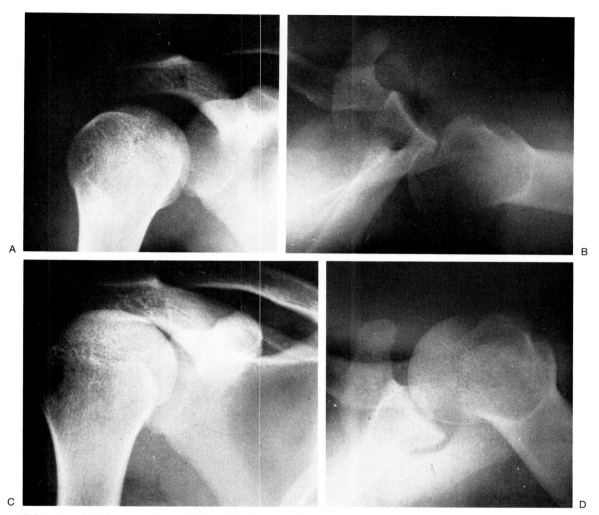

FIG. 20-35. A, Anteroposterior and, B, modified axillary views demonstrating posterior dislocation of the shoulder of an adult. On the anteroposterior view, note the widened joint space, which can easily be overlooked. The modified angled-up axillary view shows the impression defect of the anteromedial humeral head upon the posterior rim of the glenoid. Following reduction, C, anteroposterior and, D, modified axillary views demonstrate the reduced humeral head. Note the notch defect in the anteromedial aspect of the humeral head both in the dislocated shoulder and in the reduced joint. (Reprinted from Post, M., and Haskell, S.: Fractures and Dislocations of the Shoulder Girdle, Ribs, and Sternum, Chapter 8. In Practice of Surgery, Volume 2, Orthopedics, 1973 revision, with permission of the medical Department, Harper & Row, Publishers, Inc., Hagerstown, Md.)

forward, the patient tilts the affected shoulder backward over the cassette. The ray is directed perpendicularly downward over the shoulder toward the cassette.

Finally, humeral defects or impression fractures in the anteromedial portion of the humeral head may be missed if they are not sought.[150] They occur when the internally rotated humeral head is forcibly driven across the posterior glenoid rim.

TREATMENT. *Sprains of Posterior Shoulder.* Mild and moderate sprains of the posterior shoulder joint can be treated like sprains of the anterior shoulder joint. Sling immobilization for 1 to 3 weeks, respectively, for mild and moderate sprains is adequate treatment. The more severe sprain that can cause residual instability in the posterior joint should be treated like an acute posterior shoulder dislocation. When there is doubt as to whether the sprain is moderate or severe it is better to treat it as a severe sprain.

Acute Traumatic Posterior Dislocation. In treating an acute posterior dislocation it is essential to obtain relaxation of the muscles surrounding the affected joint. It is often possible to achieve this by using a slow intravenous injection of meperidine and hydroxyzine or similar medications, as described for acute anterior dislocation. When it is apparent that reduction cannot be achieved in this manner general anesthesia should be employed in order to avoid force and the chance of additional injury to the joint. The surgeon should not be deluded into thinking that recurrent posterior dislocations are easier to reduce than first-time acute dislocations. Although this is often true, it is not always the case.

Successful manipulation is best accomplished by applying gentle but firm traction to the extremity while it is in the internally rotated, adducted position. Although the humeral head can be assisted over the posterior glenoid rim, I have not found this maneuver necessary as a part of the manipulation. When a mechanical block to reduction is present because the posterior glenoid rim is impacted into a notch defect on the anteromedial head of the humerus, gentle internal rotation of the arm with the elbow flexed should be added to the maneuver to unlock the head. Immediately following the manipulation the arm is rotated into approximately 50 degrees of internal rotation to prevent backward slipping of the head (Fig. 20-36). In any case, that degree of rotation in which the joint is most stable should be used. If the patient is somnolent the extremity can be temporarily immobilized in a sling and swath, and soft towels placed between the forearm and body to prevent full internal rotation. The next day an appropriate plaster of Paris shoulder cast is applied. I have not had to maintain the humeral head in the glenoid fossa using transfixion pins through the acromion and humeral head, as suggested by Wilson and McKeever,[151] because of instability following reduction.

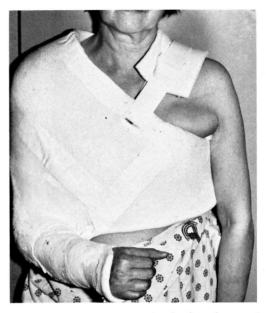

FIG. 20-36. Following a closed reduction of an acute posterior shoulder dislocation in a woman, the extremity was immobilized in a plaster spica cast with the extremity in 50 degrees of internal rotation because this was the most stable position.

Recurrent Posterior Dislocation. When recurrent posterior dislocation occurs frequently, is painful and disabling, then surgical correction is indicated. The patient may complain of a "slipping" in the shoulder as the arm is lifted and flexed in varying degrees of internal rotation. Occasionally, the patient may experience severe recurrent posterior dislocations that require the services of a surgeon.

Surgical measures to correct this condition have worked well. These include (1) the reverse Bankart in which the posterior capsule is repaired;[132,146,152] (2) a reverse Putti-Platt in which the infraspinatus is shortened or plicated, and if thought necessary, the infraspinatus-teres minor tendon structures may be employed in the plication; (3) a posterior capsulorraphy in which the long head of the biceps is transferred to the posterior glenoid rim;[125] (4) the creation of a posterior bone block or reverse Eden-Hybbinette procedure in which acromial or iliac bone grafts are used to shape the graft;[135] (5) glenoid osteotomy with which

Scott,[147] English and Macnab,[131] and Kretzler and Blue,[133] by using an opening, posterior wedge osteotomy in the glenoid neck, reported good results (Fig. 20-37); and (6) combined soft-tissue and bone procedures. In the combined procedures a poste-

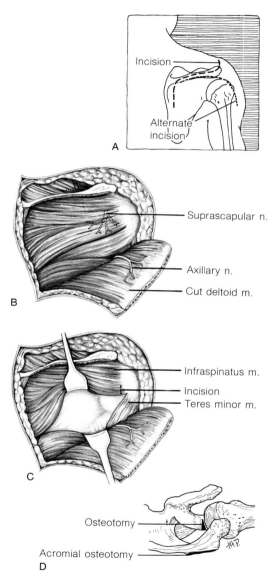

FIG. 20-37. Scott's method of posterior glenoid osteotomy. A, Dotted lines indicate alternate posterior incisions. B, Posterior portion of supraspinatus is shown after reflection of posterior deltoid from the scapular spine. C, Exposure of posterior shoulder capsule. D, Segment of posterior acromion is removed and placed into posterior osteotomy site (see text for details of operation).

rior glenoid osteotomy or a bone block can be combined with various soft-tissue reconstructions, wherein the subscapularis tendon is detached from its origin through an anterior surgical approach and attached within the defect in the anteromedial humeral head using a suture, or the Neer modification of removing a bit of bone from the lesser tuberosity with the subscapularis tendon and using screw fixation.[91] Nicola methods or modifications as advocated by May are not recommended.[139]

I prefer the method of posterior bone block or posterior glenoid osteotomy (Figs. 20-29 and 20-37), combined with capsule reconstruction whenever possible for recurrent dislocation.[129] Initially, in 1952 McLaughlin advocated transferring the cut subscapularis tendon into the defect in the anteromedial head for recurrent dislocation.[136] He subsequently retracted his suggestion, noting that a sharp distinction should be made between fixed and recurrent posterior dislocation.[137] He pointed out that subscapularis transfer into the defect was ineffectual for recurrent dislocation and recommended posterior bone block instead. For fixed posterior dislocation with a defect in the humeral head, transfer of the subscapularis tendon is worthwhile if the defect is no more than 20 to 40 percent. When the defect is larger than 40 percent subscapularis transfer into the defect is likely to fail. In this event other procedures may be considered, such as arthrodesis, a Neer humeral head replacement if the rotator muscles are functioning, or a fixed fulcrum total shoulder replacement when the rotator muscles are nonfunctioning.

For a *posterior glenoid osteotomy* (Scott[147]), the patient is positioned in a semiprone position and the extremity draped free. A posterior surgical approach is used, and the incision is extended along the whole spine of the scapula to the tip of acromion (Fig. 20-37A). The deltoid is freed from the scapular spine and acromion thereby exposing the infraspinatus and teres muscles (Fig. 20-37B). Next, the overhanging part of the acromion is excised and later used as a bone graft (Fig. 20-37D).

The interval between the infraspinatus and teres minor is identified, and the infraspinatus tendon is divided close to its insertion and retracted medially to expose the capsule (Fig. 20-37C). Care should be taken to avoid injury to the suprascapular nerve as it courses downward from the suprascapular notch into the undersurface of the infraspinatus, as excessive medial traction of this muscle may injure the nerve. Likewise, the deltoid should not be pulled below the teres minor in order to prevent injury to the axillary nerve. The posterior capsule is then opened by making a parallel incision $\frac{1}{4}$-in. lateral to the glenoid rim (Fig. 20-37C). The joint is inspected for loose bodies.

If the labrum is detached an intracapsular osteotomy can be performed by reflecting the capsule medialward. If needed, transverse medial extensions of the incision in the superior and inferior parts of the capsule permit exposure of the scapular neck. If the medial portion of the capsule and labrum is tightly adherent to the scapular neck, the capsule is not reflected, and the osteotomy is made through the capsule medial to the glenoid rim. A broad osteotome is employed, and an osteotomy is made from the supraglenoid tubercle to the origin of the long triceps head inferiorly. The blade is directed medialward to avoid cutting into the concave articulating surface of the glenoid fossa. When the osteotomy site can be opened 1.3 to 2 cm., shoulder stability is checked while the osteotomy site is held open. The denuded acromial graft is inserted into the osteotomy site until flush with the neck surface (Fig. 20-37D). Additional internal fixation is not usually needed to secure the graft.

The capsule is closed, and if desired a soft-tissue repair such as a Putti-Platt and lateral advancement of the infraspinatus may be performed. The deltoid is reattached to the acromion and spine of the scapula.

The extremity is maintained in a plaster shoulder cast with the arm in neutral or slight external rotation for 3 to 4 weeks (Fig. 20-36). Vigorous activity is not permitted for approximately 10 weeks.

Atraumatic Voluntary Dislocation. The patient who can voluntarily dislocate his shoulder posteriorly ordinarily can reduce it at will.[126] Occasionally, the help of a surgeon may be needed to aid in the reduction. Unless the condition becomes disabling surgical correction is not recommended. Surgical reconstructions in patients with psychiatric problems who voluntarily dislocate the shoulder should not be performed because they often fail.[99]

Congenital and Acquired Posterior Dislocation. Dislocations associated with birth injuries may require surgical treatment. Methods for such treatment are described under the section on Birth Trauma, Chapter 9. Other acquired conditions have been discussed by Kretzler and Blue,[133] who reported good results with glenoid osteotomy for posterior dislocation of the shoulder in cerebral palsy patients.

Still other rare congenital dislocations may be seen. These may be grouped as pure posterior dislocation or classified as a separate group. In one such case a clinical diagnosis of posterior-inferior dislocation was made in a 5-month-old infant. Roentgenograms confirmed the diagnosis (Fig. 20-38A). It was believed to be congenital in nature since there was no birth trauma and no ossification center on the dislocated side. A gentle manipulation was tried but failed to change the position of the humeral head. For the next 6 years the patient was followed clinically and the head of the humerus developed without treatment but failed to keep pace with that of the normal side. Its shape was slightly flattened. Its relationship to the glenoid fossa improved (Fig. 20-38B). More important, there was painless, functional motion. Laskin and Sedlin reported one rare case of luxatio erecta incurred during forcible manipulation of the arm of an infant with Erb-Duchenne palsy that required open reduction.[134] They reviewed the literature and found that such cases of this rare dislocation may be classified under three separate groups: (1) those with true congenital forms; (2) those secondary to birth trauma; and (3) those with dislocations resulting

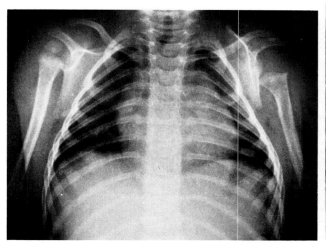
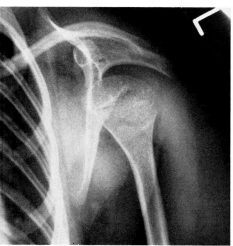

A   B

FIG. 20-38. A, A chronic posterior-inferior dislocation was diagnosed in a 5-month-old infant. There was no birth injury and no history of trauma. The diagnosis was made when the child showed restricted use of the shoulder, flattening of the normal anterior shoulder contour, but no other abnormal findings. A few attempts at gentle manipulation while the baby was under general anesthesia failed to reduce the dislocation. At 1 year of age underdevelopment of the proximal humerus with persistent posterior-inferior dislocation was noted. B, At 6 years of age note the flattened humeral head still posteriorly dislocated. The patient lacked full overhead and external rotation motion, but had suprisingly good left upper extremity function.

from long-standing brachial plexus palsies. The first group are characterized by their presence at birth, and later retardation of bony development of the shoulder (Fig. 20-38).

Chronic Unreduced Dislocations. When a posterior dislocation of the shoulder is missed initially, the surgeon may attempt closed reduction in a chronic unreduced shoulder dislocation as long as 2 weeks and perhaps as long as 4 weeks in some cases following injury. The longer the delay, the less chance is present that reduction can be effected. Moreover, the larger the defect that often locks the head on the posterior glenoid rim, the less chance exists of accomplishing a closed reduction with delay of treatment. This delay may occur because the patient has not come for treatment or the diagnosis may have been missed (Figs. 20-30 and 20-34B).

Closed manipulation must never be tried unless the patient is under general anesthesia, and force must never be used. Repeated manipulations should be avoided.

After 2 to 4 weeks open reduction is required to achieve reduction. The longer the delay in reduction, the more extensive must be the dissection of the surrounding scarred structures if open reduction is contemplated. Oyston reported a case of unreduced posterior dislocation of 3 months' duration in which an open reduction and transfer of the subscapularis into the defect were accomplished with an excellent result.[143]

If excessive stripping of the soft tissues must be performed to reduce such a dislocation as described by Neviaser using a superior approach, the end result is not likely to be satisfactory.[141] In such cases an arthrodesis, a Neer humeral replacement if the rotator muscles are functioning, or a fixed fulcrum total shoulder replacement if there are nonfunctioning rotator muscles can be considered, depending upon the circumstances. When the dislocation is long standing and there is minimal discomfort, particularly if the patient is elderly or is in a tenuous medical state, it is best left alone (Fig. 20-34B).

COMPLICATIONS. I have not encountered any complications with posterior shoulder dislocations, because neurovascular injury does not usually occur when the humeral head is displaced away from the anterior neurovascular structures.

ACROMIOCLAVICULAR JOINT

Over the years there has been great controversy and many varied methods of treatment for acromioclavicular joint dislocation. Some of the questions that the surgeon must consider before rendering treatment are (1) whether the injury should be treated surgically or conservatively; (2) if operation is decided upon which method would be best and when should it be performed; and (3) will the results of operation be better than those of conservative treatment. The vulnerability of this joint especially to athletic injuries requires answers to these questions.

ANATOMY AND FUNCTION.[177,192,197,237] The acromioclavicular joint is a diarthrodial articulation positioned between the acromial end of the clavicle and the medial side of the scapula. The superior acromioclavicular ligament is composed of parallel fibers which interlace with the aponeuroses of the trapezius and deltoid. It is stronger than the thinner inferior acromioclavicular ligament. The joint may have an articular disc but often it does not. There is usually one synovial membrane present in the joint unless a complete disc is present. In this event there may be two synovial membranes.[197] Bosworth reported that the average size of the acromioclavicular joint surface is 9 by 19 mm.[173] DePalma reported a great variation in the plane of the joint which probably relates to the degree of movement that is possible.[186-188] Codman stated there was little movement in this articulation.[181]

The other important ligament that connects the clavicle with the coracoid is the coracoclavicular ligament, composed of the trapezoid and conoid portions. They serve to strengthen the thin inferior acromioclavicular ligament.

The trapezoid ligament is broad, thick, and quadrilateral. It attaches to the superior surface of the coracoid, and runs to the oblique ridge on the inferior surface of the clavicle behind the tendon of the pectoralis minor lateral to the conoid ligament.

The conoid ligament is a dense band of fibers, conical in form, whose base is directed superiorly. The ligament attaches to the coracoid tuberosity on the undersurface of the clavicle, and runs to the base of the coracoid process medial to the trapezoid.

The function of the acromioclavicular joint permits (1) a gliding motion of the articular end of the clavicle on the acromion, and (2) rotation of the scapula on the clavicle especially during abduction of the arm. The acromion is fixed a specific distance from the sternum by the clavicle thus serving as the radius of a circle through which the acromion can move. This joint allows the scapula to change its position as it moves on the chest wall.[251] Bosworth found the average distance between the clavicle and coracoid to be 1.3 cm.,[173] and Bearden and associates reported this space varied from 1.1 to 1.3 cm.[165]

Because the clavicle serves as the connecting strut with the axial skeleton, the strength and integrity of the coracoclavicular ligament are important. Cadenat,[177] in 1917, and Watkins,[242] in 1925, reported that a traumatic disruption of the acromioclavicular ligament produces a partial acromioclavicular dislocation, whereas a more severe injury that causes a tear of the coracoclavicular ligament is necessary for a complete dislocation to occur.

Urist reported a unique series of findings obtained from experiments on cadavers.[237] First, the coracoclavicular ligaments were transected and traction was placed on the lateral clavicle. Motion was not in excess of the intact opposite side.

Second, when the superior acromioclavicular ligament and the whole joint capsule was incised in a second shoulder, incomplete disarticulation could be produced in only 50 percent of the shoulders. In this specimen the attachments of the deltoid and trapezius to the clavicle were then divided. Now when the end of the clavicle was pulled upward and posteriorly, complete disarticulation resulted, and when traction was applied upward, again only incomplete disarticulation occurred. The coracoclavicular ligaments were cut in this second shoulder specimen and complete disarticulation of the outer end of the clavicle occurred.

In a third shoulder, the trapezoid ligament was cut along with the deltoid and trapezius attachments to the clavicle, as well as the superior acromioclavicular ligaments. Traction upward or posteriorly caused complete dislocation. In a fourth experiment, the same structures were divided as were severed in the third shoulder except that the conoid ligament was cut instead of the trapezoid. The result with traction caused further upward dislocation of the acromial end of the clavicle.

In a last experiment the same structures were cut as were divided in the third and fourth experiments except that the coracoacromial ligament was cut, first alone and then in combination with the other ligaments, and no effect on the stability of the acromioclavicular joint was noted.

Urist concluded from these experiments that complete dislocation of the acromioclavicular joint occurred without rupture of the coracoclavicular ligament.[237] However, the definition of dislocation must be reviewed. If a vertical displacement of the end of the clavicle as defined by Tossy and co-workers[234] and Imatani and associates[202] is accepted, then true vertical dislocation does require the rupture of the coracoclavicular ligament. Urist's findings are correct. But it is probably the acromioclavicular ligaments that control horizontal stability. Thus, to-and-fro movement of the distal clavicle must be differentiated from true vertical upward dislocation. Moreover, he correctly concluded the importance of the capsule, the deltoid and trapezius attachments to the clavicle, and the acromion in maintaining acromioclavicular joint integrity.

Coracoclavicular Articulation. Gradoyevitch,[198] in 1939, and Nutter,[223] in 1941, described the not uncommon finding of coracoclavicular articulation occurring in 1.2 percent in a review of 1,000 random roentgenograms.[223] These articulations are believed to be true joints formed by the bony outgrowths of the clavicle at the site of the conoid attachment. Pillay believed one fourth of these joints studied in his series were true diarthrodial joints.[227] The patient with such a finding is asymptomatic. Six of twelve cases in Nutter's series were bilateral.

Roentgenograms show a triangular bony outgrowth from the undersurface of the clavicle (see Fig. 5-13). The lateral side of the outgrowth forms the articular surface with the tubercle on the upper, medial surface of the coracoid process.

Acromioclavicular Joint Motion. In a classic paper Inman, Saunders, and Abbott showed the total range of motion at the acromioclavicular joint was about 20 degrees, occurring both in the first 30 degrees of abduction and after 135 degrees of elevation of the arm.[203] Between these two points almost no motion occurred in this joint. Caldwell,[178] Kennedy and Cameron,[208] and Kennedy[207] showed that a screw placed across the coracoclavicular space, in effect, gives an arthrodesis between the coracoid and clavicle, but still allows full arm abduction. Kennedy and Cameron term this movement with such a screw in place as "synchronous scapuloclavicular rotation."[208]

CLASSIFICATION. Allman has classified sprains of the acromioclavicular joint into grades I, II, and III[156] (Fig. 20-39).

Grade I sprains result from a mild force with tearing of only a few fibers of the acromioclavicular ligament and capsule. There is no instability of the joint (Fig. 20-39B).

Grade II sprains result from a moderate force which causes rupture of the capsule and acromioclavicular ligament (Figs. 20-39C and 20-40). This injury often causes a subluxation. The coracoclavicular ligament is not ruptured.

Grade III sprains of the joint result from a severe force which ruptures both the acromioclavicular and coracoclavicular ligaments. Grade III injuries produce dislocations of the acromioclavicular joint (Figs. 20-39D and 20-41).

Rarely, a posterior displacement of the

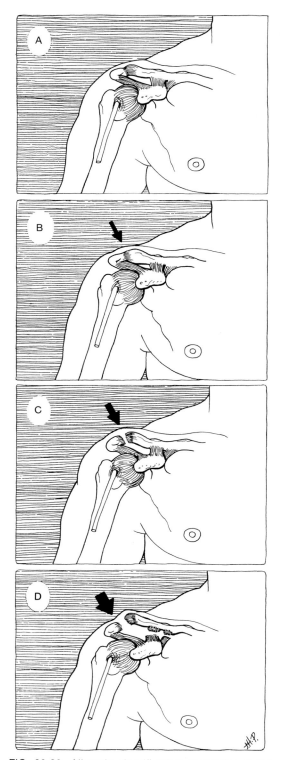

FIG. 20-39. Allman's classification of sprains of the acromioclavicular joint. A, Normal; B, grade I; C, grade II; D, grade III (see text for discussion).

lateral clavicle may occur following a blow to the distal end of the clavicle.[156] Finally, Patterson reported a case of inferior dislocation of the distal clavicle which required open reduction and a transfixion pin across the joint because the end of the clavicle locked beneath the coracoid behind the conjoined tendon.[225] He stated his belief that wide abduction and retraction of the scapula was the cause of injury, and recommended open reduction to obviate later possible neurologic deficit.

INCIDENCE OF ACROMIOCLAVICULAR JOINT INJURIES. Rowe and Marble reviewed 1603 shoulder-girdle injuries at the Massachusetts General Hospital and found 52 acromioclavicular injuries.[231] Fifteen percent were grade I, 34 percent were grade II, and 51 percent were grade III (complete dislocation). They found that most of the injuries occurred in the second decade of life, but otherwise there was an even distribution between 20 and 60 years of age. The experience at Michael Reese Hospital indicates that many more grade I and grade II injuries occur than grade III in all age groups, but that most occur in the second decade of life.

MECHANISM OF INJURY. *Direct Force.* Injuries of the acromioclavicular joint usually result from a fall onto the point of the shoulder. The harder the blow, the more severe is the injury. When this happens there is a forceful, sudden depression of the shoulder tip with the arm in slight internal rotation and abduction.[165,175]

At first the scapula is suddenly depressed and pulls its attached clavicle though the suspensory coracoclavicular ligament. With a severe force the medial part of the clavicle strikes the first rib, the latter producing an opposing resistance and causing a concentrating force at the acromioclavicular and coracoclavicular ligaments.

Indirect Force. Injury to the acromioclavicular joint may be caused through a force transmitted from a fall on the elbow or outstretched hand thereby forcing the humeral head against the undersurface of the acromion. Nielsen reviewed 101 injuries of the acromioclavicular joint and found only

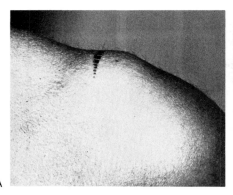
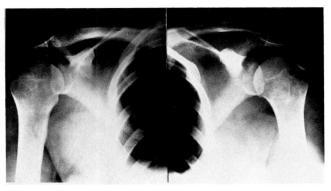

A

B

FIG. 20-40. A, A 23-year-old man fell on the point of his shoulder and sustained a grade II subluxation of the acromioclavicular joint. Note the abrasion and the degree of upward displacement of the clavicle. B, Comparison anteroposterior views of the joints with 10 pounds of weight suspended from his wrists show the degree of subluxation of the clavicle. He was treated with a harness for 25 days and the results were excellent.

5 percent was due to a fall on the outstretched hand, whereas 70 percent was caused by direct injury.[221]

PATHOLOGY. As the severity of the injury is related to increased injury to the anatomic structures comprising the acromioclavicular joint, a sequence of pathologic changes occur. Anything from a mild sprain, causing small tears of the capsular ligaments, to a severe sprain, causing a disruption of all the surrounding ligaments and tearing of the clavicular attachments of the deltoid and trapezius muscles, may occur (Fig. 20-42). Wilson and Prothero

found an incidence of 31 percent of meniscus tear in their series of 30 cases.[245] There may be associated fractures of the acromion, clavicle, or coracoid process.

DIAGNOSIS. Because extensive tearing of the ligaments may not produce visible dislocation early without stressing the extremity, it is important first to examine the patient thoroughly and take a complete history.

The patient will point to the area of pain at the acromioclavicular joint. The pain does not usually radiate, and its severity is related to the degree of injury. The arm is

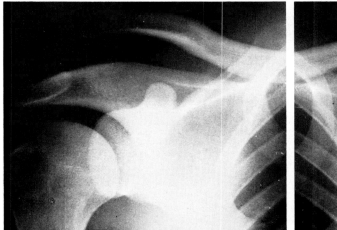
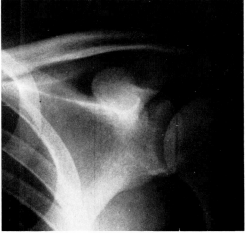

A

B

FIG. 20-41. A 22-year-old man fell on his shoulder and sustained a grade III acromioclavicular joint dislocation. Comparison films show the extent of displacement of the right clavicle without using weights.

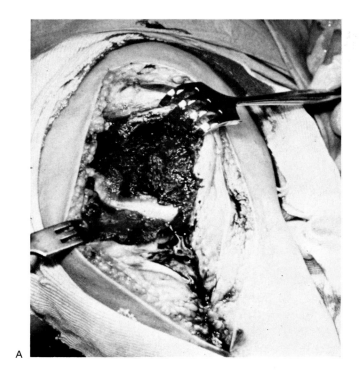

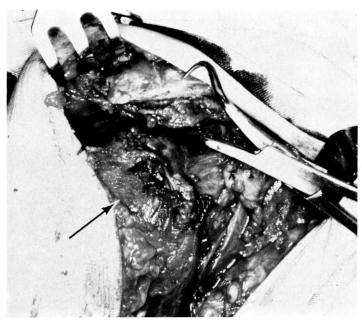

FIG. 20-42. A 25-year-old man sustained an acromioclavicular dislocation. There was an avulsion of the trapezius and deltoid aponeuroses, respectively, from their lateral clavicle attachment, leaving a denuded lateral clavicle that was discovered during operation. A, Following separation of the deltoid and trapezius, note the extensive hematoma and torn tissue about the acromioclavicular joint 4 days after injury. B, A towel clip displaces the clavicle upward. Note the extensive tearing of the meniscus. Arrow points to the avulsed deltoid. Following Dacron tape graft repair, the trapezius and deltoid were imbricated and firmly sutured to the clavicle. The result was excellent.

voluntarily splinted at the side and all movements are restricted because of pain.

Physical examination may show a swelling, an abrasion, or a deformity over the acromioclavicular joint (Fig. 20-48A). Ecchymosis may be present. Local tenderness is evident in grade I injuries and may be exquisite in grade III injuries. Tenderness may be present over the coracoid and lateral infraclavicular region.

In grade II dislocation it may be possible to palpate increased back-and-forth motion early when manipulating the clavicle from its central portion. In grade III injuries it may be possible to move the end of the clavicle from a dislocated to a reduced position and vice versa, thereby confirming the true diagnosis. Moreover, in grade III injuries the clavicle may be ballotable. If this is the case torn tissue may be interposed beneath the dislocated clavicle. This finding is especially useful after 3 weeks when the reduced clavicle stabilizes, and a positive result of ballottement at this time suggests that conservative treatment is ineffective.[237]

Active arm adduction is limited because this motion increases pain.[175] Any movement of the shoulder downward, upward, forward, or backward exacerbates the pain. Active elevation about the horizontal, in the frontal, and parasagittal planes causes pain in the last third of the movement, and does not usually exceed 140 degrees. The reason why pain is not often produced during the first 90 degrees of abduction relates to the glenohumeral motion almost entirely in this phase while the scapula is fixed. Beyond 90 degrees the scapula tilts and pain is felt by the patient. Brosgol points out this feature in differentiating glenohumeral joint injuries wherein the glenohumeral joint is splinted and the patient abducts from the beginning by tilting the scapula.[175]

If the trapezius is torn, lateral flexion of the head away from the side of injury causes pain.

Roentgenographic Examination. With the patient preferably standing or sitting on a stool, the acromioclavicular joint may appear normal on anteroposterior roentgenograms or show widening of the joint space, subluxation (Fig. 20-40B), complete dislocation (Fig. 20-41), and associated fractures of the acromion, coracoid, or lateral clavicle (Fig. 20-43). The views of both joints should be identical.[183]

In order to differentiate a grade II and grade III injury 5 to 15 pounds of weight, depending on the size of the patient, should be suspended from each wrist and anteroposterior films obtained (Fig. 20-44). When the weights are held in the hands the patient has a tendency to lift the extremity involuntarily which possibly decreases the injured joint separation. Therefore, the weights should be suspended from the wrists. Bearden and associates stated that an increase of up to 4 mm. in the coracoclavicular space, greater than the normal average distance of 1.1 to 1.3 cm., indicates partial dislocation.[165] Over a 40 to 50 percent increase in the space can be considered a complete dislocation. The normal joint

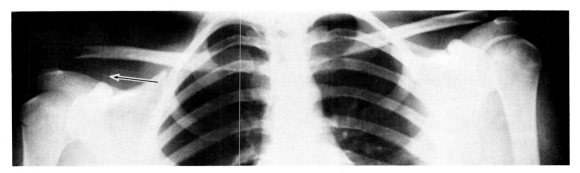

FIG. 20-43. A 14-year-old girl sustained a grade III acromioclavicular dislocation. Right shoulder shows the dislocation. Avulsion of a piece of bone from the coracoid (arrow) is not present in the left shoulder.

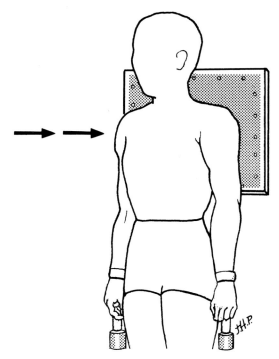

FIG. 20-44. Method for obtaining similar anteroposterior views of the acromioclavicular joints. The weights should be suspended from the wrists and not be held by the patient. Arrows indicate direction of the x-ray beam.

space itself ranges from 1 to 3 mm.[223] With joint degeneration following pin transfixion the space may narrow (see Fig. 20-52C), or become wider in subluxation.

In grade I injury the joint on the initial film is normal but later films may show subperiosteal calcification at the distal clavicle.[156] Roentgenograms of grade II sprains reveal some upward displacement of the clavicle, and grade III films show severe displacement.

Arthrography of the acromioclavicular joint is not particularly useful in diagnosing an acute injury but may have some prognostic value in the treatment of joint ligament tears.[175] I do not have experience in this technique especially since a standard study of the normal is not known.

Finally, if the surgeon is planning an operation that requires an intact coracoid for the placement of a loop or suture, Dacron tape, or screw from the clavicle to the cora-

coid, it must be predetermined that there is no fracture, and that the bone is not osteoporotic. An angled view with the x-ray tube pointed upward will disclose such an injury. If the coracoid is intact and there is a dislocation it is likely that the coracoclavicular ligament is intact and has avulsed the coracoid process or a portion of it (Fig. 20-43).

MANAGEMENT. *Closed Methods for Grades I and II Sprains.* The surgeon should establish a correct diagnosis and understand the pathologic alterations before undertaking treatment. There is general agreement that grade I and grade II sprains should be treated conservatively.

Grade I sprains should be protected until most of the pain has subsided. Immediately following the injury ice packs may be applied to the injured joint for relief of pain as tolerated. After the second day warm packs may be applied to the injured joint. Sling support is used for 4 to 10 days depending upon the symptoms. Thereafter, a gradual increase in activities is started. Full activity is not permitted for 3 to 4 weeks even if there is a full range of painless motion early.[164] I have examined young, athletic patients who have returned to full activity within the first 2 weeks after injury. Occasionally, pain has returned, thus prolonging the treatment because of zealous activity too early.

Grade II sprains are immobilized for 3 weeks (Fig. 20-40). I have tried a variety of splints including harnesses, braces, halters,[156,184,193,194,196,206,208,233,236,237,239,241] and adhesive taping methods.[229] For those surgeons who use other methods and an axillary pad beware of the roll that causes a neurapraxia of the nerves in the high medial arm. I have seen two referred cases with just such complications that took weeks to several months to resolve. Adhesive taping treatment often causes irritation and excoriation of the skin especially in warm weather. The Kenny Howard-type sling-halter advocated by Allman works satisfactorily in the cooperative patient[156] (Fig. 20-45). The other devices are troublesome and do not seem to work well in my experience.

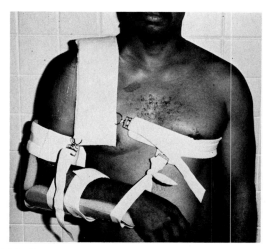

FIG. 20-45. A 45-year-old man sustained a grade III acromioclavicular dislocation that was unsuccessfully treated with adhesive taping. For this reason, he was treated with a harness device.

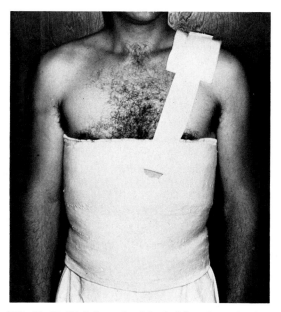

FIG. 20-46. Wolin's method for holding the reduction in a dislocated acromioclavicular joint. Note the molded cast over the iliac crests. A padded canvas strap is held with a buckle.

In accomplishing reduction in grade II subluxation in the acute phase, local anesthetic injection may be used. As a resident I was instructed in an excellent method of immobilization for grades II and III injuries many years ago by the late Dr. Irving Wolin.[246] He gave credit for the method to the late Dr. Hunkin of San Francisco. In this method a molded body cast with well-padded iliac crests is applied (Fig. 20-46). A canvas strap with felt pressure pad is applied over the end of the clavicle. In the first several days a sling also may be used if there is severe pain. The patient should be seen twice the first week, and at least once weekly thereafter in order to tighten the strap which may loosen. Roentgenograms are taken periodically to be certain that the reduction position is being maintained. This method leaves the extremity free for gentle activities and is usually well tolerated by the patient. I prefer the Wolin-Hunkin method for most cases of grades II and III sprains.[246]

After 3 weeks immobilization is stopped and gentle motion exercises are permitted depending upon the type of activity and any residual symptoms.

I have not had to perform excision arthroplasty for grade II sprains except in two cases in 20 years. The patients required an excision of the end of the clavicle lateral to the intact coracoclavicular ligament because they developed a painful, progressive arthritis of the acromioclavicular joint. Before operating upon such a joint, steroid injection therapy may be tried.

A significant number of grade III dislocations can be treated by closed methods described previously. Quigley,[230] Arner and associates,[158] Jacobs and Wade,[205] and Imatani and co-workers[202] recommended conservative treatment. In treating athletic injuries Glick recommended conservative treatment, believing normal function is regained in a short period of time despite the severity of the dislocation.[195] These authors suggest that results of closed treatment are as good as those of open treatment. Jacobs and Wade go so far as to state that it does not matter what method is employed as long as it is used correctly, because any residual symptoms depend upon the extent of tissue injury in and about the joint.[205] I concur in this statement.

I recommend a trial of conservative

treatment using a sling-halter device or preferably the Wolin-Hunkin cast-strap method for 6 to 8 weeks. The patient should be seen twice the first week and at least once a week thereafter to tighten the straps and maintain reduction. This should be confirmed by roentgenograms periodically. After 6 weeks motion exercises are gradually increased. Not until 8 to 10 weeks later is full activity allowed in order to permit adequate ligament healing (Fig. 20-47).

For those patients who cannot tolerate the strap device and in whom conservative treatment is not effective for various reasons, or in those individuals who wish to be assured that they will not have any unsightly bump open treatment is indicated. For example, an abraded area over the injured joint will prevent conservative treatment in most cases (Fig. 20-48).

Open Methods for Grade III Dislocation. When conservative treatment fails, or the patient is not a candidate for closed methods, or the patient, usually a woman, will not accept an unsightly deformity at the shoulder, open treatment is indicated (Fig. 20-48). In any event the chief goals of any treatment are to achieve stability under any kind of stress, and painless, full motion.[228] The purpose of surgical treatment is (1) to restore the anatomy of the acromioclavicular joint as near to normal as possible, (2) to maintain the reduction of the dislocation by any number of methods of internal fixation until effective ligament healing has occurred, and (3) to restore the dynamic action of any torn structures such as the deltoid and trapezius so that the chief goals are likely to be met during the acute phase of injury. In the chronic phase of injury where there is weakness and residual pain only surgical treatment will be of benefit. Whatever treatment method, conservative or surgical, is selected for each individual, success depends to a large extent on the patient's cooperation and the surgeon's exactitude to detail. It is not so much a matter of which treatment is better, but with which treatment the patient will do best. Nicoll believed that surgical treatment did not give better results than closed methods.[220] Those operations that have been found useful in treating acute and chronic grade III acromioclavicular dislocations are:

1. Coracoclavicular ligament repair, fixation, or reconstruction[91,155,164,165,208,209,214,239,245]
2. Acromioclavicular joint repair, internal fixation, or reconstruction[154,156,164,176,213,217,219]
3. Dynamic muscle transfers[161,162,189]
4. Excision of lateral clavicle[153,164,199,210,212,214,244,246]

Coracoclavicular Ligament Repair, Fixation, or Reconstruction. The evaluation of surgical procedures to treat acromioclavicular dislocations began in earnest with Cadenat in 1917, who transferred the cut end of the coracoacromial ligament from its coracoid attachment and sutured it to the remnants of the conoid, the periosteum on the posterior-superior clavicle, and the aponeurotic attachment of the trapezius.[177] Campos modified Cadenat's procedure by freeing the acromial insertion of the coracoacromial ligament after reduction and implanting it in a hole in the lateral clavicle.[179] In 1925, Watkins used a stout silk suture to hold the reduced clavicle to the

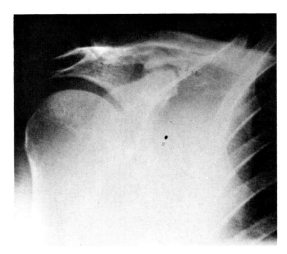

FIG. 20-47. A 27-year-old man was treated with a harness device for grade III acromioclavicular dislocation. Note the extensive calcification in the infraclavicular space. The result was excellent.

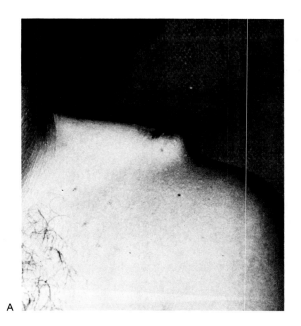

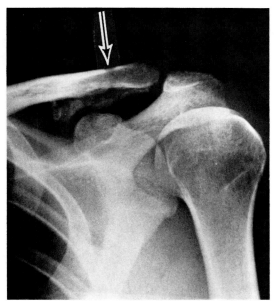

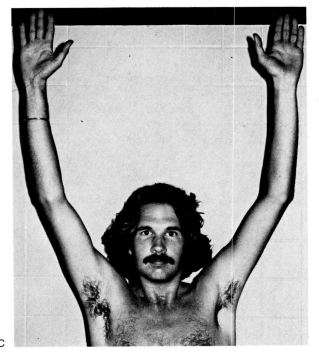

FIG. 20-48. A, A 20-year-old man sustained a grade III dislocation. He had a deep abrasion over the lateral end of the clavicle. Operation was performed 1 week later in order to allow the abrasion to heal. B, Arrow shows the hole through which a 4-mm. Dacron tape graft was placed to hold the clavicle in reduction. At 4 weeks postoperatively note the calcification in the space between the clavicle and coracoid. The trapezius and deltoid aponeuroses were plicated (see text for discussion). C, Six weeks postoperatively, note the extent of painless overhead motion. At 6 months overhead motion was complete.

coracoid, first "cleaning out the space between the coracoid and clavicle."[242] A large number of modified operations using suture, wire, fascia lata, and synthetic materials are based on Watkin's work. Carrell used fascia lata strips to hold the clavicle to the coracoacromial ligament near its coracoid attachment,[180] whereas Schneider[232] and Birkett[168] used fascia lata strips looped about the coracoid itself. Both repaired the joint using smaller fascia lata strips. Gallie reported excellent results with fascia lata strips wrapped around the coracoid and over the lateral clavicle.[191] Bowers employed heavy silk suture to repair the joint and also looped from the clavicle about the coracoid.[174] Anderson used a temporary heavy wire about the acromioclavicular joint.[157] Alldredge employed a wire loop between the clavicle and coracoid,[155] and Bearden and associates used two loops of wire between the clavicle and coracoid, first removing torn interposed tissue in the acromioclavicular joint, and then repairing any detached deltoid-trapezius muscle.[165] Vargas used a portion of the short head of the biceps looped through a hole in the clavicle.[238] Laing transferred the long biceps head through drill holes in the coracoid and clavicle to maintain reduction.[209] In a recent modification Harrison and Sisler described the use of a Dacron tube placed through a hole in the clavicle and looped about the coracoid process[200] (Figs. 20-48 and 20-49).

In 1941, Bosworth described his technique of holding the clavicle in reduction by placing a screw through the superior clavicle into the coracoid below[171] (Fig. 20-50). He used a lag screw with a flat head. In subsequent reports he did not repair the coracoclavicular ligament nor explore the joint.[172,173] Later, Kennedy and Cameron[208] and Kennedy[207] modified the technique by debriding the acromioclavicular joint, overcorrecting the clavicle, and after the insertion of a lag screw, repairing the detached trapezius and deltoid muscles. Kennedy attempted to enhance healing in the coracoclavicular space in acute cases by placing the drilled bone dust into the space, whereas in chronic cases he used refrigerated bone. Thus, any ossification obtained in the coracoclavicular space stabilizes the clavicle without interfering with the rotation of the clavicle. Kennedy and Cameron found that less favorable results were achieved with Bosworth screw fixation in

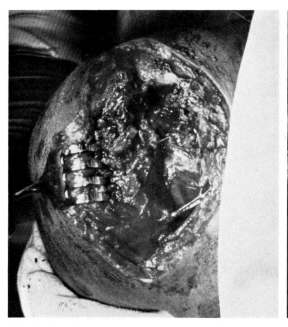
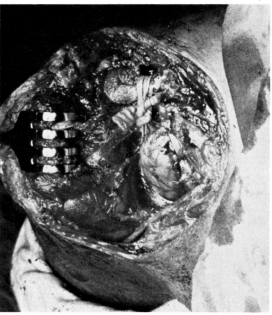

A   B

FIG. 20-49. A 25-year-old man sustained a grade III acromioclavicular dislocation that was unsuccessfully treated by closed methods. A, Retraction of the deltoid at operation shows the extent of tearing in the infraclavicular space. A 4-mm. Dacron tube was prestretched and placed through a hole in the clavicle and about the base of the coracoid (see text for discussion). B, The Dacron graft was tied and oversewn with suture to prevent loosening of the knot. Preoperative x-ray films excluded a fracture of the coracoid. Immobilization in a sling was continued for 5 weeks and gentle motion exercises were then started. The result was excellent.

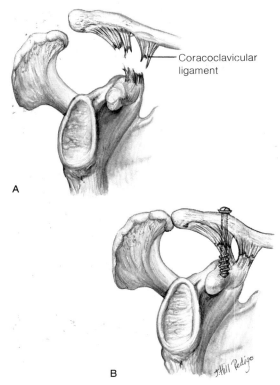

Coracoclavicular ligament

A

B

FIG. 20-50. Bosworth screw fixation method for treating acromioclavicular dislocations. Preoperative x-ray films must be obtained in order to exclude coracoid fracture.

older than in younger patients.[208] Weitzman reported on 24 cases on which he used a modified Bosworth method.[244] He reduced the dislocation under direct vision, removed the meniscus, and then inserted a lag screw across the clavicle into the coracoid. He imbricated the deltoid and trapezius muscles in the manner similar to that described by Bundens and Cook.[176] Weitzman believed his excellent to good results in 17 of 19 patients, followed clinically for more than 24 months, related to the removal of interposed soft tissues within the joint.

Acromioclavicular Repair, Internal Fixation, or Reconstruction. In 1942 Phemister reported a method of open reduction and internal dual wire fixation of the dislocated acromioclavicular joint[226] (Figs. 20-51 and 20-52). Bloom reported his series of cases.[169] I agree with his statement that 25 percent of the wires loosen and migrate toward the skin. Occasionally, they will erode through the skin. Bundens and Cook employed this method but also imbricate the trapezius and deltoid muscles over the top of the clavicle.[176] Ahstrom uses wires and a portion of the short head of the biceps to hold down the clavicle.[154] Rowe and Marble recom-

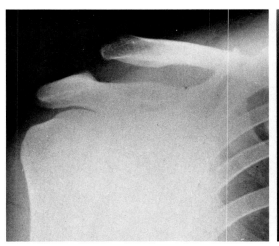

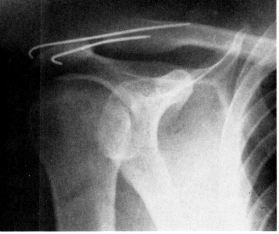

A

B

FIG. 20-51. A, Anterosuperior film of the shoulder shows an acromioclavicular dislocation. B, Following open reduction and internal fixation. The smooth pins were removed at 6 weeks. The extremity was maintained in a sling for 4 weeks. The result was excellent. (Reprinted from Post, M., and Haskell, S.: Fractures and Dislocations of the Shoulder Girdle, Ribs, and Sternum, Chapter 8. In Practice of Surgery, Volume 2, Orthopedics, 1973 revision, with permission of the Medical Department, Harper & Row, Publishers, Inc., Hagerstown, Md.)

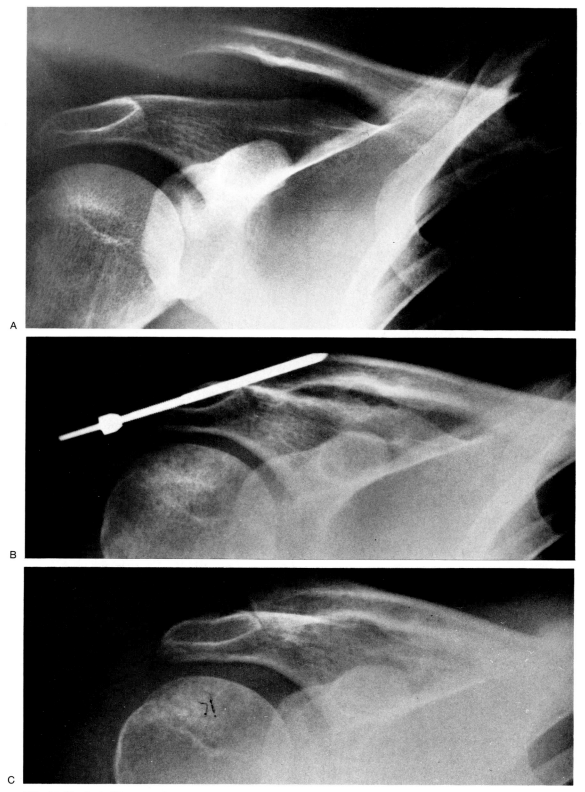

FIG. 20-52. A, A 29-year-old man sustained a grade III acromioclavicular dislocation that was unsuccessfully treated by closed methods. B, A smooth pin was used to hold the clavicle in a reduced position for 6 weeks and then removed. C, Observe the marked narrowing of the joint 3 years later. The result was excellent.

mended the use of one or two smooth wires introduced across the joint in a retrograde manner with further stabilization of the joint by using the detached coracoacromial ligament from the coracoid.[231] Neviaser described his technique of stabilizing the joint with one pin and using the detached coracoclavicular ligament[204,217-219] (Fig. 20-53A). Moshein and Elconin reported 10 cases in which they reinforced the joint ligaments by repairing the coracoclavicular ligament directly, or by utilizing the detached coracoid end of the coracoacromial ligament.[213] Weaver and Dunn[243] modified Neviaser's[217-219] coracoacromial ligament transfer by placing the cut end of the shortened ligament into the medullary canal of the clavicle (Fig. 20-53B). They believed that removal of the lateral 2 cm. of clavicle precluded symptomatic late arthritis. They

used this technique in acute and chronic cases with good results.

Dynamic Muscle Transfers. In 1965, Dewar and Barrington described their method for restoring a chronically dislocated acromioclavicular joint by transferring the coracoid tip with its conjoined tendon to the end of the clavicle, and reported good results in five patients.[189] Bailey and associates enlarged the number of indications for this method by including acute fractures of the lateral clavicle associated with rupture of the coracoclavicular ligament, and old painful injuries of the joint associated with traumatic arthritis.[161,162] The principle involves a dynamic downward pull on the clavicle by the conjoined structures.

Excision of the End of the Clavicle. In 1941 Gurd[199] and Mumford[214] independently described their methods for resection of the distal clavicle as a method of treating acromioclavicular separation. Although Gurd believed that the operation was best for complete dislocations,[199] Mumford reported that the technique was best for subluxations, and favored the use of fascial repair of the acutely torn coracoclavicular ligament.[214] In 1961 Lazcano and co-workers stated that excision of the lateral clavicle alone gave satisfactory results in eight cases and in seven additional cases when combined with other methods.[210] However, six cases showed persistent upward displacement of the clavicle which did not perturb the patients or cause symptoms. Accardo reported consistently good results by this method for acute and chronic cases.[153] Wilson and Prothero reported on several operative methods for correcting acromioclavicular dislocation and stated that excision of the distal clavicle was best in their study.[245] Weaver and Dunn report good results by resecting the lateral 2 cm. of clavicle and transposing the coracoacromial ligament from the coracoid to the medullary portion of the clavicle.[243] The detached deltoid and trapezius structures are sutured together over the clavicle. Moseley and Templeton recommended that outer clavicle excision be avoided; they concentrate on restoration

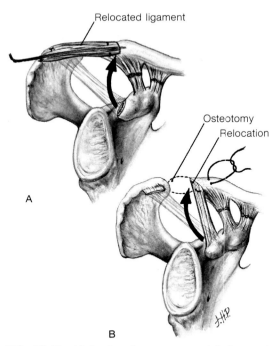

Relocated ligament

Osteotomy
Relocation

A

B

FIG. 20-53. Methods of coracoacromial ligament transfer. A, Neviaser method for repairing a grade III acromioclavicular dislocation using a smooth wire and the coracoacromial ligament. B, Weaver-Dunn's method for repairing a grade III acromioclavicular dislocation by transferring the coracoacromial ligament into the medullary canal of the clavicle after oblique osteotomy of the lateral 2 cm.

of the anatomy of the acromioclavicular joint.[212] Nielson resected the lateral clavicle 23 times in 101 cases and reported poor results.[221]

Arthrodesis. Cooper was probably one of the first to report successful arthrodesis of the "scapuloclavicular" joint for dislocation.[182] After removal of the joint cartilage, he successfully performed this operation in three patients using a silver wire to hold the clavicle in a reduced position. Caldwell reported satisfactory results in two cases with surgical fusion of the acromioclavicular joint.[178] Brosgol stated it is difficult to obtain an arthrodesis.[175] DePalma reported that such an arthrodesis diminishes shoulder abduction by at least 20 percent.[185] I have had no experience with this method.

AUTHOR'S METHODS OF TREATMENT. *Acromioclavicular Dislocation.* If the dislocated clavicle can be reduced manually or can be overcorrected, an attempt is made to treat the patient conservatively. If there is ballottement or a rubbery sensation during manipulation it indicates that there is a torn meniscus or interposed tissue, and surgery is recommended.[159] An abraded area of the skin will prevent the application of an external pressure device. In this case the skin area is left open until dry, and operation is performed as long as a week later. The very elderly or poor medical-risk patient is treated with a sling or harness as tolerated, and the probable functional and cosmetic results that can be expected are explained. For the patient who is uncooperative and in whom conservative treatment fails operation is performed.

I have seen a few cases in which the screw has pulled away from the coracoid, and so prefer other methods that do not require a second operation, albeit simple, to remove the screw or wire.

Coracoclavicular Repair.[163,200] I prefer the loop method of Harrison and Sisler, using a 4- or 5-mm. Dacron tube, especially in young patients[200] (Fig. 20-49). It is particularly well suited when there is an associated fracture of the distal clavicle. I inspect the acromioclavicular joint and remove the meniscus if it is badly torn along with any other interposed tissue. The bone should not be osteoporotic and the coracoid must be intact when using this method. The trapezius and deltoid are imbricated over the superior clavicle.

The operation is performed through a curved incision over the acromioclavicular joint which is extended downward just distal to the medial side of the coracoid process. The acromioclavicular joint is inspected and the meniscus removed if torn and displaced. Often the deltoid and trapezius attachments to the clavicle are also torn. Occasionally, the clavicle is buttonholed through the aponeuroses of these structures. An opening is made beneath the conjoined tendon inferior to the coracoid process. A $\frac{1}{4}$-in. hole is made in the lateral clavicle. A 4- or 5-mm. Dacron tube graft is prestretched. A heavy suture is placed through one end of the graft, and then through the hole in the clavicle using a curved aneurysm needle. The graft is passed beneath the coracoid in a similar manner. An assistant holds the clavicle in reduction using a pusher bar with a dull serrated edge while the surgeon ties a snug square knot (Fig. 20-49B). It is important to hold the clavicle in a reduced position using a pusher bar and not attempt reduction by tightening the Dacron tape. Each cut end of the graft is oversewn to the loop to be certain the knot does not open postoperatively. The deltoid and trapezius are then imbricated over the superior clavicle. The wound is closed.

The patient is discharged on the third postoperative day, and the extremity is kept in a sling for 2 to 3 weeks. Roentgenograms are taken immediately postoperatively as a baseline and weekly for 3 weeks, particularly if the patient uses his extremity. Activities are gradually increased. After 8 weeks full activities are permitted (Fig. 20-48).

In the event that a deep infection results, the graft may need to be removed. In one such case the Dacron graft was removed at 3 weeks. Fibrous tissue had invaded the graft. The result was good because enough scarring had occurred to hold the clavicle reduced in any event.

Acromioclavicular Joint Repair. If the dislocation is not too severe, can be easily reduced, or there is a fractured or osteoporotic coracoid, and the patient cannot be treated by closed methods, I use smooth transfixion wires to maintain the reduction of the acromioclavicular joint (Figs. 20-51 and 20-52). If the coracoid is fractured and open reduction is necessary, it is not enough merely to fix the coracoid with a screw or heavy suture, even if the coracoclavicular ligament is intact. I also recommend maintaining joint reduction with transfixion wires and repairing a torn deltoid-trapezius aponeurosis.[215,216] If the deltoid and trapezius are not torn they are not plicated unless the stability of the fixation is not secure. In this event I occasionally add the method of Neviaser and transpose the cut end of coracoacromial ligament from the coracoid to the clavicle[218] (Fig. 20-53A).

An incision is made at the lateral edge of the acromion and carried across the anterior edge of the acromion and the acromioclavicular joint medialward for 2.5 cm. (Fig. 20-54). The aponeurosis between the trapezius and deltoid is incised and the capsule is opened (Fig. 20-54B). The meniscus is removed, if torn, along with any detritus.

The clavicle is held in reduction by an assistant as a test to be certain reduction is adequate. Blind pinning will usually fail and should not be attempted. One or two $^3/_{32}$-in. smooth wires are inserted across the joint until the point strikes the superior endosteal surface of the clavicle. They are cut short beneath the skin (Fig. 20-52). Occasionally, retrograde introduction through the acromion is required for correct positioning of the pins. Threaded wires across the joint should not be used, as they tend to break easily. If smaller diameter wires are used the ends should be bent to prevent migration of the wires (Fig. 20-51). If the heavier pins with a threaded outer end are used a nut device should be added for the same reason. When the nut is small a washer should be included.

The deltoid-trapezius aponeurosis is closed, and is usually plicated at this point. Occasionally, the coracoacromial ligament

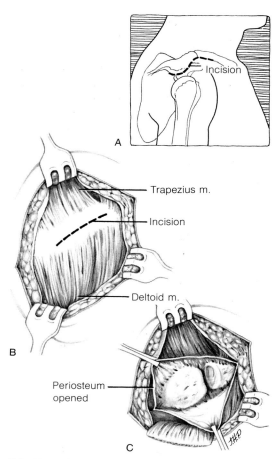

FIG. 20-54. Surgical approach used for exploring and inserting smooth transfixion wires across the acromioclavicular joint. A, Dotted line shows skin incision. B, Periosteum over clavicle is opened and the deltoid and trapezius are reflected. C, The acromioclavicular joint is exposed.

is also transposed; it should be done before closing the aponeurosis. The deltoid is elevated from the anterior outer third of the clavicle. The coracoacromial ligament is exposed, the acromioclavicular joint already having been exposed. After transfixion of the reduced joint with smooth wires, the coracoacromial attachment to the coracoid is removed with a small piece of bone. The strong broad ligament is placed over the acromion and sutured in place to the tough fascial tissue on the superior acromial surface. The rest of the ligament is folded back over the joint and anchored to a raw surface on the clavicle (Fig. 20-53A).

Aftercare includes immobilization in Velpeau position. The wires are removed after 6 weeks. The wound is inspected weekly to be sure the wires do not erode through the skin. Each week roentgenograms are taken to be certain the wires are in position, and that reduction is being maintained. If the wires loosen they can be removed earlier than the usual 6 weeks. After 4 weeks gentle exercises are started. After 8 to 10 weeks full activity is permitted.

It appears that Jacobs and Wade are generally correct in their belief that good results can be attained with almost any method of treatment.[205] However, it is important to individualize treatment for each patient, because attempting closed treatment for a patient with a torn trapezius and interposed tissue in the joint will probably lead to a poor result.

Chronically Painful Acromioclavicular Joint. For the patient who complains of local pain at the acromioclavicular joint, whether it is caused by failed treatment for acromioclavicular dislocation or subsequent painful acromioclavicular joint arthritis,[224] I prefer excision of the distal clavicle lateral to the attachment of the coracoclavicular ligament[160,240,247] (Fig. 20-55).

A transverse 4- to 5-cm. incision is made over the outer clavicle and its joint anteriorly. The aponeurosis between the trapezius and deltoid is incised and the periosteum over the lateral inch is elevated circumferentially (Fig. 20-54B and C). At least 2 cm. of distal clavicle are removed lateral to the coracoclavicular ligament using a power saw for young bone or an osteotome for the elderly patient whose bone is not as dense. The trapezius and deltoid are approximated and the wound is closed.

The patient wears a sling for 4 to 7 days, and thereafter gradually increases shoulder motion exercises until asymptomatic.

In those symptomatic cases in which the clavicle is chronically dislocated, easily moving up and down with activity of the extremity, I employ the transfer of the conjoined tendon described by Dewar and Barrington to stabilize the clavicle.[189] The cosmetic and functional results of this procedure have been good. When it appears that the distal end of the clavicle already has degenerative changes, or cannot be easily reduced without excessively close contact of one joint surface to another, I resect the distal end of the clavicle and then perform the transfer of the conjoined tendon to the lateral clavicle. As an alternative a Dacron tape can be used to hold down the clavicle.

COMPLICATIONS. A number of authors have reported complications after treatment of acromioclavicular joint injuries.[156,171,208,210,211,222,235,237,245] In observing a large number of treated cases of acromioclavicular joint injuries in 20 years at Michael Reese Medical Center I can attest to the variety of complications that have been reported. Complications that have occurred in both closed and open treatment methods are:

A. *Closed methods*
   1. Deformity
   2. Degenerative arthritis
   3. Residual subluxation with or without symptoms
   4. Calcification of soft tissues
   5. Skin irritation, ulcers due to external pressure
   6. Joint stiffness and decreased function

B. *Open methods*
   1. Wound infection
   2. Traumatic arthritis
   3. Soft-tissue calcification
   4. Metal failure
   5. Migration of pins medially or laterally
   6. Loosening of screw
   7. Inadequate reduction
   8. Inadequate fixation
   9. Iatrogenic fracture
   10. Residual deformity
   11. Pain, weakness, and loss of motion
   12. Poor cosmetic scar
   13. Anesthetic complications

Closed methods often require patients to visit the office daily in order to have the pressure straps adjusted, and still the re-

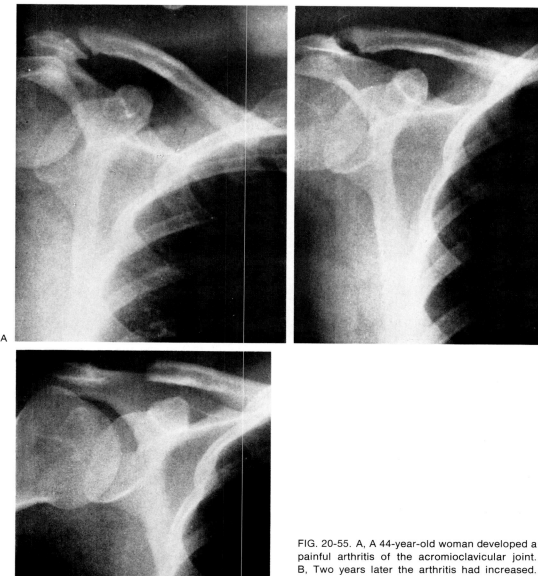

A

B

C

FIG. 20-55. A, A 44-year-old woman developed a painful arthritis of the acromioclavicular joint. B, Two years later the arthritis had increased. C, Two centimeters of lateral clavicle was resected, and results were excellent.

sulting skin maceration may preclude successful treatment. The patient cannot bathe and is generally uncomfortable. When the skin is already abraded prior to injury, conservative methods should not be attempted.

Open methods that require screw and wire fixation require a second operation. I use $^3/_{32}$-in.-diameter smooth pins across the joint with a nut device at the end to prevent medial migration (Fig. 20-52B). Smaller di-

ameter pins should be bent (Fig. 20-51). If the wires back out through the skin after the fourth postoperative week they should be removed. If it happens in the first 3 weeks and the pins protrude a little, the wound is cleansed with alcohol, a sterile dressing is applied, and the patient is observed frequently until enough healing has occurred about the joint so that they can be removed. In no event should pins that have

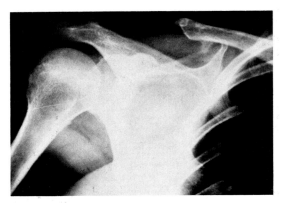

FIG. 20-56. A 52-year-old woman had had an excessive amount of lateral clavicle resected, and complained of a poor cosmetic result and weakness during abduction of the shoulder.

protruded through the skin to a marked degree be pushed back into place. They will not be secure, and this will likely cause a deeper wound infection that may require an open drainage operation.

I have seen cases of calcification and ossification of the coracoclavicular space with open and closed methods of treatment and am not impressed that this causes any great disability.[155,158]

Excessive lateral clavicle resection should be avoided, as it can cause cosmetic deformity and weak abduction (Fig. 20-56).

STERNOCLAVICULAR JOINT DISLOCATIONS

Dislocations of the sternoclavicular joint are uncommon injuries that occasionally cause disability, morbidity, and on rare occasion may threaten life. It is important to diagnose this condition early and correctly.[265]

ANATOMY AND FUNCTION. The sternoclavicular joint is a diathrodial joint and represents a double gliding joint, according to Goss.[197] It is composed of the medial end of the clavicle, the superior and lateral part of the manubrium sterni, and the first rib cartilage. The articular surface of the clavicle is considerably larger in area than that of the sternum, and has a fibrocartilaginous layer thicker than that of the sternum. The joint is

bound by the articular capsule, the anterior and posterior sternoclavicular ligaments, the interclavicular and costoclavicular ligaments, and the articular disc (Fig. 20-57).

The capsule varies in thickness, forming the thicker anterior and posterior sternoclavicular ligaments, and thinning in the other parts about the joint. The anterior sternoclavicular ligament connects the medial end of the clavicle to the manubrium sterni, and is covered by the sternal part of the sternocleidomastoid. It is related to the

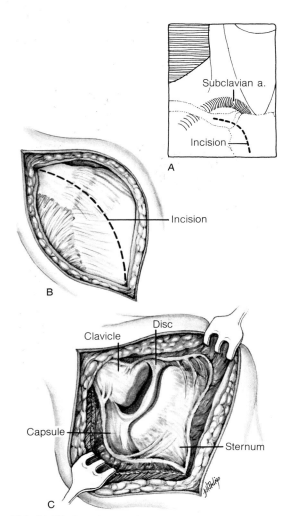

FIG. 20-57. Anterior surgical approach to the sternoclavicular joint. A, Dotted line indicates skin incision. B, Capsule is opened along the dotted line. C, The joint is exposed. Note the relationship of the articular disc to its capsule.

capsule and articular disc dorsally (Fig. 20-57B). The posterior sternoclavicular ligament also connects the sternal end of the clavicle with the manubrium sterni, and is also related to the articular disc (Fig. 20-57C).

The interclavicular ligament is a flat band that curves from the superior portion of the sternal end of the clavicle to the contralateral side of the opposite sternal end of the clavicle. The costoclavicular ligament is short, flat, strong, and rhomboid and connects the medial part of the cartilage of the first rib to the costal tuberosity on the undersurface of the clavicle. It is in relation to the origin of the subclavius and to the subclavian vein behind. Cave described the detailed anatomy of the costoclavicular ligament,[258] and Bearn showed that there is a bursa between its anterior and posterior fasciculi.[252]

The articular disc is flat, almost circular, and divides the joint. It is thick peripherally and is attached circumferentially to its surrounding ligaments (Fig. 20-57C).

There are two synovial membranes in this joint. The medial membrane is larger than the membrane in the compartment lateral to the articular disc.

DePalma showed that rarely when the articular disc is perforated there is a free communication between the medial and lateral compartments.[262] Also, because of its connection to the anterior and posterior sternoclavicular ligaments the disc serves to prevent excessive medial movement of the sternal end of the clavicle. Cave reported that the costoclavicular ligament acts to prevent upward displacement of the medial end of the clavicle,[258] whereas Bearn believed that the capsular ligament was more important in protecting against upward displacement.[252]

Bearn obtained five postmortem specimens each comprising the manubrium sterni, the upper half of the body of the sternum, both first ribs, and both clavicles.[252] He transected the sternum between the fourth and fifth costal cartilages, divided the first ribs anterior to their tubercles, and disarticulated the lateral extremities of the clavicle by cutting the conoid and trapezoid components of the coracoclavicular ligament and the capsule of the acromioclavicular joint.

The lateral end of each clavicle in the region of the conoid tubercle was loaded through a spring balance with 10-, 15-, and 20-pound weights (Fig. 20-58A). In the intact and unloaded specimen the clavicle was maintained by tension in the sternoclavicular joint capsule, the lateral clavicular end being maintained 5 to 6.25 cm. higher than the medial end. With added weights of 5 to 20 pounds the lateral clavicle depressed 2.5 to 3.8 cm. Each ligament was then sectioned either singly or in combinations.

Section of the sternoclavicular joint capsule resulted in a lower descent of the lateral end than of the medial end (Fig. 20-58B). The clavicle is now supported by the disc. When the clavicle is loaded with the divided capsule the end depresses below the level of medial end about an axis, and results in tearing of the disc from the costal cartilage. Bearn noted that division of the costoclavicular ligament and disc did not alter clavicular poise. Finally, Bearn found that section of the first costal cartilage medial to the costoclavicular ligament did not change clavicular poise.[252]

The results of this study show that clavicular poise is not merely related to trapezius muscle action but to the strong capsule. Bearn discovered that the fulcrum is placed between the undersurface of the medial end of the clavicle and the adjacent first costal cartilage, contrary to the costoclavicular ligament suggested by Cave.[258] He also found that the lateral end of the clavicle moved forward and downward during depression because of the first rib obliquity.[252] Thus, the clavicular head moved backward and upward thereby placing great strain on the posterior-superior capsule. The weaker anterior capsule explains why anterior dislocation of the sternoclavicular joint is common compared to the rare posterior dislocation.

Epiphysis of the Medial Clavicle. The sternal end of the clavicle contains an articular surface which articulates with manu-

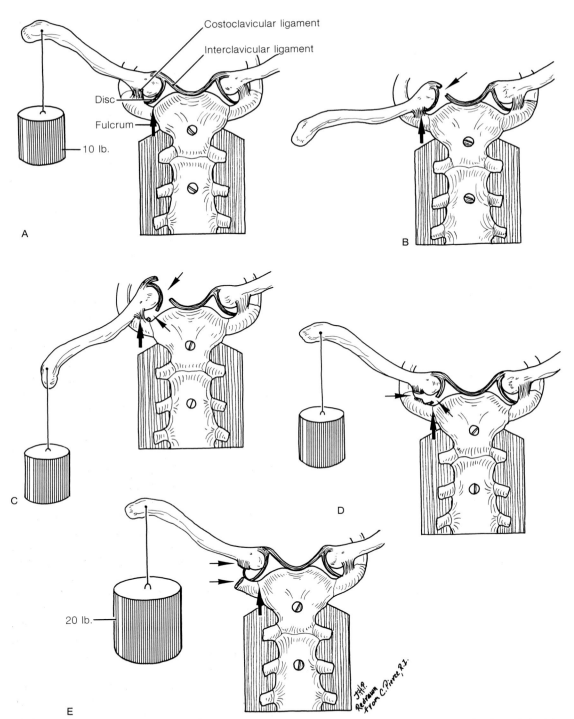

FIG. 20-58. Bearn's observations on the function of the capsule of the sternoclavicular joint. A, The lateral clavicle is normally maintained 5 to 6.3 cm. higher than the medial end. Five- to twenty-pound loading depresses the lateral clavicle 2.5 to 3.8 cm. beyond the normal. B, Capsule section of the sternoclavicular joint leads to descent of the lateral end to a level lower than the medial end. C, Capsule section with 10 pounds of loading leads to full depression of the lateral end about an axis (arrow), and tearing of the disc from the costal cartilage. D, Section of the costoclavicular ligament and disc does not change clavicular poise. E, Division of the first costal cartilage medial to the costoclavicular ligament does not alter clavicular poise. (Redrawn from Bearn, J. G.: Direct observations on the function of the capsule of the sternoclavicular joint in clavicular support. J. Anat., 101:159–170, 1967.)

490

brium sterni through the disc portion. Although the clavicle is the first bone to ossify in the body through the two primary ossification centers for the body, the secondary center for the sternal end first appears about the eighteenth to twentieth year, and may not unite until the twenty-fifth year.[197] It is important to understand this fact when treating injuries of the sternoclavicular joint in young persons.

Joint Motion. The sternoclavicular joint is the only connecting link with the axial skeleton, and has movement in every direction, although it is limited.

Inman, Saunders, and Abbott[203] and Lucas[271] showed that if the scapula is fixed it is possible to actively raise the arm to 90 degrees, but that power is significantly decreased when there is no scapular rotation. They reported that elevation of the arm is accompanied by elevation of the clavicle at the sternoclavicular joint. The movement is virtually complete at 90 degrees, when for every 10 degrees of arm elevation there are 4 degrees of clavicular elevation. Above 90 degrees, clavicular motion is slight. Inman and associates reported that there were 50 degrees of clavicular rotation during full abduction of the arm. If this rotation is hindered the arm can be actively abducted to only 120 degrees.

Movement of the sternoclavicular joint occurs between the clavicle with the articular disc and the sternum. Both the clavicle and disc move, rolling back and forth on the articular surface of the sternum, and sliding up and down. The clavicle rotates upon the articular disc, both structures also rolling upon the sternum. Thus, circumduction and motion occur in almost every direction. Shoulder elevation is limited mainly by the costoclavicular ligament, and depression is prevented by the interclavicular ligament and articular disc.

CLASSIFICATION. Allman has classified sternoclavicular sprains into four grades[156] (Fig. 20-59). Grade I sprain results in slight tearing of the fibers of the sternoclavicular

FIG. 20-59. Allman's classification of sternoclavicular sprain. A, Normal; B, grade I; grade II; D, grade III.

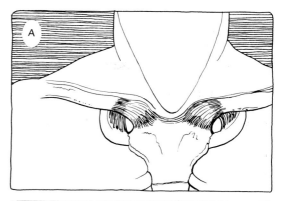
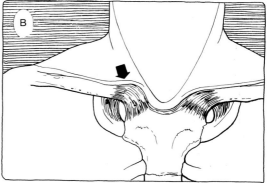
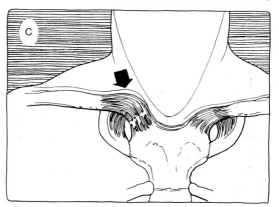
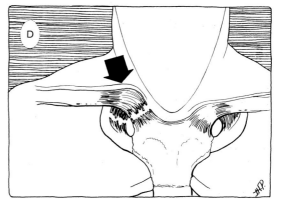

ligaments (Fig. 20-59B). There is no laxity and little pain. In Grade II injury the sternoclavicular ligaments are ruptured without concomitant tearing of the costoclavicular ligament (Fig. 20-59C). Mild deformity may be seen. Grade III sprain is accompanied by complete ruptures of the sternoclavicular and costoclavicular ligaments (Fig. 20-59D), and displacement may be anterior (see Fig. 20-61) or posterior (retrosternal) (see Fig. 20-66).

Recurrent Dislocation. After an acute traumatic dislocation that fails to heal, there may be recurrent dislocation.[263] This is most unusual and has been seen only once by me.

Chronic Dislocation. It is common for acute dislocations to become chronic after injury, usually by mutual choice of the patient and surgeon. This is most often observed in anterior dislocations that do not commonly cause disability or endanger life. Occasionally, a posterior dislocation may be missed, if not suspected. It can be left untreated if it is asymptomatic.

Voluntary Dislocation. Some patients can subluxate their sternoclavicular joint by certain overhead movements of the extremity. The condition may be associated with congenital joint laxity.

INCIDENCE. Sternoclavicular joint injuries are uncommon. Rowe and Marble found only 13 patients in a review of 1603 cases of shoulder-girdle injuries at the Massachusetts General Hospital.[231] They reported that the majority of cases occur in the second decade of life. Salvatore reported 14 cases almost evenly divided between males and females.[279]

Omer reported 82 cases of sternoclavicular dislocation in military personnel and found that 47 percent resulted from vehicular accidents and 31 percent from athletic accidents.[276] Salvatore reported that 5 of 14 cases were due to athletic accidents and automobile accidents accounted for 3 cases.[279] The great majority of cases are anterior dislocations.

MECHANISM OF INJURY. Like acromioclavicular joint dislocations, similar injuries to the sternoclavicular joint are caused most often by a fall on the point of the shoulder so that the force is directed medially.[201] In 30 percent of the cases there is a direct force applied to the clavicle.[231] Usually the clavicle is suddenly displaced upward and outward. A direct force may drive the inner clavicle posteriorly. Tyer and associates stated that the costoclavicular ligament acts as a fulcrum about which a forward motion on the outer end of the clavicle moves to create a sudden, short forceful backward movement at the inner end of the clavicle.[281] However, Bearn contradicts this view, believing the fulcrum is placed between the undersurface of the medial end of the clavicle and the adjacent first costal cartilage.[252] Paterson suggested that the angle of the sternoclavicular joint to the sagittal plane varied greatly, most joints subtending an angle of only a few degrees to the sagittal plane.[278] In two patients with retrosternal dislocation Paterson reported that each had an increased angle of 20 to 25 degrees, allowing easy posterior dislocation.[278]

PATHOLOGY. Not only are the ligaments torn at the sternoclavicular joint but the articular disc may be injured. With dislocation (grade III sprain) the costoclavicular and sternoclavicular ligaments are ruptured.

The dislocation of the adult sternoclavicular joint is quite different from the dislocation of the inner clavicle in the young person in which the thin medial epiphysis, a few millimeters thick, does not unite with the metaphysis until 22 to 25 years of age. This latter injury corresponds to a Salter-Harris type I injury (see Fig. 20-62).

DePalma showed that regressive changes in the components of the sternoclavicular joint are first manifested in the third decade of life, and progress slowly.[261] Severe changes do not occur until the seventh and eighth decades, which is in contrast to the more rapid degeneration of the acromioclavicular joint during the fourth decade.

DIAGNOSIS. Acute grade I injuries may produce minimal pain, and only slight local tenderness over the joint. There is usually no deformity. Grade II sprains produce more pain, local swelling, tenderness, and some deformity. There may be slight ballottement at the inner end of the clavicle. When an acute grade III sprain occurs and is of the anterior type there is severe tenderness and swelling and considerable pain (Fig. 20-60). Such an acute injury may allow manual reduction by extension and elevation of the shoulder and redislocation by bringing the shoulder back to a neutral position. With acute anterior dislocation the pain and tenderness may subside quickly, so that within 10 days extremity function may be almost normal although the swelling persists (Fig. 20-61).

Posterior dislocation of the sternoclavicular joint may cause moderate to severe pain, considerable local tenderness, and a visible depression or loss of normal contour over the joint if observed soon after injury (Fig. 20-62). If several hours elapse and swelling increases this valuable sign may be missed.

In either the anterior or posterior dislocations, extremity movement increases local pain. Thus, the patient supports his extremity. The head may tilt toward the affected side. Finally, the patient has increased pain when asked to lie on a flat surface, tilting the injured shoulder forward.

Retrosternal dislocation of the joint may be masked by its associated complications that can be caused by the injury (Fig. 20-62). Signs and symptoms can vary from mild tenderness to hoarseness, dyspnea, difficulty in swallowing, paralysis of the upper extremity, and cardiovascular collapse.[270,273]

Especially in retrosternal dislocation early diagnosis is important because closed reduction is seldom successful after 48 hours, and the complications can be fatal.[156,274] These disasters result from tearing of the lung, trachea, and great vessels. In such cases a pneumothorax may result and circulation to the involved extremity may be impaired causing a decreased radial pulse.

Roentgenographic Diagnosis. The sternoclavicular joints are often difficult to assess by roentgenograms. Simultaneous routine anteroposterior views should be obtained for comparison. Slight differences may disclose subtle changes in the height of the clavicle on the injured side. The medial clavicle may be displaced upward or downward (Fig. 20-63). Special oblique and axial views of both joints may better show the true relationship of the clavicle to its manubrium.[267,268,274] Some authors rely on tomograms to establish the diagnosis.[249,264,281] Although I have employed these techniques with success I find them troublesome. I now depend more upon xeroradiograms in lieu of tomograms for roentgen diagnosis. The fine detail and overlapping contours of the bone can be more easily determined by this method (Fig. 20-62C).

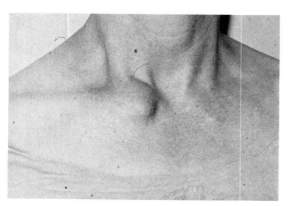
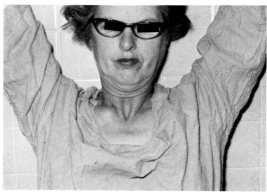

A   B

FIG. 20-60. A, A 52-year-old woman had sustained an anterior sternoclavicular joint dislocation many years before. Note the swelling of the right sternoclavicular joint. B, The injury remained untreated by the patient's choice because it did not hinder her function or cause pain.

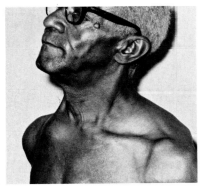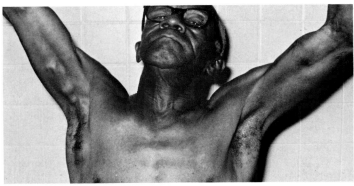

A   B

FIG. 20-61. A, A 70-year-old man sustained an anterior sternoclavicular joint dislocation. He refused treatment except for a sling the first week. B, Note the extent of painless active overhead motion 10 days after injury, and the swelling of the right sternoclavicular joint.

TREATMENT. *Traumatic Injuries.* Grade I. In the first 24 hours ice packs are applied to the joint area. The patient does not always tolerate even moderate heat after this period and in this event nothing is applied. The involved extremity is immobilized in a sling for 3 to 5 days or until there is comfort. Thereafter, activities are gradually resumed until normalcy is achieved.

Grade II. Ice packs are applied initially while analgesics are given for pain. I prefer Velpeau immobilization with or without subluxation. If there is subluxation manipulation may be attempted, often with good results. Manipulation can be performed by drawing the shoulders backward after the torso is placed on a roll positioned longitudinally along the spine. A soft figure-eight splint may be adequate along with sling immobilization of the involved extremity.[156] Some patients are more comfortable in a plaster jacket. In this case the plaster jacket is applied in much the same manner as it is for a fractured clavicle, by first manipulating the injured shoulder with the patient lying supine on a smooth, narrow plate. The plate is withdrawn following cast application. Immobilization is continued for 4 to 6 weeks. A longer period of immobilization is continued if significant tenderness persists. I have not found it necessary to operate upon a patient with a grade II injury.

Anterior Type. Grade III. Anterior dislocation can be treated closed in the vast majority of patients. An early attempt may be made to manipulate the proximal clavicle in such a way as to increase the space between the proximal clavicle and manubrium sterni.[280] I prefer to position the patient on a smooth, long narrow steel plate suspended between two tables, as described previously (see section on Clavicular Fractures). The patient's arm is abducted and extended while pressure is applied directly over the medial end of the clavicle. Soon after the injury this may be accomplished after administering an intravenous analgesic to the patient. Following manipulation a plaster of Paris body jacket is applied. The bony prominences about the shoulder should be well padded. The involved extremity is included in the cast. The cast should be molded in order to maintain extension of the shoulder. The plate is then withdrawn.

If the reduction is lost it is probably better to accept the resulting deformity rather than to attempt open reduction, especially in the elderly patient, since function is excellent anyway (Fig. 20-60). Often, the patient chooses the deformity of an anterior dislocation rather than accept closed treatment, and a sling is worn until the pain subsides (Fig. 20-61). In any event, I encourage most patients to accept treatment in the hope that reduction will later prevent adverse symptoms.

If intractable pain persists many months

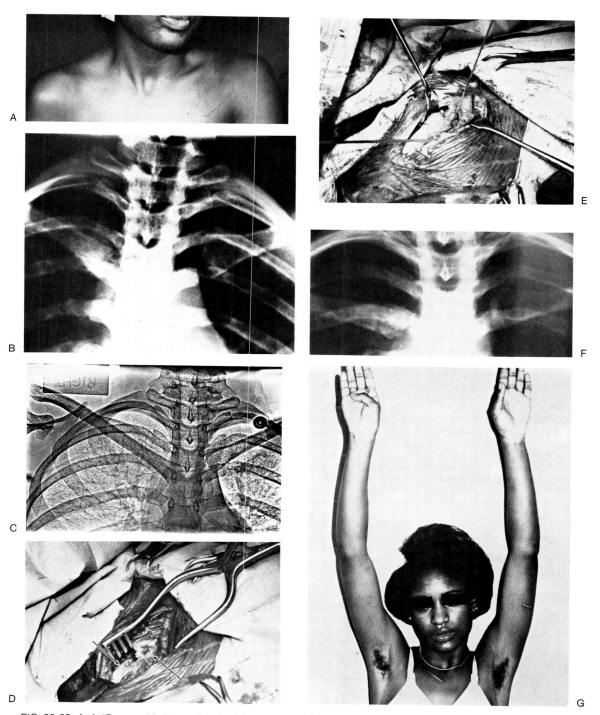

FIG. 20-62. A, A 17-year-old girl was involved in an automobile accident and had a serious pneumothorax. A chest tube was removed on the third day after injury. The patient was referred to the orthopaedic service 12 days later when she continued to complain of dysphagia and dyspnea. Note the loss of the normal contour over the right medial clavicle and the depression over the right sternoclavicular joint. B, Anteroposterior view of the clavicles shows a difference in the sternoclavicular joints. The right joint space has disappeared. C, Xeroradiogram clearly shows the retrosternal dislocation of the right joint. D, The posterior dislocation. The clavicle was buttonholed through the posterior capsule, making reduction difficult. The upper arrow points to the clavicle and the lower arrow shows the medial clavicular epiphysis (Salter-Harris type I). E, The clavicle was held by heavy stay sutures to the costal cartilage below. F, X-ray film 3 months postoperatively shows the joint alignment. G, Note the extent of painless, active overhead motion 3 months postoperatively. The result was excellent.

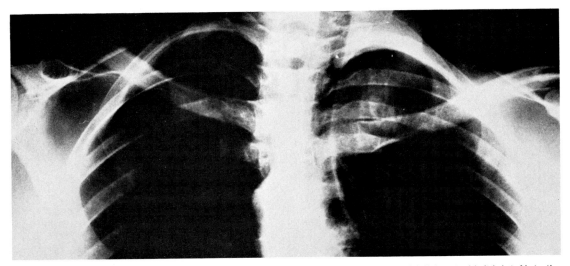

FIG. 20-63. Anteroposterior view of the sternoclavicular joints shows the anteriorly dislocated left joint. Note the inferior displacement of the left clavicle.

after injury of the anterior or posterior type, the medial end of the clavicle may be resected with good results[266] (Fig. 20-64). This may be accomplished through a straight tranverse incision (Fig. 20-65) or curvilinear incision (Fig. 20-57).

In the rare event that open reduction is elected by the surgeon for the acute injury, using a short traverse incision (Fig. 20-65) or a curvilinear incision over the sternoclavicular joint (Fig. 20-57), the reduced medial clavicle may be immobilized by Kirschner wire fixation, fascial or suture repair, or combinations of these methods. The wire should be bent subcutaneously to prevent migration, and should be removed after 6 weeks. Roentgenograms should be obtained periodically to watch for possible migration

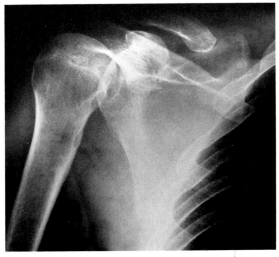
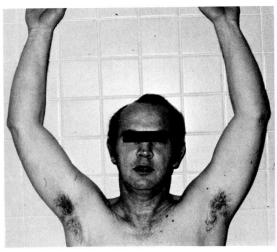

A

B

FIG. 20-64. A, A 47-year-old man sustained a posterior fracture-dislocation of the sternoclavicular joint that could not be reduced by closed or open methods. He underwent partial medial clavicle resection when he continued to complain of pain, shortness of breath, and dysphagia. B, Note the extent of motion postoperatively. The result was excellent except for a persistent causalgia-like pain in the arm postoperatively.

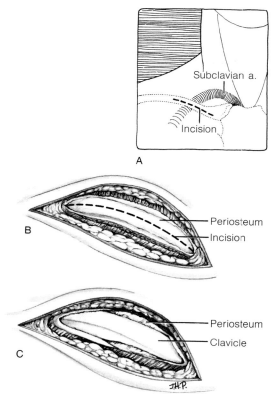

FIG. 20-65. Anterior approach to clavicle. A, Dotted line shows placement of skin incision over the medial clavicle. Note the relationship of the clavicle to the subclavian artery. B, The periosteum over the medial clavicle is opened (dotted line). C, The periosteal cover is elevated and the medial clavicle thus exposed. For resection of the medial clavicle, power saw osteotomy is preferred with cautious retrograde stripping of the periosteum and capsule from the bone.

if wire is used. If the meniscus is badly torn and displaced it should be removed. Following surgery, a figure-eight harness or plaster of Paris body jacket that includes the extremity should be employed for 5 to 6 weeks. In any event I have seldom observed a patient operated upon for anterior dislocation who was more satisfied than those patients treated conservatively even with their deformity.

Posterior Type. It is important to restate that posterior dislocation of the sternoclavicular joint may pose serious problems that can endanger life. Therefore, it is essential to take a careful history and perform a thorough physical examination of all sys-

tems. Nowhere else is the diagnostic acumen of the surgeon more needed than in this injury.

If a pneumothorax results from the injury, treatment of the lung problem must take precedence over the dislocated joint. If there is compression or tearing of great vessels, or dysphagia, the appropriate specialist should be called at once.

Most retrosternal dislocations can be treated closed. A sandbag or roll is placed between the shoulders and manipulation is performed. Again, I prefer placing the patient supine on a smooth, narrow metal plate suspended between two tables, and then manipulating the clavicle. The manipulation should be performed with an anesthetist standing by even though intravenous analgesia may suffice. If the patient is in severe pain general anesthesia may be required.

Traction is applied while the arm is abducted beyond 90 degrees and extended. The medial end of the clavicle is easily grasped between the thumb and fingertips in the first few hours after injury if the patient is thin. Occasionally, a sterile towel clip may be carefully applied through the surgically prepared skin to grasp the clavicle and pull it anteriorly. If reduction is successful often there is an audible snap. A figure-eight splint is applied. After a few days the surgeon may decide to replace this form of immobilization with a plaster of Paris body jacket if the patient is active. In any event, extension immobilization of the shoulders is maintained 4 to 6 weeks. Thereafter, gentle motion exercises of the extremity are gradually increased for an additional 6 weeks.

If closed reduction fails and the patient has symptoms, I prefer open reduction in the acute injury or resection of the medial clavicle in the chronic case of retrosternal dislocation. I have seen some patients who had a missed diagnosis or refused treatment and did well because they had no symptoms. However, in most cases I do not believe the same inaction should be allowed with retrosternal dislocation as is permitted with anterior dislocation because of the large number of symptoms and complications that can result from posterior dislocation. Therefore, when closed treatment fails open treatment is indicated.

An open reduction can be exceptionally difficult and dangerous because of the close proximity of the subclavian vein and other important structures (see Figs. 20-57 and 20-65). It may even be necessary to resect a short segment of the sternal end of the clavicle before using internal fixation methods. Occasionally, the clavicle may even be buttonholed through the posterior capsule, making open reduction even more difficult (Fig. 20-62). However, once open reduction is accomplished the medial clavicle may be held by a Kirchner wire bent at one end to prevent migration, subclavius tenodesis, fascial repair, heavy nonabsorbable suture fixation, or combinations of these methods (Fig. 20-66). I prefer soft-tissue repair with heavy sutures, tying the clavicle to the rib below because pins do not hold well in the manubrium and can migrate (Fig. 20-66). If the meniscus is badly torn and displaced it should be removed. After 6 weeks the pin should be removed, if used.

Aftercare is the same as that for the closed method, except I believe better immobilization is achieved at the operative site by applying a plaster body jacket that includes the arm a few days after surgery.

Epiphyseal Fracture of Medial End of Clavicle. Denham and Dingley reported four cases of epiphyseal separation of the medial end of the clavicle in teenage patients.[260] Three cases were anterior and one was posterior. Two anterior cases and the one posterior case were treated open with good results.

The symptoms and findings of this injury are identical to those found in anterior and posterior dislocations of the sternoclavicular joint. Unless the injury is suspected, the time of epiphyseal closure of the medial epiphysis of the clavicle understood, and the fact that the epiphysis stays with the manubrium, a poor result may follow in such cases. The thin epiphyseal structure may be mistaken for the articular disc even though it is lateral to it.

Anterior injuries may be treated closed, especially in the young teenager where molding will occur. The shoulders should be kept extended in a figure-eight splint for 3 to 4 weeks. Brooks and Henning stated that closed treatment may fail because the cephalad pull of the sternocleidomastoid, soft-tissue interposition at the fracture site, and long lever arm of the upper extremity tend to displace the medial clavicle[256] (Fig. 20-67).

In the posterior type the injury may be more ominous. If the patient has no symptoms, the injury may be treated conservatively with a figure-eight splint for 3 to 4

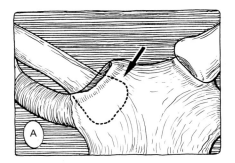

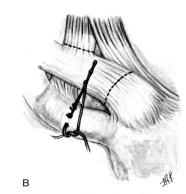

FIG. 20-66. Repair of posterior dislocation of sternoclavicular joint. A, The retrosternal clavicle dislocation (arrow) found in the patient shown in Figure 20-62. B, Result after open reduction method of fastening the reduced medial clavicle to the costochondral cartilage below. However, any similar well-executed technique will work. Dotted line over the medial clavicle shows where the clavicle may need to be resected to effect reduction for posterior dislocation, and sternocleidomastoid tendon may be transected (dotted line) in case this is required to effect reduction.

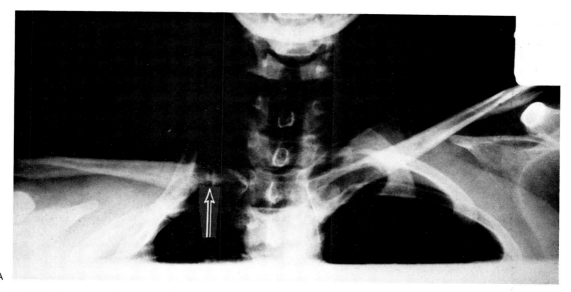

A

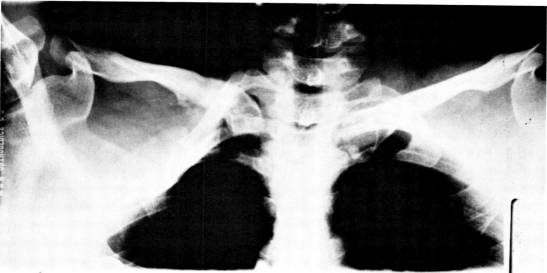

B

FIG. 20-67. A, A teenage girl had an open reduction of an anterior sternoclavicular dislocation when closed treatment failed. Arrow shows vertical hole in medial clavicle through which a heavy suture was placed to secure the clavicle to the rib cartilage below. B, Six years later note the convex deformity of the medial clavicle that was attributed to the pull of the attached sternocleidomastoid muscle. The articular surface of the clavicle remained in the previous position, determined at operation. Perhaps transection of the sternocleidomastoid tendon may have avoided this bone deformity. Nevertheless, the result was satisfactory.

weeks. However, when the patient has severe symptoms the injury should be treated open with internal fixation (see Fig. 20-62). The surgeon should respect the growth plate and remember that in contrast to a retrosternal dislocation in a mature adult in whom treatment is aimed at getting a torn capsule and ligaments to heal about a reduced medial clavicle, the epiphyseal separation in a young person will heal more easily because there is raw bone on the displaced medial clavicle and a slender film of bone on the lateral side of the thin epiphyseal plate that is retained with the manubrium. Holding the two opposing surfaces of raw bone in reduction will give an excellent result (Fig. 20-62). Moreover, it may be necessary to resect up to a centimeter or more of length of the medial clavicle in order to effect reduction. This should not affect healing of the growth plate to its new raw surface on the medial clavicle because the epiphyseal plate stays with the manubrium.

Chronic Dislocation. Chronic, unreduced anterior and posterior dislocation need not be treated if the patient has no symptoms. When symptoms are present, most likely with the posterior type, I believe partial medial clavicle resection is indicated. Lunseth and associates reviewed their methods of managing symptomatic chronic or recurrent sternoclavicular dislocation.[272] They reflect the clavicular head of the pectoralis major subperiosteally.[272] A flap over the joint is turned upward. The superior part of the sternal portion of the pectoralis major and sternal head of the sternocleidomastoid are sharply dissected from the sternum. The plane between pectoralis major and subclavius is exposed. Care is taken to avoid injury to the subclavian vessels beneath the subclavius tendon. The sternoclavicular joint is inspected, and if the meniscus is severely damaged or blocking reduction of the clavicle, it is removed along with any osteophytes. Reduction is then accomplished.

Two 4-mm. holes are made in the anteroinferior and anterosuperior medial clavicle. The freed subclavius tendon is placed in the inferior hole and brought out the superior hole. The tendon is sutured upon itself with heavy synthetic material. In the last three of their five patients they used a threaded Steinmann pin through the joint to ensure postoperative stability of the joint. They also perform a snug capsular repair of the anterior sternoclavicular ligament.

A stockinet Velpeau bandage is used for at least 2 weeks and a sling for 4 weeks, and light exercises are resumed at 6 weeks. The end of the pin is left subcutaneously and later removed. The fifth case failed following a drinking bout. The authors stress that most cases do not need surgical treatment.

COMPLICATIONS. Except for the lump or occasional pain that follows degenerative changes it is most unusual to observe complications with anterior dislocations of the sternoclavicular joint. On the other hand, numerous and serious complications may follow retrosternal dislocation. Still other complications may arise after operation. For example, Pate and Wilhite reported the migration of a wire from the sternoclavicular joint into the heart.[277]

Bonnin reported 11 patients with spontaneous subluxation of the sternoclavicular joint.[254] Bremner described 12 patients, all middle-age women, with monarticular non-infectious subacute arthritis of the sternoclavicular joint.[255] These patients complained of a gradual onset of a lump over the sternoclavicular joint, the right side in 11 of the 12, and all dominant on the side of involvement. Sixty percent of the patients had erosion of the articular surfaces of the sternoclavicular joint, but never subluxation. These conditions should be differentiated from traumatic dislocations.[248]

Retrosternal Dislocation. Complications of retrosternal dislocation are:

1. Pressure or rupture of the trachea[278]
2. Pneumothorax and laceration of superior vena cava[282]
3. Pressure on subclavian artery and great vessels[269,282]
4. Compression on right common caroid artery[269]
5. Dysphagia[278,282]
6. Dyspnea[270,279,281]
7. Brachial plexus compression[274]

It is obvious after reviewing these complications that the surgeon must not underestimate the seriousness of retrosternal dislocation.

In addition to the direct complications resulting from retrosternal dislocation, Brown reported a 30 percent incidence of surgical complications in 10 cases, including two broken pins, and another in which the pin migrated through the manubrium and entered the pulmonary artery almost causing death.[257] If the major vessels behind the clavicle are injured and must be exposed, a portion of the clavicle may be removed in order to obtain control of the vessels above and below the vascular lesion.[190] Clark, Milgram, and Yawn reported a fatal cardiac tamponade due to migration of a wire from the right sternoclavicular joint.[259]

Omer reported 15 patients operated upon for sternoclavicular dislocation.[276] Two of five patients with metal internal fixation had pin breakage with recurrent dislocation, one patient had pin migration into the mediastinum with recurrent dislocation, and two patients developed osteomyelitis. Three other patients, with soft-tissue reconstructions, had recurrent dislocation with drainage, recurrent dislocation, and subsequent arthritis with extremity weakness, respectively.

Recurrent Dislocation. I have examined patients with recurrent anterior dislocation of the sternoclavicular joint who had relatively no symptoms. I do not think these patients require surgical treatment in most instances. In some, partial resection is indicated if surgery is needed. Bankart reported four cases wherein he reconstructed these joints using a fascial repair technique.[250]

Complete Dislocation of Clavicle. I have never seen such a case, but have been advised by reliable orthopaedists who have practiced in India that they have observed such cases incurred from the bite of a camel, the clavicle being pulled completely away from its two joints and periosteum.[275] Beckman reviewed the literature in 1923 and found that in one series of reported cases 3 of 13 cases occurred in children 13 to 14 years of age, but the majority occurred in men in the prime of life.[253]

Beckman described two mechanisms of injury and believed that the clavicle was well developed in these cases even in children because they did not first fracture.[253] Either the force of the injury caused the shoulder to be pressed together while a torsion of the body occurred around the opposite fixed clavicle, or a direct blow was received on the external posterior aspect of the shoulder as in a fall from a height. Beckman achieved a good result by surgical repair in the case of a 13-year-old boy, restoring the clavicle within its periosteal soft-tissue sleeve.[253] In his review of the literature up to that time of those cases treated conservatively, a good functional result was achieved in 66 percent of the cases, and ideal healing occurred in 40 percent of the cases.

REFERENCES

Anterior Glenohumeral Dislocations

1. Adams, J. C.: Recurrent dislocations of the shoulder. J. Bone Joint Surg., 30-B:26–38, 1948.
2. Adams, J. C.: The humeral head defect in recurrent anterior dislocations of the shoulder. Br. J. Radiol., 23:151–156, 1950.
3. Allman, F.: Presentation, The American Academy of Orthopedic Surgeons, Committee on Sports Medicine, Course on Athletic Injuries of the Upper Extremities. Eugene, Oregon, July, 1974.
4. Augustine, R. W.: Repair of dislocation of the shoulder using modern Magnuson technique. Am. J. Surg., 91:736–741, 1956.
5. Badgley, C. E., and O'Connor, G. A.: Combined procedure for the repair of recurrent anterior dislocation of the shoulder. J. Bone Joint Surg., 47-A:1283, 1965.
6. Bailey, R. W.: Acute and recurrent dislocation of the shoulder. J. Bone Joint Surg., 49-A:767–773, 1967.
7. Baker, D, M., and Leach, R. E.: Fracture-dislocation of the shoulder. Report of three unusual cases with rotator cuff avulsion. J. Trauma, 5:659–664, 1965.
8. Bankart, A. S. B.: Recurrent or habitual dislocation of the shoulder joint. Br. Med. J., 2:1132–1133, 1923.
9. Bankart, A. S. B.: Dislocation of the shoulder joints. In Robert Jones' Birthday Volume. A Collection of Surgical Essays. London, Oxford University Press, 1928.
10. Bankart, A. S. B.: The pathology and treatment of recurrent dislocation of the shoulder joint. Br. J. Surg., 26:23–29, 1938.
11. Bateman, J. E.: Gallie technique for repair of recurrent dislocation of the shoulder. Surg. Clin. North Am., 43:1655–1662, 1963.

12. Bateman, J. E.: The Shoulder and Neck. Philadelphia, W. B. Saunders Co., 1972.

13. Bennett, G. E.: Old dislocations of the shoulder. J. Bone Joint Surg., 18:594–606, 1936.

14. Blazina, M. E., and Satzman, J. S.: Recurrent anterior subluxation of the shoulder in athletes—A distinct entity. J. Bone Joint Surg., 51-A:1037–1038, 1969.

15. Bonnin, J. G.: Transplantation of the tip of the coracoid process for recurrent anterior dislocation of the shoulder. J. Bone Joint Surg., 51-B:579, 1969.

16. Bonnin, J. G.: Transplantation of the coracoid tip. A definitive operation for recurrent anterior dislocation of the shoulder. Proc. R. Soc. Med., 66:755–758, 1973.

17. Bost, F., and Inman, V. T.: The pathologic changes in recurrent dislocation of the shoulder. A report of Bankart's operative procedure. J. Bone Joint Surg., 24:595–613, 1942.

18. Boyd, H. B., and Hunt, H.: Recurrent dislocation of the shoulder. J. Bone Joint Surg., 47-A:1514–1520, 1965.

19. Brav, E. A.: An evaluation of Putti-Platt reconstruction procedure for recurrent dislocation of the shoulder. J. Bone Joint Surg., 37-A:731–741, 1955.

20. Brav, E. A.: Ten years experience with Putti-Platt reconstruction procedure. Am. J. Surg., 100:423–430, 1960.

21. Brav, E. A., and Jefferess, V. H.: Simplified Putti-Platt reconstruction for recurrent shoulder dislocation. A preliminary report. West. J. Surg. Obstet. Gynecol., 60:93–97, 1952.

22. Brockbank, W., and Griffiths, D. L.: Orthopaedic surgery in the 16th and 17th centuries. J. Bone Joint Surg., 30-B:365–375, 1948.

23. Caird, F. M.: The shoulder joint in relation to certain dislocations and fractures. Edinb. Med. J., 32:708–714, 1887.

24. Christophe, K.: A functioning false shoulder joint following an old dislocation. J. Bone Joint Surg., 21:916–917, 1939.

25. Cotton, F. J., and Morrison, G. M.: Recurrent dislocation of the shoulder. New Engl. J. Med., CCX, 1070, 1934.

26. Cowan, D. J., and Shaw, P. C.: Two cases of anterior subluxation of the shoulder locking in abduction. J. Bone Joint Surg., 46-B:108–109, 1964.

27. Cozen, L.: Congenital dislocation of the shoulder and other abnormalities. Arch. Surg., 35:956–966, 1937.

28. Crosby, E. H.: A surgical procedure for repair of recurrent dislocation of the shoulder joint. A preliminary report. J. Bone Joint Surg., 28:809–812, 1946.

29. Day, A. J., MacDonell, J. A., and Peterson, H. E.: Recurrent dislocation of the shoulder. Clin. Orthop., 45:123–126, 1966.

30. De Anquin, C. E.: Recurrent dislocation of the shoulder—Roentgenographic study. J. Bone Joint Surg., 47-A:1085, 1965.

31. DePalma, A. F.: Recurrent dislocation of the shoulder joint. Ann. Surg., 132:1052–1065, 1950.

32. DePalma, A. F.: Factors influencing the choice of a modified Magnuson procedure for recurrent anterior dislocation of the shoulder—With a note on technique. Surg. Clin. North Am., 43:1647–1649, 1963.

33. DePalma, A. F., Cooke, A. J., and Prabhakar, M.: The role of the subscapularis in recurrent anterior dislocation of the shoulder. Clin. Orthop. 54:35–49, 1967.

34. Dickson, J. W., and Devas, M. B.: Bankart's operation for recurrent dislocation of the shoulder. J. Bone Joint Surg., 39-B:114–119, 1957.

35. Downing, F. H.: The operative treatment for anterior dislocation of the shoulder. J. Bone Joint Surg., 51-A:811–812, 1969.

36. du Toit, G. T., and Roux, D.: Recurrent dislocation of the shoulder. A 24-year study of the Johannesburg stapling operation. J. Bone Joint Surg., 36-A:1–12, 1956.

37. Eden, R.: Zur Operation der Habituellen Schulterluxation Unter Mitteilung eines Neuen Verfahrens Bei Abriss am Inneren Phannenrande. Deutsch. Ztschr. Chir., 144:269–280, 1918.

38. Eyre-Brook, A. L.: Recurrent dislocation of the shoulder. Lesions discovered in seventeen cases. Surgery employed and intermediate report on results. J. Bone Joint Surg., 30-B:39–48, 1948.

39. Gallie, W. E., and LeMesurier, A. B.: An operation for the relief of recurring dislocations of the shoulder. Trans. Am. Surg. Assoc., 45:392–398, 1927.

40. Gallie, W. E., and LeMesurier, A. B.: Recurring dislocation of the shoulder. J. Bone Joint Surg., 30-B:9–18, 1948.

41. Giannestras, N. J.: Magnuson-Stack procedure for recurrent dislocation of the shoulder. Surgery, 23:794–798, 1948.

42. Golding, C.: Radiology and orthopedic surgery. J. Bone Joint Surg., 48-B:320–332, 1966.

43. Grieg, D.: On true congenital dislocation of the shoulder. Edinb. Med. J., 4:157–175, 1923.

44. Hays, M. B.: Glenoid osteotomy for treatment of recurrent dislocations of the shoulder. J. Bone Joint Surg., 51-A:811, 1969.

45. Hejna, W. F., Fossier, C. H., Goldstein, T. B., and Ray, R. D.: Ancient anterior dislocation of the shoulder. J. Bone Joint Surg., 51-A:1030–1031, 1969.

46. Helfet, A. J.: Coracoid transplantation for recurring dislocation of the shoulder. J. Bone Joint Surg., 40-B:198–202, 1958.

47. Henderson, M. S.: Habitual or recurrent dislocation of the shoulder. Surg. Gynecol. Obstet., 33:1–7, 1921.

48. Henderson, M. S.: Tenosuspension operation for recurrent or habitual dislocation of the shoulder. Surg. Clin. North Am., 5:997–1007, 1949.

49. Hermodsson, L.: Rontgenologische Studien Über die Traumatischen und Habituellen Schultergelenk-Verrenkungen Nach Vorn und Nach Unten. Acta Radiol. (Suppl.), 20:1–173, 1934.

50. Hill, H. A., and Sachs, M. D.: The grooved defect of the humeral head. A frequently unrecognized complication of dislocations of the shoulder joint. Radiology, 35:690–700, 1940.

51. Hindmarsh, J., and Lindberg, A.: Eden-Hybbinette's operation for recurrent dislocation of the humero-scapular joint. Acta Orthop. Scand., 38:459–478, 1967.

52. Hobart, M. H.: Open reduction of an old dislocation of the head of the humerus: Importance of complete mobilization of the head. A report of two cases. J. Bone Joint Surg., 17:199–210, 1935.

53. Hussein, M. K.: Kocher's method is 3,000 years old. J. Bone Joint Surg., 50-B:669–671, 1968.

54. Hybbinette, S.: De la Transplantation d'un fragment osseux pour remedier aux luxations recidivantes de l'epaule; Constatations et resultats operatores. Acta Chir. Scand., 71:411–445, 1932.

55. Ilfeld, F. W., and Holder, H. G.: Recurrent dislocation of the shoulder joint. J. Bone Joint Surg., 25:651–658, 1943.

56. Kazár, B., and Relovszky, E.: Prognosis of primary dislocation of the shoulder. Acta Orthop. Scand., 40:216–224, 1969.

57. Lam, S. J. S.: Irreducible anterior dislocation of the shoulder. J. Bone Joint Surg., 48-B:132–133, 1966.

58. Leslie, J. T., and Ryan, T. J.: The anterior axillary incision to approach the shoulder joint. J. Bone Joint Surg., 44-A:1193–1196, 1962.

59. Levy, L. J.: Anterior axillary incision in the repair of recurrent dislocation of the shoulder. J. Bone Joint Surg., 49-A:204, 1967.

60. Lombardo, S. J., Kerlan, R. K., Jobe, F. W., Carter, V. S., Blazina, M. E., and Shields, C. L.: The modified Bristow procedure for recurrent dislocation of the shoulder. J. Bone Joint Surg., 58-A:256–261, 1976.

61. McLaughlin, H. L.: Trauma. Philadelphia, W. B. Saunders Co., 1959.

62. McLaughlin, H. L.: Recurrent anterior dislocation of the shoulder. Am. J. Surg., 99:628–632, 1960.

63. McLaughlin, H. L., and MacLellan, D. I.: Recurrent anterior dislocation of the shoulder II. A comparative study. J. Trauma, 7:191–201, 1967.

64. Magnuson, P. B.: Treatment of recurrent dislocation of the shoulder. Surg. Clin. North Am., 25:14–20, 1945.

65. Magnuson, P. B., and Stack, J. K.: Recurrent dislocation of the shoulder. J.A.M.A., 123:889–892, 1943.

66. May, V. R., Jr.: A modified Bristow operation for anterior recurrent dislocation of the shoulder. J. Bone Joint Surg., 52-A:1010–1016, 1970.

67. Morrey, B. F., and Janes, J. M.: Recurrent anterior dislocation of the shoulder. Long term follow-up of the Putti-Platt and Bankart procedures. J. Bone Joint Surg., 58-A:252–256, 1976.

68. Moseley, H. F.: The use of metallic glenoid rim in recurrent dislocation of the shoulder. Can. Med. Assoc. J., 56:320–321, 1947.

69. Moseley, H. F.: The basic lesions of recurrent anterior dislocation. Surg. Clin. North Am., 43:1631–1634, 1963.

70. Moseley, H. F., and Overgaard, B.: The anterior capsular mechanism in recurrent anterior dislocation of the shoulder. J. Bone Joint Surg., 44-B:913–927, 1962.

71. Myers, O. R.: Experience with capsulorrhaphy for recurrent dislocation of the shoulder. J. Bone Joint Surg., 28:253–261, 1946.

72. Nash, J.: The status of Kocher's method of reducing recent anterior dislocation of the shoulder. J. Bone Joint Surg., 16:535–544, 1934.

73. Neviaser, J. S.: An operation for old dislocation of the shoulder. J. Bone Joint Surg., 30-A:997–1000, 1948.

74. Neviaser, J. S.: The treatment of old unreduced dislocations of the shoulder. Surg. Clin. North Am., 43:1671–1678, 1963.

75. Nicola, T.: Recurrent anterior dislocation of the shoulder. J. Bone Joint Surg., 11:128–132, 1929.

76. Nicola, T.: Recurrent dislocation of the shoulder—Its treatment by transplantation of the long head of the biceps. Am. J. Surg., 6:815, 1929.

77. Nicola, T.: Anterior dislocation of the shoulder. The role of the articular capsule. J. Bone Joint Surg., 24:614–616, 1942.

78. Nicola, T.: Acute anterior dislocation of the shoulder. J. Bone Joint Surg., 31-A:153–159, 1949.

79. Osmond-Clarke, H.: Habitual dislocation of the shoulder. The Putti-Platt operation. J. Bone Joint Surg., 30-B:19–25, 1948.

80. Øster, A.: Recurrent anterior dislocation of the shoulder treated by the Eden-Hybbinette operation. Follow-up on 78 cases. Acta Orthop. Scand., 40:43–52, 1969.

81. Palmer, I., and Widén, A.: The bone block method for recurrent dislocation of the shoulder joint. J. Bone Joint Surg., 30-B:53–58, 1948.

82. Perthes, G.: Über Operationen bei Habituell Schulterluxation. Deutsch. Ztschr. Chir., 85:199–227, 1906.

83. Pettersson, G.: Rupture of the tendon aponeurosis of the shoulder joint in anterio-inferior dislocation. A study on the origin. Acta Chir. Scand., Vol. 10 (Suppl.), 77:1–187, 1942.

84. Plummer, W. W., and Potts, F. N.: Two cases of recurrent anterior dislocation of the shoulder. J. Bone Joint Surg., 7:190–198, 1925.

85. Poppen, N. K., and Walker, P. S.: Normal and abnormal motion of the shoulder. J. Bone Joint Surg., 58-A:195–200 1976.

86. Rang, M.: Anthology of Orthopaedics. Edinburgh, E. S. Livingstone, Ltd., 1966.

87. Reeves, B.: Experiments on the tensile strength of the anterior capsular structures of the shoulder

region. J. Bone Joint Surg., 50-B:858–865, 1965.

88. Reeves, B.: Arthrography of the shoulder. J. Bone Joint Surg., 48-B:424–435, 1966.

89. Reich, R. S.: Trauma dislocation of the shoulder. J. Bone Joint Surg., 14:73–84, 1932.

90. Robertson, R., and Stark, W. J.: Diagnosis and treatment of recurrent dislocation of the shoulder. J. Bone Joint Surg., 29:797–800, 1947.

91. Rockwood, C. A., and Green, D. P.: Fractures, Vol. I. Philadelphia, J. B. Lippincott Co., 1975.

92. Rowe, C. R.: Prognosis in dislocations of the shoulder. J. Bone Joint Surg., 38-A:957–977, 1956.

93. Rowe, C. R.: Acute and recurrent dislocations of the shoulder. J. Bone Joint Surg., 44-A:998–1008, 1962.

94. Rowe, C. R.: Anterior dislocation of the shoulder. Surg. Clin. North Am., 43:1609–1614, 1963.

95. Rowe, C. R.: The results of operative treatment of recurrent anterior dislocations of the shoulder using a modified Bankart procedure. Surg. Clin. North Am., 43:1663–1666, 1963.

96. Rowe, C. R.: Complicated dislocations of the shoulder. Guidelines in the treatment. Am. J. Surg., 117:549–553, 1969.

97. Rowe, C. R., and Pierce, D.: The enigma of voluntary recurrent dislocation of the shoulder. J. Bone Joint Surg., 47-A:1670, 1965.

98. Rowe, C. R., and Sakellarides, H. T.: Factors related to recurrences of anterior dislocations of the shoulder. Clin. Orthop., 20:40–48, 1961.

99. Rowe, C. R., Pierce, D. S., and Clark, J.: Voluntary dislocation of the shoulder. A preliminary report on a clinical, electromyographic, and psychiatric study of 26 patients. J. Bone Joint Surg., 55-A:445–460, 1973.

100. Saha, A. K.: Anterior recurrent dislocation of the shoulder. Treatment by latissimus dorsi transfer with follow-up in 22 cases. J. Int. Coll. Surg., 39:361–373, 1963.

101. Saha, A. K.: Anterior recurrent dislocation of the shoulder. Acta Orthop. Scand., 39:479–493, 1967.

102. Saha, A. K.: Dynamic stability of the glenohumeral joint. Acta Orthop. Scand., 42:491–505, 1971.

103. Schulz, T. J., Jacobs, B., and Patterson, R. L.: Unrecognized dislocations of the shoulder. J. Trauma, 9:1009–1023, 1969.

104. Sweeney, H. J., Mead, N. C., Dawson, W. J., and Fitzsimmons, P.: Fourteen Years' Experience with the Modified Bristow Procedure for Recurrent Anterior Dislocation of the Shoulder. Read at the Annual Meeting of the American Academy of Orthopedic Surgeons. San Francisco, Calif., March 5, 1975.

105. Symeonides, P. P.: The significance of the subscapularis muscles in the pathogenesis of recurrent anterior dislocation of the shoulder. J. Bone Joint Surg., 54-A:476–483, 1972.

106. Watson-Jones, R.: Dislocation of the shoulder joint. Proc. R. Soc. Med., 29:1060–1062, 1936.

107. Watson-Jones, J. R.: Note on recurrent dislocation of the shoulder joint superior approach causing the only failure in 52 operations for repair of the labrum and capsule. J. Bone Joint Surg., 30-B:49–52, 1948.

108. Watson-Jones, J. R.: Recurrent dislocation of the shoulder (Editorial). J. Bone Joint Surg., 30-B:6–8, 1948.

109. Watson-Jones, J. R.: Fractures and Joint Injuries, 2 vols., ed. 4. Baltimore, Williams & Wilkins Co., 1957.

110. Zimmerman, L. M., and Veith, I.: Great Ideas in the History of Surgery, 2nd rev. ed. New York, Dover Publications, Inc., 1967.

111. Barnes, R.: Traction injuries of the brachial plexus in adults. J. Bone Joint Surg., 31-B:10–16, 1949.

112. Blom, S., and Dahlback, L. P.: Nerve injuries in dislocations of the shoulder joint and fractures of the neck of the humerus. Acta Chir. Scand., 136:461–466, 1970.

113. Bonney, G.: Prognosis in traction injuries of the brachial plexus. J. Bone Joint Surg., 41-B:4–35, 1959.

114. Brown, F. W., and Navigato, W. J.: Rupture of the axillary artery and brachial plexus palsy associated with anterior dislocation of the shoulder. Clin. Orthop., 60:195–199, 1968.

115. Curr, J. F.: Rupture of the axillary artery complicating dislocation of the shoulder. J. Bone Joint Surg., 52-B:313–317, 1970.

116. Gariepy, R., Derome, A., and Laurin, C. A.: Brachial plexus paralysis following shoulder dislocation. Can. J. Surg., 5:418–421, 1962.

117. Gibson, J. M. C.: Rupture of the axillary artery following anterior dislocation of the shoulder. J. Bone Joint Surg., 44-B:114–115, 1962.

118. Gryska, P. F.: Major vascular injuries—Principles of management in selected cases of arterial and venous injuries. N. Engl. J. Med., 266:381–385, 1962.

119. Jardon, O. M., Hood, L. T., and Lynch, R. D.: Complete avulsion of the axillary artery as a complication of shoulder dislocation. J. Bone Joint Surg., 55:189–192, 1973.

120. Johnston, G. W., and Lowry, J. H.: Rupture of the axillary artery complicating anterior dislocation of the shoulder. J. Bone Joint Surg., 44-B:116–118, 1962.

121. Milton, G. W.: The mechanism of circumflex and other nerve injuries in dislocation of the shoulder and the possible mechanism of nerve injuries during reduction of dislocation. Aust. N.Z. J. Surg., 23:25–30, 1953–55.

Posterior Glenohumeral Dislocations

122. Arndt, J. H., and Sears, A. D.: Posterior dislocation of the shoulder. Am. J. Roentgenol., 94:639–645, 1965.

123. Bell, H. M.: Posterior fracture-dislocation—A method of closed reduction. J. Bone Joint Surg., 47-A:1521–1524, 1965.

124. Bloom, M. H., and Obata, W. G.: Diagnosis of posterior dislocation of the shoulder with use of Velpeau axillary and angle-up roentgenographic views. J. Bone Joint Surg., 49-A:943–949, 1967.

125. Boyd, H. B., and Sisk, T. D.: Recurrent posterior dislocation of the shoulder. J. Bone Joint Surg., 54-A:779–786, 1972.

126. Budd, F. W.: Voluntary bilateral posterior dislocation of the shoulder joint. Clin. Orthop., 63:181–183, 1969.

127. Carter, C., and Sweetman, R.: Recurrent dislocation of the patella and of the shoulder. Their association with familial joint laxity. J. Bone Joint Surg., 42-B:721–727, 1960.

128. Cave, E. F.: Fractures and Other Injuries. Chicago, Year Book Publishers, 1961.

129. Detenbeck, L. C.: Posterior dislocations of the shoulder. J. Trauma, 12:183–192, 1972.

130. Dimon, J. H., III: Posterior Dislocations of the Shoulder. J. Trauma, 12:183–192, 1972.

131. English, E., and Macnab, I.: Recurrent posterior dislocation of the shoulder. J. Bone Joint Surg., 17:147–151, 1974.

132. Hindenach, J. C. R.: Recurrent posterior dislocation of the shoulder. J. Bone Joint Surg., 29:582–586, 1947.

133. Kretzler, H. H., and Blue, A. R.: Recurrent posterior dislocation of the shoulder in cerebral palsy. J. Bone Joint Surg., 48-A:1221, 1966.

134. Laskin, R. S., and Sedlin, E. D.: Luxatio erecta in infancy. Clin. Orthop., 80:126–129, 1971.

135. Lindholm, T. S.: Recurrent posterior dislocation of the shoulder. Acta Chir. Scand., 140:101–106, 1974.

136. McLaughlin, H. L.: Posterior dislocation of the shoulder. J. Bone Joint Surg., 34-A:584–590, 1952.

137. McLaughlin, H. L.: Posterior dislocation of the shoulder. J. Bone Joint Surg., 44-A:1477, 1962.

138. McLaughlin, H. L.: Locked posterior subluxation of the shoulder—Diagnosis and treatment. Surg. Clin. North Am., 43:1621–1622, 1963.

139. May, H.: Nicola operation for posterior subacromial dislocation of the humerus. J. Bone Joint Surg., 25:78–84, 1943.

140. Neviaser, J. S.: Posterior dislocations of the shoulder; Diagnosis and treatment. Surg. Clin. North Am., 43:1623–1630, 1963.

141. Neviaser, J. S.: The treatment of old unreduced dislocations of the shoulder. Surg. Clin. North Am., 43:1671–1678, 1963.

142. Nobel, W.: Posterior traumatic dislocation of the shoulder. J. Bone Joint Surg., 44-A:523–538, 1962.

143. Oyston, J. K.: Unreduced posterior dislocation of the shoulder treated by open reduction and transposition of the subscapularis tendon. J. Bone Joint Surg., 46-B:256–259, 1964.

144. Pear, B. L.: Bilateral posterior fracture dislocation of the shoulder—An uncommon complication of a convulsive seizure. N. Engl. J. Med., 283:135–136, 1970.

145. Pear, B. L.: Dislocation of the shoulder, x-ray signs (Correspondence). N. Engl. J. Med., 283:1113, 1970.

146. Rowe, C. R., and Yee, L. K.: A posterior approach to the shoulder joint. J. Bone Joint Surg., 26:580–584, 1944.

147. Scott, D. J., Jr.: Treatment of recurrent posterior dislocation of the shoulder by glenoplasty. Report of 3 cases. J. Bone Joint Surg., 49-A:471–476, 1967.

148. Scourgall, S.: Posterior dislocation of the shoulder. J. Bone Joint Surg., 39-B:726–732, 1957.

149. Warrick, C. K.: Posterior dislocation of the shoulder joint. J. Bone Joint Surg., 30-B:651–655, 1948.

150. Warrick, C. K.: Posterior dislocation of the shoulder joint. Br. J. Radiol., 38:758–761, 1965.

151. Wilson, J. C., and McKeever, F. M.: Traumatic posterior (retroglenoid) dislocation of the humerus. J. Bone Joint Surg., 31-A:160–172, 1949.

152. Zadik, F. R.: Recurrent dislocation of the shoulder joint. J. Bone Joint Surg., 30-B:531–532, 1948.

Acromioclavicular Joint Dislocations

153. Accardo, N. J.: The Gurd-Mumford procedure for acromioclavicular dislocations. Bull. Tulane U. Med. Fac., 20:41–46, 1960.

154. Ahstrom, J. P., Jr.: Surgical repair of complete acromioclavicular separation. J.A.M.A., 217:785–789, 1971.

155. Alldredge, R. H.: Surgical treatment of acromioclavicular dislocation. J. Bone Joint Surg., 47-A:1278, 1965.

156. Allman, F. L., Jr.: Fractures and ligamentous injuries of the clavicle and its articulation. J. Bone Joint Surg., 49-A:774–784, 1967.

157. Anderson, M. E.: Treatment of dislocations of the acromioclavicular and sternoclavicular joints. J. Bone Joint Surg., 45-A:657–658, 1963.

158. Arner, O., Sandahl, U., and Öhrling, H.: Dislocation of the acromioclavicular joint—Review of the literature and report of 56 cases. Acta Chir. Scand., 113:140–152, 1957.

159. Aufranc, O. E., Jones, S. N., and Harris, W. H.: Complete acromioclavicular dislocation. J.A.M.A., 180:681–682, 1962.

160. Badgley, C. E.: Sports injuries of the shoulder girdle. J.A.M.A., 172:444–448, 1960.

161. Bailey, R. W.: A dynamic repair for complete acromioclavicular joint dislocation. J. Bone Joint Surg., 47-A:858, 1965.

162. Bailey, R. W., O'Connor, G. A., Tilus, P. D., and Baril, J. D.: A dynamic repair for acute and chronic injuries of the acromioclavicular area. J. Bone Joint Surg., 54-A:1802, 1972.

163. Barnhart, J. M., Fain, R. H., Dewar, F. P., and Stein, A. H.: Acromioclavicular joint injuries. Clin. Orthop., 81:199, 1970.

164. Bateman, J. E.: Athletic injuries about the shoulder in throwing and body-contact sports. Clin. Orthop., 23:75–83, 1962.

165. Bearden, J. M., Hughston, J. C., and Whatley,

G. S.: Acromioclavicular dislocation: Method of treatment. J. Sports Med., 1:5–17, 1973.

166. Beckman, T.: A case of simultaneous luxation of both ends of the clavicle. Acta Chir. Scand., 56:156–163, 1923.

167. Behling, F.: Treatment of acromioclavicular separations. Orthop. Clin. North Am., 4:747–757, 1973.

168. Birkett, A. N.: The result of operative repair of severe acromioclavicular dislocation. Br. J. Surg., 32:103–105, 1944–45.

169. Bloom, F. A.: Wire fixation in acromioclavicular dislocation. J. Bone Joint Surg., 27:273–276, 1945.

170. Bonnin, J. G.: Complete Outline of Fractures. London, William Heinemann, 1941.

171. Bosworth, B. M.: Acromioclavicular separation. New method of repair. Surg. Gynecol. Obstet., 73:866–871, 1941.

172. Bosworth, B. M.: Acromioclavicular dislocation: End results of screw suspension treatment. Ann. Surg., 127:98–111, 1948.

173. Bosworth, B. M.: Complete acromioclavicular dislocation. N. Engl. J. Med., 241:221–225, 1949.

174. Bowers, R. F.: Complete acromioclavicular separation. Diagnosis and operative treatment. J. Bone Joint Surg., 17:1005–1010, 1935.

175. Brosgol, M.: Traumatic acromioclavicular sprains and subluxation. Clin. Orthop., 20:98–107, 1961.

176. Bundens, W. D., and Cook, J. I.: Repair of acromioclavicular separations by deltoid-trapezius imbrication. Clin. Orthop., 20:109–114, 1961.

177. Cadenat, F. M.: The treatment of dislocations and fractures of the outer end of the clavicle. Int. Clin., 1:145–169, 1917.

178. Caldwell, G. D.: Treatment of complete permanent acromioclavicular dislocation by surgical arthrodesis. J. Bone Joint Surg., 25:368–374, 1943.

179. Campos, O. P.: Acromioclavicular dislocation. Am. J. Surg., 43:287–291, 1939.

180. Carrell, W. B.: Dislocation at the outer end of clavicle. J. Bone Joint Surg., 10:314–315, 1928.

181. Codman, E. A.: The Shoulder, ed. 1. Boston, Thomas Todd & Co., 1934.

182. Cooper, E. S.: New method of treating long-standing dislocations of the scapuloclavicular articulation. Am. J. Med. Sci., 41:389–392, 1861.

183. Copher, G. H.: A method of treatment of upward dislocation of the acromial end of the clavicle. Am. J. Surg., 22:507–508, 1933.

184. Currie, D. I.: An apparatus for dislocation of the acromial end of the clavicle. Br. Med. J., 1:570, 1924.

185. DePalma, A. F.: Degenerative Changes in the Sternoclavicular and Acromioclavicular Joints in Various Decades. Springfield, Ill., Charles C Thomas, 1957.

186. DePalma, A. F.: Surgical anatomy of the acromioclavicular and sternoclavicular joints. Surg. Clin. North Am., 43:1540–1550, 1963.

187. DePalma, A. F.: Surgery of the Shoulder, ed. 2. Philadelphia, J. B. Lippincott Co., 1973.

188. DePalma, A. F., Callery, G., and Bennett, G. A.: Variational Anatomy and Degenerative Lesions of the Shoulder Joint. American Academy of Orthopaedic Surgeons Instructional Course Lectures, 6:255–281, 1949.

189. Dewar, F. P., and Barrington, T. W.: The treatment of chronic acromioclavicular dislocation. J. Bone Joint Surg., 47-B:32–35, 1965.

190. Elkin, D. C., and Cooper, F. W., Jr.: Resection of the clavicle in vascular surgery. J. Bone Joint Surg., 28:117–119, 1946.

191. Gallie, W. E.: Dislocations. N. Engl. J. Med., 213:91–98, 1935.

192. Gardner, E., and Gray, D. J.: Prenatal development of the human shoulder and acromioclavicular joints. Am. J. Anat., 92:219–276, 1953.

193. Giannestras, N. J.: A method of immobilization of acute acromioclavicular separation. J. Bone Joint Surg., 26:597–599, 1944.

194. Gibbens, M. E.: An appliance for conservative treatment of acromioclavicular dislocation. J. Bone Joint Surg., 28:164–165, 1946.

195. Glick, J.: Acromioclavicular dislocation in athletes. Orthop. Rev., No. 4, 1:31–34, 1972.

196. Goldberg, D.: Acromioclavicular Joint Injuries: Modified Conservative Form of Treatment. Amer. J. Surg., 71:529–531, 1946.

197. Goss, C. M. (Ed.): Gray's Anatomy, 29th Am. ed. Philadelphia, Lea & Febiger, 1974.

198. Gradoyevitch, B.: Coracoclavicular joint. J. Bone Joint Surg., 21:918–920, 1939.

199. Gurd, F. B.: The treatment of complete dislocation of the outer end of the clavicle. An hitherto undescribed operation. Ann. Surg., 113:1094–1098, 1941.

200. Harrison, W. E., and Sisler, J.: Acromioclavicular Separation Treated by Dacron Vascular Graft Loop Beneath the Coracoid and Through the Clavicle. Scientific Exhibit. American Academy of Orthopaedic Surgeons. Dallas, Texas, January 17–22, 1974.

201. Hoyt, W. A., Jr.: Etiology of shoulder injuries in athletes. J. Bone Joint Surg., 49-A:755–766, 1967.

202. Imatani, R. J., Hanlon, J. J., and Cady, G. W.: Acute, complete acromioclavicular separation. J. Bone Joint Surg., 57-A:328–332, 1975.

203. Inman, V. T., Saunders, J. B., and Abbott, L. C.: Observations on the function of the shoulder joint. J. Bone Joint Surg., 26:1–30, 1944.

204. Inman, V. T., McLaughlin, H. D., Neviaser, J., and Rowe, C.: Treatment of complete acromioclavicular dislocation. J. Bone Joint Surg., 44-A:1008–1011, 1962.

205. Jacobs, B., and Wade, P. A.: Acromioclavicular joint injury. End result study. J. Bone Joint Surg., 48-A:475–486, 1968.

206. Jordan, H. H.: An improved abduction splint for the upper extremity. J. Bone Joint Surg., 26:600–601, 1944.

207. Kennedy, J. C.: Complete dislocation of the acromioclavicular joint. J. Trauma, 8:311–318, 1968.

208. Kennedy, J. C., and Cameron, H.: Complete dislo-

cation of the acromioclavicular joint. J. Bone Joint Surg., 36-B:202–208, 1954.

209. Laing, P. G.: Transplantation of the long head of the biceps in complete acromioclavicular separations. J. Bone Joint Surg., 41-A:1677–1678, 1969.

210. Lazcano, M. A., Anzel, S. H., and Kelly, P. J.: Complete dislocation and subluxation of the acromioclavicular joint. End results in 73 cases. J. Bone Joint Surg., 43-A:379–391, 1961.

211. Mazet, R. J.: Migration of a Kirschner wire from the shoulder region into the lung. Report of two cases. J. Bone Joint Surg., 25-A:477–483, 1943.

212. Moseley, H. F., and Templeton, J.: Dislocation of acromioclavicular dislocation, utilizing the coracoacromial ligament. J. Bone Joint Surg., 51-B:196, 1969.

213. Moshein, J., and Elconin, K. B.: Repair of acute acromioclavicular dislocation, utilizing the coracoacromial ligament. J. Bone Joint Surg., 51-A:812, 1969.

214. Mumford, E. B.: Acromioclavicular dislocation. J. Bone Joint Surg., 23:799–802, 1941.

215. Murray, G.: Fixation of dislocations of the acromioclavicular joint and rupture of the coracoclavicular ligament. Can. Med. Assoc. J., 43:270–273, 1940.

216. Murray, G.: The use of longitudinal wires in the treatment of fractures and dislocations. Am. J. Surg., 67:156–167, 1945.

217. Neviaser, J. S.: Acromioclavicular dislocation treated by transference of the coracoacromial ligament. Bull. Hosp. Joint Dis., 12:46–54, 1951.

218. Neviaser, J. S.: Acromioclavicular dislocation treated by transference of the coracoacromial ligament. Arch. Surg., 64:292–297, 1952.

219. Neviaser, J. S.: Acromioclavicular dislocation treated by transference of the coracoacromial ligament. Clin. Orthop., 58:57–68, 1968.

220. Nicoll, E. A.: Miners and mannequins (Annotation). J. Bone Joint Surg., 36-B:171–172, 1954.

221. Nielsen, W. B.: Injury to the acromioclavicular joint. J. Bone Joint Surg., 45-B:207, 1963.

222. Norrell, H., and Llewellyn, R. C.: Migration of a threaded Steinmann pin from an acromioclavicular joint into the spinal canal. A case report. J. Bone Joint Surg., 47-A:1024–1026, 1965.

223. Nutter, P. D.: Coracoclavicular articulation. J. Bone Joint Surg., 23:177–179, 1941.

224. Oppenheimer, A.: Arthritis of the acromioclavicular joint. J. Bone Joint Surg., 25:867–870, 1943.

225. Patterson, W. R.: Inferior dislocation of the distal end of the clavicle. J. Bone Joint Surg., 49-A:1184–1186, 1967.

226. Phemister, D. B.: The treatment of dislocation of the acromioclavicular joint by the open reduction and threaded-wire fixation. J. Bone Joint Surg., 24:166–168, 1942.

227. Pillay, V. K.: Significance of the coracoclavicular joint. J. Bone Joint Surg., 49-B:390, 1967.

228. Powers, J. A., and Bach, P. J.: Acromioclavicular

separations—Closed or open treatment. Clin. Orthop., 104:213–223, 1974.

229. Pridie, K.: Dislocation of acromioclavicular and sternoclavicular joints. J. Bone Joint Surg., 41-B:429, 1959.

230. Quigley, T. B.: Injuries to the acromioclavicular and sternoclavicular joints sustained in athletics. Surg., Clin. North Am., 43:1551–1554, 1963.

231. Rowe, C. R., and Marble, H. C.: Fractures and Other Injuries. Edited by E. F. Cave. Chicago, Year Book Publishers, Inc., 1958.

232. Schneider, C. C.: Acromioclavicular dislocation: Autoplastic reconstruction. J. Bone Joint Surg., 15:957, 1933.

233. Spigelman, L.: A Harness for acromioclavicular separation. J. Bone Joint Surg., 51-A:585–586, 1969.

234. Tossy, J. D., Mead, N. C., and Sigmond, H. M.: Acromioclavicular separations: Useful and practical classification for treatment. Clin. Orthop., 28:111–119, 1963.

235. Tristan, T. A., and Daughteridge, T. G.: Migration of a metallic pin from the humerus into the lung. N. Engl. J. Med., 270:987–989, 1964.

236. Trynin, A. H.: Conservative treatment for complete dislocation of the acromioclavicular joint. J. Bone Joint Surg., 16:713–715, 1934.

237. Urist, M. R.: Complete dislocation of the acromioclavicular joint. The nature of the traumatic lesion and effective methods of treatment with an analysis of 41 cases. J. Bone Joint Surg., 28:813–837, 1946.

238. Vargas, L.: Repair of complete acromioclavicular dislocation, utilizing the short head of the biceps. J. Bone Joint Surg., 24:772–773, 1942.

239. Varney, J. H., Coker, J. K., and Cawley, J. J.: Treatment of acromioclavicular dislocation by means of a harness. J. Bone Joint Surg., 34-A:232–233, 1952.

240. Wagner, C.: Partial claviculectomy. Am. J. Surg., 85:259–265, 1953.

241. Warner, A. H.: A harness for use in the treatment of acromioclavicular separation. J. Bone Joint Surg., 19:1132–1133, 1937.

242. Watkins, J. T.: An operation for the relief of acromioclavicular luxations. J. Bone Joint Surg., 7:790–792, 1925.

243. Weaver, J. K., and Dunn, H. K.: Treatment of acromioclavicular injuries, especially complete acromioclavicular separation. J. Bone Joint Surg., 54-A:1187–1198, 1972.

244. Weitzman, G.: Treatment of acute acromioclavicular joint dislocation by a modified Bosworth method. J. Bone Joint Surg., 49-A:1167–1178, 1967.

245. Wilson, F. C., Jr., and Prothero, S. R.: Results of operative treatment of acute dislocation of the acromioclavicular joint. J. Trauma, 7:202–209, 1967.

246. Wolin, I.: Acute acromioclavicular dislocation. J. Bone Joint Surg., 26:589–592, 1944.

247. Worchester, J. N., and Green, D. P.: Osteoarthritis of the acromioclavicular joint. Clin. Orthop., 58:69–73, 1968.

Sternoclavicular Joint Dislocations

248. Bachmann, M.: Swelling of the sternoclavicular joint. Israel Med. J., 17:65–72, 1958.
249. Baker, E. C.: Tomography of the sternoclavicular joint. Ohio State Med. J., 55:60, 1959.
250. Bankart, A. S.: An operation for recurrent dislocation (subluxation) of the sternoclavicular joint. Br. J. Surg., 26:320–323, 1938.
251. Bateman, J. E.: The Shoulder and Neck. Philadelphia, W. B. Saunders Co., 1972.
252. Bearn, J. G.: Direct observation on the function of the capsule of the sternoclavicular joint in clavicular support. J. Anat., 101:159–170, 1967.
253. Beckman, T.: A case of simultaneous luxation of both ends of the clavicle. Acta Chir. Scand., 56:156–163, 1923.
254. Bonnin, J. G.: Spontaneous subluxation of the sternoclavicular joint. Br. Med. J., 2:274–275, 1960.
255. Bremner, R. A.: Monarticular, noninfective subacute arthritis of the sternoclavicular joint. J. Bone Joint Surg., 41-B:749–753, 1959.
256. Brooks, A. L., and Henning, G. D.: Injury to the proximal clavicular epiphysis. J. Bone Joint Surg., 54-A:1347–1348, 1972.
257. Brown, J. E.: Anterior sternoclavicular dislocation—A method of repair. Am. J. Orthop., 31:184–189, 1961.
258. Cave, A. J. E.: The nature and morphology of the costoclavicular ligament. J. Anat., 95:170–179, 1961.
259. Clark, R. L., Milgram, J. W., and Yawn, D. H.: Fatal aortic perforation and cardiac tamponade due to a Kirschner wire migrating from the right sternoclavicular joint. South. Med. J., 67:316–318, 1974.
260. Denham, R. H., Jr., and Dingley, A. F., Jr.: Epiphyseal separation of the medial end of the clavicle. J. Bone Joint Surg., 49-A:1179–1183, 1967.
261. DePalma, A. F.: The role of the disks of the sternoclavicular and acromioclavicular joints. Clin. Orthop., 13:222–233, 1959.
262. DePalma, A. F.: Surgical anatomy of acromioclavicular and sternoclavicular joints. Surg. Clin. North Am., 43:1541–1550, 1963.
263. Duggan, N.: Recurrent dislocation of sternoclavicular cartilage. J. Bone Joint Surg., 13:365, 1931.

264. Elting, J. J.: Retrosternal dislocation of the clavicle. Arch. Surg., 104:35–37, 1972.
265. Ferry, A., Rook, F. W., and Masterson, J. H.: Retrosternal dislocation of the clavicle. J. Bone Joint Surg., 39-A:905–910, 1957.
266. Gurd, F. B.: Surplus parts of skeleton; Recommendation for excision of certain portions as means of shortening period of disability following trauma. Am. J. Surg., 74:705–720, 1947.
267. Heinig, C. F.: Retrosternal dislocation of the clavicle: Early recognition, x-ray diagnosis and management. J. Bone Joint Surg., 50-A:830, 1968.
268. Hobbs, D. W.: Sternoclavicular joint: A new axial radiographic view. Radiology, 90:801–802, 1968.
269. Howard, F. M., and Shafer, S. J.: Injuries to the clavicle with neuromuscular complications. J. Bone Joint Surg., 47-A:1335–1346, 1965.
270. Kennedy, J. C.: Retrosternal dislocation of the clavicle. J. Bone Joint Surg., 31-B:74–75, 1949.
271. Lucas, D. B.: Biomechanics of the shoulder joint. Arch. Surg., 107:425–432, 1973.
272. Lunseth, P. A., Chapman, K. W., and Frankel, V. H.: Surgical treatment of clavicular joint. J. Bone Joint Surg., 57-B:193–196, 1975.
273. Lusskin, R., Weiss, C. A., and Winer, J.: The role of the subclavius muscle in the subclavian vein syndrome (costoclavicular syndrome) following fracture of the clavicle: A case report with a review of the pathophysiology of the costoclavicular space. Clin. Orthop., 54:75–83, 1967.
274. McKenzie, J. M. M.: Retrosternal dislocation of the clavicle, a report of two cases. J. Bone Joint Surg., 45-B:138–141, 1963.
275. Maini, P. S.: Personal communication.
276. Omer, G. E.: Osteotomy of the clavicle in surgical reduction of anterior sternoclavicular dislocation. J. Trauma, 7:584–590, 1967.
277. Pate, J. W., and Wilhite, J.: Migration of a foreign body from the sternoclavicular joint to the heart—A case report. Am. Surg., 35:448–449, 1969.
278. Paterson, D. C.: Retrosternal dislocation of the clavicle. J. Bone Joint Surg., 43-B:90–94, 1961.
279. Salvatore, J.: Sternoclavicular joint dislocation. Clin. Orthop., 58:51–55, 1968.
280. Stein, A. H.: Retrosternal dislocation of the clavicle. J. Bone Joint Surg., 39-A:656–660, 1957.
281. Tyer, H. D. D., Sturrock, W. D. S., and Callow, F. McC.: Retrosternal dislocation of the clavicle. J. Bone Joint Surg., 45-B:132–137, 1963.
282. Worman, L. W., and Leagus, C.: Intrathoracic injury following retrosternal dislocation of the clavicle. J. Trauma, 7:416–423, 1967.

21

Tumors of the Shoulder

WILLIAM F. ENNEKING
ROBERT ROY

Tumors of the shoulder region occur in all age groups and span the entire spectrum of biologic aggressiveness. This chapter will consider the pathology and surgical management of the more common benign and malignant intraosseous tumors as well as the common soft-tissue sarcomas of the shoulder region. Only those surgical modalities that preserve a functional extremity will be considered. The indications and techniques of shoulder disarticulation and forequarter amputation are presented elsewhere. No effort is made to present detailed descriptions of the roentgenologic and microscopic characteristics of each lesion since this information is readily available in several well-illustrated texts.[1,4,6] Rather, the more practical aspects of tumor pathology are stressed. This brief survey of the pathology is followed by a presentation of the basic principles involved in the diagnostic evaluation and surgical management of these tumors and their application is illustrated with selected cases.

Although the entire gamut of benign and malignant neoplasms may occur about the shoulder, certain entities have a predilection for this region. Figure 21-1 illustrates the subdivisions of tumors commonly encountered in the shoulder region. There are three benign intraosseous lesions: unicameral bone cyst, osteochondroma or exostosis, and benign epiphyseal chondroblastoma. The malignant lesions of bone encompass three categories: metastatic car-

cinomas, those sarcomas arising from bone marrow elements, and the sarcomas arising from connective tissue elements. The important soft-tissue sarcomas are liposarcoma, fibrosarcoma, rhabdomyosarcoma, and malignant Schwannomas. Schwannomas usually arise in the brachial plexus and their envelopment of the brachial vessels makes radical resection unfeasible. In this event, forequarter amputation usually offers the only hope of complete tumor eradication.

PATHOLOGIC CONSIDERATIONS

Benign Lesions

UNICAMERAL BONE CYST. Unicameral bone cyst develops during the period of skeletal growth and is most often found in the proximal humerus.[3] Although the cause remains unknown, roentgenographic appearance and anatomic location usually make diagnosis rather straightforward.[7] The lesion appears radiographically as an ovoid osteolytic lesion that is markedly radiolucent (Fig. 21-2). The defect usually is first detected just below the epiphyseal plate. The metaphyseal spongiosa is replaced by a cystic cavity containing a straw-colored fluid under increased hydrostatic pressure (Fig. 21-3). This fluid accounts for the marked radiolucency which contrasts with the ground-glass appearance of fibrous dysplasia. Also, unicameral bone cyst does

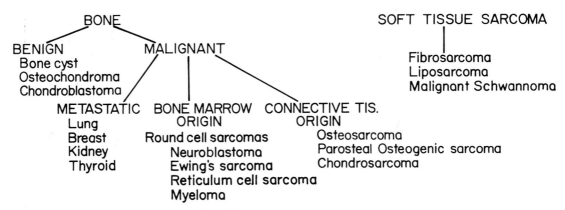

FIG. 21-1. Common tumors about the shoulder.

not exhibit any periosteal layering of new bone unless a pathologic fracture has occurred. These two features—the marked radiolucency, as opposed to the ground-glass appearance, and the absence of periosteal new bone formation—help to distinguish the bone cyst from the occasionally problematic lesions of monostotic fibrous dysplasia or eosinophilic granuloma, respectively.

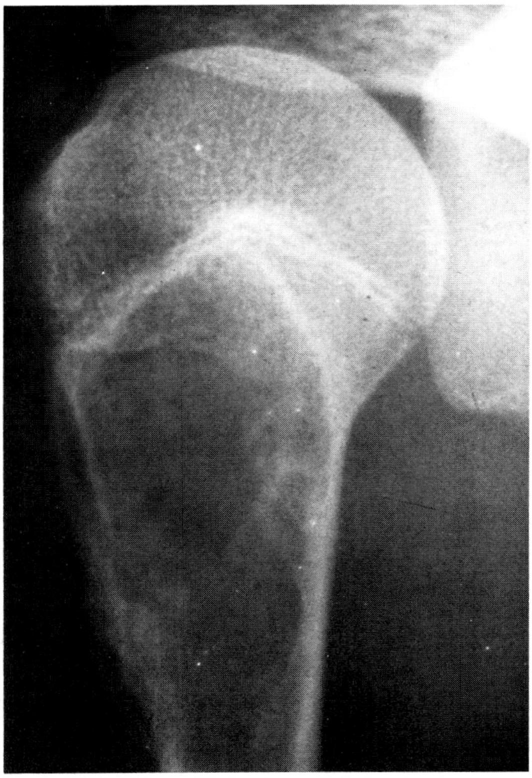

The solitary bone cyst often remains asymptomatic and undetected until the child sustains a pathologic fracture. The associated pain then leads to roentgenographic evaluation. A biopsy specimen at this point may present a confusing histologic picture of extremely active mesenchymal tissue laying down new bone. If the pathologist is unaware of the clinical setting and roentgenographic appearance of the lesion, he might be misled on histologic grounds to entertain a diagnosis of osteogenic sarcoma.

The surgeon must be wary of the confusing appearance that results from biopsy of any lesion with a recently superimposed pathologic fracture. If biopsy of such a lesion is indicated, it is best to do so within the first 48 hours after injury or to defer biopsy for 6 to 8 weeks until the fracture callus matures. A delay of 6 to 8 weeks permits separation of the orderly arrangement of maturing callus from the disorganized pattern of osteogenic sarcoma. The child who sustains repeated pathologic fractures or whose lesion fails to heal after pathologic fracture is best treated by operative intervention. The cyst should be thoroughly curetted to remove all traces of the lining from its scalloped walls and then packed with autogenous bone graft (Fig. 21-4). If the lesion is large cortical struts of

FIG. 21-2. An anteroposterior roentgenogram of a latent simple cyst in a 15-year-old girl.

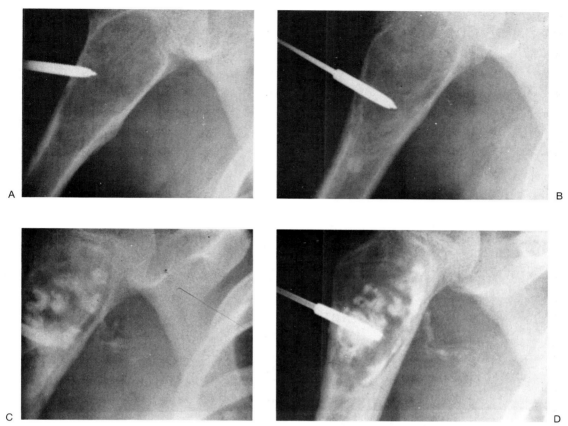

FIG. 21-3. A series of roentgenograms were made of the simple cyst shown in Figure 21-2. A, A threaded watertight trochar was inserted into the cavity. The pressure of the fluid was 42 cm. of water, the meniscus of the fluid in the manometer pulsated in concert with apical heart rate, and the pressure was increased 3.5 cm. by a Valsalva maneuver. B, An injection of radiopaque dye was begun. C, One second later, the dye is rapidly being taken up during drainage. D, Another second later, the drainage is shown clearly. This series of films demonstrates the increased pressure of the cystic fluid and the close relationship between the fluid and the venous circulation.

bone are needed to provide initial mechanical stability.

Preoperative prediction of the chances of eradicating these bone cysts is possible. Jaffe and Lichtenstein were the first to separate these bone cysts into active and latent stages. The active stage has a 50 percent recurrence rate. Three features distinguishing the active cysts are (1) that the cyst is in a juxtaepiphyseal location, whereas the latent cyst has been left behind as the epiphyseal plate grows away from the cyst; (2) that the patient is 10 years old or younger; and (3) that the cyst wall is thin and does not exhibit the scattered giant cells, hemosiderin, and cholesterol deposits seen in the thickened lining of the latent cyst (Fig. 21-5).

OSTEOCHONDROMA. The osteochondroma, or exostosis, is an outgrowth of bone and cartilage which may arise from any epiphysis or apophysis. Some consider the lesion as simply an outgrowth of the epiphyseal plate and not a neoplasm in the strict sense of the word. Exostoses grow by proliferation of their cauliflowerlike cartilaginous cap. The chondrocytes mature, degenerate, undergo matrix calcification, and subsequently are invaded by vascular mesenchymal buds of tissue. These fingers of tissue lay down trabeculae of immature bone on the scaffold of calcified matrix. This se-

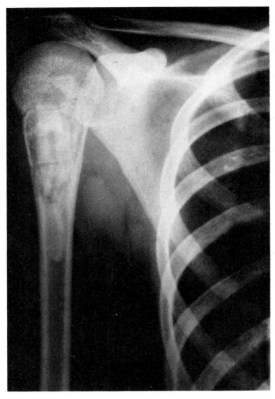

FIG. 21-4. An anteroposterior roentgenogram taken 1 year after adequate grafting of the simple bone cyst shown in Figures 21-2 and 21-3.

quence mimics epiphyseal enchondral ossification, albeit in a somewhat less orderly fashion.

Exostoses continue to grow throughout the period of normal skeletal growth. When epiphyseal growth ceases, the lesion also stops growing. However, its cartilaginous cap persists indefinitely. Eighty percent of all the exostoses of the upper extremity arises at the proximal humeral epiphysis or scapular apophyses. The lesions either are broad based (sessile) or have a slender stalk of bone that is continuous with the cortical shaft. A sagittal section of the cartilaginous cap reveals a rim of cartilage no thicker than 5 mm. During periods of rapid growth, as in adolescence, the rim can be as thick as 1 cm. and have many binucleated chondrocytes. This biologic activity is reflected by an increase in radio-scan activity. However,

once skeletal growth has ceased, a cartilaginous rim greater than 5 mm. should be regarded with extreme suspicion, as it suggests chondrosarcomatous change.

The chance of a solitary exostosis evolving into a chondrosarcoma is extremely small, probably less than 2 percent. The same is not true of patients with multiple hereditary exostoses. These individuals have approximately a 50 percent chance of transmitting this disease to their offspring and a greater chance of chondrosarcomatous degeneration. The typical osteochondroma remains asymptomatic unless one of three problems arises: (1) the lesion's anatomic location leads to compression of an adjacent neural structure; (2) the bulk of the osteochondromatous mass interferes with the joint's range of motion; or (3) the exostosis elicits a painful bursa over its cartilaginous cap. If any of these three problems arises, simple excision is indicated. Any exostosis that begins to enlarge after skeletal growth has ceased and is "hot" on radioisotope scanning should be suspected of being a potential low-grade chondrosarcoma and should be treated as such by regional excision early in its evolution.

BENIGN EPIPHYSEAL CHONDROBLASTOMA. Chondroblastoma is a benign cartilaginous tumor which arises in a secondary center of ossification at a time when there is an open epiphyseal plate. It occurs frequently about the knee and hip, but the classic location is the proximal humeral epiphysis. In fact, it was the shoulder region where Codman first described the lesion in 1931, and called the tumor an epiphyseal chondromatous giant cell tumor.[2] The lesion is still frequently referred to as Codman's tumor.

The patient usually complains of a dull aching pain in the shoulder and may have a sympathetic effusion. Ninety percent of the lesions appears in persons between 5 and 25 years of age. Their radiographic appearance showing a round or ovoid osteolytic lesion eccentrically located in the epiphysis and sometimes extending across the open plate into the metaphysis is characteristic. Usually a small amount of reactive bone rings the lesion, and about 50 percent of the le-

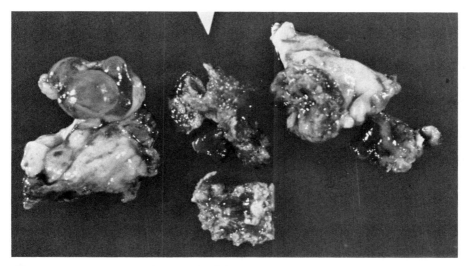

FIG. 21-5. The gross appearance of the material lining the latent cyst shown in Figures 21-2 through 21-4.

sions exhibits stippled calcifications within the lytic area (Fig. 21-6).

Histologically, the lesion consists of immature chondroblasts, fibrous tissue, multinucleated giant cells, and islands of mature cartilage. Foci of the cartilaginous matrix are often calcified, accounting for the radiographic appearance of stippling.

There have been isolated reports of malignant change, mostly some years after inadequate therapeutic irradiation. If the lesion is treated with curettage, recurrence is uncommon. The surgeon should resist the temptation of easy access to the lesion via arthrotomy, which potentially contaminates

the joint with tumor cells and leads to subsequent synovial implants. Aggressive recurrences with involvement of contiguous tissue planes are not unknown (Fig. 21-7). Such recurrences are better managed by radical local resection whenever feasible, rather than by repeated attempts at curettage (Fig. 21-8). The principles apply in the management of the adult counterpart of chondroblastoma, i.e., giant cell tumor.

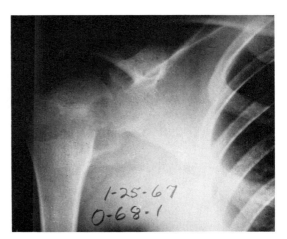

FIG. 21-7. The roentgen appearance of a chondroblastoma that had been curetted and grafted on two previous occasions. This second recurrent lesion had invaded the metaphysis, inferior capsule of the shoulder, cavity of the joint, and the subscapularis muscle.

FIG. 21-6. The roentgenographic appearance of an untreated chondroblastoma in a 15-year-old boy.

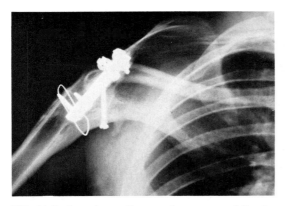

FIG. 21-8. A postoperative roentgenogram of the fusion employed to gain control of the recurrent chondroblastoma shown in Figure 21-7 after radical local resection. The patient is now 20 years old, had played high school football, and works as a telephone line repairman.

Malignant Lesions

The sarcomas in the shoulder region of primary concern to the surgeon are those that arise from the connective tissue and include osteosarcoma, chondrosarcoma, and soft-tissue sarcomas. The gross and microscopic pathologic appearances of these lesions reveal certain characteristics which have practical application in planning their surgical treatment.

Sarcomas are disseminated via the blood stream, and viable tumor emboli reach the lung where some survive and develop into pulmonary metastases. Many of the mechanisms and factors that control this dissemination and subsequent development of metastases are being unraveled by tumor biologists and immunopathologists. As these mechanisms are elucidated it is hoped that the tumor-host relationship can be manipulated in favor of host survival.

Complete surgical excision of the primary lesion remains the initial definitive treatment, with or without adjunctive radiotherapy, chemotherapy, or immunotherapy. The surgeon is obliged to remove the primary sarcoma completely, and in certain carefully selected cases this objective can be achieved without sacrificing the extremity. To most patients, preservation of a functional upper extremity is even more impor-

tant than preservation of a lower extremity. The overriding importance of the upper extremity both functionally and psychologically is readily apparent from the reactions of the patients undergoing amputation and the orthopaedic surgeons called upon to do the surgery. Despite their recent mechanical sophistication, upper extremity prostheses lack sensation and the proprioceptive feedback essential to coordinated manual dexterity. Even when the patient has to relinquish all shoulder motion he still has a normal elbow and, most importantly, his own normal hand.

Shoulder disarticulation or forequarter amputation can be supplanted by radical resection in cases of less biologically aggressive sacomas without compromising the primary objective, namely, complete ablation of the tumor. Three important criteria used to determine potential resectability of a sarcoma are (1) the lesion's precise anatomic location and extent; (2) its mode of local growth or spread; and (3) the tumor's degree of biologic aggressiveness. For example, the classic osteosarcoma of the proximal humerus infiltrates the metaphyseal latticework of cancellous bone and quickly penetrates the cortex, extending out into the soft tissues in all directions. This sarcoma is very aggressive with a high incidence of early metastasis. These characteristics usually preclude local resection and are in direct contrast to the less common parosteal or juxtacortical osteosarcoma which is slow growing and late to metastasize.

The parosteal osteosarcoma tends to wrap itself around the shaft of the bone leaving a plane of uninvolved soft tissue discernible between the cortical shaft and the enveloping tumor mass. It pushes the neighboring soft tissues ahead of itself, eliciting a pseudocapsule at the tumor-host interface. These characteristics of the parosteal osteogenic sarcoma make it an ideal lesion for early local radical resection supplemented, when necessary, by a shoulder fusion of a somewhat foreshortened extremity.

The chondrosarcomas of the shoulder

region, like the parosteal osteosarcoma, are slow growing and late to metastasize. As they progress, they too displace rather than invade adjacent soft tissues. The diagnosis of a malignant cartilaginous tumor cannot be safely made on microscopic criteria alone. The presence of mitotic fingers and binucleated chondrocytes is helpful and suggestive, but the pathologist must also consider the history, roentgen findings, and the gross appearance of the lesion's cut surface. Chondrosarcoma found in the scapula is the most common sarcoma and usually is the consequence of a previous exostosis. In contrast, chondrosarcoma of the proximal humerus is characteristically central in location, and less frequently a complication of enchondromata.

It may be judicious to consider all cartilaginous lesions in the shoulder region (much as those in the pelvic region) that become painful or increase in size in the skeletally mature individual as chondrosarcomas. By remaining well beyond the clearly defined pseudocapsule, it is usually possible to resect the tumor locally without spilling tumor into the wound. Contamination with chondrosarcomatous cells results in a high incidence of local recurrence. This phenomenon is not infrequently seen in old biopsy sites or surgical scars after a previous inadequate operation.

Of the sarcomas arising in soft tissue, fibrosarcoma, rhabdomyosarcoma, and liposarcoma are frequently amenable to total ablation by radical resection when the lesions are detected early and when the tumors do not encroach on essential neurovascular structures. Fibrosarcomas arising in bone are usually much more aggressive than those arising in soft tissues, infiltrating the cancellous bone and intermedullary canal, much like an osteogenic sarcoma. These primary intraosseous fibrosarcomas are often not suitable lesions for radical local resection. However, many of the patients with low-grade soft-tissue fibrosarcomas and the aggressive fibromatoses (extra-abdominal desmoids) that arise in the pectoral girdle are excellent candidates for radical local resection. Dissection of many

of these soft-tissue sarcomas in our laboratory reveals a common tendency to progress locally by creeping along fascial planes or between the muscle fascicles and replacing the perimysium. Adequate excision necessitates resection of the entire muscle mass en bloc from its origin to its insertion without visualizing the tumor. The minimum line of dissection must be one anatomic plane removed from the lesion, staying well outside of the pseudocapsule or reactive "rind" that the lesion frequently evokes from the neighboring tissues.

The metastatic lesions and round cell sarcomas should be considered in the differential diagnosis of intraosseous lesions in the shoulder region. Even when clinically evident, they should receive the same prebiopsy examination as the primary lesions. Although they may be best managed by nonsurgical means, i.e., radiotherapy and/or chemotherapy, such information may be of great value in planning treatment fields and gauging response to therapy. In this instance, the function of the surgeon is to obtain the biopsy specimen and stabilize the humerus when indicated. Many patients with round cell sarcomas often sustain pathologic fractures or have such an extensive lesion that a pathologic fracture is imminent. Frequently, these patients live for many months, and sometimes years, with their tumors under radiotherapeutic and chemotherapeutic control. The quality of life during these months is greatly improved if the patient can be provided with a stable, painfree, and functional upper extremity. Such skeletal stabilization often requires intramedullary fixation augmented with methyl methacrylate bonding. Recent information suggests that the therapeutic effect of radiotherapy/chemotherapy may be enhanced by surgically removing the bulk of the primary lesion with function-conserving excisions rather than with extensive radical operation.

Such operative intervention offers the opportunity to reduce significantly the total tumor cell mass. For solitary round cell lesions, such a reduction may be of more than just theoretical importance in the patient's chemotherapy and chance of survival.

DIAGNOSTIC CONSIDERATIONS

The preparation of patients for open biopsy and definitive surgical treatment involves a complete history and physical examination, and a special effort must be made to detect any subtle signs or symptoms of neural or vascular compromise. Special diagnostic procedures are a routine part of the initial evaluation. When arteriography and/or radioisotope scanning is employed in the patient who previously had had a biopsy, there is an unavoidable diminution in the yield of helpful information. Since simple biopsy alters the vascular pattern of the area, the arteriographer cannot distinguish what findings are due to the primary lesion and what are secondary to the healing response of the surgical biopsy or superimposed pathologic fracture. The ideal time to gather all possible information about the lesion is before surgical biopsy, and the information should include the following:

1. In addition to conventional roentgenograms of the lesion, tomograms often provide important supplemental data. The surgeon should also carefully scrutinize the standard chest film for signs of metastatic lesions, using tomograms to examine questionable areas.
2. The use of radioisotope scanning has been most helpful, since scanning is a more sensitive method of detecting additional osseous lesions than is the usual skeletal survey. The areas of increased uptake on the total body scan are then examined with cone-down roentgen techniques. Some scans may also be useful when soft-tissue sarcomas lie adjacent to radiologically normal bone; i.e., if the underlying bone is hot it is occultly involved by or contiguous with tumor. The ^{99m}Tc scan has also shown a manyfold increase in uptake activity in the exostosis that

has undergone chondrosarcomatous change as compared to the uptake by other exostoses in patients with multiple hereditary exostoses.

3. Perhaps the most helpful of all preoperative studies in precisely locating tumors is the angiogram. Its usefulness is enhanced when performed by a radiologist with expertise in selective catheterization, who uses vasodilating agents such as tolazoline (Priscoline) and high-pressure injection of contrast medium. The angiographer can preoperatively determine better than anyone else (a) the exact anatomic extent of the lesion into the soft tissues, (b) whether there is major vessel displacement, and (c) the presence of otherwise occult satellite lesions in the adjacent soft tissues. These factors are more valuable in assessing the relative biologic aggressiveness of the lesion than the simple detection of neoplastic vascular patterns.

Once these studies have been completed, the surgeon needs to review all pertinent data with the pathologist who will perform the frozen section examination. The patient also needs to be aware of all diagnostic possibilities and contemplated modes of surgical management, including the occasional intraoperative necessity of abandoning the intended radical local resection and converting the procedure to an amputation. When the surgeon has developed good rapport with his patient, the patient will usually give his consent even for the possible amputation, knowing that his surgeon will make every effort to remove the sarcoma and preserve a functional limb if at all possible.

THERAPEUTIC CONSIDERATIONS

Figure 21-9 indicates the relationship between the biologic behavior of the lesions and the usual surgical management. Such surgical management of these tumors must be rationally based upon the information derived from the preoperative evaluation

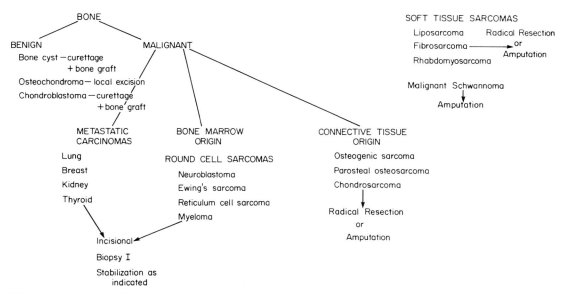

FIG. 21-9. Treatment of common tumors about the shoulder.

and biopsy as well as being individually suited to each patient. The two basic types of biopsies employed are incisional and excisional.

Incisional biopsy involves the removal of a portion of the lesion for microscopic identification. A portion of the surrounding soft tissue or bone immediately adjacent to the lesion should also be removed, so that the pathologist can examine the morphologic response of the host tissues to the tumor. This tumor-host interface often provides clues to the biologic aggressiveness of the tumor.

An excisional biopsy involves removal of the entire lesion as a single intact unit with a narrow margin of pseudocapsule and/or surrounding soft tissues. It, of itself, is not an adequate therapeutic operation for a malignant tumor. Local excision, meaning removal of the lesion plus an envelope of reactive and/or normal tissue that grossly appears to remove the lesion totally but leaves behind portions of the anatomic structure harboring the lesion, is attractive from the function-preserving aspect. It leads to an unacceptably high (about 50 percent) local recurrence rate.

Recently, the term "radical local resection" is used to define the surgical process in which the entire lesion with any potentially contaminated tissues (old biopsy tracts) is removed en bloc with an enveloping layer of the surrounding non-neoplastic tissues, and which totally removes both the lesion and the involved structure(s) of origin in both the transverse and longitudinal dimensions. The dissection is carried through tissue on the other side of the fascial plane that separates the involved tissue from the uninvolved tissue. All structures within the intervening fascial plane must be removed. The dissection thus remains at all times one anatomic plane removed from the structure(s) of origin. Therefore, the operative field is theoretically never contaminated with neoplastic tissue.

In numerous instances when these principles are applied, the location and the histogenesis of the lesion require such sacrifice of major nerves, vessels, and additional tissue that an adequate procedure can only be accomplished by an amputation proximal to the involved structures. In other situations a more functional result may be obtained by radical local resection and reconstruction. The local recurrence rate with resections (as defined) is comparable to that following amputation in the region of the shoulder (about 5 percent).

In the operating room, the upper extremity is prepared and draped in such a fashion that any of the alternative procedures, including forequarter amputation, can be performed. A second layer of drapes is used to isolate the biopsy region. The biopsy incision should be made in such a manner that it can be resected later as part of the specimen, without compromising the flaps needed for wound closure of the radical local resection or forequarter amputation. The biopsy itself should be carried out without soft-tissue stripping or undermining in order to minimize the area of potential wound contamination with tumor.

Once the pathologist has adequate biopsy material to determine that the lesion is definitely sarcomatous and not a radiosensitive neoplasm, the biopsy wound is tightly closed and sprayed with a plastic sealing agent. The outer drapes are discarded as are the biopsy instruments, gloves, and gowns. The incision for the definitive surgery is then designed to include the biopsy tract with the resected specimen. This points up the care with which the original incision should be planned so as to make its subsequent removal possible without amputation. If radical local resection is carried out, staying one anatomic plane away from the lesion, once the specimen is removed the pathologist and surgeon should section the mass with its enveloping tissues and check any questionable margins by examination of frozen section. If residual tumor is identified, these areas can be resected to the next anatomic plane. The reconstructive aspect of the operation is then carried out as indicated.

The following diagrams and cases are presented to demonstrate the most commonly executed resection-reconstruction procedures for malignant lesions about the shoulder.

RADICAL LOCAL RESECTION OF SHOULDER AND RECONSTRUCTION WITH ARTHRODESIS. A young woman had had an excisional biopsy of a painless mass about the proximal humerus at 22 years of age (Fig. 21-10A). A diagnosis of "osteoma" was made without further treatment. Four years later a local recurrence was treated by local excision through a second incision. A diagnosis of parosteal osteosarcoma was made. Three years later she was seen for a second local recurrence. This recurrence was noted at the insertion of the shoulder capsule, and a combination of arthrography and angiography demonstrated intra-articular extension without displacement of major vessels, nerves, or soft tissues.

The shoulder was removed en bloc including the deltoid, subscapularis, rotator cuff, proximal humerus, lateral scapula, and the overlying skin and subcutaneous tissue through which the previous two incisions had been made (Fig. 21-10B). The relationship of the recurrence to the insertion of the capsule and the intra-articular extension is shown in Figure 21-10C. Obviously, resection of only the proximal humerus would have predisposed to recurrence in the capsule; hence, the necessity of removing the scapular portion of the joint extracapsularly. The amount removed distally was dictated by the previous sites and incisions. The distal humerus was fused to the remaining scapula (Fig. 21-10D). The patient is free from disease and does all her own housework (Fig. 21-10E).

Comment. Lesions of the proximal humerus or the neck of the scapula that have invaded the cavity of the joint have been implanted into the capsule or cavity by previous operation. If pericapsular tissues are involved, en bloc resection of the joint and enveloping musculature is required to achieve "one plane away" resection (Fig. 21-11). Following such resection, the amount of musculature removed makes prosthetic replacement injudicious because instability, dislocation, and weakness are common problems. On the other hand, fusion of the remaining portion of the scapula furnishes the patient with a stable, painless shoulder and the range of motion that accompanies shoulder arthrodesis. In our experience, this has proven to be a much more satisfactory procedure, particularly in young active people.

Resection of as much as one third of the proximal humerus and/or the lateral third

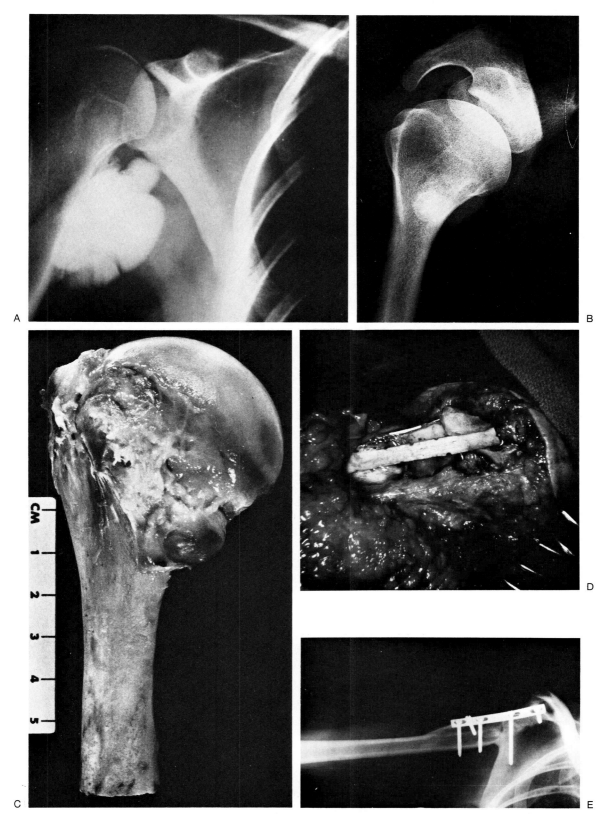

FIG. 21-10. A, Painless mass about the proximal humerus of 22-year-old woman. The shoulder was removed en bloc. B, Roentgenogram of specimen showing extent of the procedure. C, Gross specimen. D, Operative view of scapula, humerus, fixing plate, and onlay tibial autogenous graft. E, Roentgenogram obtained 8 years postoperatively.

LOCATION

RESECTION BED

RECONSTRUCTION

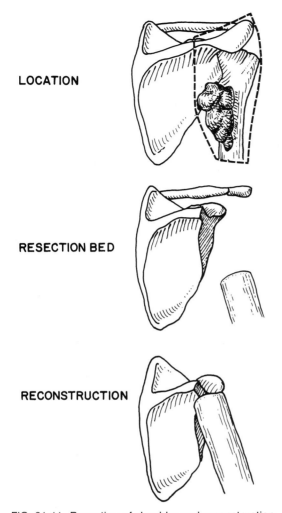

FIG. 21-11. Resection of shoulder and reconstruction with arthrodesis.

of the scapula is satisfactory for such a procedure. The shortening thus produced is not obvious cosmetically and function is not compromised. If the lesion requires more extensive resection of bone, the gap may be filled with autogenous cortical bone grafts. The midshaft of the fibula is the best source of graft material. Late fatigue fractures of such grafts are quite common but generally heal and allow satisfactory function when treated conservatively. Homogenous cortical grafts of this magnitude are slow to unite and sustain fatigue fractures more frequently than similar ones through the use of autogenous grafts. For these reasons such grafts are to be avoided if at all possible.

Obviously, lesions that involve major neurovascular structures about the shoulder or are of the histogenic type, in which occult invasion of contiguous structures is common, are not amenable to such resections and require amputation more proximally. Thus, the need for careful scanning, angiography, and biopsy prior to selecting the definitive procedure is important.

RADICAL LOCAL RESECTION OF THE PROXIMAL HUMERUS AND ARTHROPLASTY. A 23-year-old woman with multiple heritable exostoses noted painful enlargement of a long-standing mass about her left shoulder. Roentgenograms demonstrated progressive peripheral growth. The lesion was "hot" on scintillation scanning in contrast to her other exostoses. Angiography demonstrated neovasculature about the lesion as well as normal planes between the lesion and the major neurovascular structures (Fig. 21-12A). The proximal half of the humerus was resected and the cut surface of the specimen demonstrated satisfactory margins about a histologically low-grade chondrosarcoma (Fig. 21-12B).

Reconstruction was accomplished by obtaining a comparable segment of her ipsilateral fibula which fortuitously had by scan a "cold" benign exostosis of a configuration comparable to that on the humeral head (Fig. 21-12C). The transplant was secured distally by cross bolts and proximally articulated with the glenoid (Fig. 21-12D). The soft tissues (remaining deltoid, subscapularis, and rotator cuff stump) were sutured to the fibular exostosis. The extremity was immobilized in 60 degrees of abduction for 3 months in a shoulder plaster of Paris spica cast and then guarded rehabilitation begun. At the fifth postresection month, the fibula was solidly united to the distal humerus and the patient could actively abduct 45 degrees (Fig. 21-12E). Six months postoperatively the bolts were removed, union was verified by direct inspection, and the patient started vigorous activity. The cosmetic appearance and range of active abduction are shown in

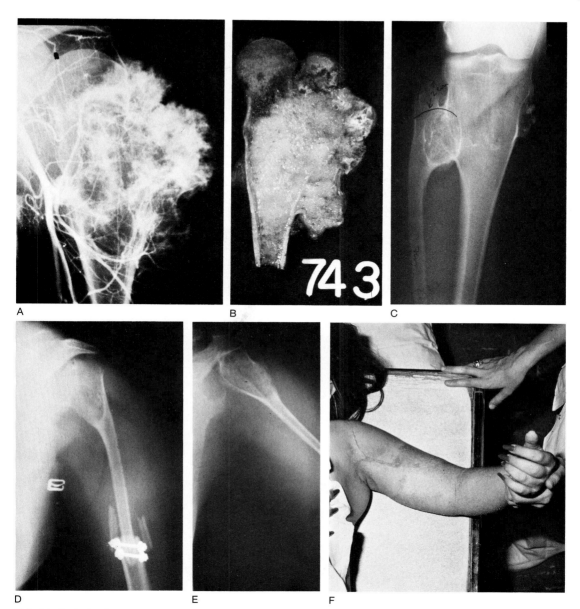

FIG. 21-12. A, Angiogram of neovasculature about a mass in the left shoulder of a young woman. B, Cut surface of gross specimen. C, Roentgenogram of patient's fibula with exostosis. D, Roentgenogram of transplant held by cross bolts. E, Five months postoperatively, there is union of the fibular graft and humerus. F, Appearance and active range of motion.

Figure 21-12F. Function of the hand and elbow were normal.

Comment. This case demonstrates the result of arthroplasty when there is no need to resect the scapular portion of the shoulder joint. The same type of result may be obtained with an artificial custom-made prosthesis. Motion and stability are provided for by the cuff of remaining musculature. The cuff can be preserved in lesions with little propensity to metastasize when adequately resected but such tumors are prone to recur if inadequately excised or curetted. In this unusual case, additional soft-tissue attachment to the segmental replacement was possible with a "customized" autogenous graft.

Another more commonly employed reconstruction is shown in Figure 21-13. In this method portions of both fibulae were onlaid to the remaining distal humerus, and the proximal fibular heads were bolted together in such a way that the articular cartilage of the fibular head faced the glenoid. The long head of the biceps was passed through the fibular head as in the Nicola procedure, and the soft tissues were reapproximated to the grafts.

In general, giant cell tumor and chondrosarcoma are lesions that require resection when they do not invade the joint, and in this instance, permit resection-arthroplasty with safety.

The function of these arthroplasties is a trade-off with resection-fusion. They are cosmetically more acceptable, although they limit range of motion (60 degrees or less of abduction) and are less powerful and more painful than fusions. Thus, the surgeon must realistically adapt the chosen procedure to the patient's life-style.

RADICAL LOCAL RESECTION OF SOFT-TISSUE SARCOMA AND SOFT-TISSUE REPAIR. A 32-year-old man was seen 1 year after he had had an excisional biopsy of a liposarcoma. In the ensuing interval he had developed a firm recurrent lesion. The original procedure had not penetrated the fascia of the underlying deltoid muscle. The appearance and site of this recurrence is shown in Figure 21-14A. Roentgenograms showed no involvement of the underlying humerus. The humerus was not hot when scanned, and soft-tissue views suggested a superficial bilobed mass at the sulcus between the deltoid and triceps muscle (Fig. 21-14B). Angiograms demonstrated the lesion to extend deeply into the deltoid, to be supplied by the circumflex humeral vessels, and to have no component near the major neurovascular structures (Fig. 21-14C).

A radical local resection of the entire deltoid muscle and the proximal half of the triceps including circumflex humeral vessels, axillary nerve, and subscapular vessels

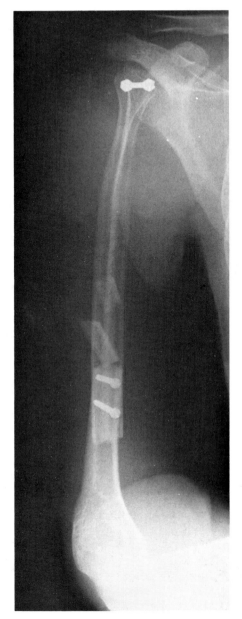

FIG. 21-13. Commonly employed method of reconstruction (see text for discussion).

was performed. Figure 21-14D shows the relationship of the excised scar, skin, and deeper tissues, and Figure 21-14E shows the deep margin of the lesion and its pseudocapsule within the deltoid muscle. Four years postoperatively the patient was still clinically free from disease and had good range of motion (Fig. 21-14F).

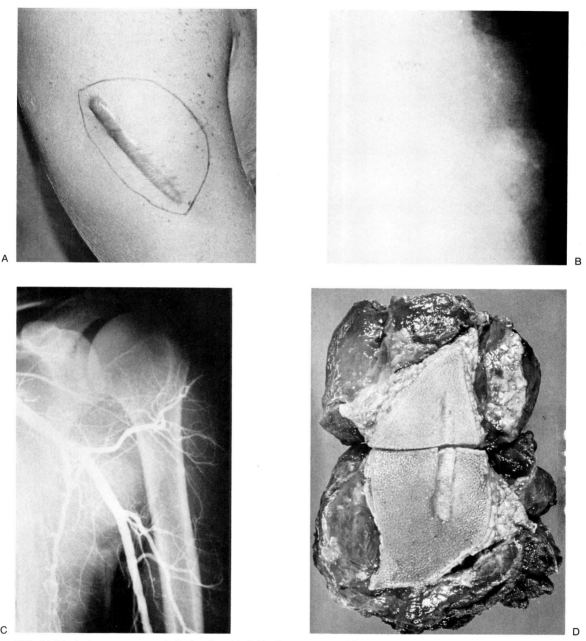

FIG. 21-14. A, Appearance and site (outlined in ink) of recurrence of liposarcoma in a young man. B, Roentgenogram of bilobed mass at sulcus between deltoid and triceps muscles. C, Angiogram of the lesion. D, Gross specimen.

Comment. Lesions that can be conclusively demonstrated preoperatively not to involve the anatomic planes adjacent to bone or joint can be adequately managed without skeletal sacrifice (Fig. 21-15). A hot scan in the underlying bone inevitably means recurrence if the lesion is blindly dissected subperiosteally from the bone. Shoulder stability and functional abduction were restored in this instance by suturing the trapezius to the rotator cuff of the shoulder.

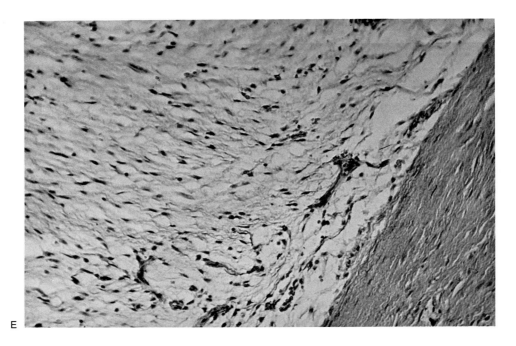

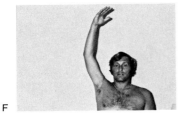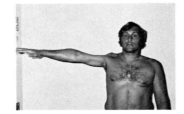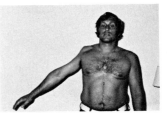

FIG. 21-14. (Cont'd). E, Microscopic appearance of lesion (hematoxylin and eosin, X 100). F, Range of motion 4 years postoperatively.

A patient who has had an incisional biopsy, and then 5 to 7 days later is found to have an inadequately excised malignant lesion, presents a dilemma for the surgeon. Should he observe the patient until the almost inevitable recurrence is clinically palpable and well localized and accept the risk of metastasis during this 6- to 24-month interval before undertaking the next procedure? Should he radically reexcise the wound without really knowing where the hematoma from the prior biopsy has potentially seeded the tissues, and thus not know what is an adequate procedure? Should he amputate control of the primary lesion? Should he hope that radiotherapy/chemotherapy will be justification in lieu of an inadequate operation without any certain

knowledge of the efficacy of such treatment? Our practice has been to take a middle course. Eight to twelve weeks after biopsy, when the vascular and skeletal reaction to the previous procedure has in the main subsided, a combination of scanning, angiography, and careful examination is employed to establish the ostensible disease-free margins. Data from these examinations are used as guidelines for a decision of radical local resection versus amputation at that time. Examination of tissue obtained surgically has frequently shown that residual disease is identifiable grossly and microscopically, that margins are adequate, and that a more extensive resection has been done than would have been required had the diagnosis been ascertained by fro-

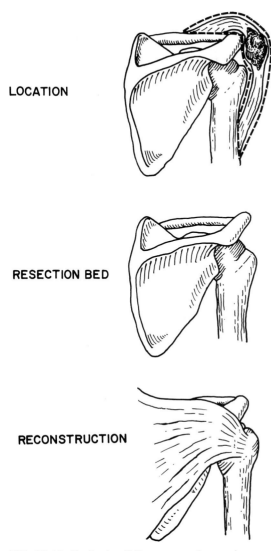

LOCATION

RESECTION BED

RECONSTRUCTION

FIG. 21-15. Radical soft-tissue resection and reconstruction.

zen section and the resection been carried out on the basis of preoperative studies. This has been even more striking when the patient has received postbiopsy radiotherapy, as both the studies and surgical observations are further obfuscated. The results of such an approach have been a low incidence of further recurrence (less than 10 percent) and survival rates comparable to those in patients treated initially who have not shown recurrence.

RADICAL LOCAL RESECTION OF THE SCAPULA

WITH FLAIL SHOULDER. A 34-year-old woman had a 3-year history of a slowly progressive deformity about the right shoulder caused by an apparent mass deep to the scapula (Fig. 21-16A). An excisional biopsy of a walnut-size lesion along the lateral border of the scapula had been performed 4 years earlier. Figure 21-16B shows the edge of a low-grade fibrous lesion infiltrating the adjacent skeletal muscle. On physical examination while the scapula was fixed to the thorax the extremity had no vascular or neurologic deficit. A plain roentgenogram demonstrated the lesion filling the area between the chest wall and scapula and intimately involving the lateral aspect of ribs 3 to 5 (Fig. 21-16C). It did not involve or displace major vascular structures (Fig. 21-16D).

A radical local resection of the overlying skin, posterior parascapular musculature, scapula subscapular musculature, ribs 3, 4, and 5, and parietal pleura was performed. Figure 21-16E shows a coronal surface of the specimen. The overlying skin, fat, and superficial muscles have been removed and the relationship of the lesion to the more superficial serratus anterior, scapular blade, and infraspinatus muscle can be seen. On the deep surface can be seen pleura and the cross section of the involved ribs. In Figure 21-16F, the magnitude of the defect prior to reconstruction of the thoracic wall is shown. The extremity was suspended from the distal end of the clavicle by looping the tendon of the biceps through a drill hole. Four years postoperatively, the patient had normal functions of the hand, wrist, and elbow. She could shrug the shoulder and had passive abduction to 70 degrees, but no active shoulder motion (Fig. 21-16G and H).

Comment. A flail shoulder with an otherwise functional upper extremity is of obvious advantage over the limb with a prosthetic replacement following shoulder disarticulation or thoracoscapular amputation. This type of resection again must be selected only when there is conclusive evidence that the histogenesis and anatomic location permit an adequate radical resection (Fig. 21-17). In our experience, attempts

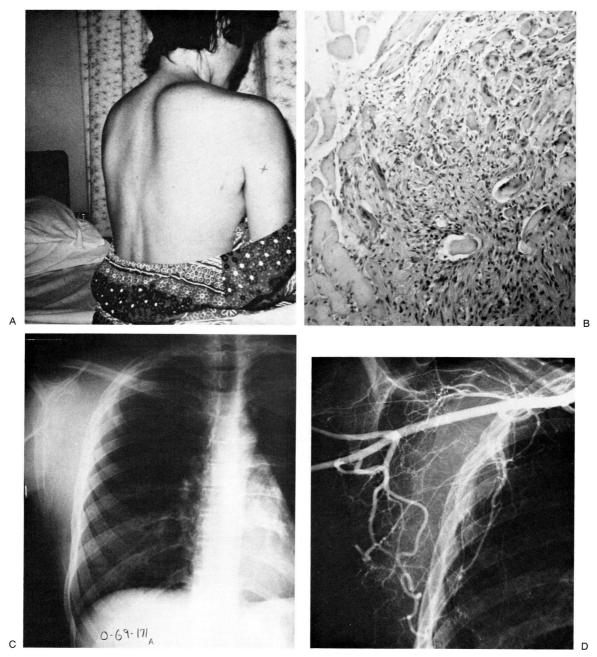

FIG. 21-16. A, Posterior displacement of the scapula. B, Microscopic appearance of the fibrous lesion. C, Roentgenogram of lesion filling area between chest wall and scapula. D, Angiogram of lesion.

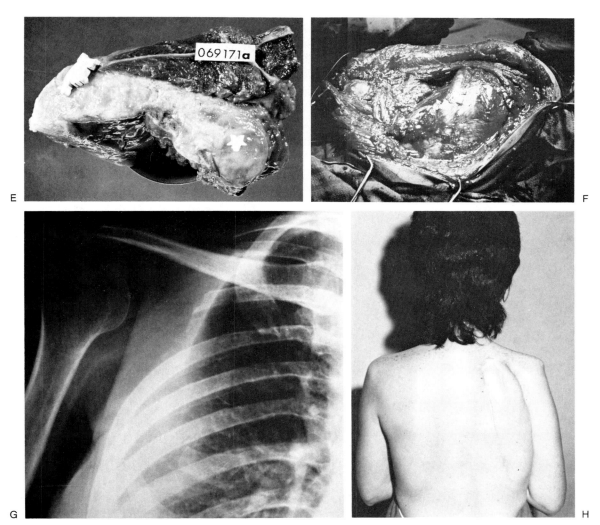

FIG. 21-16. (Cont'd). E, Gross specimen. F, Extent of the defect at operation. G, Roentgenogram of shoulder 4 years postoperatively. H, Physical appearance of shoulder 4 years postoperatively.

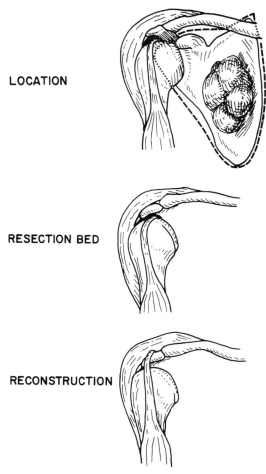

LOCATION

RESECTION BED

RECONSTRUCTION

FIG. 21-17. Radical resection of scapula in flail shoulder.

to preserve remnants of the scapula to anchor total shoulder replacements and the like lead to a high incidence of recurrence while the function is not appreciably improved. Compromising adequate margins for token or questionable gains in function,

in most instances, ultimately does not serve the patient's best interests.

At this point in time, definitive surgical excision, following the principles outlined, remains the primary treatment for sarcomas when there is no clinical evidence of metastasis. If adequate local control is obtained by the operative procedure, the patient's survival depends mainly upon whether or not occult pulmonary micrometastases have been established prior to surgery. Survival rates indicate that such micrometastases are present in a high percentage of cases. It remains to be seen whether adjunctive therapy, be it chemotherapy, radiation therapy, immunotherapy, or a combination of these, will be capable of suppressing such minute foci. There is some early inconclusive evidence that such may be the case. A logical extension of that thought would be whether such adjunctive treatment might also permit more limited surgical control of the primary lesion with preservation of better function. There are considerably fewer data in this regard. It is recognized that the efficacy of any adjunctive therapy is related to the quantitative amount of disease present. What the absolute numbers of cells are for any given tumor is unknown. It would thus seem that limited or inadequate operation for sarcoma might well be as detrimental to the patient's survival as it has been, previously, to achieve local control. In other words, although adjunctive therapy holds promise, there is no current assurance that it can be substituted for inadequate operation. Assuredly, there is no place for a poorly planned operation for sarcoma that is not based on sound biologic principles.[5]

REFERENCES

1. Ackerman, L., and Spjut, H.: Tumors of Bone and Cartilage. Washington, D.C., Armed Forces Institute of Pathology, 1962.
2. Codman, E. A.: Epiphyseal chondromatous giant cell tumors of the upper end of the humerus. Surg. Gynecol. Obstet., 52:543, 1931.
3. Cohen, J.: Etiology of simple bone cysts. J. Bone Joint Surg., 52-A:1493, 1970.
4. Edeiken, J., and Hodes, P.: Roentgenologic Diagnosis of Diseases of Bone, 2 Vols., 2nd ed. Baltimore, Williams & Wilkins, 1973.
5. Enneking, W. F.: Principles of Musculoskeletal Pathology. Gainesville, Fla., Storter Printing Company, 1970.
6. Jaffe, H. L.: Tumors and Tumorous Conditions of the Bones and Joints. Philadelphia, Lea & Febiger, 1958.
7. Jaffe, H. L., and Lichtenstein, L.: Solitary unicameral bone cysts. Arch. Surg., 34:1004, 1942.

22

Miscellaneous Lesions of the Shoulder

MELVIN POST

A number of pathologic lesions can cause disability of the shoulder and ultimately adversely affect normal hand function. Some of these conditions will be reviewed.

UNICAMERAL BONE CYST OF PROXIMAL HUMERUS

Although the true cause of unicameral bone cyst remains an enigma, some advances in understanding its pathogenesis and treatment have been made. Because of the high incidence of solitary bone cyst in the proximal humerus and the disability it can cause, it is important to recognize and correctly treat such lesions.

PATHOLOGIC ANATOMY. Since Bloodgood first recognized solitary bone cyst as a separate entity in 1910,[3] documentation of its pathology has been well described.[8,10,11] At operation gross findings reveal an expanded cortical wall which may be attenuated or quite thickened and hard, depending upon the activity and age of the lesion. The expansion is usually fusiform (Fig. 22-1). The periosteal cover peels easily from the surface cortex. When the cortex is thin it is easy to push the point of a heavy gauge needle into the cyst cavity.

The cavity may be filled with air or a fluidlike material, depending upon the character of the cyst wall lining. The fluid contents of the cyst may range from a watery fluid to a gelatinous material to a serous liquid when a delicate material containing an areolar connective tissue with a paucity of cells is present.[11] Experience in treating such lesions shows that the fluid may be colorless, varying shades of yellow, or red from the bleeding of a recent trauma. Cohen reviewed the kinds of cystic fluids that are present in lesions and their theories of production.[5]

The cyst wall lining can vary from a few micra to a centimeter,[11] but more often is only 1 to 2 mm. thick.[8] Johnson and Kindred also described a parietal nubbin that projected into the cyst cavity or lay in the adjacent bone marrow.[11] They found that a lipomatous element was predominant in more than half the 200 specimens studied at the Armed Forces Institute of Pathology. They termed the nubbin an angiomyxofibrillar lipoma and related it to four elements of primitive mesenchymal tissue. Importantly, the authors believed that failure to eliminate the nubbin of tissue at operation could account for recurrence after surgical obliteration of the cavity.[11]

INCIDENCE. Johnson and Kindred found

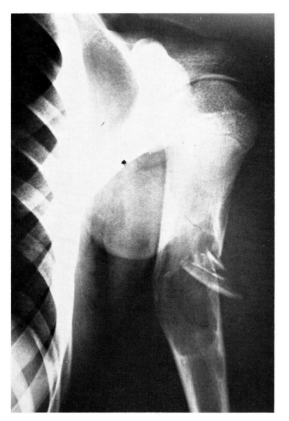

FIG. 22-1. A 9-year-old boy developed a pathologic fracture of the proximal humerus when he fell. Note the fusiform shape of the cyst cavity and the expanded and thinned cortex. The fracture healed, and the patient eventually underwent curettage and bone grafting with excellent results.

the age range to be from 8 months to 70 years, with the majority of cases occurring in patients younger than 40 years of age.[11] In 1954 Garceau and Gregory found that 75 percent of cases in their patients occurred in the proximal humerus and femur.[8] Jaffe and Lichtenstein,[10] in 1942, and Tachdjian,[14] in 1972, reported that about 50 percent of the cases occurred in the proximal shaft of the humerus. Neer and associates pointed out that unicameral bone cysts occurred most often in the proximal humerus where 80 percent of the bone growth occurs.[13] Thus, the lesion seems to be related to where bone growth is greatest.

Most cysts are discovered in patients in the first 20 years of life, the greatest fre-

quency being noted in those between 9 and 14 years of age, and males predominating 2:1 over females.[8] The same authors found that 20 of 26 patients who had failed surgical treatment were under 10 years of age.[8] Neer and co-workers confirmed that true recurrence following surgical treatment is significantly more frequent in patients younger than 10 years of age.[13] They also discovered that age served as a more reliable prognostic sign than the proximity of the cyst to the growth plate when evaluating the possibility of recurrence following surgical treatment.

PATHOGENESIS. Jaffe and Lichtenstein believed bone cysts were caused by an inflammatory mechanism.[10] They were the first to stress that these lesions grow away from the epiphyseal plate with maturation, although Neer and associates showed that cysts remained close to the growth plate in 30 (73 percent) of 41 conservatively treated patients.[13] Garceau and Gregory agreed that during the active phase the cyst is displaced away from the epiphyseal plate.[8]

Cohen postulated an attractive theory that the cause of simple cysts was related to a blockage of the interstitial fluid drainage in an area that is rapidly growing and remodeling.[5,6] He reported two cases in which the cysts were injected with radiopaque dye.[6] He believed these cases showed an obstruction to the venous drainage. Because fluid is incompressible, the hydrodynamic pressure within the cyst cavity can exceed that of the surrounding well-drained interstitial tissue and thereby lead to enlargement of the cyst cavity. Garceau and Gregory showed that 15 percent of their cases after fracture went on to resolution[8] (Fig. 22-2), a statement that is consistent with Cohen's idea that relief of cyst cavity pressure may possibly allow resolution of the cyst.

Broder reported two cases in children in which early lesions were inadvertently discovered and then followed through various stages.[4] He believed that the resulting cysts were preceded by lesions that resembled nonossifying fibromas containing foci of fibrous tissue, and consistent with the idea

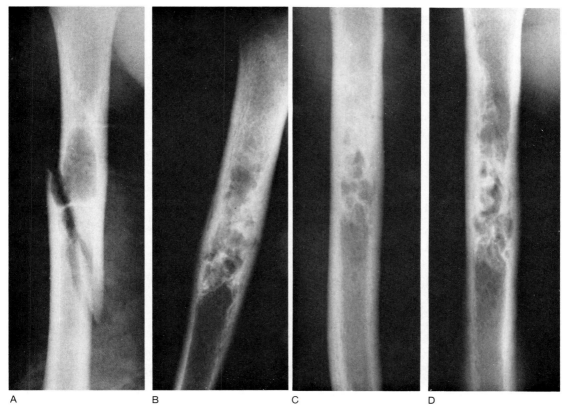

A B C D

FIG. 22-2. A, A 14-year-old boy sustained a pathologic fracture through a cyst in the proximal humerus. The extremity was immobilized in a hanging cast. The fracture healed. B, When the boy was 16 years old, the cyst had entered the latent phase and seemed to be healing. C, Anteroposterior and, D, lateral views of the shaft at the age of 18 years show progressive healing of the cyst. Although the patient had no symptoms, he was forewarned of the possibility of another fracture.

that there is vascular obstruction of the cystic lesion.

DIAGNOSIS. Unicameral bone cysts can remain asymptomatic and then be discovered accidentally, or only when some complication such as a pathologic fracture occurs (Fig. 22-3). At other times the initial complaint may be pain, and there may be tenderness over the site of the lesion. It is unusual for pain to radiate to another area or to decrease active shoulder motion.

Roentgenographic diagnosis is indispensable for establishing the true nature of the lesion. Certainly the roentgen and pathologic features and the clinical history must be correlated to differentiate a cyst from an aneurysmal bone cyst, or rarely a sarcomatous lesion of the scapula that I have seen in one case. Other conditions that should be considered in the differential diagnosis are fibrous dysplasia, nonossifying fibroma, giant cell tumor, enchondroma, osteitis fibrosa cystica secondary to hyperparathyroidism, neurofibroma, and lipoma.[8]

Roentgen findings may show (1) destruction of the medullary bone and inner cortex, (2) subperiosteal new bone causing the appearance of an expansion, (3) an expansile defect at the metaphysis, (4) trabecular lines in the cyst wall giving the impression of multiloculation, (5) a thin, dense cyst wall which may separate from the medullary cavity, and (6) migration of the cyst from the epiphyseal plate.

TREATMENT. Although a large percentage of the total cases of solitary bone cyst does

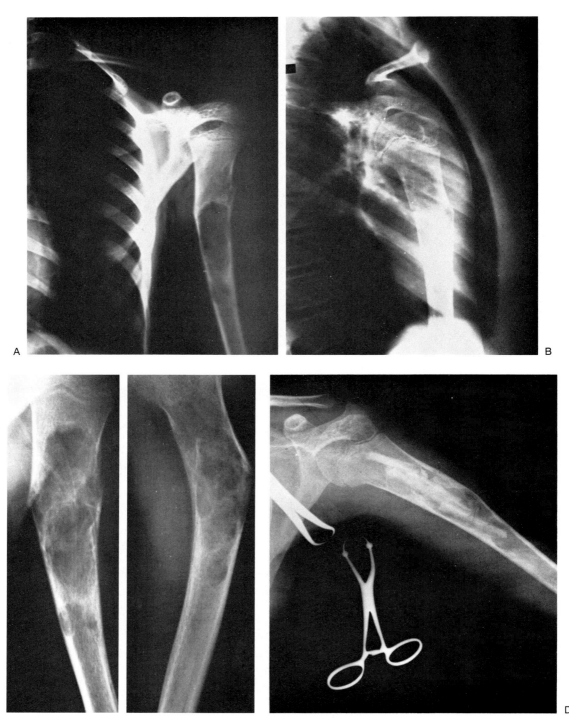

FIG. 22-3. A, Anteroposterior and, B, lateral views of a 6-year-old boy who sustained a pathologic fracture through a cyst of the proximal humerus. C, The child was treated in a sling and swath and the fracture allowed to heal. Note the degree of angulation at the healed fracture after 12 weeks. D, A large cortical window was made in the cortex, the cyst wall was thoroughly curetted, and the cavity was packed with autogenous tibial bone 6 months after injury. Note the placement of the most proximal bone graft at operation where the cyst lining was also found and removed.

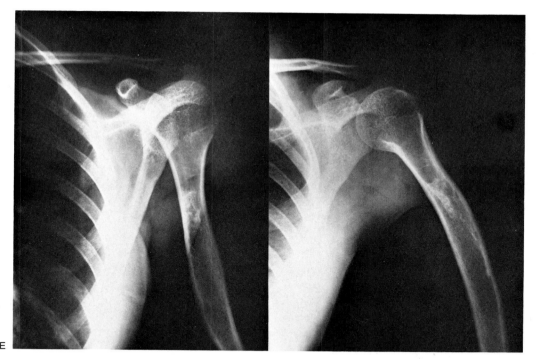

E

FIG. 22-3 continued. E, At 12 years of age, note complete healing of the cyst cavity. The result was excellent.

require surgical treatment, some cysts can be treated conservatively because occasionally they heal following a pathologic fracture especially in the older child (Fig. 22-2). Fahey and O'Brien showed that of 9 patients with cysts treated conservatively, 6 cysts healed whereas 3 did not.[7] They also showed that 34 of their 40 cases had a pathologic fracture. Seven of 15 active cysts with fracture and 11 of 19 latent cysts with fracture were treated conservatively for 6 months or longer after fracture. Two active and 4 latent cysts, or 6 of 18 cysts with pathologic fracture, all in the humerus, healed without operation. However, it required 10 years for one cyst to heal. Baker studied 45 cases and found that pathologic fractures occurred in 30 (66 percent).[2] He stated that occasionally a cyst will heal following pathologic fracture but such a fracture did not appear to provide a greater than normal chance that such a cyst will heal. Moreover, when a cyst appears to be healing it may recur months or years later. Neer and co-workers stated that in selected cases it is reasonable to observe a cyst in the proximal humerus, a nonweight-bearing bone, especially when the lesion is adjacent to the growth plate.[12] Curettage of such lesions next to the epiphyseal plate may cause injury (Fig. 22-4). In any event, the cyst may not grow away from the growth plate and eventually should be treated surgically if judgment determines there is danger of pathologic fracture. Whenever possible I prefer to operate upon cystic lesions after they grow away from the plate. If pathologic fracture occurs, I prefer to wait until the fracture heals to determine the actual extent of the lesion by serial roentgenographic studies.

Surgical Treatment. In 1942 Jaffe and Lichtenstein showed that curetting the cyst wall and filling the cavity with autogenous bone chips yielded a cure in most cases, especially when the cyst was inactive.[10]

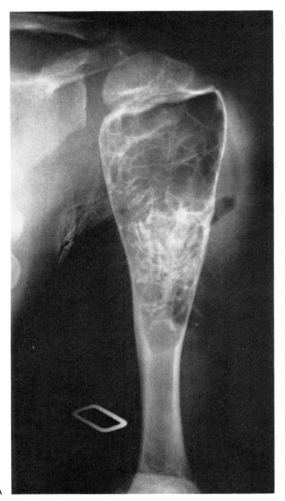
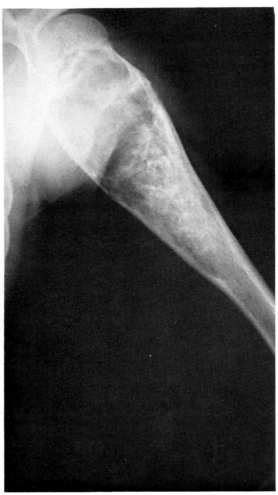

A   B

FIG. 22-4. A, A 7-year-old child complained of a tender area in his left arm. A large cyst was found adjacent to the growth plate. It was observed for 6 months but did not grow away from the epiphysis. B, Soon afterward it was curetted through a large window and then packed with autogenous bone, shown here 12 months later. The cyst persisted. Moreover, the arm was growing at a reduced rate due to the cyst involvement of the epiphysis and possible surgical injury to the growth plate. The arm had shortened and the result was poor. Observe that the cyst still is adjacent to the epiphysis.

Baker expressed a similar viewpoint.[2] Agerholm and Goodfellow believed that curettage and filling the cyst cavity with bone chips was an uncertain method of treatment and led to a significant number of reoperations.[1] They used subperiosteal excision of the whole cyst-bearing portion of the shaft and reported their method of partial diaphysectomy in three successful cases. After partial shaft excision they filled the subperiosteal space with finely minced bone chips and repaired the periosteal sleeve for three quarters of its length. The patient's used their arms normally in 8 weeks.

Gartland and Cole performed subperiosteal diaphysectomy of the proximal humerus on 14 patients with cysts in both the active and latent phases who were above and below the age of 10 years, and reported no recurrences. They agreed with Agerholm and Goodfellow[1] that children return to full activity within 8 weeks postoperatively.

Neer and associates believed that the recurrence rate following curettage and bone grafting was reduced by using large windows (two thirds the circumference of the cyst) to evacuate completely and then fill the periosteal sleeve and cavity with autogenous bone. This method was in agreement with that of Fahey and O'Brien,[7] who relied on subtotal resection of the shaft and bone grafting to effect cure of active cysts having repeated pathologic fractures without a tendency to become latent or for progressive enlargement of the cyst. They subdivided the latent stage into latent primary and latent secondary stages. The former was defined as one in which the distance between the nearest epiphyseal plate and the cyst did not exceed one third of the length of the shaft. The latent secondary cyst was one in which the distance between the cyst and the nearest growth plate exceeded one third of the length of the diaphysis. This was in accord with the concept of Jaffe and Lichtenstein that the cyst has a capacity for continued growth when it resides in the metaphyseal region.[10] Fahey and O'Brien also recommended subtotal resection and bone graft for latent primary cysts, and for cysts that recurred after previous curettage, believing that conventional lesser resection and curettage with bone graft cured latent secondary cysts.[7] Using these criteria and subtotal resection methods, they reported cure in 19 of 20 cases.

Author's Treatment.   With the initial discovery of a cyst without pathologic fracture, if the lesion is located 3 cm. from the proximal growth plate, and the cortices are not too thinned and therefore less likely to fracture easily, the cyst is observed. If it enlarges or expands and the cortex becomes attenuated, surgical treatment is recommended, especially if the patient is younger than 10 years of age.

In the event that the cyst causes an acute pathologic fracture, the fracture is allowed to heal and a determination is made later whether or not surgery is needed to effect a cure. When the lesion is close to the epiphysis and surgical intervention is contemplated, I prefer to wait until the cyst grows away from the growth plate (Fig. 22-5). If it does not and is enlarging, then I proceed with a subtotal resection and autogenous bone graft, taking care to avoid injury to the epiphysis. I frequently use pin markers above and below the cyst to define the true extent of the lesion. I make every attempt to curette the entire cyst wall thoroughly before inserting an autogenous iliac or tibial bone graft.

Occasionally, the cyst tends to heal without surgical intervention (Fig. 22-2). However, most active cysts do tend to refracture and should be surgically treated.

For small cysts initially discovered after the patient is 10 years of age, especially when the cysts have migrated 3 cm. or more from the proximal growth plate indicating that they are latent, less active cysts, I practice a less radical procedure, but still open a large enough cortical window to curette the cyst wall adequately, and then use an autogenous bone graft (Fig. 22-6). For the uncooperative child I recommend a plaster shoulder spica for 4 to 6 weeks or longer. Most surgically treated cysts are stable in 8 weeks.

I employ subtotal resection and an autogenous bone graft for a large cyst, especially if it is active, and for recurrent cysts after previous conventional curettage and bone graft operation. Recurrence can be recognized by a cavity that returns and enlarges, whose cortex expands and thins, and is likely to fracture.[12]

Only in children under 10 years of age with recurrence after previous subtotal resection is segmental diaphysectomy recommended. In principle, if the entire cyst wall is removed through an adequate cortical window and the cavity packed with autogenous bone graft I have found that recurrence is unlikely.

POLYMYOSITIS AND DERMATOMYOSITIS

Polymyositis and dermatomyositis are unusual disorders characterized by diffuse inflammation and degeneration of striated

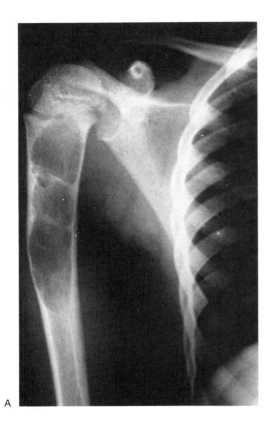

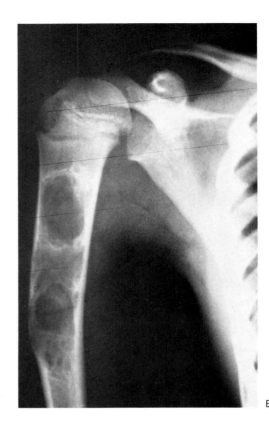

A

B

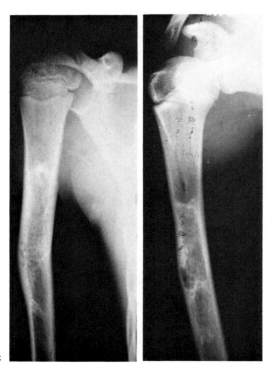

C

FIG. 22-5. A 6-year-old girl sustained a pathologic fracture through a cyst of the humerus. A, An anteroposterior view shows an undisplaced spiral fracture. The cyst was adjacent to the growth plate. B, The cyst did not heal, but did migrate away from the growth plate after 1 year. The patient's activities were restricted. At operation a large cortical window was made by removing about one third of the circumference the length of the cyst. Pins above and below the cyst were used as markers to determine the extent of the lesion. The cyst wall was extensively curetted, and packed with autogenous tibial bone graft. C, Two views show healing of the cyst $6\frac{1}{2}$ years postoperatively. There was no recurrence and the result was excellent.

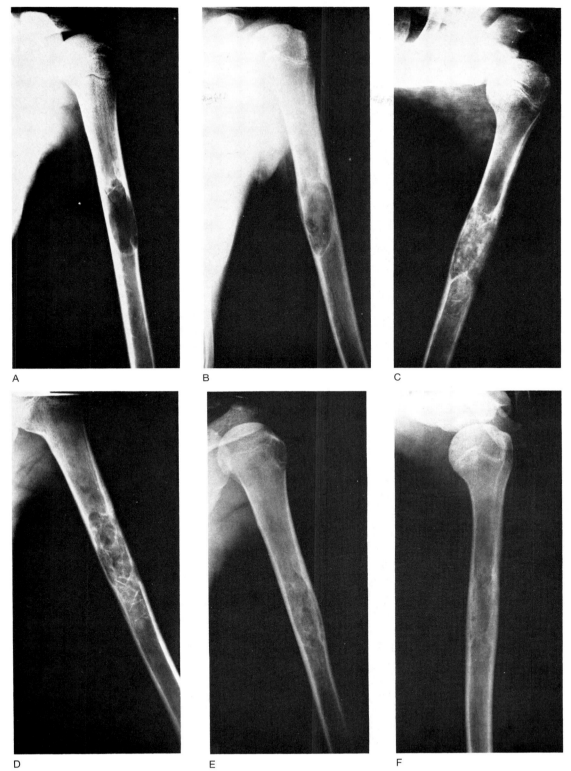

FIG. 22-6. A, A 12-year-old girl sustained a pathologic fracture through a cyst of the humerus. B, The fracture was allowed to heal and was observed for several months. C and D, The patient had one small refracture even though the cyst appeared to be latent. Shortly afterward a conventional curettage of the cyst wall and autogenous iliac bone graft was performed. The extremity was kept in a plaster shoulder spica for 5 weeks and a sling for 2 weeks. E and F, Healing of the cyst is shown 18 months later. After 5 years postoperatively there has been no recurrence. The result was excellent.

muscle causing symmetric weakness and eventual atrophy of muscle. The cause of polymyositis remains unknown since it was first described by Wagner in 1863.[21] Even though the origin is unknown the disease is ordinarily grouped with the collagen or connective tissue diseases since it may involve tissues other than the muscles, including the skin (dermatomyositis). Arundell and co-workers have shown that males over 40 years of age with dermatomyositis have a 50 percent chance of developing a malignant neoplasm. The sequelae of this disease have serious implications in shoulder function.

INCIDENCE. Polymyositis and dermatomyositis can occur at any age from infancy to the eighth decade. Females are affected twice as often as are males.[16] The disease is not particularly rare. Rose and Walton reported 89 new cases in a 12-year period in an area with a population of 3.3 million people.[19]

CLASSIFICATION. Unverricht first categorized the subgroup dermatomyositis in 1887.[20] Pearson stated that it has been recognized only in the last decade and that most cases of myositis do not manifest any dermal lesions.[17] Thus, Pearson pointed out the wide variation in the clinical and pathologic features making any classification difficult.[17] He classified polymyositis into six types: type I, adult polymyositis; type II, typical dermatomyositis; type III, typical dermatomyositis, occasionally polymyositis, with malignant change; type IV, childhood dermatomyositis; type V, acute myolysis; type VI, polymyositis in conjunction with Sjögren's syndrome. Pearson believed this classification offered a guide for the prognosis of favorable types that respond best to treatment.[17]

PATHOLOGY. The site for muscle biopsy should be selected where the muscle is neither too weakened nor atrophic, but it should not have normal strength. A proximal muscle is chosen, preferably the deltoid. If in doubt as to the involvement of the muscle, electromyography should be performed to sample the muscle before biopsy. A special muscle clamp should be employed to maintain the "normal" length of the muscle fibers.

In any event, there may be no inflammatory changes even in typical cases. When inflammatory changes do occur they may vary considerably. Essentially, extensive primary muscle fiber degeneration may occur and may be associated with necrosis. Chronic inflammatory cells may be seen and are predominantly lymphocytes. In time interstitial fibrosis may occur.[17] In children and adults clinical and pathologic features of the proximal muscles make differentiation of polymyositis from muscular dystrophy difficult.

DIAGNOSIS. Numerous, diverse symptoms of multiple systems, singularly or together, are the hallmark of this condition. Muscular, dermal, articular, or other symptoms may be manifested.[17] Moreover, chronic cases may demonstrate exacerbations and remissions, making predictability of the course of the disease difficult.

Muscle weakness is observed in all cases of polymyositis. In subacute or chronic cases weakness is slow to appear and first affects the lower limbs. During this stage the disease may be confused with muscular dystrophy. After weakness appears in the pelvic girdle muscles, weakness may appear in the shoulder girdle muscles, and the patient may find it impossible to lift light objects overhead or even to comb the hair. Weakness during abduction of the arms against gravity may gradually increase, and eventually the patient may become confined to a wheelchair. Even weakness in the anterior neck muscles may prevent the patient from raising the head from a pillow. In some early cases, muscle pain, tenderness, and even induration are present. A skin rash of dermatomyositis may be seen. Pain is most often manifest about the shoulder girdle and upper arms, and forearms.

Contractures do not usually occur early, but may be seen in advanced disease and cause contractures at the elbows and in the wrist flexors (Fig. 22-7A). Muscle atrophy gradually increases but does not usually occur to the extent seen with advanced dystrophy. Calcinosis of the muscles may be seen after acute myositis and occurs most often in children (Fig. 22-7B).

The rash of dermatomyositis is observed in 40 percent of the patients. The usual rash appears as a dusky erythematous eruption over the face in "butterfly" fashion. It may appear on the neck, shoulders, and on the front and back of the upper chest and proximal arms. In severe, acute cases the rash over the shoulders and arms may show edematous skin lesions.

Symptoms of Raynaud's disease such as cyanosis or blanching of the fingers may occur commonly but are not usually severe. A variety of other symptoms may occur including neurologic, visceral, and gastrointestinal symptoms.

The most common variety of the disease is type I, occurring in 35 percent of the cases and primarily in women. Dermal lesions may not be seen. On the other hand, joint pain and findings such as joint effusion may be manifested. Type II (typical dermatomyositis) is seen in 25 percent of the cases in which proximal muscle weakness and a diffuse skin rash are commonly observed. Type III (dermatomyositis with malignant alteration) almost always occurs in patients older than 40 years of age and in a variety of different tissues.

Type IV (childhood dermatomyositis) may be serious and disabling (Fig. 22-7). Most children demonstrate a rash, although in a rare case it may be absent (Fig. 22-7A). This type is commonly observed in patient's between 4 and 10 years of age. Proximal muscle weakness predominates over that of the distal muscles. Pain and stiffness are moderate. In some children weakness may be progressive over weeks to months. However, the evolution of the condition is variable with weakness progressing rapidly and leading to severe disability or to a more gradual loss of muscle strength. There may be joint contractures and muscle atrophy, especially of the arms. In the advanced stage, subcutaneous calcifications (calcinosis universalis) may be seen (Fig. 22-7B).

Type V (acute myolysis) is acute and often fatal, and constitutes 3 percent of all the cases.[17] There is generalized muscle weakness of the proximal and distal muscles. Severe muscle pain is common.

Type VI (polymyositis in Sjögren's syndrome) includes hypofunction of the lacrimal glands and hypertrophy of the salivary glands with a decrease in production of salivary secretions. When muscle weakness does occasionally occur in this type, it progresses slowly and involves the proximal muscles of the limbs. This type comprises 5 percent of all the cases.

Laboratory Findings. The sedimentation rate may be elevated, whereas the results of most other laboratory tests are normal. In acute cases the neutrophils may be elevated. The only other abnormalities are observed in the serum and urine levels of creatine and creatinine, but these are not specific for myositis and should not be relied upon for diagnosis. The serum proteins are abnormal in 50 percent of the cases. Serum enzyme elevations are valuable for diagnosis and prognosis. Accordingly, the levels of transaminases, creatine phosphokinase, or aldolase enzymes should be studied but are not pathognomonic for diagnosis.[18] Although these enzymes also are elevated in muscular dystrophy they do not respond to treatment as they do in polymyositis.

TREATMENT. Conservative treatment in the acute stage of polymyositis is indicated and includes bed rest and moist heat applied to painful, tender muscles. Corticosteroids are administered. These drugs alter the course of the disease.[17] Determination of serial serum enzyme levels allows for an early prognosis. When the abnormal levels diminish toward normal, a reversal of symptoms (muscle weakness) will usually occur. At this point the steroid dosage (prednisone for instance) is slowly decreased. A certain number of all types of polymyositis or dermatomyositis patients may not respond favorably to corticosteroids. In this situation immunosuppressive therapy plus low dose prednisone is beneficial.[17]

During the early stage of disease, active and passive exercises are prescribed to preserve normal joint motion. Once contrac-

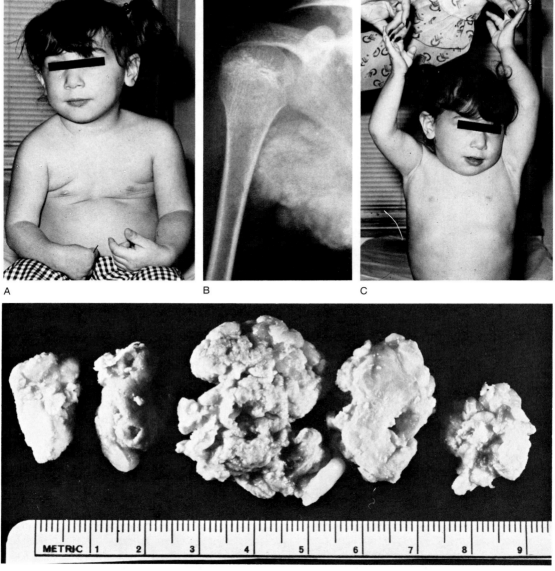

FIG. 22-7. A, A 6-year-old child with dermatomyositis (type IV) complained of pain in both upper arms. She exhibited shoulder and wrist joint contractures as shown. B, Anteroposterior roentgenogram of the shoulder shows a large calcific mass filling the axilla. C, After excision of the calcified mass from each axilla, pain disappeared, overhead shoulder motion increased, and wrist extension improved. D, Gross specimen from the right axilla shows calcinosis cutis. The mass was enclosed in a cyst whose wall measured 1 mm. in thickness.

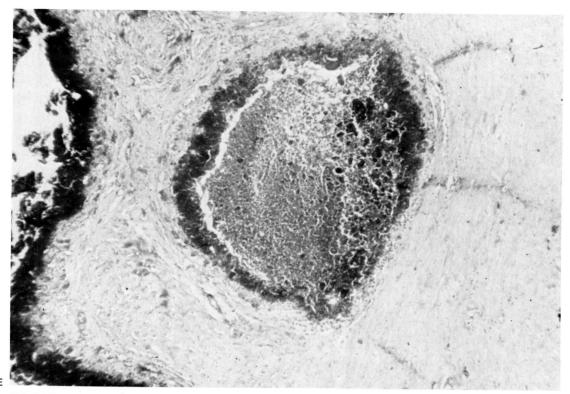

E

FIG. 22-7 continued. E, Microscopic section revealed calcified areas and foreign body granulomatous reactions seen in dermatomyositis. Note the fibrous septa ($\times$ 575 magnification).

tures develop the joint(s) should be immobilized in a functional position in padded splints. If soft-tissue calcifications are thought to be responsible for contractures in the advanced stage, these calcified masses should be resected when the prognosis for longevity is present (Fig. 22-7). These surgical procedures not only lessen joint contracture but can improve circulation to the muscles and skin.

SOLITARY OSTEOCHONDROMA

Solitary osteochondroma is the most common benign tumor of bone. It is characterized by its usual metaphyseal location on the long bones, and in nearly half the cases the femur and humerus are involved. Dahlin reported 22 scapular lesions in a total of 272 cases.[22] Almost half the lesions occurs in patients younger than 20 years of age at the time of their excision and 38 percent occurs in patients in the second decade of life.[22] Jaffe agreed that the great

majority of cases occurred in those in the second decade of life, and the lesions are discovered when the patients are admitted to the hospital for treatment.

DIAGNOSIS. Symptoms are related to the size of the tumor (Fig. 22-8). It is usually discovered in the proximal humerus when a "lump" which is ordinarily painless is felt on the affected bone. However, the mass can interfere with function of the extremity or cause pressure phenomenon on the overlying soft parts. At times, the tumor may be traumatized, thereby calling attention to the lesion.

The lesion is easily recognized on roentgenograms, appearing as a projection beyond the normal cortex. The projection may have a broad base or be pedunculated, varying greatly in size. Irregular zones of calcification may be visible, especially in the cartilage cap. The lesion often arises at the site of a tendon insertion, and its growth is directed along the line of tendon pull. Serial roentgenograms will often demonstrate the

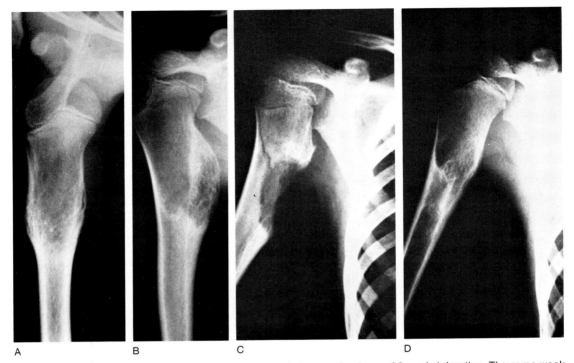

A   B   C   D

FIG. 22-8. A 9-year-old girl complained of a tender mass in her proximal arm of 6 weeks' duration. The same week her identical twin underwent an above-knee amputation for osteosarcoma of the proximal tibia. A, Anteroposterior and, B, lateral views of the proximal humerus demonstrate a broad-based projection of the medial humerus. Trabeculation is seen throughout the tumor. The osteochondroma with its periosteal cover was excised. The neurovascular structures were stretched over the apex of the tumor. The extremity was immobilized in a spica cast. C, On the eighth day postoperatively the patient fell down and sustained an oblique fracture. Spica cast immobilization was maintained for 6 weeks. D, Anteroposterior film shows the healed bone 1 year later. Now 3 years after operation, both she and her sister are well.

growth of the lesion. The lesion commonly becomes quiescent with closure of the epiphysis.

Rarely, the solitary lesion demonstrates a malignant change and must be differentiated from multiple osteochondroma, a hereditary disorder with an 11 to 20 percent incidence of malignant transformation in which the lesions are distributed over the skeleton.[23]

TREATMENT. The presence of a solitary osteochondroma alone is not a reason for surgical excision. Excision is recommended if the lesion creates clinical difficulty or disfigurement, or suddenly shows unusual growth. When the solitary lesion is removed the whole lesion including its periosteal cover over the cartilaginous cap should be extirpated without stripping the periosteum (Fig. 22-8). If the humerus is unduly weakened the extremity must be appropriately immobilized.

OSTEOGENESIS IMPERFECTA

Osteogenesis imperfecta is a congenital disorder wherein the bone is fragile, thereby allowing easy breakage, but heals without difficulty. The disease was first described by Ekman in 1788.[25] The disease is inherited as an autosomal dominant and affects all races. It is now considered a disorder of the connective tissue in which there is a defect in the normal maturation of collagen.

The most commonly accepted classification was devised by Fairbanks who distinguished three types: Type I is the thick bone type in which the patient is dwarfed and shows other serious manifestations. The bones at birth are short and wide, but the cortex is thin and the spongiosa expanded. Although fractures are common, deformity is less severe than it is in the slender bone type. The limbs appear stunted as in achondroplasia. Type II is the slender, fragile bone type seen in prenatal infants who survive more than a few months, and in all postnatal ones (Fig. 22-9). The skeleton is osteoporotic. It is the most common type. Bending occurs in the long bones without fracture, leading to gross deformity. Most of these children cannot walk. Moreover, upper extremity deformity may be so severe that hand function may be greatly impaired. Type III is the cystic type in which the bone may have a honeycomb appearance. It is seen at birth and progresses. Cystic changes with aging occur to a greater degree in the lower than in the upper extremities.

DIAGNOSIS. There are no pathognomonic signs or diagnostic tests that permit a diagnosis. The diagnosis is made on clinical and roentgenographic grounds. A wide spectrum of severity of fractures occurs in this disease, regardless of the type. The effects of the disorder may be so minimal that no treatment is indicated. In my experience, those patients who reach early adult years seem to have a lesser number of fractures than in the early years of life. Regardless of the severity of the disease, growth is retarded.[24]

Patients with osteogenesis imperfecta have other abnormalities that adversely affect health. They can show a hypermetabolic state and an increased risk of malignant hyperthermia induced by anesthetic agents. Solomons and Millar pointed out that there is early osteoporosis and deafness.[28] These patients have a natural resistance to malignant neoplasms and seem to cope well psychologically with their affliction.

TREATMENT. Once the diagnosis is established, the child's parents soon understand the importance of handling the child gently, always protecting the child from injury. Despite this care fractures do occur even with splinting and bracing. After a point, bracing is no longer effective.

In 1959 Sofield and Millar reported their fragmentation and rod techniques for managing osteogenesis imperfecta patients.[27] Various modifications of these techniques, including the use of telescoping rods, have been employed to allow for growth.

The indications for fragmentation and insertion of a rod are primarily to prevent fracture and deformity of a long bone, and thus the severe crippling effects of fracture with the attendant risk of conservative treatment in such cases. Those patients who have had rods inserted have fewer fractures, have less hospitalization, are happier, and have less deformity than those treated conservatively.[29]

It is much more difficult to approach the humerus surgically with safety than bones of the lower extremity, for example. The humerus may be devoid of a medullary cavity for almost its whole length, and may be so wide in only one diameter as to make insertion of a rod ineffective at times. In fact, the length of the humerus may appear as a wide flat length of shaft (rib shaped). The same holds true for the forearm bones, making insertion of a rod nearly impossible at times, or impractical. Nevertheless, at least for the humerus it is worthwhile to attempt to insert a rod (Fig. 22-9).

To insert a rod in the humerus, the entire length of the bone should be exposed. Blind pinning is not recommended and can be dangerous. As many osteotomy cuts are made in the humerus with an oscillating saw blade as are necessary to achieve a straight bone. Care must be exercised to avoid crushing the shaft when holding the bone with instruments. The largest diameter rod possible should be used to lessen the risk of bending or breaking.

Once a rod is correctly inserted, it is easier to insert a rod the entire length of the shaft later. The growth of the bone should be observed, or else severe deformity will develop over the end of the rod. Thus, telescoping rods have been used.

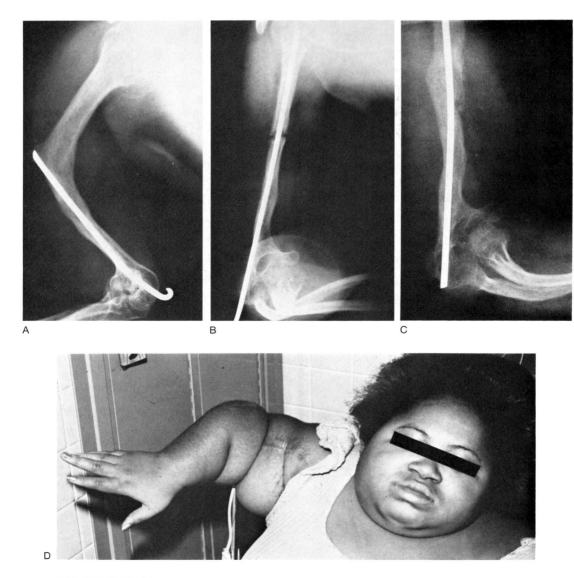

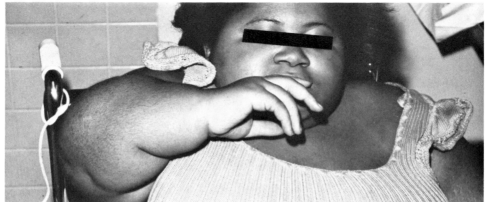

FIG. 22-9. A, A 19-year-old girl with type II osteogenesis imperfecta sustained bending of the midhumerus over the end of rod placed there 6 years before. She had great difficulty reaching out and was severely disabled. B, A single osteotomy was performed in the midhumerus and a new rod was inserted from below with difficulty. Five months postoperatively there was delayed union, and an iliac bone graft was performed. C, Note the healing 4 months later. D and E, The patient could now reach out and touch her face. Deformity in the forearm bones is apparent. The result was quite satisfactory.

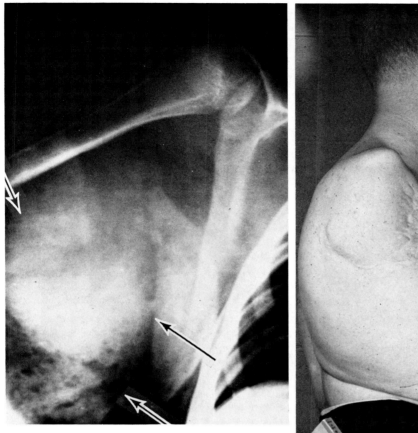
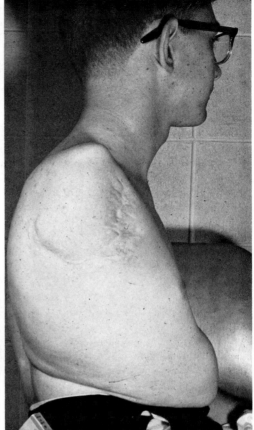

A

B

FIG. 22-10. A, A 17-year-old boy with factor VIII deficiency developed a football-size hemophilic pseudotumor. The lesion (arrows) involved the neurovascular bundle. A shoulder disarticulation was necessary to save his life before the advent of concentrates. B, Note the shoulder 7 years after operation. He was still well 15 years later without recurrence and used an upper extremity prosthesis.

I have observed delayed union or nonunion only once after inserting a rod (Fig. 22-9). The fact is that most fractures and osteotomies heal easily. Whatever the dangers and difficulties in these operations, they are outweighed by the excellent results and long periods without symptoms brought about by these procedures.

HEMOPHILIC PSEUDOTUMOR

The most catastrophic complication of hemophilia that can befall a patient with the condition is the formation of a pseudotumor. Any hemophilic tumor that increases in volume, causes bone erosion, causes neurologic deficit, displaces other tissues and organs, or leads to a loss of normal function of tissues and organs regardless of site of origin is considered to be a pseudotumor.[30] It may be so destructive that it must be surgically eradicated as early as possible (Fig. 22-10). Once removed, the patient must be observed thereafter for recurrence locally or elsewhere.

REFERENCES

1. Agerholm, J. C., and Goodfellow, J. W.: Simple cysts of the humerus treated by radical excision. J. Bone Joint Surg., 47-B:714–727, 1965.
2. Baker, D. M.: Benign unicameral bone cyst. A study of forty-five cases with long-term follow up. Clin. Orthop., 71:140–151, 1970.
3. Bloodgood, J. C.: Benign bone cysts, ostitis fibrosa, giant cell sarcoma and bone aneurism of the long pipe bones. A clinical and pathological study with the conclusion that conservative treatment is justifiable. Ann. Surg., 52:145–185, 1910.
4. Broder, H. M.: Possible precursor of unicameral bone cysts. J. Bone Joint Surg., 50-A:503–507, 1968.
5. Cohen, J.: Simple bone cysts. Studies of cyst fluid in six cases with a theory of pathogenesis. J. Bone Joint Surg., 42-A:609–616, 1960.
6. Cohen, J.: Etiology of simple bone cyst. J. Bone Joint Surg., 52-A:1493–1497, 1970.
7. Fahey, J. J., and O'Brien, E. T.: Subtotal resection and grafting in selected cases of solitary unicameral bone cyst. J. Bone Joint Surg., 55-A:59–68, 1973.
8. Garceau, G. J., and Gregory, C. F.: Solitary unicameral bone cysts. J. Bone Joint Surg., 36-A:267–280, 1954.
9. Gartland, J. J., and Cole, F. L.: Modern concepts in the treatment of unicameral bone cysts of the proximal humerus. Orthop. Clin. North Am., 6:487–498, 1975.
10. Jaffe, H. L., and Lichtenstein, L.: Solitary unicameral bone cyst with emphasis on the roentgen picture, the pathologic appearance and the pathogenesis. Arch. Surg., 44:1004–1025, 1942.
11. Johnson, L. C., and Kindred, R. G.: The anatomy of bone cysts. J. Bone Joint Surg., 40-A:1440, 1958.
12. Neer, C. S., Francis, K. C., Johnston, A. D., and Kiernan, H. A.: Current concepts on the treatment of solitary unicameral bone cyst. Clin. Orthop., 97:40–51, 1973.
13. Neer, C. S., Francis, K. C., Marcove, R. C., Terz, J., and Carbonara, P. N.: Treatment of unicameral bone cyst. A follow-up study of one hundred seventy-five cases. J. Bone Joint Surg., 48-A:731–745, 1966.
14. Tachdjian, M. O.: Pediatric Orthopaedics. Philadelphia, W. B. Saunders Co., p. 509, 1972.

Polymyositis and Dermatomyositis

15. Arundell, F. D., Wilkinson, R. D., and Haserick, J. R.: Dermatomyositis and malignant neoplasms in adults. Arch. Derm. Suph., 82:772–775, 1960.

16. Pearson, C. M.: Polymyositis; Clinical forms, diagnosis and therapy. Postgrad. Med., 31:450–458, 1962.
17. Pearson, C. M.: Polymyositis and dermatomyositis. In Arthritis and Allied Conditions, 8th ed. Edited by J. L. Hollander and D. J. McCarty. Philadelphia, Lea & Febiger, 1972, Chapter 53.
18. Rose, A. L., and Walton, J. N.: Polymyositis: A survey of 89 cases with particular reference to treatment and prognosis. Brain, 89:747–768, 1966.
19. Rose, A. L., Walton, J. N., and Pearce, G. W.: Polymyositis: An ultramicroscopic study of muscle biopsy material. J. Neurol. Sci., 5:457–472, 1967.
20. Unverricht, H.: Polymyositis acuta progressiva. Z. Klin. Med., 12:533–549, 1887.
21. Wagner, E.: Fall einer seltnen Muskelkrankheit. Arch. Heilk., 4:282–283, 1863.

Solitary Osteochondroma

22. Dahlin, D. C.: Bone Tumors. Springfield, Ill., Charles C Thomas, 1957.
23. Jaffe, H. L.: Tumors and Tumorous Conditions of the Bones and Joints. Philadelphia, Lea & Febiger, 1958.

Osteogenesis Imperfecta

24. Albright, J. A., and Grunt, J. A.: Studies of patients with osteogenesis imperfecta. J. Bone Joint Surg., 43-A:1415–1425, 1971.
25. Ekman, D. J.: Medical Doctorate Thesis at Uppsala, 1788.
26. Fairbanks, Sir T.: An Atlas of General Affections of the Skeleton. Baltimore, Williams & Wilkins, 1951.
27. Sofield, H. A., and Millar, E. A.: Fragmentation, realignment and intramedullary rod fixation of deformities of the long bones in children. J. Bone Joint Surg., 41-A:1371–1391, 1959.
28. Solomons, C. C., and Millar, E. A.: Osteogenesis imperfecta—New perspectives. Clin. Orthop., 96:299–303, 1973.
29. Williams, P. F., Cole, W. H. J., Bailey, R. W., Dubow, H. I., Solomons, C. C., and Millar, E. A.: Current aspects of the surgical treatment of osteogenesis imperfecta. Clin. Orthop., 96:288–298, 1973.

Hemophilic Pseudotumor

30. Post, M., and Telfer, M. C.: Surgery in hemophilic patients. J. Bone Joint Surg., 57-A:1136–1145, 1975.

23

Amputation About the Shoulder Girdle

ROBERT D. KEAGY

This chapter reviews the techniques that have been found useful in amputations about the shoulder.[9] Ablative surgery at this level can be classified as transverse amputation or intercalary resection:

Transverse amputations
 Shoulder disarticulation
  Functional—less than 2 in. of humerus below the anterior axillary fold
  Anatomic—glenohumeral disarticulation
 Forequarter amputation

Intercalary resections
 Scapulectomy
 Shoulder resection (Tikhor-Linberg procedure)

Intercalary resections preserve the elbow, forearm and hand, but a flail shoulder, variable loss of shoulder contour, and sometimes considerable change in length of the extremity severely compromise the patient's static appearance. The patient's performance capability is greatly reduced, and his action patterns appear strange to the inexperienced observer.

Resections at the shoulder girdle level can be caused by trauma or the need to rid the patient of a malignant neoplasm, infection, or complication of radiotherapy. It would be most unusual for deformity or neurologic or vascular disease to require resection at this level. When such problems are distal in a limb, the surgeon can choose a proximal anatomic site where a standard procedure can be done with ease. When the lesion is at the shoulder girdle level, the surgeon must perform the procedure between the lesion distally and the lungs and neck vessels proximally. Standard procedures can be described, but the exigencies necessitating these amputations require the surgeon to be unbounded by the constraints of standard approaches.

The random residues of trauma seldom supply sufficient skin to allow standardized skin flap formation or wound closure. Trauma producing or requiring amputation at the shoulder is frequently associated with other wounds of the thorax or avulsion of masses of tissue. Providing a neat scar by shifting skin flaps frequently taxes one's surgical ingenuity. Such flaps may be irregular and insufficient for closure. Split-thickness skin grafts may be required. The amputation specimen may be a source of skin grafts in such cases.

Similarly, because of the treacherous borders of an infiltrating malignant tumor, the surgeon may not see the tumor at the time of amputation. The primary goal in tumor surgery must be adequate resection. This requires that some normal tissue be excised with the tumor. Skin flaps and muscle resection must provide for this border of normal tissue. Formalized amputations with standard flaps are appropriate only when the resection is sufficiently proximal to the malignant lesion so that these flaps would not be involved in the malignant process. Only occasionally, with small lesions or with those of limited malignant involvement, can flaps be fashioned from overlying tissues. The hairy skin of the axilla can be unsightly and is the most dispensable. Flaps must not displace the female breast. Split-thickness grafts are well tolerated on the thorax but not on the acromion. Generally, elective scars should be kept as low on the thorax as possible, and the placing of unnecessary scars near the brachial plexus or over the acromion should be avoided.

The selection of the original level or procedure should be in terms of initial adequacy of tumor control. Resection should not be done at any level with the thought that if a tumor recurs, then higher or radical resection can be done. This is not conservative. Forequarter amputation performed for tumor recurrence after less radical operations often fails.

The term "forequarter amputation" is used here to refer to amputation of the entire upper extremity with the scapula and most of the clavicle. The term "interscapulothoracic" amputation is considered synonymous.

The classification of shoulder disarticulations includes the truly anatomic glenohumeral disarticulation and those amputations that retain the humeral head and proximal metaphysis but leave a residual stump with less than 2 in. of bony length distal to the anterior axillary fold. Except in children, these short stumps do not permit fitting with an above-elbow prosthesis. Therefore, these procedures are classified as shoulder disarticulations from a functional and prosthetic standpoint.

Scapulectomy is a resection of the scapula. Scapulectomy is not often a sufficient procedure for the control of tumor. It can be used for the patient who resolutely refuses more effective amputation or for pal-

liation in a patient in whom systemic spread of malignant alteration has already been demonstrated.

Intercalary shoulder resection (the Tikhor-Linberg procedure[5,10]) removes the scapula, upper end of the humerus, and the lateral clavicle. It has been termed "interscapulothoracic resection" by Linberg[5] and by Moseley.[7] The title "en bloc resection of the shoulder girdle" was used by Janecki and Nelson.[4] The indications for this procedure include the residuals of radiation therapy to the shoulder girdle and chronic severe infection of the glenohumeral joint. Like scapulectomy, the procedure is indicated only when the neurovascular bundle is not involved.

All these procedures are best done with the patient lying on the sound side. The entire involved extremity should be draped so as to permit its free manipulation. The thorax should be draped so that free access is available from the midline posteriorly to the midline anteriorly, and from the angle of the jaw superiorly to the level of the inferior angle of the scapula inferiorly. If the assault is to include the sternal end of the clavicle, the surgeon should be prepared to make an emergency incision into the chest that may be required if the subclavian or innominate vein is torn. Ordinarily, blood loss is easily controlled, but hypotensive anesthesia can reduce the loss to nil.

KINESIOLOGY OF INTERCALARY RESECTIONS

Amputation of an upper extremity is a major functional and psychic forfeit. The body image needs of a few patients will not tolerate the loss of a hand. In the most severe of these situations the intercalary resections may be indicated. To legitimize scapulectomy or intercalary shoulder resection, there should be some hope of sparing the median, ulnar, and radial nerves, as well as the axillary artery and veins.

From the biomechanical standpoint, the function of the shoulder girdle is to provide the proximal stability and the muscular power to achieve stable, purposive hand placement. The key requirement is the ability to fix the glenohumeral joint on the thorax and, from this stable base, to drive the humerus. When the hand is moved forward by any mechanism (e.g. elbow flexion), gravity tends to extend the shoulder. This extensor movement is ordinarily controlled by the shoulder flexors and scapular stabilizing muscles.

The intercalary loss of the bony structures of the glenohumeral joint or the loss of power in the stabilizing musculature of the shoulder results in the inability to place the hand in space. Thus scapulectomy, intercalary shoulder resection, and an upper brachial plexus lesion produce the same dysfunction. There is, subsequently, a hand present in form but severely limited in function, not because grasp and release or sensation is gone, but because the hand cannot be placed in space and may dangle helplessly alongside the thigh, swing flaccidly as the patient turns, or flap when the patient runs. Although elbow flexion is possible, the hand moves upward along the trunk as the elbow moves backward. The patient cannot move the hand forward, and can only use the hand to hold light objects or to fasten clothing at the midline in front.

When contemplating these intercalary procedures, it is important to explain to the patient exactly what the limitation of function in the remaining hand will be. A full understanding that the presence of a hand is not synonymous with normal upper extremity function may help the patient to accept a more definitive procedure.

Prosthetic devices for amputations at this level are of minimal functional value at present. Some cosmetic symmetry can be achieved prosthetically, but little functional value can be attained. The prostheses are frequently such a nuisance that they are not worn. Forequarter amputees do use a cosmetic shoulder cap device to permit normal clothing to be worn.

SHOULDER DISARTICULATION

For an individual of ordinary size, at least 2 in. of bony length distal to the anterior

axillary fold are required to permit useful fitting with an above-elbow prosthesis. A fleshy individual requires more bony length, whereas a slender child requires less. If the residual limb cannot be fitted for function with an above-elbow prosthesis, the amputee has a functional shoulder disarticulation whether some of the humerus is present or not. However, preservation of the humeral head maintains the fullness of the shoulder contour so that the patient can wear clothes well. This is of sufficient import that one should conserve the humeral head whenever possible.

The shoulder disarticulation amputee will seldom wear a functional prosthesis of the body-powered type, especially when the stump is fleshy or badly scarred anteriorly or superiorly. However, the residual mobility of the shoulder girdle permits the use of the acromion to operate switches within the shoulder cap of currently experimental electrically powered prostheses.

If the humeral segment is longer than the surgical neck, some consideration must be given to muscle balance because the rotator cuff will tend to abduct and flex the humeral remnant, resulting in a stump that is both unusable and unsightly. In general, the deltoid should be used to cover the humerus when resection is above the deltoid insertion.

Under optimal conditions, the flap for disarticulation at the glenohumeral joint is the same as that for a resection at the surgical neck. The wound may be as limited as that indicated in Figure 23-1 or as generous as that shown in Figure 23-2.

The anterior incision is begun over the infraclavicular fossa. It should be medial to the coracoid since a scar over the coracoid may be tender. The incision for the lateral flap is made parallel to the deltopectoral groove and the medial margin of the anterior deltoid, is carried across the arm at the level of the deltoid insertion, and then is curved proximally to the posterior axillary fold, following the medial edge of the posterior deltoid.

The incision for the medial flap is made with the patient's arm abducted and de-

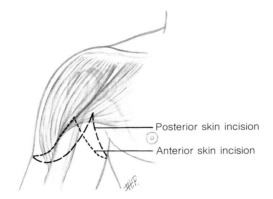

FIG. 23-1. Incision for amputation through the surgical neck of the humerus.

parts from the anterior incision so as to cross the axilla to join the lateral incision at the posterior axillary fold. The selective level of this flap is determined by how much skin is available on the lateral flap and by how much of the humerus is to be resected. If a large lateral flap is available and the humerus is to be disarticulated, the medial wound can be on the medial axilla.

The deltoid is sectioned 1 cm. proximal to its insertion. When feasible, the deltoid is elevated with the lateral flap. Elevation of the deltoid flap clearly exposes the axillary nerve and facilitates its definition and conservation (see Fig. 23-8B). As the axillary

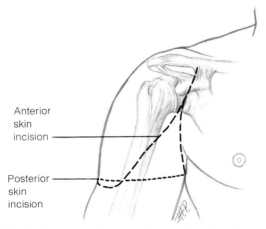

FIG. 23-2. Incision for anatomic shoulder disarticulation.

nerve is followed through the quadrilateral space, it is convenient to section the triceps and posterior rotator cuff.

The pectoralis major is sectioned near its insertion. With the pectoralis muscle reflected medially, the interval between the pectoralis minor and the coracobrachialis is identified and dissection is continued proximally to expose the axillary vessels and nerves. Section of these vessels and the several nerves is performed so that the ligations and neuromas will lie medial and deep to the lateral margin of the pectoralis minor. The axillary nerve should be spared if possible.

The coracobrachialis and the short head of the biceps are sectioned about 2 cm. distal to the proposed site of bone resection. The long head of the biceps is cut at the line of bone resection.

The latissimus dorsi and the teres major are sectioned near their insertions. The humerus is then sectioned at the surgical neck, or the rotator cuff and capsule are transected to disarticulate the humerus. If the humerus is transected distal to the surgical neck, the teres and latissimus should be reattached distally to avoid the flexion-abduction deformity that is produced by an unopposed rotator cuff.

If the joint is disarticulated, there is no special treatment required for the cartilage of the glenoid fossa. The rotator cuff edges should be sutured together over the glenoid fossa to help fill the gap beneath the acromion. The deltoid (which may be shortened), the pectoralis major, teres, and latissimus are sutured together (to cover the coracoid, if possible), the wound is drained, and the skin is closed. A bulky compression dressing is applied.

If surgical exigencies require release of the pectoralis minor from the coracoid, or prevent reattachment of the pectoralis major to the posterior muscles, the scapula will ride upward and posteromedially, rotated by the unopposed pull of the trapezius and serratus anterior muscles. This migration destroys the symmetry of the shoulders in an unsightly way. Therefore, every effort should be made to reattach the pectorales so as to provide "level" symmetry to the shoulder contours.

Vasconcelos describes shoulder disarticulation as a "bad operation," and indicates that it is an "orthopedic failure," to be performed only in exceptional cases.[11]

The residual after disarticulation is more unsightly than the residual after resection at the surgical neck of the humerus because removal of the humeral head leaves the acromion projecting prominently. This prominence is not quite enough to fill out the shoulder of a garment. At the same time, the acromion is not adequately capable of bearing the weight of a functioning prosthesis and is not useful either for suspension or as a power source for a body-powered prosthesis. Additionally, the coracoid is prominent when the humeral head is removed. Scars over the acromion or coracoid are troublesome and often require special relief even for a light cosmetic shoulder cap. However, the acromion is the most mobile point of the shoulder girdle and the best structure with which to operate electric switches inside a shoulder cap socket suspended on the thorax. Such prostheses are available only on an experimental basis.

Shoulder disarticulation is not a good operation for attempted cure of malignant tumor of the proximal humerus because the operative field is too near the tumor. The surgeon must avoid the trap of seeming to be conservative as an apparent favor to the patient when, in fact, the operative field is likely to be involved by the tumor.

In some situations, resection of the entire deltoid and section of the pectoralis major, latissimus, and teres major medial to the axillary fold reduce the chance of opening the tumor, but a bony, high-riding, troublesome stump results. The patient is left with both an awkward stump and a reduced chance of surgical cure. Surgery for palliation or for tumors of limited malignant change may occasionally justify this, but surgery "for cure" usually demands wider margins of normal tissue, absolute avoidance of the risk of "uncovering" the tumor or dissecting through some undetected tumorous extension, and should offer a greater opportunity for lymphatic resection (Fig. 23-3).

SCAPULECTOMY

The incision for scapulectomy may vary considerably, but it must always provide for adequate access to the superior medial and superior lateral angles of the scapula. If a biopsy has been performed, the resection should include the skin and deep tissues around the biopsy site. (A well-planned biopsy accomplished without lateral undermining can minimize this problem.) One must achieve access to the three angles of the scapula and totally extirpate the biopsy field. The skin tolerates extensive undermining and large flaps can be raised. A gently curvilinear incision will usually permit exposure of the entire scapular insertion of the trapezius and all three borders of the bone (Fig. 23-4). It is uncommon to need a T-shaped, or triradiate, incision. The nature of the pathologic lesion will determine whether the muscles should be resected subperiosteally or further from the bone.

Simply detaching the latissimus from the inferior angle permits the scapula to be tilted upward so that the scapulocostal space can be investigated from below.

The vertebral border of the scapula is freed next. The inferior and middle trapezius are detached from the spine of the scapula to expose the rhomboids for section (see Fig. 23-8A and B). The superior trapezius is resected from the scapular spine, the acromion, and the distal clavicle. The levator scapulae is sectioned. This initial muscular dissection should move along briskly. It is easy to do a blunt digital dissection, followed by dissection with a knife or scissors. The branches of the superficial cervical and descending scapular vessels can now be definitively controlled. The omohyoid muscle and suprascapular vessels and nerve are also exposed for control.

The scapula can now be lifted away laterally from the thorax. The brachial plexus is identified along with the axillary vessels (see Fig. 23-8C). The surgeon must remember to combine palpation with vision. The axillary,

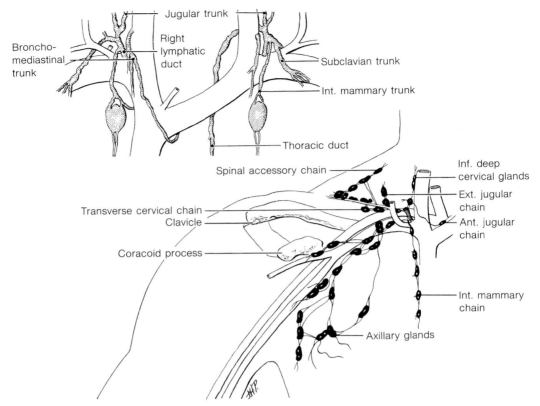

FIG. 23-3. Lymph node chains about the shoulder girdle.

thoracodorsal, and radial nerves can be identified, if desired. Decisions concerning subperiosteal elevation of the spinati and serratus anterior are usually made preoper-

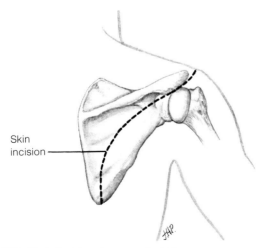

FIG. 23-4. Incision for scapulectomy.

atively. Most commonly, these muscles should be removed with the bone. It is occasionally possible to preserve the acromion and the continuity of the superior trapezius-deltoid suspensory system.

The axillary border of the scapula is approached next. The deltoid is transected from the spine of the scapula and from the acromion, if the scapula is to be totally resected. The teres major and the long head of the triceps are transected. The subscapular artery is controlled. Care must be taken to preserve the axillary and radial nerves. The scapula can then be freed, either by disarticulation of the acromioclavicular joint and detachment of the coracoclavicular ligaments or, more conveniently, by severance of the clavicle just medial to the coracoclavicular ligaments. By raising the scapula away from the chest, the pectoralis minor, coracobrachialis, and short head of the biceps can be detached from the coracoid. The rotator cuff is easily transected by rotating the humerus, leaving a stub of tendons.

De Palma describes a technique wherein the rotator cuff is sectioned at the level of the neck of the scapula, so that with the scapula removed the cut end of the distal cuff can be sutured about the distal clavicle.[2] This suspends and stabilizes the humerus to preserve the outline of the shoulder for an improved cosmetic result.

Metastatic malignant neoplasm of the scapula is best managed by radiotherapy rather than by resection, as pointed out by Pack and Baldwin.[8]

De Nancrede indicates, after extensive experience, that scapulectomy is rarely the operation of choice for cancerous conditions when "cure" is the goal of surgery.[1]

INTERCALARY SHOULDER RESECTION

The goal of intercalary shoulder resection (Tikhor-Linberg shoulder resection[5,10]), like that of scapulectomy, is to achieve massive removal of the musculoskeletal elements of the shoulder girdle while preserving the distal limb. The neurovascular structures supplying the hand and forearm must be free of tumor involvement. The scapula, distal clavicle, and proximal humerus are resected with all of the intrinsic shoulder muscles. Variable amounts of the biceps, triceps, pectorales, and latissimus are resected. The skin over the deltoid and scapular areas can be removed. A connecting pedicle consisting of the axillary vessels, the brachial plexus, and the axillary skin is preserved. Closure requires a juryrigged suspension of the distal arm to the remnant of the clavicle or to the chest. Considerable proximal telescoping is possible to achieve closure. Advantages of this procedure over scapulectomy include the more extensive resection and, since the hand and elbow are closer to the face, the patient is more likely to be able to use the hand for facial self-care and feeding activity.

The operation is performed with the patient lying on the uninvolved side. The entire upper extremity and chest are prepared and draped so that the upper extremity is free for manipulation. The incision for shoulder resection resembles a folded tennis racquet (Fig. 23-5). The "handle" is along the clavicle. The anterior limb is made downward along the deltopectoral groove to the midpoint of the medial edge of the biceps, then turned distally for an inch or two, and then curved upward to cross the lateral surface of the arm at the mid-deltoid level. From this point, the posterior limb of the racquet is curved from the mid-deltoid area downward and medially toward the inferior angle of the scapula, where it again is curved upward to join the handle near the acromioclavicular joint.

The deep dissection can be done from either an anterior or a posterior approach. The anterior approach starts with resection of the clavicle, somewhat like the anterior (Berger) technique of forequarter amputation (see Fig. 23-7). The posterior approach is similar to that used for scapulectomy, or to the posterior (Littlewood) technique of forequarter amputation[6] (see Fig. 23-8). The brachial plexus is preserved (the lateral

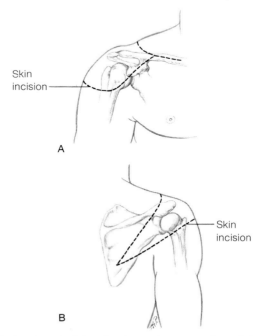

FIG. 23-5. Incision for intercalary resection of the shoulder. A, Anterior aspect. B, Posterior aspect.

cord may be sacrificed, but only if necessary), and the major vessels are conserved. The transverse cervical, suprascapular, circumflex scapular, circumflex humeral, and thoracoacromial arteries are ligated.

After detachment of the scapulothoracic muscles and the deltoid, the biceps and triceps are cut. The humerus is then transected at the surgical neck or somewhat lower. The biceps, triceps, and deltoid (if it is salvaged) are attached to the thorax and the trapezius to suspend the arm as well as possible.

The wound must be drained extensively, and the forearm and hand are supported in a Velpeau or similar type of dressing.

FOREQUARTER AMPUTATIONS

The two general approaches to the scapulothoracic procedure are related to where the surgeon chooses to start: the anterior approach, so well described by Berger in 1887 that it is called the Berger technique, and the posterior approach, advocated by Littlewood in 1922 and known as the Littlewood technique.[6] The anterior technique is more direct but is definitely more time-consuming than is the posterior approach.

When the tumor does not involve the scapula and the space between the subscapularis and the serratus can be safely used, the anterior approach is acceptable. When there is doubt about this, the posterior approach should be used, as this easily permits the serratus anterior to be lifted off the ribs with the scapula.

ANTERIOR APPROACH (BERGER TECHNIQUE). Vasconcelos describes the anterior (Berger) technique as occurring in two consecutive "sessions," the first session having two stages and the second session having three stages. These are as follows:

1st Session
  1st stage—partial resection of the clavicle
  2nd stage—isolation and section of the subclavian vessels

2nd Session
  1st stage—incision of the contour and section of the antero-inferior flap; section of the pectoralis minor and latissimus dorsi
  2nd stage—incision and upward detachment of the postero-superior flap and trapezius
  3rd stage—section of the muscles inserting on the margins of the scapula: the omohyoid, serratus anterior, levator scapulae, and the rhomboids.

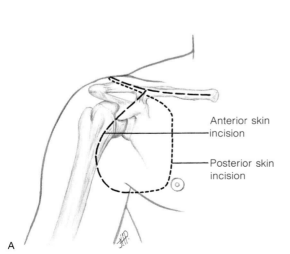

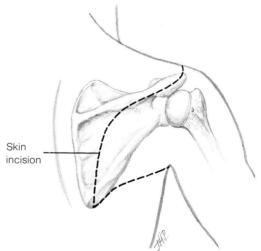

A   B

FIG. 23-6. Incision for forequarter amputation. A, Anterior aspect. B, Posterior aspect.

The incision is outlined in Figure 23-6. Pertinent anatomy is illustrated in Figure 23-7.

The wound is developed to form an anterior-inferior and a posterior-superior flap through a racquet-shaped incision with the handle on the clavicle. The anterior rim of the racquet is made from the clavicle downward along the deltopectoral groove, curved under the pectoralis, and continued posteriorly across the medial side of the arm to the posterior axillary fold. It is then made downward along the axillary fold to the inferior angle of the scapula, upward toward the acromioclavicular joint, then curved medially to join the initial incision.

The clavicular wound is deepened through the skin, fat, and platysma to expose the clavicle and clavicular head of the pectoralis major. The pectoralis major is detached from the clavicle. The exposure of the clavicle is completed subperiosteally to the site of medial resection, which should be 3 cm. lateral to the sternoclavicular joint.

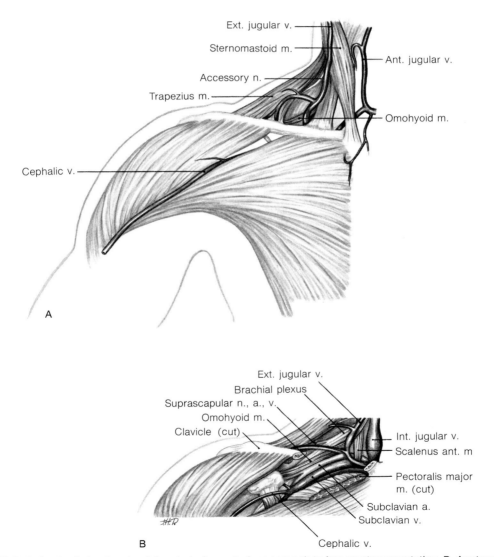

FIG. 23-7. A, Anatomic landmarks at the start of an anterior approach to forequarter amputation. B, Anatomy after removing a portion of the clavicle.

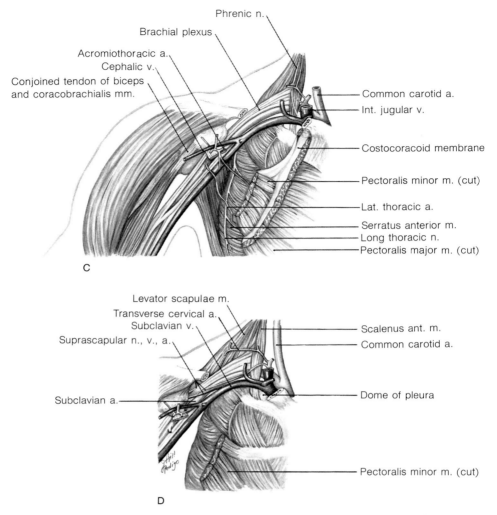

Phrenic n.
Brachial plexus
Acromiothoracic a.
Cephalic v.
Conjoined tendon of biceps
and coracobrachialis mm.
Common carotid a.
Int. jugular v.
Costocoracoid membrane
Pectoralis minor m. (cut)
Lat. thoracic a.
Serratus anterior m.
Long thoracic n.
Pectoralis major m. (cut)

C

Levator scapulae m.
Transverse cervical a.
Subclavian v.
Suprascapular n., v., a.
Scalenus ant. m.
Common carotid a.
Subclavian a.
Dome of pleura
Pectoralis minor m. (cut)

D

FIG. 23-7 continued. C and D, Details of anatomy as seen during the anterior approach for forequarter amputation.

Resection of only the middle third of the clavicle leaves a long stump of clavicle medially with the sternomastoid attached. This muscle pulls the stump of clavicle upward and may cause an unsightly prominence.

The clavicle should be resected with a Gigli saw in an oblique superomedial direction so that the remnant of the clavicle will be beveled appropriately. The dissection of the medial end of the clavicle must be done most carefully because the subclavian vein is closely applied and adherent (this is why the Gigli saw is the safest instrument to use). Total removal of the clavicle by disarticulation from the sternum is indicated only when a full-scale lymph node dissection is needed in the management of malignant tumors that have lymphatic dissemination. Even when this is desired, resection of the clavicle with subsequent removal of the medial stump is easier and safer than disarticulation.

After transecting the clavicle medially, the shaft is turned laterally and transected lateral to the site of the deltopectoral groove with a saw or rongeur. The arm can then be abducted and externally rotated to "offer up the contents of the axilla on the scapula, as on a plate."[3]

A plane of fascia and periosteum containing the omohyoid muscle above, the subclavius muscle, the costocoracoid membrane, and the pectoralis minor muscle is now exposed. This plane of fascia is called the omohyoid fascia above the clavicle, and the costocoracoid fascia below the clavicle. The omohyoid fascia is penetrated by the external and anterior jugular veins. The costocoracoid fascia is penetrated by the cephalic vein, the lateral anterior thoracic nerve, and the anterior branches of the thoracoacromial trunk. There are three choices of route through the plane: through the omohyoid fascia, through the costocoracoid membrane (following the lateral anterior thoracic nerve to the axillary artery), or by the middle route, excision of the subclavius muscle.

Immediately deep to the subclavius muscle is the important suprascapular artery which is ligated and transected.

The inferior approach through the costocoracoid membrane is probably easiest. The lateral anterior thoracic nerve leads easily to the lateral side of the axillary artery. Blunt dissection upward and medially permits an item-by-item division of the costocoracoid membrane, the subclavius muscle, the omohyoid fascia, and the omohyoid muscle.

The brachial plexus and the axillary subclavian vessels are thus exposed. The first part of the axillary artery or the third part of the subclavian artery can then be doubly ligated. Dissection of the axillary or subclavian vein should be done carefully because the vein is quite fragile and densely adherent to the first rib and costoclavicular ligaments. Extensive hemorrhage and air embolism have been reported as complications of the venous dissection.

The nerves can be simply transected. It is not necessary to inject them with local anesthetic, nor is it useful to ligate them. With careful management, the neuromas will be between the scalenes, out of harm's way. The nerves should not be pulled so hard as to avulse their roots from the spinal cord.

The transverse cervical or superficial cervical artery and the descending scapular arteries appear as the nerves are traced to the margins of the scalenes. These arteries, as well as the suprascapular artery, are sometimes quite large, particularly if the tumor is very vascular.

With the blood supply secured and the nerves sectioned, the anterior descending loop of the skin incision is deepened, and the pectorales major and minor are transected as far distally as is compatible with safe avoidance of the tumor. The arm is drawn forward and adducted (thereby abducting the scapula) to permit the posterior skin incision to be deepened and the skin flap to be turned back from the scapula.

The muscular dissection proceeds well if a finger is passed along the acromion deep to the trapezius and the muscle severed with a scissors. The levator scapulae and the rhomboids are similarly cut. The serratus anterior is sectioned. The latissimus is separated from the inferior pole of the scapula and sectioned as far laterally as is reasonable. The limb is now free.

The pectorales, trapezius, and latissimus muscles are attached to the chest and each other as well as one can. The skin flaps are trimmed and closed over a suction drain. A light compression dressing is applied.

POSTERIOR APPROACH (LITTLEWOOD TECHNIQUE).[6] An advantage of the posterior approach is that first the nerves, then the axillary artery, and finally the vein are exposed. However, the vein is deep in the wound and may be difficult to visualize. If the clavicle is sectioned before the vein is controlled, careless retraction may rip the vein disastrously.

The incision is ultimately the same as that for the anterior approach, but the posterior limb is developed first (see Fig. 23-6). The large scapular skin flap is elevated to the medial border of the scapula. The latissimus is detached from the inferior angle of the scapula (and from its lateral humeral attachment, if convenient) (Fig. 23-8A and B). This allows the inferior pole of the scapula to be lifted and the scapulothoracic space inspected. The trapezius is dissected away by passing a finger or curved hemostat beneath it and cutting the muscle free of the spine and the scapula. Usually the middle of

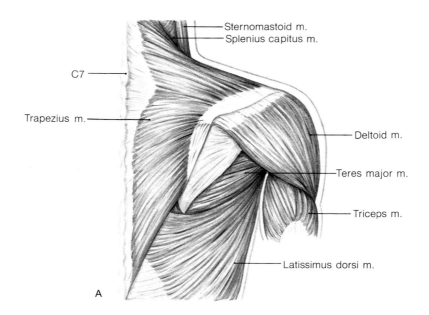

A

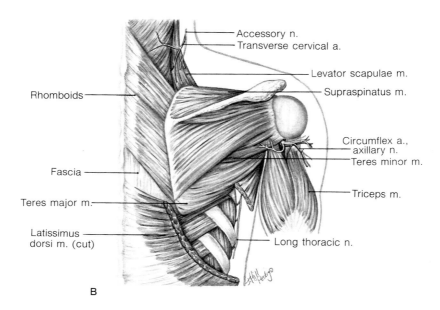

B

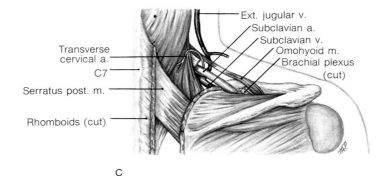

C

FIG. 23-8. A and B, Details of anatomy pertinent to scapulectomy, intercalary shoulder resection, or posterior approach to forequarter amputation. C, Posterior view of the first part of the axillary artery and vein after cutting the brachial plexus.

the superior belly of the trapezius is cut directly across to its easily palpable anterior edge. The rhomboids and levator scapulae are sectioned. The transverse cervical and suprascapular vessels can be definitively controlled. The scapula can be rolled forward to facilitate identification of the major neurovascular structures in their fibrofatty bed. The omohyoid and its fascia are anterior. The neurovascular structures lie on the belly of the first digitation of the serratus anterior. The serratus is severed near its scapular insertion if the subscapular space is free of disease. This is best performed by inserting a finger between the subscapularis and the serratus from below as a guide for the knife.

The scalenus covers the first rib, so that the rib can only be palpated. It is the second rib that can be seen. The nerve to the serratus anterior can be seen on the scalenus medius and is easily saved. The cords of the brachial plexus cover the artery. The elements of the plexus can be sectioned item by item. The artery can then be divided. The vein must be carefully approached. It is easy to identify but not to isolate. Care must be taken.

Lymph node dissection (see Fig. 23-3) may be added as indicated.

The subsequent dissection and clavicular section are relatively simple. Wound closure is the same regardless of how the procedure was started.

REFERENCES

1. De Nancrede, C. B. G.: The end results after total excision of the scapula for sarcoma. Ann. Surg., 50:1–22, 1909.
2. De Palma, A. F.: Scapulectomy and a method of preserving the normal configuration of the shoulder. Clin. Orthop., 4:217–224, 1954.
3. Henry, A. K.: Extensile Exposure. Baltimore, Williams & Wilkins Co., 1957.
4. Janecki, C. J., and Nelson, C. L.: En bloc resection of the shoulder girdle: Technique and indications. J. Bone Joint Surg., 54-A:1754–1758, 1972.
5. Linberg, B. E.: Interscapulo-thoracic resection for malignant tumors of the shoulder joint region. J. Bone Joint Surg., 10:344–349, 1928.
6. Littlewood, H.: Amputations at the shoulder and at the hip. Br. Med. J., 1:381, 1922.
7. Moseley, H. F.: The forequarter amputation. Edinburgh, E. & S. Livingstone, Ltd., 1957, p. 49.
8. Pack, G. T., and Baldwin, J. C.: The Tikhor-Linberg resection of the shoulder girdle, a case report. Surgery, 38:753–757, 1955.
9. Slocum, D. B.: Atlas of Amputations. St. Louis, C. V. Mosby Co., 1949.
10. Tikhor, P. T.: Tumor Studies. Russia, 1900.
11. Vasconcelos, E.: Modern Methods of Amputation. New York, Philosophical Library of New York, 1945.

24

Prosthetic Restoration for Shoulder Amputations

ROBERT G. THOMPSON

MARK HAJOST

Shoulder disarticulations and scapulo-thoracic amputations are employed, respectively, as life-saving measures for malignant tumors involving the proximal humerus and shoulder joint, or for progressive uncontrolled infections of the shoulder joint area. These amputations are severe, mutilating procedures, made necessary by the seriousness of the primary pathologic lesion (Fig. 24-1).

Prior to World War II patients with amputations at these high levels were rarely fitted with prostheses, since available artificial limbs were cumbersome, heavy, and functionally inadequate. With the advent of lighter plastic sockets, Bowden control cables, simplified harnesses, and the practicability of external power, the fitting of prostheses at these amputation levels became more feasible.[1] At these high levels of amputation control sites for such prostheses are few.

Recently, considerable interest has been generated toward finding efficient sources of external power to activate prostheses for these high levels of amputation. For example, in Europe efforts have concentrated on pneumatic prostheses activated by carbon dioxide. Noteworthy success has been achieved in Heidelberg, Germany, where a large number of children afflicted with phocomelia have been treated with such devices. In the United States, research has been directed toward achieving more efficient use of available body power and control, with electricity as the prime source of external power.

The patient with a shoulder disarticulation has lost the function of the hand, forearm, and elbow, and lacks active shoulder-joint motion. Significantly, the patient retains the ability to elevate, abduct, adduct, forward flex, and extend the scapuloclavicular segment of the remaining shoulder. The forequarter (scapulothoracic) amputee loses not only all of the functions of the patient with a shoulder disarticulation, but also shoulder elevation and scapular abduction and adduction. This additional loss drastically reduces control site possibilities for the operation of an efficient functional prosthesis. Common experience has shown that the required increased complexity of control motions and the minimal or diminished function which results generally decrease patient acceptance of functional prostheses for these amputation levels. Furthermore, the greater the number of mechanical substitutions (for normal structures), the less is the likelihood for patient acceptance. Since tolerance of gadgets decreases with increasing numbers of substi-

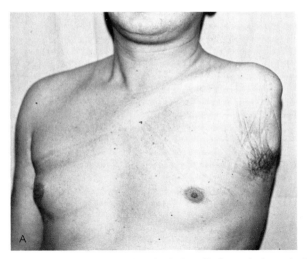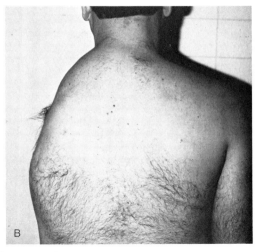

FIG. 24-1. A, Shoulder disarticulation. B, Scapulothoracic (forequarter) amputation.

tutions and closely related control functions required to operate the prosthesis, prostheses are often rejected.

PROSTHETIC REQUIREMENTS

INTERFACE (SOCKET). The interface (socket) of a prosthesis for a shoulder disarticulation generally has a proximal section (providing distal arm stability) that rests on the superior border of the scapula, protected by its overlying muscle mass, and the clavicle (Fig. 24-2). The socket also includes anterior and posterior wings, providing rotational stability and suspension. Obviously, an intimately fitted interface is necessary to minimize excursion and power loss through unwanted motion at the amputation site. Since the acromion and lateral clavicle are preserved, there is no need for a socket filler. The interface can be contoured closely to the shoulder thereby permitting a cosmetically acceptable shoulder appearance. If the shoulder disarticulation stump has prominent bony structures, the cast of the true anatomic parts is modified to protect the bony prominence rather than attempting later to pad the areas with soft foam material.

The interface for the scapulothoracic, or forequarter, amputation prosthesis is larger than the one for shoulder disarticulation in order to obtain reasonable stability on the sloping chest wall. At the same time, considerable filler is needed to obtain symmetric shoulder outline (Fig. 24-3). Filler material may be urethane foam or other light substances to keep the weight of the prosthesis to a minimum. Because of the great loss of body structures, of necessity the interface must be bulky. Whenever the trunk surface is covered with a large plastic surface, as represented by this prosthetic interface, the area for body heat radiation is reduced. In this event methods for socket ventilation must be considered.

SHOULDER MECHANISMS. A number of shoulder joints are now available either without motion or with motion possible in six planes. Currently, there is no known method for providing externally powered abduction, adduction, flexion, or extension of artificial shoulder joints. Thus, all prosthetic shoulder joints are positioned passively.

Shoulder disarticulation prostheses may utilize a simple bulkhead connection between the interface and the humeral segment that allows only passive flexion and extension. Other types of bulkhead shoulder joints allow not only flexion and extension but also passive abduction and adduction. In an effort to increase the range and planes of motion, other kinds of shoulder

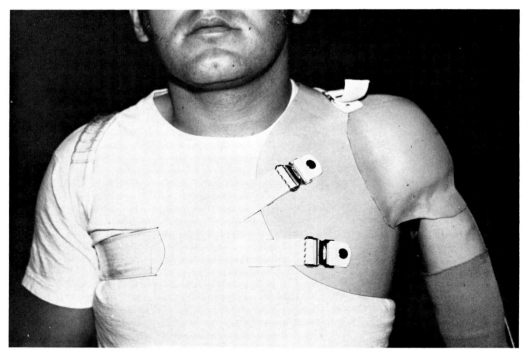

FIG. 24-2. Typical interface (socket) of a prosthesis for shoulder disarticulation amputation. Note chest harness providing stability.

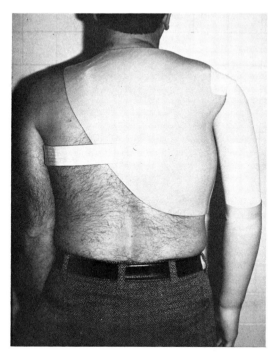

FIG. 24-3. Forequarter amputation interface (socket). Note large areas of body surface enclosed by plastic socket.

joints have been developed: (1) Hinge joints, similar to that used for the elbow joint in a short below-elbow amputee, provide passive abduction and adduction at the shoulder joint (Fig. 24-4). (2) Four-way shoulder joints allow abduction and adduction, as well as shoulder flexion and extension (Fig. 24-5). These joints, however, require frequent adjustment to maintain the degree of joint friction that is present in a new prosthesis. (3) An orthogonal cylinder joint has been developed at the Northwestern Prosthetics Research Laboratory to improve the stability of the multi-axis shoulder joint. This joint gives four planes of motion and requires less frequent adjustment (Fig. 24-6).

ELBOW MECHANISMS. Presently, there are two practical systems available for the elbow. The first is an automatic locking elbow mechanism, which has been successfully used in the standard above-elbow amputees, and provides for eleven different locking positions, from full extension to full flexion. This mechanism is operated by a

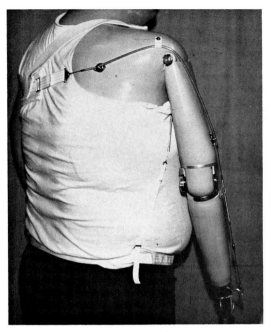

FIG. 24-4. Single-plane shoulder joint allowing passive abduction and adduction.

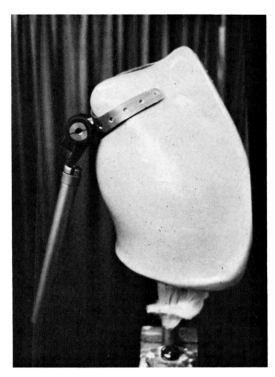

FIG. 24-6. Improved shoulder joint allowing passive range of motion in four planes, and with improved retention of stability.

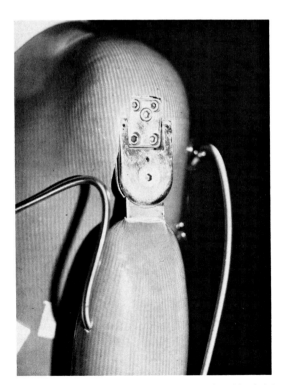

FIG. 24-5. Two-plane (four-way) motion shoulder joint allowing passive flexion, extension, abduction, and adduction.

lanyard which requires a $3/8$-in. excursion of the control cable in order to lock or unlock the joint.[1] It also requires a functional body control site (Fig. 24-7). With a shoulder disarticulation amputation, the patient retains active shoulder elevation on the amputated side permitting the elbow lock lanyard to be attached to a waist belt. Thus, the necessary excursion is obtained by shoulder elevation on the amputated side. This is probably the most commonly used control mechanism for this elbow unit.

The forequarter amputee, however, does not have shoulder elevation on the amputated side, and so other control sites are required. In some instances, this has depended on a "nudge" control, a small device placed on the interface near the patient's chin, and actuated by the patient's leaning laterally forward to depress the mechanism with his chin (Fig. 24-8). This technique has, however, lost favor. It is being replaced by a waist belt with lanyard excursion obtained

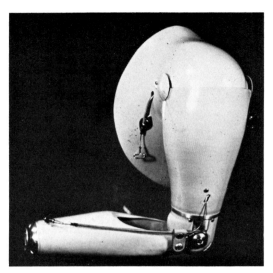

FIG. 24-7. Automatic locking elbow joint. Note control lanyard on anterior portion of interface (socket).

by elevating the shoulder on the contralateral side.

Another available elbow joint is actuated by external electric power. An early model of an electric elbow was referred to as the "Boston arm"; however, this design was heavy and required the use of a heavy battery pack (adding to the load), and five skin-contact sites. Simplified electric elbow designs have appeared and, at present, the most useful appears to be the Veterans Administration Prosthetic Center (VAPC) elbow joint actuated by an off-and-on switch (Fig. 24-9). The electric elbow joint still needs further refinement.

Common patient complaints over the present generation of electric elbows are that they are too noisy and, in most instances, too slow to react to the patient's needs. However, for the bilateral shoulder disarticulation amputee, electric elbows are a definite necessity because of the paucity of body control sites to provide either flexion of the elbow joint or locking of the elbow mechanism (Fig. 24-10). For the bilateral amputee, however, the slowness of operation and/or the noise of operation does not appear to be a significant problem, con-

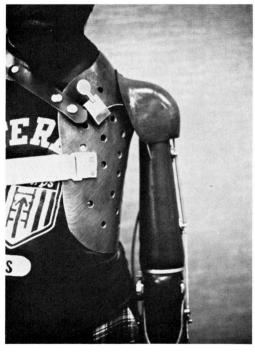

FIG. 24-8. Nudge control for elbow lock on anterior proximal portion of interface (socket).

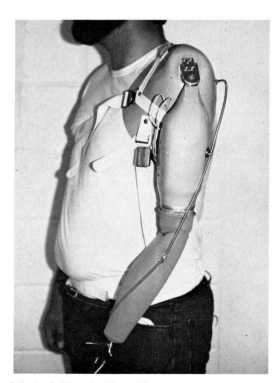

FIG. 24-9. Electric elbow. Note anterior placement of switch mechanism operated by shoulder elevation against a fixed-point waist belt.

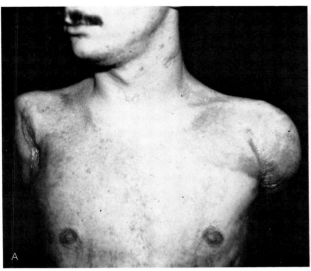
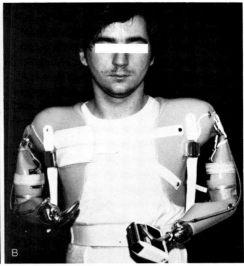

FIG. 24-10. A, Bilateral shoulder-level amputation: the right, a true shoulder disarticulation; the left, a prosthetically designated shoulder disarticulation with retention of the humeral head. B, Prosthetic fitting of bilateral shoulder disarticulation. Note electric elbows operated by anteriorly placed switches activated by shoulder elevation.

sidering the improvement in function that the patient is able to obtain.

Other variations in the arm, elbow, and forearm replacement may employ modular construction, usually with passive elbow flexion, and provide for manual locking by the opposite hand. This technique sets free a control site which may operate a functional terminal device (Fig. 24-11).

WRIST UNITS. Wrist units may be either oval or round which allows quick interchange of a hand or hook. In practice in addition to providing a wrist unit, a wrist flexion device allows the patient to operate his terminal device close to the midline. This unit is often used with unilateral amputation, but is definitely needed for the bilateral shoulder-level amputee.

TERMINAL DEVICES. Because the terminal device for a forequarter or shoulder disarticulation amputee has to be light, aluminum finger hooks are preferred. If a hand is required, it can be either a cosmetic nonfunctioning hand or a cosmetic glove-covered functioning hand. However, the cosmetic functional hand requires so much cable excursion and power that its operative efficiency is low. Because the patient

with these levels of amputation deficiencies generally has minimal power available to operate terminal devices, the device most often used is an aluminum hook, such as a Dorrance 5XA. To accommodate the considerable amputee interest in functional cosmetic hands, the attention of research institutions in the field of upper limb pros-

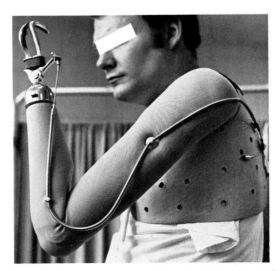

FIG. 24-11. Modular arm with passively operated elbow joint and body control terminal device.

thetics has turned to the use of electrically controlled functional hands. Such hands are now commercially available and can be switch or myoelectrically activated, utilizing myoelectricity from the trapezius muscle for opening and the pectoral muscles for closing the fingers.

PROSTHETIC CONTROL TECHNIQUES

Because of the reduction in available body-powered control sites, high levels of amputation provide either rudimentary body control of the elbow and terminal device, or by sophisticated but not as yet completely reliable myoelectric techniques, fair control of the terminal device and elbow. Most of the body control prostheses require a chest strap for interface stability.

The chest strap also provides an origin point for a control cable that allows several functions (Fig. 24-12). There are minimal problems involved in the use of a chest strap in the male, but in the female because of the mammary glands (small or large) the chest strap may require modification to a sturdy brassiere to which the ends of the chest strap are attached. Chest excursion, obtained through either the chest strap or the brassiere, provides a certain degree of control cable excursion which may be insufficient for optimum elbow flexion and/or terminal device operation. Cable excursion can be increased by an excursion amplifier; however, by increasing the cable travel, one must be aware that the power available is always reduced in proportion to the improvement in excursion (Fig. 24-13). The chest strap and/or brassiere mechanism may provide dual control utilizing a single cable to provide elbow flexion when the elbow mechanism is unlocked, and terminal device operation when the elbow is locked (Fig. 24-14). It is obvious that this type of control presents problems; namely, if the patient has an object in his terminal device and attempts to flex his forearm against the weight of the object he will find that rather than flexing his forearm he may inadvertently open his terminal device, thus dropping the object held in the hook fingers.

Further improvement in the dual control mechanism is necessary, and at present the Northwestern Prosthetic Laboratory has a "live lift lock" mechanism under development which may obviate this problem. In order for the dual control (single-cable) system to work satisfactorily, a second control

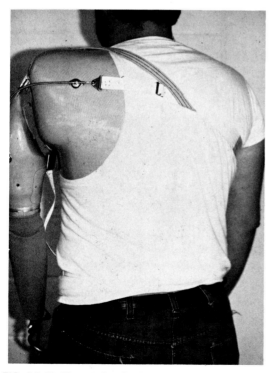

FIG. 24-12. Harnessing for body control terminal device. Note single-cable take-off from chest harness.

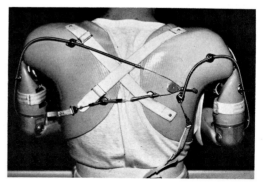

FIG. 24-13. A cable excursion amplifier providing increased excursion but decreased power of the terminal device.

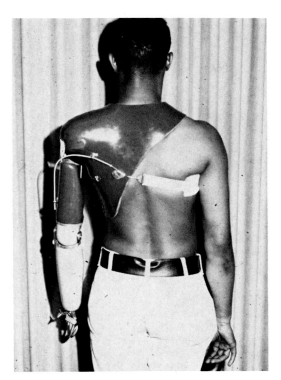

FIG. 24-14. Dual control system operated by chest harness. The single cable provides elbow flexion when elbow is unlocked. When elbow is locked, excursion of the same cable allows opening of the terminal device.

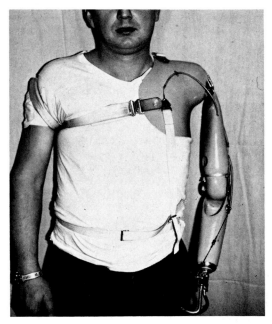

FIG. 24-15. Note location of elbow lock lanyard attached to waist belt. Shoulder elevation against the fixed point of the waist belt provides excursion of the lanyard.

source is required to lock and unlock the elbow joint. In the patient with a shoulder disarticulation, this may be achieved by elevating the shoulder, the lanyard being harnessed at two points: one to a waist belt which provides a stationary point, and the second to the anterior socket which is raised when the shoulder is elevated, thus producing adequate excursion of the elbow lock lanyard (Fig. 24-15).

As a means of further refining control of these types of prostheses, a triple control has been used in some amputees. A chest strap provides socket stability and activates the terminal device. A loop about the contralateral shoulder connected by a second cable to the forearm lift mechanism provides elbow flexion (Fig. 24-16). This so-called triple control technique requires a neuromuscularly able individual who can effectively separate scapular abduction and

shoulder motion from chest expansion. Frustration often occurs, and because of the resultant poor ability to operate his prosthesis the patient may abandon its use.

To simplify and improve operation of the triple control prosthesis, myoelectric control has been utilized but the patient must have adequate pectoral and trapezius muscles for useful electromyographic signals. External skin contact electrodes can be implanted in the interface (socket) over the area of these two muscle groups, thus permitting an on-off operation of a cosmetic electric hand. Considerable training is required to effect smooth operation of the terminal device. Optimal sites for electrodes are chosen only after an evaluation by a qualified, responsible prosthetist. The patient may also be fitted with an electric elbow mechanism activated by a switch mechanism which can be actuated either by shoulder elevation on the amputated side or by a shoulder control loop mechanism on the contralateral side (Fig. 24-17).

When all is said and done, however, the

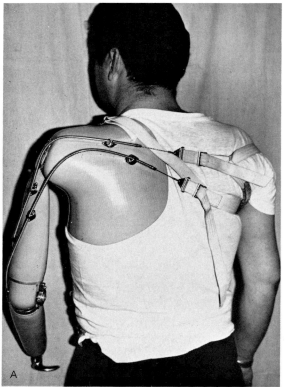
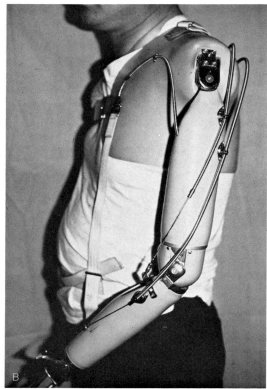

FIG. 24-16. A, Triple control utilizing a shoulder loop (superior cable) with scapular abduction as motivating force. A second cable (inferior cable) activated by chest excursion operates terminal device. B, Triple control. Note superior cable providing elbow flexion, inferior posterior cable to operate terminal device, and elbow lock mechanism activated by shoulder elevation (third cable).

patient with this level of amputation may decide that the effort of obtaining functional control of his prosthesis is not worth the effort, and may compromise on a purely cosmetic interface with a fixed or solid

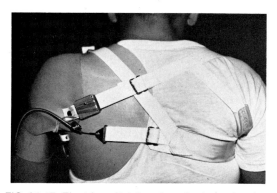

FIG. 24-17. Electric switch for elbow flexion-extension activated by shoulder abduction. Chest excursion cable provides terminal device operation.

shoulder joint, a modular elbow and forearm construction covered by a soft cosmetic cover, and a cosmetic passive nonfunctional hand (Fig. 24-18).

PRESCRIPTION PRINCIPLES

In view of the patient's requirement for a fairly large prosthesis, the first admonition to the prosthetist is that he make the prosthesis as light as possible. These amputees are not likely to be heavy-duty users, and therefore, great strength will not be required in the sockets, arm, or forearm components. Experience has shown that the use of available body power provides quicker prosthetic response with less complication, providing body power can be harnessed for simple and efficient usage.

In the patient with a forequarter amputa-

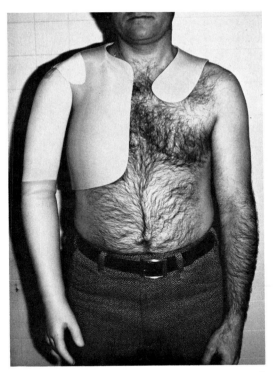

FIG. 24-18. A cosmetic arm for a scapulothoracic amputee providing shoulder contour and sleeve filling.

tant, wherever possible, to minimize the area of interface in order to allow more exposure of body surface for heat removal. If this is not feasible sufficient socket ventilation is required.

Nowhere in the upper limb is training in the use of a prescribed prosthesis more important than in the shoulder disarticulation and forequarter amputee. Control site motion must be taught and spontaneous prosthetic function mastered by the patient with the least frustration and the greatest efficiency possible. Because available body sources of power vary considerably with the levels of amputation, it is sometimes necessary to try several control sites and methods of control in order to attain the most functional prosthesis. Where body control sites are not sufficient, consideration should be given to the use of external power, particularly for operation of elbow mechanisms and/or terminal devices.

Each prosthesis is a custom-made device involving considerable trial and error, particularly as it relates to harnessing, in order to make it as efficient as possible. These high level amputees require the most sophisticated and dedicated prosthetic service that is obtainable. When experience with myoelectric control improves, and as sophistication of electromyographic signal pick-up amplification is gained, so too will the functional level of these amputees likewise increase. The unilateral shoulder disarticulation amputee has one remaining functional extremity which can provide the minimum of comforts, such as self-feeding and simple dressing; however, at present, even the most sophisticated bilateral prosthesis does not provide adequate ability to provide self-toilet care. Considerably more research is indicated before this optimal level of prosthetic usage is obtained. However, owing to the small numbers of such amputees, and the increased cost of research in the field, the development of such a "toilet care" arm is proceeding slowly.

tion or a bilateral shoulder disarticulation, the use of external power will generally add to the functional use of any prosthesis. Particularly in the bilateral shoulder disarticulation amputee, electric-powered elbows are most beneficial, whereas in the single shoulder disarticulation amputee it is less desirable to have external power for the elbow or the terminal device. There is no question, however, that external power for terminal devices will be used to a greater degree, when an electrically powered hook, as an alternative to the electric hand, is available. Such a terminal device is presently undergoing research and development at the Northwestern University Prosthetic Laboratory, as well as at the Veterans Administration Prosthetic Center (VAPC).

Because of the need for rotational stability, large sockets are required. It is impor-

REFERENCE

1. Orthopedic Appliance Atlas, Volume 2. American Academy of Orthopaedic Surgeons, 1960.

Index

Page numbers in *italic* refer to illustrations; page numbers followed by "T" refer to tables.